Register Now f

Access to You

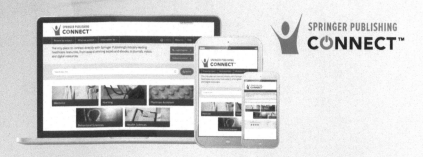

Your print purchase of *Gynecologic Oncology Handbook, Third Edition,* **includes online access to the contents of your book—** increasing accessibility, portability, and searchability!

Access today at:
http://connect.springerpub.com/content/book/978-0-8261-5598-6 or scan the QR code at the right with your smartphone. Log in or register, then click "Redeem a voucher" and use the code below.

KCA4Y9EH

Scan here for quick access.

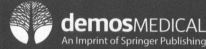
demosMEDICAL
An Imprint of Springer Publishing
View all our products at springerpub.com/demosmedical

Gynecologic Oncology Handbook

Gynecologic Oncology Handbook

An Evidence-Based Clinical Guide

Third Edition

Michelle F. Benoit, MD, FACOG, FACS
Seattle, Washington

M. Yvette Williams-Brown, MD, MMSc, FACOG
Associate Professor of Obstetrics and Gynecology
Department of Women's Health; and
Courtesy Associate Professor
Department of Oncology
The University of Texas at Austin Dell Medical School
Austin, Texas

Creighton L. Edwards, MD
Professor and Raymond H. Kaufman, MD and Patricia Ann
  Kaufman Endowed Chair in Obstetrics and Gynecology
Department of OB-GYN
Division of Gynecologic Oncology
Baylor College of Medicine
Houston, Texas

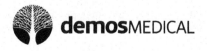 **demos**MEDICAL

Springer Publishing Company, LLC
11 West 42nd Street, New York, NY 10036
www.springerpub.com
connect.springerpub.com/

Acquisitions Editor: David D'Addona
Compositor: Exeter Premedia Services Private Limited

ISBN: 978-0-8261-5597-9
ebook ISBN: 978-0-8261-5598-6
DOI: 10.1891/9780826155986

23 24 25 26 / 5 4 3 2 1

Medicine is an ever-changing science. Research and clinical experience are continually expanding our knowledge, in particular our understanding of proper treatment and drug therapy. The authors, editors, and publisher have made every effort to ensure that all information in this book is in accordance with the state of knowledge at the time of production of the book. Nevertheless, the authors, editors, and publisher are not responsible for any errors or omissions or for any consequence from application of the information in this book and make no warranty, expressed or implied, with respect to the content of this publication. Every reader should examine carefully the package inserts accompanying each drug and should carefully check whether the dosage schedules therein or the contraindications stated by the manufacturer differ from the statements made in this book. Such examination is particularly important with drugs that are either rarely used or have been newly released on the market.

Library of Congress Cataloging-in-Publication Data is available

Publisher's Note: New and used products purchased from third-party sell-ers are not guaranteed for quality, authenticity, or access to any included digital components.

Printed in the United States of America by Hatteras, Inc.

"First learn stand, then learn fly."

We are dedicating the third edition of this handbook to our mentor, Dr. Alan Kaplan. He taught us mastery, protocol, and perseverance. As a founding member of the Society of Gynecologic Oncology, he had the foresight to develop this amazing subspecialty in women's medicine. He never strayed from being a gentleman, while constantly advocating for the health of his patients and the betterment of his fellows. He taught us discipline, balance in life, and humility—and from that we hope we are the better physicians.

—Michelle and Yvette

We would also like to thank Jayson Field, MD, and Paiman Ghafoori, MD, for their efforts and contributions.

Contents

List of Tables

List of Figures

Preface

This handbook is structured to provide comprehensive care for the gynecologic cancer patient. It is directed toward clinicians at all levels of training and the chapters are tiered in this fashion. Basic diagnosis, workup, staging, and treatment are outlined first. Specific surgical and adjuvant therapies that reflect the current standards of care are then recommended. Finally, the evidence-based medicine is summarized in support of recommended treatments. Thus, the medical student can have a dedicated overview, the resident can refer to directed patient-care protocols, and the fellow and practicing physician can support their clinical decisions with easily accessible literature.

This updated third edition furthers the content to include the latest cancer-screening information, new surgical technology and platforms, novel cytotoxic chemotherapy, in addition to targeted and immuno-therapy treatments, vaccination information, and the most current clinical trial outcomes. The ninth edition American Joint Committee on Cancer staging guidelines[1] have also been incorporated, providing accurate instructions for staging to keep the reader at the forefront of medicine. With this additional information, we continue to provide a comprehensive and contemporary reference for clinical practice.

It is our honor to assemble this handbook for our friends and colleagues. We again acknowledge the dedication it has taken from the physicians, support staff, and especially our patients, to design and participate in the trials that have advanced our knowledge of these difficult gynecologic cancers. We hope the information provided herein can continue to guide high-quality care and reflect our commitment to the subspecialty.

REFERENCE

1. Olawaiye AB, Mutch DG, Bhosale P, et al. AJCC Cancer Staging System: Cervix Uteri (Version 9 of the AJCC Cancer Staging System). American College of Surgeons; 2020.

1 Cancer Screening, Prevention, and Preinvasive Gynecologic Disease

CERVICAL CANCER SCREENING

Between 1955 and 1992, the incidence and death rates of cervical cancer in the United States decreased by more than 60% due to the implementation of widespread screening.[1] Nevertheless, cervical cancer remains a significant gynecologic cancer in the United States and worldwide, disproportionally affecting women along racial/ethnic and socioeconomic lines.

The Human Papilloma Virus

HPV has been found to cause over 90% of cervical cancers. It is a DS circular DNA virus. The virus is organized into three regions: the upstream regulatory regions, the early region containing genes E1–E7, and the late region containing genes L1–L2.

- The early, or E, region proteins are related to viral gene regulation and cell transformation:

  E1: ATP-dependent helicase for replication
  E2: Transcriptional regulatory activities, regulates E6/7
  E3: Ubiquitin ligases
  E4: Structural proteins, expressed in late stages; these proteins disrupt the intermediate filaments and cornified cell envelopes, facilitate the release of assembled virions, and produce koilocytosis
  E5: Stimulates cell growth, complexes with EGFR and is lost during cancer development
  E6: Binds to and degrades p53, preventing cell death and promoting viral replication
  E7: Binds to and inactivates tumor suppressor protein, Rb; cooperates with activated Ras; and activates cyclins E and A
  E6 and E7: These are the two primary oncoproteins of HPV

- The late, or L proteins are necessary for the virion capsid production:
  L1: Major capsid
  L2: Minor capsid
- HPV infection occurs in the basal epithelial cells in the lower reproductive tract. HPV binds to alpha 6 integrin on the host cell, stimulating mitosis when normally dormant. The basal cells then divide with the potential for malignant transformation.
- HPV can be detected by either viral DNA, viral RNA, or by using cellular markers. Detection of HPV DNA is either by PCR or hybridization. HPV RNA detection methods look for expression of E6/E7 by detecting mRNA. Finally, a dual stain on a Pap test can identify viral proteins or cellular proteins, such as p16 or Ki-67, by IHC to determine HPV infection.
- Transmission is mostly via sexual contact and the majority of persons are infected with HPV shortly after the onset of sexual activity. HPV has also been detected in 3% of sexually naïve persons. The use of condoms reduces the rate of HPV infection by 50%. Fomite transmission has not been definitively documented.
- Most exposures produce a transient productive viral infection. One third of women develop low-grade cytological changes. Most changes clear spontaneously within 2 Y. Less than 20% of women are still HPV+ at 2 Y. Long-term or persistent infections occur in fewer than 10% of women at 2 Y. Rates of HPV infection differ by age: If older than 29 Y, there is a 31% infection rate; if younger than 29, there is a 65% rate of infection.

Screening Recommendations

The 2018 U.S. Preventive Services Task Force, endorsed by the ASCCP (formerly known as the *American Society of Colposcopy and Cervical Pathology*), ACOG, and SGO, recommended screening for cervical cancer beginning at age 21, regardless of sexual history. Persons with a cervix (including those who have had a supracervical hysterectomy) aged 21–29 are recommended to have screening with cytology alone every 3 Y. For those 30 to 65, screening is recommended with any of the following: cervical cytology every 3 Y, HPV testing alone every 5 Y (using a test approved by the FDA for stand-alone testing) or co-testing every 5 Y (cytology and HPV testing).

The American Cancer Society differs in that they recommend screening starting with primary HPV testing at the age of 25, as well as cotesting or cytology alone when primary HPV testing is not available.

The aforementioned screening recommendations are for routine screening for immunocompetent individuals who are asymptomatic and do not apply for follow-up of prior abnormal screening results.

In addition to HPV testing and cytology, WHO also recommends visual inspection with acetic acid (VIA) as an acceptable method for screening in low resource areas.

- End screening: Discontinuation of screening is recommended for persons with an intact cervix who are aged 65 Y and older and who have had three or more consecutive normal Pap tests (cytology) or two consecutive negative cotests, or two consecutive negative HPV tests within a 10-Y period. Screening should not be restarted including for a new partner. For individuals who have had a total hysterectomy (removal of the body of the uterus and cervix) performed for benign indications, screening can be discontinued.

- Changes are being considered for those who are older than 65 Y as 20% of cervical cancers occur in this subset of women.[2] Given that women diagnosed with CIN3 at 50 Y or older are at a 7 times higher risk of developing cervical cancer, continued screening for dysplasia at older ages, along with overall surveillance, is necessary in those with a history of dysplastic lesions. Women are also living longer and deaths from cancer are preventable if cancer is found at an early stage. Population-based incidence rates also need to account for hysterectomy-adjusted rates to accurately reflect cervical cancer incidence. Finally, consideration of health disparities in high-risk populations should highlight focus areas for increased screening, with verification of the adequacy of negative prior screening within 10 Y for all populations.

- Indefinite annual screening is recommended for women with a history of intrauterine DES exposure.

- For HIV-positive women: Screening should begin within 1 Y of sexual activity or within the first Y of HIV diagnosis if already sexually active, but no later than 21 Y of age. Annual cytologic testing without HPV testing should continue up to age 29. If three consecutive annual cytology-alone tests are negative, follow-up cytology testing should occur at 3-Y intervals. For those over the age of 30, annual screening should continue with cytology alone or cotesting. After three negative annual cytology-alone tests, follow-up screening can be every 3 Y. Women who have one negative cotest result can have their next cervical cancer screening in 3 Y: cervical cancer screening should continue throughout their lifetimes and not be discontinued.

- Women with a history of an abnormal Pap test: a) who are over age 65 Y should continue screening until there are three or more consecutive normal Pap tests (cytology) or two consecutive negative cotests, or two consecutive negative HPV tests within in a 10-Y period. b) Women with a history of cervical HSIL (–IN 2/3) should continue HPV-based surveillance every 3 Y for 25 Y after diagnosis and/or treatment. c) Women with a history of hysterectomy due to cervical HSIL (–IN 2/3) or AIS should continue HPV-based screening every 3 Y for 25 Y after surgery. Continued surveillance beyond 25 Y is acceptable for women with a longer life expectancy. d) Women with a history of cervical cancer should continue annual screening indefinitely with cytology alone. For individuals with a limited life expectancy, discontinuation of screening can be reasonably considered.

PAP Test

The widespread use of the Pap test (cytology), introduced in the 1950s, resulted in a significant decrease in the rates of cervical cancer.

- The FN rate of Pap smears is between 6% and 25%. The conventional Pap smear has a sensitivity of 51% and a specificity of 98%.[3] The rate of cervical cancer following a negative normal Pap test is 7.5/100,000 women/Y; for all women with HPV-negative testing there are 3.8 cervical cancers/100,000 women/Y. For women who are both HPV negative and Pap cytology negative, the rate is 3.2 cervical cancers/100,000 women/Y.

- The Bethesda system of Pap smear reporting has three basic components: descriptive interpretation, statement of adequacy, and categorization of the interpretation (optional). The adequacy communicates the quality of the specimen. There are three optional interpretive categories: within normal limits, benign cellular changes, and epithelial cell abnormality.

- Epithelial cell abnormalities can be divided into either squamous or glandular cell changes:
  - Squamous cell cytology abnormalities are reported as LSIL, HSIL, squamous cell carcinoma, or ASC. ASC is divided into ASC-US (the risk of cervical HSIL [-IN 2/3] is 7%–17%) or ASC-H (the risk of cervical HSIL [-IN 2/3] is 40% and the risk of invasive cancer is 0.1%).
  - Glandular cell cytology abnormalities include AGC, AIS, and AC. AGC is divided into AGC–not further classified, or AGC–favor neoplasia.

HPV Testing

HPV testing can be used as a co-test or stand-alone test in cervical cancer screening; HPV testing increases the sensitivity of detecting cervical histopathology, including AC (Table 1.1).

- ATHENA study using HPV as first-line screening test: The 3-Y cumulative incidence rates (CIRs) of cervical HSIL (-IN 3+) in cytology-negative women was 0.8% (95% CI: 0.5%–1.1%); it was 0.3% (95% CI: 0.1%–0.7%) in HPV-negative women, and 0.3% (95% CI: 0.1%–0.6%) in cytology- and HPV-negative women. The sensitivity for cervical HSIL (-IN 3+) of cytology was 47.8% compared to 61.7% for the hybrid strategy (cytology if 25–29 Y old and co-testing with cytology and HPV if >30 Y old) and 76.1% for HPV as a primary test. Specificity for cervical HSIL (-IN 3+) was 97.1%, 94.6%, and 93.5%, respectively. HPV as the sole and primary screen test detects significantly more cases of cervical HSIL (-IN 3+) in women older than 25 Y than either cytology or the hybrid strategy, although it requires more colposcopies.[4]

Table 1.1 HPV-Based Cervical Cancer Screening Tests*

Marker	Test Name	Manufacturer	Target M	Target HPV Genotypes	HPV Genotyping	Technology
HPV DNA	Amplicor	Roche	L1	13 carcinogenic	No	PCR
	careHPV	QIAGEN	Full genome	13 carcinogenic and HPV66	No	Hybridization
	Cervista	Hologic	L1	13 carcinogenic and HPV66	Partial (HPV16 and HPV18)	Hybridization
	CLART	Genomica	L1	13 carcinogenic and 22 noncarcinogenic	Yes	PCR
	COBAS 4800	Roche	L1	13 carcinogenic and HPV66	Partial (HPV16 and HPV18)	Real-time PCR
	eHC	QIAGEN	Full genome	13 carcinogenic, HPV66, and HPV82	Partial (HPV types 16, 18, and 45)	Hybridization
	GP5+/6+ EIA	Not commercialized	L1	13 carcinogenic and HPV66	No	PCR
	HC2	QIAGEN	Full genome	13 carcinogenic	No	Hybridization

(continued)

Table 1.1 HPV-Based Cervical Cancer Screening Tests* *(continued)*

Marker	Test Name	Manufacturer	Target M	Target HPV Genotypes	HPV Genotyping	Technology
	HPV QUAD	Autogenomics	E1	13 carcinogenic and HPV66	Partial (HPV types 16, 18, 31, 33, and 45)	PCR
	High-risk-HPV Dx PCR	BioRad	n/a	13 carcinogenic and HPV66	No	PCR
	Infinity HPV	Autogenomics	E1	13 carcinogenic and 13 noncarcinogenic	Yes	PCR
	InnoLiPA	Innogenetics	L1	13 carcinogenic and 15 noncarcinogenic	Yes	PCR
	Linear array	Roche	L1	13 carcinogenic and 24 noncarcinogenic	Yes	PCR
	Multiplex HPV genotyping kit	Multimetrix	L1	13 carcinogenic and 11 noncarcinogenic	Yes	PCR

Papillocheck	Greiner	E1	13 carcinogenic and 11 noncarcinogenic	Yes	PCR
RT HPV	Abbott	L1	13 carcinogenic and HPV66	Partial (HPV16 and HPV18)	Real-time PCR
n/a	Becton Dickinson	n/a	13 carcinogenic and HPV66	Partial (HPV types 16, 18, 31, 45, 51, 52, and 59)	Real-time PCR
HPV RNA Aptima	GenProbe	E6/E7 mRNA	13 carcinogenic and HPV66	No	TMA
NucliSENS EasyQ HPV	BioMerieux	E6/E7 mRNA	HPV types 16, 18, 31, 33, and 45	Yes	NASBA
OncoTect	Invirion/InCellDx	E6/E7 mRNA	13 carcinogenic	n/a	In situ hybridization
PreTect Proofer	Norchip	E6/E7 mRNA	HPV types 16, 18, 31, 33, and 45	Yes	NASBA

(continued)

Table 1.1 HPV-Based Cervical Cancer Screening Tests* *(continued)*

Marker	Test Name	Manufacturer	Target M	Target HPV Genotypes	HPV Genotyping	Technology
HPV protein	E6 protein	Arbor Vitae	E6	HPV types 16, 18, and 45	n/a	Immunoassay
	Cytoactiv	Cytoimmun	L1	Carcinogenic types, not specified	n/a	Immunostain
Cellular protein	CINtec plus	mtm Laboratories	p16INK4a/ Ki-67	n/a	n/a	Immunostain
	ProExC	Becton Dickinson	MCM2/ Top2A	n/a	n/a	Immunostain
FISH	oncoFISH	Ikonisys	3q/TERC	n/a	n/a	FISH

*Cross-hybridization with noncarcinogenic HPV types described.

*Source:*Schiffman M, Wentzensen N, Wacholder S et al. Human papillomavirus testing in the prevention of cervical cancer. *J Natl Cancer Inst.* March 2, 2011;103(5):368–383.[13]

Management Guidelines

In 2019, the ASCCP released risk-based guidelines that replaced the 2012 cytology algorithms, which previously focused on management based primarily on results of current testing. Screening utilizing HPV testing alone or in combination with cytology is superior to cytology screening alone; therefore, the incorporation of HPV test results into risk determination and management was an important part of the updated management strategy. Further, CIN3+ (CIN3, AIS, and invasive cervical cancer [ICC]) was used as the main clinical endpoint for cancer risk estimates. Guidelines can be accessed from the website https://asccp.org using the web application or through their mobile app. There are three fundamental concepts that are important to understand regarding the current risk-based management of cervical cancer screening results.

1. Equal management for equal risk. The benchmark for screening is to determine which patients are at risk for cervical precancer (CIN3+). From prior management strategies, a cytology result of LSIL was the threshold for colposcopy. Statistically, a patient with LSIL from a Pap test will have a 4% risk of CIN3+.
2. The longer a high-risk HPV infection has been present, the higher the risk of CIN3+. Most HPV infections are undetectable in 1 to 3 Y. Followed over time, women who had persistently positive HPV testing, and especially those with high-risk types (HPV 16), had the highest risk of CIN3+.
3. Management is based on risk of CIN3+, not simply the results of a current screening test. Although current screening test results are important, past history and prior test results influence a patient's current risk and subsequent management.

HPV Vaccination

- The HPV **prophylactic** vaccination is recommended for both females and males between the ages of 9 and 46 Y old.
  - There is hope that this vaccine will decrease the global incidence rates of head and neck and anogenital cancers.
  - Initial vaccines consisted of the L1 capsids either with the quadrivalent vaccine for HPV 6, 11, 16, and 18; or the bivalent vaccine for HPV 16 and 18.
  - The nonavalent HPV vaccine includes HPV types 6, 11, 16, 18, 31, 33, 45, 52, and 58. In a randomized phase III trial, vaccine or placebo were given at day 1, month 2, and month 6. Tissue was obtained by biopsy or definitive therapy (conization). Efficacy against high-grade disease, related to all vaccine HPV types, was 97%. Efficacy against cervical HSIL (-IN 2/3) was 96%. Efficacy against vulvar HSIL (-IN 2/3) or vaginal HSIL (-IN 2/3) was 100%. The nonavalent vaccine was approved December 10, 2014.

○ The CDC recommends a two-dose abbreviated HPV vaccine 6 to 12 months apart for persons aged 9 to 15 Y. Adolescents who receive their two shots less than 5 months apart or persons who receive the vaccine series after the age of 15 require a third dose of the HPV vaccine. This is based on data demonstrating that two doses of HPV vaccine in young adolescents aged 9 to 14 Y produce an immune response similar to or higher than the response in young adults aged 16 to 26 Y who receive the standard three-dose series over a 6-month time period.

○ VIVIANE study: This was a randomized controlled trial of 5,747 women over the age of 25 Y vaccinated with the three-shot bivalent HPV series; of this population, 15% had documented prior HPV infection. At month 84, in women seronegative for the corresponding HPV type in the according-to-protocol cohort for efficacy, vaccine efficacy against 6-month persistent infection or cervical HSIL (-IN 1+) associated with HPV 16/18 was significant in all age groups combined (90.5%, 96.2% CI: 78.6–96.5). Vaccine efficacy against HPV 16/18-related cytological abnormalities (ASC of undetermined significance and LSIL) and cervical HSIL (-IN 1+) was also significant. Significant cross-protective efficacy against 6-month persistent infection with HPV 31 (65.8%, 96.2% CI: 24.9–85.8) and HPV 45 (70.7%, 96.2% CI: 34.2–88.4) was noted. In the total vaccinated cohort, vaccine efficacy against cervical HSIL (-IN 1+) irrespective of HPV was significant (22.9%, 96.2% CI: 4.8–37.7). Thus, in women older than 25 Y, the HPV 16/18 vaccine continues to protect against infections, cytological abnormalities, and lesions associated with HPV 16/18 and cervical HSIL (-IN 1+) irrespective of HPV type, and infection with nonvaccine types HPV 31 and HPV 45 over a 7-Y follow-up period.[7]

○ There are data to support that the nonavalent vaccine will prevent up to 90% of cervical cancers instead of the prior 70% protection provided by the quadrivalent vaccine.

● There is a possible **therapeutic** effect of the HPV vaccine:

○ From the FUTURE I and FUTURE II trials, a retrospective analysis of these two randomized trials in patients aged 20 to 45 who were treated for cervical HSIL (-IN 2/3) by LEEP: 360 were vaccinated, 377 were not. There was a 2.5% recurrence rate in the vaccination group and a 7.2% recurrence rate in the control group. This demonstrated a 64.9% reduction in high-grade disease of the cervix in women who underwent a surgical procedure for cervical HSIL (-IN 2/3) and were vaccinated. The vaccine was given prior to their excisional procedure. The HR for recurrence was 2.84 (95% CI: 1.3–6.0; $p < 0.01$) even after evaluating for positive endocervical cytology and positive margin status. This post hoc analysis was not specifically designed to address the question of a therapeutic benefit.[5,8–18]

PREINVASIVE DISEASE

The LAST project developed terminology for lower anogenital tract preinvasive disease to create a unified histopathological nomenclature with a single set of diagnostic terms. It is recommended for all HPV-associated preinvasive squamous lesions regardless of anatomic site or sex/gender and has been adopted by the WHO.[5]

The LAST project and the WHO recommend reporting intraepithelial histopathology as a two-tier diagnosis. Therefore, preinvasive pathology from the cervix, anus, vulva, and vagina is classified as cervical–SIL, anal-SIL, vulvar-SIL, and vaginal-SIL, respectively. Intraepithelial neoplasia is further categorized as LSIL (-IN 1) or high-grade (HSIL) (-IN 2/-IN 3). However, the 2019 risk-based ASCCP guidelines for cervical cancer screening relies on the three-tier nomenclature (CIN 1, 2 or 3).

Cervical SILs

- Characteristics: Cervical SILs are asymptomatic; Pap smear screening (cytology) or positive high-risk HPV testing are the main means of detection. The median age at diagnosis has ranged from 23 Y in the ALTS trial[19] to 34 Y old in a Norwegian population. Risk factors for cervical SIL are HPV infection, immunosuppression, smoking, a history of STDs, and multiple sexual partners. The use of oral contraceptives is also linked to an increased risk of HPV infection. The use of oral contraceptives was previously thought to be only a marker for exposure more than a cause; however, studies suggest that the hormones in OCP may cause changes in cervical cells that make them more susceptible to infection.[20]

- Immunosuppression can significantly contribute to increased rates of dysplasia and cancer. For those infected with HIV, the relative risk for cervical cancer is five times higher.[21] The risk of invasive cancer varies by CD4 count: HIV-infected women with baseline CD4+ T-cells of ≥350, 200 to 349, and less than 200 cells per microliter had a 2.3, 3.0, and 7.7 times increase in the incidence of invasion, respectively, compared with HIV-uninfected women (p(trend) = 0.001).[22] The standardized incidence ratio for ICC is 9.2 for HIV-infected patients.[23]

- For immunosuppressed solid organ transplant patients, the RR for cervical SIL is 13.6.[24] The RR of a transplant patient having ICC is 5.[25]

- Cervical intraepithelial lesion terminology is two-tiered: LSIL (-IN 1) is categorized as a low-grade lesion and HSIL (-IN 2/3) is combined into the category of high-grade lesions. Classification is made according to the amount of epithelium involved: Cervical LSIL (old CIN 1) demonstrates atypia in the lower third of epithelium; cervical HSIL (old CIN 2/3) demonstrates atypia from the middle third to throughout the entire epithelium. The microscopic appearance is nuclear atypia, disorganization/depolarization, parakeratosis, and abnormal mitotic figures. Most lesions occur in the transformation zone. There is no distinction between cervical HSIL (-IN 3) and CIS; thus, it is recommended that CIS terminology not be used.

- Biomarker interpretation: p16 IHC is recommended when the differential diagnosis is between -IN 2/-IN 3 and a precancer mimic or if the pathologist is entertaining a H&E morphologic interpretation of -IN 2. p16 IHC may also be used as an adjunct to biopsy specimen assessment when interpreted as -IN 1 that is high risk for missed high-grade disease due to a prior cytologic interpretation of HSIL, ASC-H, or (AGC [NOS]). If there is difficulty in stratifying LSIL from HSIL, p16 IHC can be performed on the specimen, and if positive, then the lesion is categorized as HSIL. Those results with a prior -IN2 diagnosis can have p16 IHC staining: If that staining is negative it would then fall to the lower LSIL category and, if p16 positive, upgraded into the HSIL category.

- **Colposcopy:** Microscopic evaluation of the cervix at 8x to 25x can visualize tissue abnormalities. Application of 3% to 5% topical acetic acid (vinegar) for 3 to 5 minutes can dehydrate the surface cells and unmask tissue changes such as acetowhite epithelium and atypical vessels. Directed biopsy can sample these areas for cervical SIL (-IN 1,2,3). If no abnormalities are seen, then an ECC and random or four-quadrant biopsies can be performed, with highest yield from the transformation zone. An adequate colposcopy is visualization of the entire cervix, its transformation zone, and the vaginal fornices. An ECC should usually be done if the patient is not pregnant. Histologic confirmation with biopsy should occur before ablative therapy is performed (i.e., cryotherapy).

- Treatment of cervical LSIL (-IN 1) can vary. In the ALTS trial for cervical cancer study, 41% of cervical LSIL (-IN 1) diagnoses were downgraded to normal and 13% were upgraded to cervical HSIL (-IN 2/3). In one study, 90% of women with LSIL (-IN 1) spontaneously regressed in 24 months.[26] If cervical LSIL (-IN 1) is diagnosed after a Pap test that showed HSIL or ASC-H, more aggressive management should be considered. If cervical SIL (-IN 1) is diagnosed after an ASC-US or LSIL Pap, HPV testing every 12 months or repeating a Pap smear in 6 months can be considered. If cervical LSIL (-IN 1) persists for 2 Y, an LEEP can be considered. Before using any ablative (cryo or laser) therapy, a negative ECC should be obtained (Table 1.2).

- Management of cervical HSIL (-IN 2/3) diagnosed at colposcopic biopsy:
  - Surveillance: Surveillance can be offered for women of reproductive age with cervical HSIL (-IN 2, 2/3), given that the patient is reliable, and had an adequate colposcopy. Cure rates with treatment are about 90%, whereas spontaneous regression rates are about 40%. Thus, treatment is primarily recommended as ablative techniques in women ages 21 to24. Surveillance is colposcopy and cytology every 6 months up to 24 months if colposcopy

Table 1.2 Risk of Progression to Cervical -IN3

Lesion	Regression (%)	Persistent (%)	Progress to Cervical -IN3 (%)
LSIL (-IN1)	57	32	11
HSIL (-IN 2)	43	35	22
HSIL (-IN 3)	32	35	NA

is adequate. Routine screening may resume after two normal cytology tests and colposcopy examinations followed by a normal cytology test and negative HR HPV test a Y later.

- ○ Ablation therapy: Some authors caution the use of excisional therapy in reproductive-aged women due to risk of adverse reproductive outcomes (preterm labor, cervical stenosis, and infertility).
  - ▪ Cryotherapy: Criteria for application are adequate colposcopy, the lesion is completely visible, it does not cover more than 75% of the ectocervix, and the lesions can be covered with the cryoprobe. Due to risk of cryotherapy failure, this procedure is not recommended in women over age 40.
  - ▪ Topical Imiquimod has shown promising results for regression, see Notable Trials text.
- ○ Laser: The same criteria should be met as for cryotherapy, but laser can be used for lesions larger than 2 cm, for multifocal lesions, or both, with or without vaginal involvement.
- ○ Excisional therapy: May be used for primary treatment or if criteria for ablation are not met. For the conization procedure, it is necessary to remove 5 to 7 mm of cervical stroma and perform an ECC. There may be evidence of skip lesions and multifocality, especially in glandular lesions; so one should, therefore, not solely remove the acetowhite lesion.
  - ▪ LEEP: This is an office-based procedure.
  - ▪ CKC: If there is suspicion for malignancy and margin status is important, if there has been prior cervical treatment, or if cervical atrophy is present, a CKC is recommended. This is a general anesthesia-based procedure. Pitressin or epinephrine injected at the time of the procedure will help reduce EBL.
- HPV vaccination after conization has shown lower recurrence rates of CIN2/3.
- Follow-up after treatment for cervical HSIL (-IN 2/3) is based on categorization into low or high risk groups.
  - ○ Low risk is LEEP or CKC with negative margins or those who had ablative therapies. Follow-up consists of cytology plus HR HPV testing in 12 and 24 months; colposcopy for any abnormality; if

all are normal, cytology plus HR HPV testing in 3 Y; if cytology and HPV testing at 3 Y are normal, routine screening for 20 Y. Annual co-testing or annual cytology until two negative annual tests is another option.

○ High risk includes those with LEEP- or CKC-positive margins or those with positive postprocedure ECC. Follow up is cytology and ECC at 4 to 6 months (preferred), but repeat excision is acceptable. If re-excision is not possible, then hysterectomy is acceptable. There are data to support the spontaneous resolution of positive margins in 56% of women.[27]

• Additional indications for conization beyond treatment of cervical-HSIL (-IN 2/3), and a positive ECC are evaluation of microscopic invasive cancer, treatment of Stage IA1 cervical cancer, evaluation of significant cytologic/histologic discrepancy, and evaluation of an unsatisfactory colposcopic exam. CKC may be a more favorable procedure for glandular lesions.

• The addition of a postconization ECC to cone biopsy for AIS of the cervix provides prognostic information. Women who have both a negative ECC and negative cone margin have a 14% risk of residual AIS and, if they desire fertility, can be managed conservatively. A positive ECC postcone or internal positive margin has significant risk of residual disease and 12% to 17% will have cancer.[28]

• Notable Trials

○ The relevance of random biopsy at the transformation zone when colposcopy is negative: The ATHENA study screened 47,000 plus women with cytology and HR HPV DNA genotyping. Colposcopy was performed in all women with abnormal cytology or positive HPV results. A single random biopsy was taken at the SCJ if colposcopy was adequate and no lesions were seen. This single random biopsy increased the detection of high-grade disease, diagnosing cervical HSIL in 20.9% (-IN 2) and 18.9% of (-IN 3).[29]

○ Alternative treatment to LEEP/CKC with imiquimod: 59 patients with cervical HSIL (-IN 2/3) were randomized to a 16-week treatment of self-applied vaginal suppositories of imiquimod or placebo. Imiquimod is a topical immune response modulator, is a toll-like 7 receptor agonist affecting the upregulation of interferon alpha and activation of the DC. The suppository dose was 6.25 mg, one suppository per week for weeks 1 and 2, in weeks 3 and 4 two suppositories per week, then three suppositories per week until 16 weeks, suspending application during the first 3 days of menses. Dose modification was to 3.125 mg. The main outcome was regression to cervical LSIL (-IN 1) or less. Secondary outcomes were complete histologic remission, HPV clearance, and tolerability. Histologic regression was observed in 73% versus 39%, $p = 0.009$. Complete remission was 47% in the imiquimod group compared to placebo 14%, $p = 0.008$. All patients at baseline tested HPV positive and HPV clearance rates increased in the imiquimod group 60%, versus 14% in the placebo group, $p <0.001$. No high-grade side effects were observed.[30]

o Trichloroacetic acid has been investigated in the treatment of 241 women with cervical HSIL (-IN 2/3) and 179 with cervical LSIL (-IN 1). The regression rate was 87.7% for cervical HSIL (-IN 2/3) and 82.3% for cervical LSIL (-IN 1). Clearance of HPV 16/18 was found in 73.5% of cervical HSIL (-IN 2/3) and 75% of cervical LSIL (-IN 1). Topical 85% trichloroacetic acid was applied to the ectocervix and a saturated cotton swab was inserted into the distal cervical canal one time.[31]

o Imiquimod: A phase II trial of 90 women with CIN 2/3 who were randomly assigned to imiquimod 5%, 250 mg weekly directly applied to the cervix for 12 weeks followed by LEEP vs the control without imiquimod treatment. The primary outcome was histologic regression to CIN 1 or less on LEEP specimens. Results were stratified by HPV type and G 2/3. Of the 49 women enrolled in the imiquimod group 61% had histologic regression compared to 41% in the control group. In the PP population, histologic regression compared with 23% in the control group ($p =.001$). Surgical margins were negative for CIN2/3 in 95% of the imiquimod group and 70% of the control group ($p =.004$). AE rates were 74% in the imiquimod groups, which included G 2 abdominal pain vaginal ulcer, vaginal pruritus with swelling, and moderate pelvic pain.[32]

o In 2018, 51.1% of U.S. adolescents were vaccinated. Recurrent CIN2 at 5 Y was 16.5% versus 1.9% in women vaccinated after conization. After vaccination, the incidence of CIN3 recurrence was reduced 68%.[33]

AIS

• Glandular precancerous changes include AIS. This is histologically represented as crowding of cells, atypia, pseudostratification, and increased mitotic activity. To distinguish atypia versus AIS, the degree of mitotic activity and pseudostratification should be taken into account. To diagnose an invasive lesion, atypical glands extend beyond the depth normally involved by endocervical glands, which is approximately 5 to 6 mm from the surface.[34]

o The mean age of diagnosis is 35 to 37 Y, with an average interval between AIS and early invasive cancer being 5+ Y. Fifty-five percent of patients with AIS have a coexisting squamous lesion.

o A cytologic diagnosis of AGC results in an AIS diagnosis in ~4% of patients, and invasive AC in 2%. When AIS is diagnosed on biopsy, 15% of patients will have an invasive AC. HPV infection with subtypes 16/18 is a major risk factor and vaccination has shown a decrease in incidence (HPV Impact Monitoring Project).

- ○ When histologic diagnosis of AIS is obtained, an excisional procedure (conization or LEEP) should be performed.

- ○ If negative margins and fertility are not desired, then a simple hysterectomy can be performed. If hysterectomy margins are positive, surveillance per ASCCP risk-based management guidelines should be followed.

- ○ If fertility preservation is desired, then surveillance with Pap and HPV co-testing with ECC every 6 months for 3 Y then annually for 2 Y, should be performed. If co-testing and ECC are negative throughout the first 5 Y, a surveillance interval extension to every 3 Y indefinitely can then proceed. Hysterectomy can be considered after fertility is no longer desired or indefinite surveillance can continue if HPV tests are negative.

- ○ If the LEEP/cone has positive margins, a repeat LEEP/cone should be performed if feasible. If margins on the repeat excisional procedure are negative, simple hysterectomy can proceed. If margins on the repeat procedure are positive, simple hysterectomy can proceed or modified radical hysterectomy can be considered. After hysterectomy, surveillance per ASCCP risk-based management guidelines should occur.

- ○ An adequate specimen for an excisional procedure is intact and non fragmented (no top-hat) and the length of the specimen should be at least 1cm. It can increase to 2cm for those done with childbearing. An ECC should also be performed. LEEP versus CKC showed no difference in residual disease (9.1 vs. 11%) although LEEP specimens had a higher rate of positive margins at 44%, versus 29%. For patients whose Pap/cytology shows AIS or AGC-favor neoplasia, but biopsy and ECC are negative, an excisional procedure is recommended. Rates of recurrence for AIS is 2.6% if negative margins, but up to 19% with positive margins.

- ○ Radical hysterectomy for microinvasive AC has not been shown to have a survival benefit so simple hysterectomy is acceptable with less morbidity. The risk of LN metastasis is 1% to 3%, far less than practice-changing benchmarks at 5%.

Vulvar SILs

- **Characteristics**: Vulvar SIL (prior VIN) can present with pruritus, a mass, lesion, or hyperpigmentation. They can also be asymptomatic. The median age at diagnosis is 46 Y old. Vulvar SILs are classified according to the amount of epithelium involved: Vulvar LSIL (-IN 1) demonstrates atypia in the lower third of epithelium, vulvar HSIL (-IN 2/3) demonstrates atypia from the middle third of epithelium to throughout the entire epithelium. Of vulvar HSIL patients who receive treatment, 3% to 4.8% can still progress to cancer. Of untreated patients, 88% have been found to develop invasive disease;[35,36] 12% to 23% of women with vulvar HSIL (-IN 3) are found to have invasive disease at the time of -IN 3 excision;[37] however, most of these diagnoses have less than 1-mm DOI. One third of invasive cancers have coexisting vulvar HSIL (-IN 3). Solitary lesions have the highest risk of progression. Spontaneous regression has occurred with a range of 10% to 56%. But, because this is a precancerous lesion, treatment is the standard of care. Recurrence is higher when associated with positive margins, ranging from 17% to 46%. It is important to remember that L/H-SIL is a histologic biopsy diagnosis, not a screening diagnosis.

- Risk factors for vulvar SIL are a history of other genital tract dysplasia (25% have another lower reproductive tract dysplasia), smoking, immunosuppression, HPV infection, and a history of other STDs.

- The Vulvar Oncology Subcommittee of the ISSVD classifies VIN into three categories congruent with the LAST Project. Terminology for vulvar SIL is *vulvar LSIL*, *vulvar HSIL*, and *DVIN*[5]

  o LSIL of the vulva: vulvar LSIL (prior VIN1) flat condyloma, or HPV effect

  o HSIL of the vulva

    ▪ VIN usual type: This encompasses the former VIN 2/3 subtypes of warty, basaloid, and mixed types. The microscopic appearance of the basaloid type is thickened epithelium with a flat, smooth surface, numerous mitotic figures, and enlarged hyperchromatic nuclei.

    ▪ VIN warty type: The warty type is condylomatous in appearance and microscopically, cells contain numerous mitotic figures with abnormal maturation. The usual type is the most common, typically occurring in younger, premenopausal women. Risk factors include HPV, smoking, and immunosuppression. Lesions are often multifocal.

    ▪ DVIN differentiated type: This encompasses the former category of simplex type. These lesions comprise less than 5% of VIN. They typically occur in postmenopausal women and are associated with lichen sclerosis, but not HPV. Lesions are usually unifocal and p53 positive. This lesion is probably a precursor to HPV-negative vulvar cancer.[38]

- Most often vulvar SILs are found on the vulva between 3 and 9 o'clock, in non–hair-bearing areas. The lesions are often multifocal and can be macular, papular, warty, white, red, gray, or brown. Diagnosis is with colposcopy and biopsy using 3% to 5% acetic acid applied to the perineum for 5 minutes.

- Treatment is varied. Wide local excision with 5-mm margins (skinning vulvectomy) is appropriate, as is CO_2 laser ablation, or CUSA. Topical treatment for vulvar HSIL can be with 5-FU (5% 5-FU cream once daily per week; may increase to two or three times weekly as tolerated by the patient as this medication can cause a significant chemical burn) or imiquimod 5% cream (three times a week, e.g., Monday, Wednesday, Friday, but may decrease frequency to once per week if significant vulvar swelling reaction occurs). Imiquimod should not be used in immunocompromised patients.

- Recurrent disease is common, approaching 50% if margins are positive, versus 15% if negative margins are obtained.

- Wound complications after resection of VIN are commonly due to tension, obesity, and smoking. If any of these risk factors can be mitigated, it is recommended. Antibacterial IV therapy has not been shown to affect wound disruption.[39]

- Benign lesions can mimic vulvar dysplasia. It is imperative to biopsy these lesions to confirm the histologic diagnosis prior to any treatment.

  o Warty lesions are of three main types: condyloma acuminatum, sessile plaques, and keratotic verruca vulgaris. Of patients with vulvar warts, 22% to 32% have concomitant cervical SIL (-IN 1/2/3); therefore, screening colposcopy of the entire lower genital tract is recommended. Treatment can be with topical solutions, such as imiquimod or TCA; laser ablation; CUSA; or surgical resection.

  o Micropapillomatosis labialis is asymptomatic and can appear as small areas of mucosal papillomas. No HPV DNA has been isolated in these lesions. Treatment is not necessary.

  o Lichen sclerosis can present with pruritus. The vulvar skin is paper thin and biopsy shows blunted rete pegs. Treatment is with clobetasol steroid cream to the perineum twice daily for 6 weeks. To promote thickening of the vulvar skin, applying a 2% compounded testosterone cream twice weekly may also be useful. There is an increased risk for malignant transformation to a well-differentiated squamous cell cancer with this lesion.

  o Hyperplastic dystrophy can also present with pruritus. Biopsy shows thickened and widened rete pegs and hyperkeratosis. Treatment is with 1% hydrocortisone cream to the perineum twice daily.

Notable Studies

  o Wound complication rates after vulvar excisions for premalignant lesions: A retrospective cohort study of 537 women who underwent vulvar surgery for premalignant lesions between 2007-2017 took part in this study. The primary outcome was a composite wound complication rate that included breakdown or infection within a 2m postoperative period. Wound complications occurred in 154 (28.7%) patients who had a mean age of 52y; most patients were white (83.1%), cigarette smokers (65.2%), had no prior vulvar treatment (54.4%), and had a preoperative diagnosis of VIN2/3 (70.0%). In multivariate analysis, smoking (OR 1.64, 95% CI, 1.14-2.38) and primary vs. repeat vulvar surgery (OR 1.99, 95% CI, 1.31-3.01) were associated with increased risk. There was no difference between women who received preoperative antibiotics and those who did not (30.4% vs 27.4%, p=0.45), although the mean length of wound separation in the antibiotic group was shorter (1 vs 2 cm, p=0.03). Wound complications after vulvar excisions are likely related to tension which is responsible for wound separation rather than infection.)[39]

Vaginal Squamous Intraepithelial Neoplasia

- Most patients are asymptomatic. Occasionally, patients complain of vaginal discharge or postcoital or PMPB. Most lesions are found because of an abnormal Pap smear.

- Risk factors are HPV infection, other genital tract dysplasia, and immunosuppression.

- Vaginal SIL is classified into two tiers: vaginal LSIL (-IN 1) demonstrates atypia in the lower third of the epithelium, and vaginal HSIL (-IN 2/3) demonstrates atypia into the middle third of the epithelium up to the entire epithelium. Microscopic abnormalities include nuclear atypia, cellular depolarization, parakeratosis, and abnormal mitotic figures.

- The most common location of vaginal dysplasia is the posterior vaginal fornix. Vaginal SIL is often multifocal. Diagnosis is made with colposcopic directed biopsy after application of 3% to 5% acetic acid to the vaginal mucosa.

- There are data to suggest an association of vaginal SIL in posthysterectomy women in whom surgery was done for cervical dysplasia: 5% developed vaginal SIL within 10 Y.

- Treatment can be with laser ablation, surgical excision, or topical suppository creams: 5% 5-FU cream can be used. There are many regimens, but our recommended dosing for 5-FU is once weekly for 10 weeks. This may be decreased to once every 2 to 3 weeks if the patient becomes symptomatic due to development of a vaginal chemical burn. Monthly maintenance dosing can be considered. Recurrence rates range from 0% to 38%. Compounded 2.5% imiquimod cream can also be applied via an intravaginal applicator every other night for 16 weeks. It may be necessary to decrease the dosing frequency to once per week if significant vaginal swelling reaction occurs.

- No large long-term follow-up studies have been done to evaluate the risk of vaginal SIL and progression to vaginal cancer. One study from Finland evaluated 23 patients and showed a 78% rate of regression, 13% persistence, and 8% progression to cancer. Another study evaluated vaginectomy specimens and showed a 28% incidence of cancer.[40] An 18% incidence of recurrence was demonstrated after vaginectomy.

SILs and HIV

- Cervical dysplasia in women with HIV has a more negative outcome. Screening for cervical cancer in HIV-positive women is recommended annually for 3 Y beginning within 1 Y of onset of sexual activity or within the first Y after HIV diagnosis (if already sexually active), but no later than 21 Y old. If three consecutive normal Pap smears are obtained, every 3-Y cytology can follow. If over 30 Y old, co-testing can occur. Cervical cancer screening should continue throughout the patient's lifetime and should not be discontinued. In HIV-positive women, cervical-SIL was found in 14% of women with a normal Pap versus 3% if HIV negative. Of posthysterectomy, HIV-positive women with no prior abnormal Paps, 30% had abnormal vaginal cuff cytology, 29% confirmed vaginal-SIL 2/3 —lending consideration to Pap testing in this population.[41]

- Current guidelines suggest measuring a baseline (pretreatment) viral load. A drug is considered efficacious if it lowers the viral load by at least 90% within 8 weeks. The viral load should continue to drop to less than 50 copies within 6 months. The viral load should be measured within 2 to 8 weeks after treatment is started or changed, and every 3 to 4 months thereafter. Anyone with a viral load over 100,000 should be offered treatment, as should anyone with an AIDS-defining illness or a CD4 count less than 200.

- HAART includes at least three active antiretroviral medications. Typically, two drugs are a nucleoside or NRTI plus a third medication. This third medication can be a NNRTI, a PI, or another NRTI such as abacavir (Ziagen).

- If cervical LSIL (-IN 1) is diagnosed, some clinicians treat immediately. Others may delay treatment if the Pap was a non-HSIL Pap prior to biopsy confirmation of cervical-LSIL (-IN 1). It is important to check the viral load and CD4 counts. If there is a high viral load and a low CD4 count, delay in treatment can be detrimental. For a diagnosis of cervical HSIL (-IN 2/3), conization should be performed.

- Analysis of two large studies HERS and WIHS showed that there was a 45% immediate failure rate/disease persistence at 6 months for HIV-positive women treated for cervical HSIL (-IN 2/3) by LEEP. For those who had a normal Pap smear at 6 months, there was a 56% recurrence rate. The median recurrence-free period was 30 months. Sixty percent of persistent or recurrent disease was low grade. Seventy-three percent of patients in this study were not on HAART.[42]

- Conization margins are very important in HIV-positive patients. Those patients with positive margins had 100% recurrence versus a 30% to 50% recurrence with negative margins. This is compared to an 8% to 15% recurrence rate in HIV-negative women with negative margins. There is an association with a decreased recurrence rate with the use of HAART and higher CD4 counts in two studies (one for each factor). If the CD4 is greater than 500, 30% were found to regress.

- Seven percent of HIV-positive women with condyloma in the perineal or perirectal area can develop vulvar-SIL (-IN 2/3) within a 3-Y period. HIV-positive women are 7 times more likely to develop vulvar SIL than HIV-negative women.
- HPV vaccination is recommended for HIV-infected persons per routine guidelines.
- HIV in cervical cancer: Data from 1996 to 2016 compared the incidence and OSS for Women Living with HIV (WLH) with cervical AC and SCC cervical cancer subtypes vs women without HIV. There were 54,852 women with cervical AC or SCC, (35 AC, 507 SCC) in WLH. The rate of cervical SCC was 3.6 times higher (95% CI, 3.31–3.94) in WLH and 1.47 times higher (95% CI, 1.03–2.05) for AC. The risk for SCC was higher among women who acquired HIV through injection drug use versus heterosexual transmission (aRR, 1.44; 95% CI, 1.17-1.78). Conversely, the risk of cervical AC did not differ significantly among WLH by race or method of HIV acquisition. The 5YOS was similar for cervical AC and SCC in WLH. WLH had a higher risk for death for both cervical AC (HR 2.52; 95% CI, 1.53-4.12) and SCC (HR, 2.02; 95% CI, 1.79–2.29).[43]

Uterine Precancer/Endometrial Intraepithelial Neoplasia
- Symptoms are usually PMPB.
- Imaging can assist in determining risk of cancer. EMS thickness on pelvic US is the best imaging test (Figure 1.1).

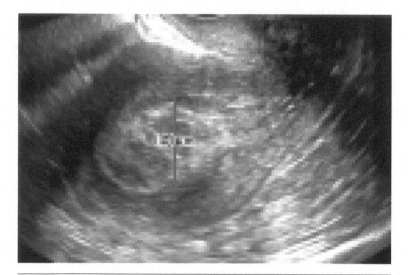

Figure 1.1 US demonstrating thickened EMS.

- ○ EMS thickness is set at an upper limit of 4 mm for postmenopausal women. All women with PMPB should be considered for sampling, but the risk of cancer is less with a smaller EMS.[44]
- ○ EMS thickness is not a 100% reliable screening method for patients with PMPB, however, as 27.6% of patients with type II cancers had an EMS ≤ 5 mm. Patients with continued PMPB and an EMB that was negative or nondiagnostic should undergo further evaluation with a method not previously used (SIS, hysteroscopy with directed sampling, or D&C).[45]
- Diagnosis is by tissue sampling. Sampling methods can include EMB, cytology retrieved at time of sonohysterography, hysteroscopy and directed biopsy, or D&C. If CAH or EIN is found on EMB, D&C can be used to reliably rule in or out G1 cancer.[46]
- Management by general OB/GYNS or referral to subspecialty is acceptable given that, although up to 42% of patients may have a G1 endometrioid cancer, 2% to 5% of patients will have a tumor in need of staging by Mayo criteria, and Mayo criteria can overestimate the percent needing LND (basing LND on tumor size alone). Complete pelvic and/or SLND is low yield given the low rate of metastasis, is not cost-effective, and can have adverse outcomes to include lymphedema.[47–51]
- There are two means of categorizing uterine precancer:
  - ○ WHO-94 schema: There is risk of progressing to cancer if left untreated see Table 1.3.
  - ○ EIN schema: This is the preferred terminology per ACOG/SOG
    - Benign: benign endometrial hyperplasia (prior WHO-94: simple hyperplasia and complex hyperplasia)
    - **EIN** (premalignant): atypical endometrial hyperplasia of more than 1 mm in size (this includes the prior WHO-94 categories of simple and CHs with atypia)
    - Malignant endometrial AC endometrioid type well differentiated (G 1 cancer)
- As per GOG 167, the risk of concurrent uterine cancer found at the time of hysterectomy performed for CAH was 42.6%:[52]

Table 1.3 WHO-94 Schema With Risk of Progressing to Cancer if Left Untreated (%)

Simple hyperplasia	1
CH	3
Simple hyperplasia with atypia	9
CH with atypia	27

- **Surgical treatment** for EIN: Hysterectomy can be performed with/ without a BSO in patients with confirmed premalignant disease and is considered effective treatment.
- **Medical treatment** for EIN: Medical treatment may be acceptable for patients who desire future fertility or for those with medical comorbidities prohibiting surgical management. Progesterone counterbalances the mitogenic effects of estrogens and induces secretory differentiation. Options include:
  - MPA 10 to 20 PO mg/day, or cyclic 12 to 14 days/month
  - Depot medroxyprogesterone 150 mg IM every 3 months
  - Micronized vaginal progesterone 100 to 200 mg/day or cyclic 12 to 14 days/month
  - Megestrol acetate 40 to 600 PO mg/day
  - Levonorgestrel IUD:
    - Mirena IUD: Contains 52 mg in steroid reservoir to be replaced every 6 Y; releases 20 mg daily: this declines to a rate of 14 mg daily after 5 Y, still in the range of clinical effectiveness.
    - Skyla IUD: Contains 13.5 mg in a steroid reservoir to be replaced every 3 Y. It releases 15 mcg daily and declines to 5 mcg daily after 3 Y.
    - Liletta IUD: Contains 52 mg levonorgestrel in steroid reservoir, replaced every 3 Y.
    - Kyleena IUD: Contains 19.5 mg levonorgestrel in a steroid reservoir, to be replaced every 5 Y.
- Regression rates for EIN or G1 cancer with medical treatment:
  - With MPA:
    - 10 PO mg daily 12 to 14 days/month, for 3 months: 80% to 90%.[53]
    - 10 PO mg daily for 6 months: EIN and G1 endometrioid AC
      - 65.8% CR for EIN
      - 48.2% CR for G1 cancer
      - 28% persistent or PD
      - 23% had a CR followed by recurrence
  - With Mirena IUD varying degrees of response have been found:
    - Response is up to 90% if simple or CH, but only 67% if EIN.
    - Response is 90% in EIN and 54% in G1 endometrioid cancer[54]
    - ORR for 12 months of use is 58%: ORR is 85% in those with EIN, and 33% RR in those with G1 cancer.[55]
- Notable Trials:
  - Meta-analysis: In this study, 344 women (77.7%) demonstrated a response to hormonal therapy. Median follow-up was 39

months, and a durable CR was seen in 53.2%. The CR rate was significantly higher for those with hyperplasia than for those with cancer (65.8% vs. 48.2%, p = .002). The median time to CR was 6 months (range, 1–18 months). Recurrence after an initial response was noted in 23.2% with hyperplasia and 35.4% with cancer (p = .03). Persistent disease was observed in 14.4% of women with hyperplasia and 25.4% of women with cancer (p = .02). During the respective study periods, 41.2% of those with hyperplasia and 34.8% with a history of cancer obtained pregnancy (p = .39), with 117 live births reported.[56]

- Medical management was given to 153 women (PO or IUD) for endometrial hyperplasia or cancer due to inappropriate surgical candidacy or desire for fertility preservation. The average age at diagnosis was 49.6 Y. Patients with hyperplasia were compared to patients with cancer. The patients who had hyperplasia responded at a higher rate than those with cancer, showing a CR of 66% to70% compared to a rate of 6% to13% for those with cancer. Eleven percent to 23% of patients with hyperplasia had an initial response but subsequently recurred, compared to 19% to 30% of those with cancer. For those patients with hyperplasia, 11% to 19% did not respond to medical management at all, compared to 57% to 75% of those with cancer, (p <.001). In those patients with cancer, the levonorgestrel-IUD, when compared to oral progesterone regimens, did demonstrate a difference in response. In those patients with hyperplasia, outcomes were significantly different only during the 9- 12-month posttreatment follow-up period, where systemic hormone therapy demonstrated a better response with less disease persistence or progression compared to the levonorgestrel-IUD. Three women were able to conceive.[57]

- Treatment was given to 344 women with CH or CAH who were treated either with IUD or oral progestins over a 12-Y period with a median follow-up of 58.8 months. Those with CH treated with an IUD had a 12.7% relapse, those treated with oral progestins had a 30.3% relapse. A BMI ≥35 yielded an HR of 18.93 for failure to regress. Oral progestins used were: norethisterone 5 mg TID, medroxyprogesterone 10 mg daily for 10 months, or Megace 180 mg daily or BID. Relapse was associated with DM, EMS greater than 9 mm, or BMI greater than 35, but was not associated with CAH versus CH.[58]

- Preoperative predictors of endometrial cancer at time of hysterectomy for EIN or CAH: This was a retrospective cohort study of women undergoing hysterectomy for pathologically confirmed EIN. In this study, 169 patients with EIN were reviewed, 87 (51.5%) had a final diagnosis of EIN/other benign disease, and 82 (48.5%) were diagnosed with endometrial cancer. No medical diagnoses were found to be associated with concurrent endometrial cancer. Preoperative imaging results showed that a thicker average EMS was present in cancer patients compared to noncancer patients at the time of hysterectomy (15.7 mm; SD, 9.5) versus 12.5 mm; SD, 6.4; p = .01). An EMS ≥2 cm was associated with 4.0-time higher odds of concurrent endometrial cancer (95% CI, 1.5–10.0), when controlling for age. Of the cancer cases, 87% were staged T1a (Nx or N0). About 44% of cancer patients with an EMS of ≥2 cm met the "Mayo criteria" for LND compared to 22% of endometrial cancer patients with an EMS <2 cm. It is important to consider that Mayo criteria tends to overestimate the need for LND and, eliminating tumor size as a component, reduces the FPs/need for LND in up to 40% of cases.[59,60]

Serous Tubal Intraepithelial Carcinoma

- STIC is a precursor lesion to high-grade pelvic serous carcinoma that usually presents in the distal fimbriated end of the fallopian tube (Figure 1.2).
- The incidence of STIC at RRBSO in women identified to have HBOC is 0.8% to9% with occult cancer ranges from 2.3% to 4.7%
- Treatment of STIC when incidentally found is long-term follow-up versus second look/staging with washings, biopsies of the peritoneum, and omentum in addition to completion BSO if not already done.
- Treatment of occult HGSTOC after RRBSO can be comprehensive surgical staging +/– LND, followed by three to six cycles of chemotherapy, or chemotherapy alone, given that 9% can recur with peritoneal disease.
- Outcomes of incidentally detected ovarian cancers diagnosed at time of RRSO in *BRCA* mutation carriers:[61] In this study, 548 patients with *BRCA* mutations underwent RRSO and 26 had an incidental cancer identified at the time of surgery. Of these 16 tumors were thought to be ovarian and 10 of primary tubal origin. Of these, 38% were stage I, eight stage II, eight stage III. All patients with cancer underwent complete surgical staging and 92% received adjuvant platinum/taxane treatment with two stage IA not receiving chemotherapy, neither of which had recurrence. Eight patients overall recurred at a median of 67.3 months with 5Y PFS being 72% and 5Y DSS 96%.
- BRCA1/2 presenting for RRSO with prevalence of invasive and in-situ carcinoma with follow-up:[62] Between 2000 and 2016, 527 patients undergoing RRSO were reviewed. Of these patients, 68% were BRCA1, 31.6% were BRCA2, and 0.4% had both mutations. HGS carcinoma was the most common finding with isolated STIC identified in 0.8%, 2 BRCA1 carriers with isolated STIC at RRSO developed peritoneal serous carcinoma >7 Y later. SEE-FIM pathology protocol

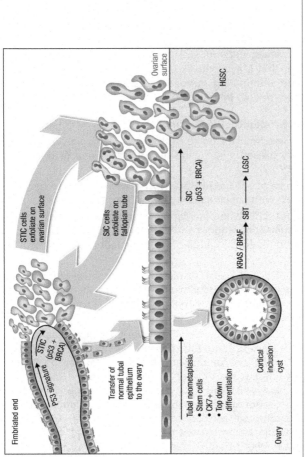

Figure 1.2 Development of HGSCs and LGSCs.

Source: Reproduced with permission from Prat J, D'Angelo E, Espinosa I. Ovarian carcinomas: at least five different diseases with distinct histological features and molecular genetics. *Hum Pathol.* 2018;80:11-27. doi: 10.1016/j.humpath.2018.06.018

was followed after 2009. The prevalence of HGSC was 2.3% (12/527); 59% of these were of tubal origin. Two of the BRCA1 carriers with isolated STIC at RRSO developed peritoneal serous carcinoma >7 Y later. Identical TP53 mutations in the peritoneal serous carcinoma and the preceding STIC demonstrated a clonal origin. Those who underwent surgery after the recommended age had a higher rate of carcinoma, thus undergoing RRSO at the proposed age is suggested.

TUBO-OVARIAN CANCER SCREENING

Screening Test

A good **screening test** is both sensitive (high probability of detecting disease) as well as specific (high probability that those without disease will be found to not have disease). An ideal screening test has a sensitivity of 100% and a specificity of 95%. Screening tests are typically not designed to diagnose disease; rather, they identify subjects who need further diagnostic tests or procedures. A PPV of 10% or greater is the goal of any screening test. This means that one diagnosis per 10 interventions is needed for the test to be considered worthwhile.

CA-125

CA-125 alone has a sensitivity of 83%, specificity of 59%, PPV of 16%, and NPV of 97%.

HE4

HE4 alone has a sensitivity of 78%, specificity of 95%, PPV of 80%,; and NPV of 99%. It has no sensitivity for borderline tumors.

Risk of Malignancy Index

- The risk of malignancy index (RMI) incorporates US findings with menopausal status (M) and the CA-125 level. It is written as: RMI = $U \times M \times$ CA-125. A score of either 0, 1, or 3 is given to the U. $U = 0$ for an US with no features of malignancy. $U = 1$ for an US score of 1. $U = 3$ for an US score of 2 to 5. A score of either 1 or 3 is given for menopausal status. $M = 1$ for premenopausal women or $M = 3$ for postmenopausal women.[63]
- On US, 1 point is given for each of the following morphologies: multiloculation, solid components, bilaterality, ascites, or intra-abdominal metastasis. The stated sensitivity is 81%, specificity is 85%, PPV is 48%, and NPV is 96%. If the calculated level of RMI is greater than 200, referral to a gynecologic oncologist is recommended.

Morphology Index

- The Ueland morphology index assesses ovarian tumors based on tumor volume and wall structure. When the morphology index is less than 5, most adnexal masses are found to be benign with a NPV of 99%. If the morphology index is greater than 5, the PPV has been stated at 40%.[64]

- The Kentucky University Algorithm has identified women at higher risk for OC. A baseline US is obtained. If it is abnormal, it is repeated within 6 weeks. If the repeat US is found to still be abnormal, a CA-125 is drawn and the morphology index is calculated. The stated sensitivity is 85%, the specificity is 98%, the PPV is 14%, and the NPV is 99%. Disease was found at an earlier stage (i.e., stage migration) if there was strict adherence to these guidelines. 64% of cancers were found at Stage I.[65]

Risk of Ovarian Malignancy Algorithm

- The combination test of HE4 and CA-125 is called the *predictive probability algorithm or ROMA*. This predictive algorithm is calculated for premenopausal and postmenopausal women separately, using the following equations. To calculate the algorithm, the assay values obtained from the HE4 EIA and CA-125 II assays are inserted into the applicable equation.
  - Premenopausal woman:
    $PI = -12.0 + 2.38 \times LN\,(HE4) + 0.0626 \times LN\,(CA\text{-}125)$
  - Postmenopausal woman:
    $PI = -8.09 + 1.04 \times LN\,(HE4) + 0.732 \times LN\,(CA\text{-}125)$
- To calculate the ROMA value (the predictive probability), insert the calculated value for the PI into the following equation: ROMA value $\% = \exp(PI)/(1 + \exp(PI)) \times 100$

The following cutoff points were used to provide a specificity level of 75%:

- Premenopausal women:
  - ROMA value $\geq 13.1\%$ = HiR of finding EOC
  - ROMA value $< 13.1\%$ = LoR of finding EOC
- Postmenopausal women:
  - ROMA value $\geq 27.7\%$ = HiR of finding EOC
  - ROMA value $< 27.7\%$ = LoR of finding EOC

This test is stated to have a sensitivity of 94%, specificity of 75%, PPV of 58%, and NPV of 97%.

Risk of Ovarian Cancer Algorithm

The ROCA represents the slope of serial CA-125 levels drawn over a period of time and correlated with patient age. If there is greater than 1% change in the slope of the line, a TVUS is recommended. The U.K. ROCA study showed a PPV of 19% and a specificity of 99.8%.

Copenhagen Index

The CPH-I uses the following variables: serum HE4, serum CA-125, and patient age instead of menopausal status, omitting US characteristics. Comparison of CPH-I, ROMA, and RMI demonstrated an AUC of 0.951,

0.953, and 0.935, respectively. Using a sensitivity at 95%, the specificities for CPH-I, ROMA, and RMI in the validation cohort were 67.3%, 70.7%, and 69.5%, respectively, in the validation study. The coefficients are CPH-I = $-14.0647 + 1.0649 \times \log2(HE4) + 0.6050 \times \log2(CA\text{-}125) + 0.2672 \times age/10$. The predicted probability is $= e^{(CPH\text{-}I)}/(1 + e^{(CPH\text{-}I)})$.[66]

OVA-1 Test

The OVA-1 test uses five well-established biomarkers: prealbumin, apolipoprotein A-1, beta$_2$-microglobulin, transferrin, and CA-125. A proprietary algorithm is used to determine the likelihood of malignancy in women with a pelvic mass for whom surgery is planned. The sensitivity is stated to be 92.5%, with a specificity of 42.8%, PPV of 42.3%, and NPV of 92.7%. It is important to remember not to perform this test if the patient has a rheumatoid factor ≥ 250 IU/L or has a triglyceride level >450 mg/dL.

Ovarian Cancer Symptom Index

The OCSI associates specific symptoms with OC. These symptoms are pelvic/abdominal pain, urinary urgency/frequency, increased abdominal size/bloating, and difficulty eating/feeling full. These symptoms become significant when present for less than 1 Y and when they occur greater than 12 days/month. The overall sensitivity was 64% and specificity 88%. For women who are found to have early-stage disease, the sensitivity is stated to be 56.7%, and for women with advanced-stage disease it is 79.5%. When age-stratified, the specificity is stated at 90% for women greater than 50 Y old and 86.7% for women less than 50 Y old.[67]

- The OCSI in combination with a CA-125 has also been used to risk stratify adnexal masses. The combination of CA-125 and the SI has been shown to identify 89.3% of women with cancer, 80.6% of early-stage cancers, and 95.1% of late-stage cancers. The FP rate was 11.8%.[68]
- The OCSI in combination with both CA-125 and HE4 has been found to have a sensitivity of 95% and specificity of 80%. If any two of the three tests were positive, a sensitivity of 84% and specificity of 98.5% were found. When all three tests were used, the specificity was 98.5% and the sensitivity was 58%.[69]

The UKCTOCS

Between 2001 and 2005, The UKCTOCS evaluated 202,562 postmenopausal women aged 50 to 74 Y between 2001 and 2005 who were randomized in a 1:1:2 ratio to one of the following: annual multimodal screening with CA-125 and US (MMS), annual transvaginal USS, or no screening. In the study, 101,299 received no treatment, 50,623 had annual screening with TVUS, and annual CA-125 (interpreted as a ROCA) with TVUS as a second-line test (50,624; designated multimodal screening, MMS). MMS screening was performed using the ROCA algorithm, including serial CA-125 level and US risk factors to include size, volume, and complexity of ovarian cyst. If US was abnormal, a repeat US was scheduled either at 3 months or 6 weeks depending on complexity assessment. Women predisposed to hereditary cancer syndromes were excluded. The primary outcome was death due to HGTOC (WHO 2014 criteria) by June 30, 2020. The sensitivity, specificity, and PPVs for all primary ovarian type cancers in 2009 were 89.4%, 99.8%, and 43.3% for MMS, and 84.9%, 98.2%, and 5.3% for TVUS screening. In the MMS arm, 2.9 surgeries were needed per cancer detected, compared to 35.2 in the TVUS group. In the follow-up study published in 2015, the primary outcome was death due to TOC. At a median follow-up of 11.1 Y, OCs were diagnosed in 630 (no screening), in 338 (MMS), and 314 (TVUS) women. The mortality reduction over Y 0 to 14 using the Cox model was 15% with MMS, and 11% with TVUS, which were **not significant compared to no screening**. This mortality reduction was made up of an 8% relative reduction in mortality during Y 0 to 7 (**NS**), and 23% relative reduction in mortality during Y 7 to 14 in the MMS versus no screening, and of 2% (**NS**) and 21%, respectively, in the TVUS group versus the no-screening group. The total number of surgeries was not reported but 488 benign surgical outcomes (FPs) were documented in the MMS group, 1,634 FP surgeries in the TVUS group, with surgical complications of 3.1% in the MMS group and 3.5% in the TVUS group. **Prevalent cases of cancer were also removed** from the analysis. In addition, 792 women in the no-screening group, 466 in the MMS group, and 441 in the US group had a BSO outside of the trial, again confounding the results. The overall ratio of women who had surgery resulting in benign pathology to cancer was 1:2 (792/645) in the no screening group, 2:7 (954:354) in the MMS group, and 6:4 (2075:324) in the TVUS group. There was no total number of women reported who screened positive, so the number of surgeries needed for FP screens is unknown.[70,71] Final data review in 2021 distilled the result that screening in normal populations cannot be recommended[72]. The median follow-up was 16.3 Y. In the study, 50,625 (25·0%) were included in the MMS group, 50,623 (25·0%) in the USS group, and 101,314 (50%) in the no screening group. 2,055 women overall were diagnosed with tubal or OC: 522 (1.0%) in the MMS group, 517 (1.0%) in the USS group, and 1016 (1.0%) in the no screening group. A 47.2% (95% CI: 19.7-81.1) increase in stage I and 24.5% (−41.8 to −2.0) decrease in stage IV disease incidence in the MMS group was seen compared to no screening. The incidence of stage I or II disease was 39.2% (95% CI: 16.1-66.9) higher in the MMS group than in the no-screening group, whereas the incidence of stage III or IV disease was 10.2% (−21.3-2.4) lower. In the study, 1,206 women died of disease: 296 (0.6%) in the MMS group, 291 (0.6%) in the USS group, and 619 (0·6%) in the no-screening group. No significant reduction in ovarian and tubal cancer deaths was observed in the MMS ($p = .58$) or USS ($p = .36$) groups compared with the no-screening group. The decrease in stage III/IV disease incidence in the MMS group did not significantly reduce ovarian and tubal cancer deaths, thus screening in normal-risk women cannot be recommended.

The PLCO Trial

This study compared CA-125 levels and US imaging versus observation in 78,216 women aged 55 to 74 with annual TVUS for 4 Y and CA-125 for 6 Y. In the study, 42 of 61 OCs were found, but 28 (67%) of these were advanced stage. The PPV was 1.1%; the number needed to treat was 20:1. Fifteen percent of patients had serious complications related to surgery. There was no evidence of stage migration. Additional data discovered in this trial revealed that 14% of postmenopausal women had simple ovarian cysts, at an 8% incidence; and 32% of these cysts spontaneously regressed. A 15-Y follow-up reviewed mortality benefit between arms. Again, 39,105 women were randomized to the intervention arm and 39,111 were in the usual-care arm. Median follow-up was 14.7 Y in each arm and maximum follow-up 19.2 Y in each arm. A total of 187 (intervention) and 176 (usual care) deaths from OC were observed, for a risk ratio of 1.06 (95% CI: 0.87–1.30). Risk ratios were similar for study Y 0 to 7 (RR = 1.04), 7 to 14 (RR = 1.06) and over 14 Y (RR = 1.09). The risk ratio for all-cause mortality was 1.01 (95% CI: 0.97–1.05). OC-specific survival was not significantly different across trial arms ($p = .16$). Conclusion: Extended follow-up of women in the PLCO Trial indicated no mortality benefit from screening.[73,74]

Japan Screening Study

Shizuoka Cohort Study of OC Screening: This was a prospective randomized controlled trial of OC screening. Asymptomatic postmenopausal women were randomly assigned between 1985 and 1999 to an intervention group ($n = 41,688$) or a control group ($n = 40,799$) in a 1:1 ratio. The mean follow-up was 9.2 Y. Women in the intervention group had annual pelvic US and serum CA-125. Women with abnormal US findings and/or raised CA-125 values were referred for surgical investigation by a gynecological oncologist. Twenty-seven cancers were detected in the 41,688 screened women. Eight more cancers were diagnosed outside the screening program. Detection rates of OC were 0.31 per 1,000 at the prevalent screen and 0.38 to 0.74 per 1,000 at subsequent screens; detection increased with successive screening rounds. Among the 40,779 control women, 32 women developed OC. The proportion of stage I OC was higher in the screened group (63%) than in the control group (38%), which did not reach statistical significance ($p = .2285$).[75]

Serial US of Ovarian Abnormalities

In a prospective TVUS study, 39,337 women were included. Ovarian masses were categorized into (a) normal, (b) simple unilocular cysts, (c) cysts with septations uni- and multiloculated, (d) cysts with solid areas, and (e) solid masses. Septated complex masses without solid areas or papillary projections had a 40% spontaneous resolution rate with a mean time to resolution of 12 months. Indications for surgical evaluation in this screened population were complexity of abnormality increased to cystic with solid area or mostly solid; an increase in volume greater than 50 cm^3 associated with constant or increasing complexity; or if newly reported regional pain occurred after a second abnormal US. Resolution of ovarian masses did occur when followed serially. Resolution by category: Unilocular cyst(s), 32.8% resolved at a mean of 55.6 weeks; cyst(s) with septation(s), 43.9% resolved at a mean of 53.0 weeks; cyst(s) with solid area(s), 76.5% resolved at a mean of 7.8 weeks; solid mass, 80.6% resolved at a mean of 8.7 weeks. LoR = unilocular and cysts with septations. HiR = cysts with solid area or solid mass. Thus, it is helpful to have more than one US. Surgery was performed on 557 patients of 39,337 participants with 85 malignancies identified. The PPV for cancer rose from 8% to 25% by reducing FP results.[76]

Serial USS for Those With a Family History of OC

Annual US for women with a family history of OC aged 25 or older and for all asymptomatic women over 50 was performed from 1987 to 2017. In the study, 46,101 women were screened in a prospective cohort trial. Women who had a persistent abnormal screen underwent tumor morphology indexing, serum biomarker analysis, and surgery. Seventy-one invasive epithelial OCs and 17 LMP tumors were detected. The DSS for screen-detected cancers was higher than in those women who were clinically detected, and directly related to earlier stage at detection (stage migration). The stage distribution for screen-detected invasive epithelial OCs was stage I-30 (42%), stage II-15 (21%), stage III-26 (37%), and stage IV-0 (0%). Follow-up varied from 9.2 months to 27 Y (mean 7.9 Y). DSS at 5, 10, and 20 Y for women with invasive EOC detected by screening was 86±4%, 68±7%, and 65±7%, respectively, versus 45±2%, 31±2%, and 19±3%, respectively (p <.001). Twenty-seven percent of screen-detected malignancies were type I and 73% were type II.[77]

GOG 199

GOG 199 was a prospective study of women with confirmed genetic risk of OCs. At enrollment, women could choose to have OC screening or undergo risk-reducing surgery to include BSO. The study enrolled 2,605 women: There were 1,030 (40%) women in the surgical group and 1,575 (60%) elected to be in the screening group. The primary study outcomes was review of ovarian and breast cancer incidence, also including use of the ROCA. Nine neoplastic tubal lesions from 966 RRSO were identified, 8 of which occurred in *BRCA* mutation carriers.[78,79]

Opportunistic Salpingectomy in Low-Risk Women

No difference was found in ovarian function in premenopausal women undergoing hysterectomy versus hysterectomy and bilateral salpingectomy for benign disease. This was determined by assessment of AMH, FSH, antral follicle count, mean ovarian diameter, and peak systolic velocity on postoperative laboratories and imaging. There was no difference in operative time, postoperative stay, time to return to normal activity, and postoperative Hg. Up to 700,000 women have a tubal ligation each Y. This procedure can provide significant risk reduction opportunity.[80]

OC Risk

OC risk after salpingectomy was evaluated in a population-based cohort study on women with prior surgery for benign indications compared to the unexposed population analyzed. The risk reductions for prior hysterectomy was HR = 0.79, sterilization HR = 0.72, hysterectomy with BSO HR = 0.06, USO compared to BSO 0.35; all CI did not cross 1. BSO had a 50% lower chance of OC, than USO[81].

Women who have any abdominal surgery and have completed childbearing could have opportunistic bilateral salpingectomy/salpingo-oophorectomy as an adjunct to surgery (i.e., appendectomy, cholecystectomy, hysterectomy). Fifteen percent of OCs could be prevented annually by BSO at time of hysterectomy. A staged surgery to preserve ovarian function can be performed by bilateral salpingectomy: Using bilateral salpingectomy, a study in Denmark reduced the risk of ovarian-type cancer by 42%, and a Swedish study by 65%.[82,83]

Changing CA-125 "Normals"

Future "screening" could focus on detection of advanced-stage OC when the disease burden is low enough that surgical debulking can primarily achieve no residual disease followed by IP chemotherapy. By making low-volume advanced-stage OC (stage IIIA/IIIB) the target, rather than stage I, the threshold for CA-125 could be raised to 70 U/mL. This would reduce the sensitivity for detecting all OCs from 75% to 70%, but increase the specificity from 95% to 99%. The PPV of a CA-125 at 70 U/mL is then 5%. If the cutoff were raised to 100 U/mL, the sensitivity would be reduced to 60%, but specificity increased to 99.9% and the PPV would increase to 31%.[84]

Screening Pelvic Examination in Adult Women

The ACP recommends against performing screening pelvic examinations in asymptomatic nonpregnant adult women. They cite three cohort studies of 5,633 women, including the negative results of PLCO assessing the diagnostic accuracy of a pelvic exam in asymptomatic women between the ages 51 to 58. Only four cases of OC were identified in 1 Y, with a PPV 0% to 3.5%. Examination- related "harms" were pain or discomfort ranging from 11% to 60%; and 10% to 80% for fear, embarrassment, or anxiety. Care should be taken with interpretation of this study.[85]

REFERENCES

1. https://www.ncbi.nlm.nih.gov/books/NBK537348/
2. Dilley S, Huh W, Blechter B, et al. It's time to re-evaluate cervical cancer screening after age 65. *Gynecol Oncol.* 2021;162(1):200–202. doi: 10.1016/j.ygyno.2021.04.027

3. Nanda K, McCrory DC, Myers ER, et al. Accuracy of the papanicolaou test in screening for and follow-up of cervical cytologic abnormalities: a systematic review. *Ann Intern Med.* 2000;132(10):810–819. doi: 10.7326/0003-4819-132-10-200005160-00009

4. Wright TC, Stoler MH, Behrens CM, et al. Primary cervical cancer screening with human papillomavirus: end of study results from the ATHENA study using HPV as the first-line screening test. *Gynecol Oncol.* 2015;136(2):189–197. doi: 10.1016/j.ygyno.2014.11.076

5. Darragh TM, Colgan TJ, Cox JT, et al. The lower anogenital squamous terminology standardization project for HPV-associated lesions: background and consensus recommendations from the college of american pathologists and the american society for colposcopy and cervical pathology. *Arch Pathol Lab Med.* 2012;136(10):1266–1297. doi: 10.5858/arpa.LGT200570

6. Schiffman M, Vaughan LM, Raine-Bennett TR, et al. A study of HPV typing for the management of HPV-positive ASC-US cervical cytologic results. *Gynecol Oncol.* 2015;138(3):573–578. doi: 10.1016/j.ygyno.2015.06.040

7. Wheeler CM, Skinner SR, Del Rosario-Raymundo MR, et al. Efficacy, safety, and immunogenicity of the human papillomavirus 16/18 AS04-adjuvanted vaccine in women older than 25 years: 7-year follow-up of the phase 3, double-blind, randomised controlled VIVIANE study. *Lancet Infect Dis.* 2016;16(10):1154–1168. doi: 10.1016/S1473-3099(16)30120-7

8. Wright TC, Stoler MH, Behrens CM, et al. The ATHENA human papillomavirus study: design, methods, and baseline results. *Am J Obstet Gynecol.* 2012;206(1):46. doi: 10.1016/j.ajog.2011.07.024

9. Siebers AG, Klinkhamer P, Arbyn M, et al. Cytologic detection of cervical abnormalities using liquid-based compared with conventional cytology: a randomized controlled trial. *Obstet Gynecol.* 2008;112(6):1327–1334. doi: 10.1097/AOG.0b013e31818c2b20

10. ASCUS-LSIL Traige Study (ALTS) Group. Results of a randomized trial on the management of cytology interpretations of atypical squamous cells of undetermined significance. *Am J Obstet Gynecol.* 2003;188(6):1383–1392. doi: 10.1067/mob.2003.457

11. ASCUS-LSIL Traige Study (ALTS) Group. A randomized trial on the management of low-grade squamous intraepithelial lesion cytology interpretations. *Am J Obstet Gynecol.* 2003;188(6):1393–1400. doi: 10.1067/mob.2003.462

12. Katki HA, Schiffman M, Castle PE, et al. Benchmarking CIN 3+ risk as the basis for incorporating HPV and pap cotesting into cervical screening and management guidelines. *J Low Genit Tract Dis.* 2013;17(5 Suppl. 1):S28–35. doi: 10.1097/LGT.0b013e318285423c

13. Melnikow J, Nuovo J, Willan AR, et al. Natural history of cervical squamous intraepithelial lesions: a meta-analysis. *Obstet Gynecol.* 1998;92(4 Pt 2):727–735. doi: 10.1016/s0029-7844(98)00245-2

14. Schiffman M, Wentzensen N, Wacholder S, et al. Human papillomavirus testing in the prevention of cervical cancer. *J Natl Cancer Inst.* 2011;103(5):368–383. doi: 10.1093/jnci/djq562

15. Huh WK, Ault KA, Chelmow D, et al. Interim guidance for use of primary HR HPV testing for cervical cancer screening. *Gynecol Oncol.* 2015;136:178–182.

16. Lammé J, Pattaratornkosohn T, Mercado-Abadie J, et al. Concurrent anal human papillomavirus and abnormal anal cytology in women with known cervical dysplasia. *Obstet Gynecol.* 2014;124(2 Pt 1):242–248. doi: 10.1097/AOG.0000000000000370

17. Kang WD, Choi HS, Kim SM. Is vaccination with quadrivalent HPV vaccine after loop electrosurgical excision procedure effective in preventing recurrence in patients with high-grade cervical intraepithelial neoplasia (CIN2-3)? *Gynecol Oncol.* 2013;130(2):264–268. doi: 10.1016/j.ygyno.2013.04.050

18. Teoh D, Musa F, Salani R, et al. Diagnosis and management of adenocarcinoma in situ: A society of gynecologic oncology evidence-based review and recommendations. *Obstet Gynecol.* 2020 Apr;135(4):869–878. doi: 10.1097/AOG.0000000000003761. https://www.acog.org/clinical/clinical-guidance/practice-advisory/articles/2021/04/updated-cervical-cancer-screening-guidelines

19. Castle PE, Gravitt PE, Wentzensen N, et al. A descriptive analysis of prevalent vs incident cervical intraepithelial neoplasia grade 3 following minor cytologic abnormalities. *Am J Clin Pathol.* 2012;138(2):241–246. doi: 10.1309/AJCPNTK6G2PXWHOO

20. Moreno V, Bosch FX, Muñoz N, et al. Effect of oral contraceptives on risk of cervical cancer in women with human papillomavirus infection: the IARC multicentric case-control study. *Lancet.* 2002;359(9312):1085–1092. doi: 10.1016/S0140-6736(02)08150-3

21. Grulich AE, van Leeuwen MT, Falster MO, et al. Incidence of cancers in people with HIV/AIDS compared with immunosuppressed transplant recipients: a meta-analysis. *Lancet.* 2007;370(9581):59–67. doi: 10.1016/S0140-6736(07)61050-2

22. Abraham AG, D'Souza G, Jing Y, et al. Invasive cervical cancer risk among HIV-infected women: a north american multicohort collaboration prospective study. *J Acquir Immune Defic Syndr.* 2013;62(4):405–413. doi: 10.1097/QAI.0b013e31828177d7

23. Fordyce EJ, Wang Z, Kahn AR, et al. Risk of cancer among women with AIDS in new york city. *AIDS Public Policy J.* 2000;15(3–4):95–104.

24. Porreco R, Penn I, Droegemueller W, et al. Gynecologic malignancies in immunosuppressed organ homograft recipients. *Obstet Gynecol.* 1975;45(4):359–364.

25. Chin-Hong PV, Kwak EJ. AST infectious diseases community of practice. human papillomavirus in solid organ transplantation. *Am J Transplant.* 2013;13:189–200.

26. Schlecht NF, Platt RW, Duarte-Franco E, et al. Human papillomavirus infection and time to progression and regression of cervical intraepithelial neoplasia. *J Natl Cancer Inst.* 2003;95(17):1336–1343. doi: 10.1093/jnci/djg037

27. Sawaya GF, Smith-McCune K. Cervical cancer screening. *Obstet Gynecol.* 2016;127(3):459–467. doi: 10.1097/AOG.0000000000001136

28. Tierney KE, Lin PS, Amezcua C, et al. Cervical conization of adenocarcinoma in situ: a predicting model of residual disease. *Am J Obstet Gynecol.* 2014;210(4):366. doi: 10.1016/j.ajog.2013.12.030

29. Huh WK, Sideri M, Stoler M, et al. Relevance of random biopsy at the transformation zone when colposcopy is negative. *Obstet Gynecol.* 2014;124(4):670–678. doi: 10.1097/AOG.0000000000000458

30. Grimm C, Polterauer S, Natter C, et al. Treatment of cervical intraepithelial neoplasia with topical imiquimod: A randomized controlled trial. *Obstet Gynecol*. 2012;120(1):152–159. doi: 10.1097/AOG.0b013e31825bc6e8

31. Geisler S, Speiser S, Speiser L, et al. Short-term efficacy of trichloroacetic acid in the treatment of cervical intraepithelial neoplasia. *Obstet Gynecol*. 2016;127(2):353–359. doi: 10.1097/AOG.0000000000001244

32. Fonseca BO, Possati-Resende JC, Salcedo MP, et al. Topical imiquimod for the treatment of high-grade squamous intraepithelial lesions of the cervix: A randomized controlled trial. *Obstet Gynecol*. 2021;137(6):1043–1053. doi: 10.1097/AOG.0000000000004384

33. Lichter K, Krause D, Xu J, et al. Adjuvant human papillomavirus vaccine to reduce recurrent cervical dysplasia in unvaccinated women: a systematic review and meta-analysis. *Obstet Gynecol*. 2020;135(5):1070–1083. doi: 10.1097/AOG.0000000000003833

34. Teoh D, Musa F, Salani R, et al. Diagnosis and management of adenocarcinoma in situ: A society of gynecologic oncology evidence-based review and recommendations. *Obstet Gynecol*. 2020;135(4):869–878. doi: 10.1097/AOG.0000000000003761

35. Jones RW, Rowan DM. Vulvar intraepithelial neoplasia III: a clinical study of the outcome in 113 cases with relation to the later development of invasive vulvar carcinoma. *Obstet Gynecol*. 1994;84(5):741–745.

36. Sideri M, Jones RW, Wilkinson EJ, et al. Squamous vulvar intraepithelial neoplasia: 2004 modified terminology, ISSVD vulvar oncology subcommittee. *J Reprod Med*. 2005;50(11):807–810.

37. Modesitt SC, Waters AB, Walton L, et al. Vulvar intraepithelial neoplasia III: occult cancer and the impact of margin status on recurrence. *Obstet Gynecol*. 1998;92(6):962–966. doi: 10.1016/s0029-7844(98)00350-0

38. Bornstein J, Bogliatto F, Haefner HK, et al. The 2015 international society for the study of vulvovaginal disease (ISSVD) terminology of vulvar squamous intraepithelial lesions. *Obstet Gynecol*. 2016;127(2):264–268. doi: 10.1097/AOG.0000000000001285

39. Mullen MM, Merfeld EC, Palisoul ML, et al. Wound complication rates after vulvar excisions for premalignant lesions. *Obstet Gynecol*. 2019;133(4):658–665. doi: 10.1097/AOG.0000000000003185

40. Ireland D, Monaghan JM. The management of the patient with abnormal vaginal cytology following hysterectomy. *BJOG:An International Journal of O&G*. 1988;95(10):973–975. doi: 10.1111/j.1471-0528.1988.tb06499.x. http://www.blackwell-synergy.com/toc/bjo/95/10

41. Smeltzer S, Yu X, Schmeler K, et al. Abnormal vaginal pap test results after hysterectomy in human immunodeficiency virus-infected women. *Obstet Gynecol*. 2016;128(1):52–57. doi: 10.1097/AOG.0000000000001457

42. Massad LS, Fazzari MJ, Anastos K, et al. Outcomes after treatment of cervical intraepithelial neoplasia among women with HIV. *J Low Genit Tract Dis*. 2007;11(2):90–97. doi: 10.1097/01.lgt.0000245038.06977.a7

43. Rositch AF, Levinson K, Suneja G, et al. Epidemiology of cervical adenocarcinoma and squamous cell carcinoma among women living with human immunodeficiency virus compared with the general population in the united states. *Clin Infect Dis*. 2022;74(5):814–820. doi: 10.1093/cid/ciab561

44. ACOG committee opinion no. 440: the role of transvaginal ultrasonography in the evaluation of postmenopausal bleeding. *Obstet Gynecol.* 2009;114(2 Pt 1):409–411. doi: 10.1097/AOG.0b013e3181b48feb

45. Billingsley CC, Kenne KA, Cansino CD, et al. The use of transvaginal ultrasound in type II endometrial cancer. *Int J Gynecol Cancer.* 2015;25(5):858–862. doi: 10.1097/IGC.0000000000000423

46. Suh-Burgmann E, Hung YY, Armstrong MA. Complex atypical endometrial hyperplasia: the risk of unrecognized adenocarcinoma and value of preoperative dilation and curettage. *Obstet Gynecol.* 2009;114(3):523–529. doi: 10.1097/AOG.0b013e3181b190d5

47. Lim SL, Moss HA, Secord AA, et al. Hysterectomy with sentinel lymph node biopsy in the setting of pre-operative diagnosis of endometrial intraepithelial neoplasia: A cost-effectiveness analysis. *Gynecol Oncol.* 2018;151(3):506–512. doi: 10.1016/j.ygyno.2018.09.020

48. Shalowitz DI, Goodwin A, Schoenbachler N. Does surgical treatment of atypical endometrial hyperplasia require referral to a gynecologic oncologist? *Am J Obstet Gynecol.* 2019;220(5):460–464. doi: 10.1016/j.ajog.2018.12.010

49. Glassman D, Emerson J, Quddus MR. Is universal SLN sampling indicated in EIN. *SGO Annual Meeting Poster 467 2020 Toronto.*

50. Sullivan MW, Philp L, Kanbergs AN, et al. Lymph node assessment at the time of hysterectomy has limited clinical utility for patients with precancerous endometrial lesions. *Gynecol Oncol.* 2021;162(3):613–618. doi: 10.1016/j.ygyno.2021.07.004

51. Benoit MF, Ward KK. Uterine cancer normogram to predict lymph node metastasis: comparison to the mayo algorithm and an external validation of a model in a north american population. *EJGO.* 2020;41(5):681. doi: 10.31083/j.ejgo.2020.05.5401

52. Trimble CL, Kauderer J, Zaino R, et al. Concurrent endometrial carcinoma in women with a biopsy diagnosis of atypical endometrial hyperplasia: a gynecologic oncology group study. *Cancer.* 2006;106(4):812–819. doi: 10.1002/cncr.21650

53. The american college of obstetricians and gynecologists committee opinion no. 631. endometrial intraepithelial neoplasia. *Obstet Gynecol.* 2015;125(5):1272–1278. doi: 10.1097/01.AOG.0000465189.50026.20

54. Westin S et al. SGO annual meeting abstract 41, march 2016. gynecol oncol vol 141, supplement 1, june 2016. challenging the paradigm of progesterone-only therapy for early endometrial cancer: results of a prospective trial of the levonorgesterel intrauterine system pages 18-19 westin SN, sun CCL, broadus N et al. 2016.

55. Westin S, Sun C, Broaddus R, et al. Prospective phase II trial of the levonorgestrel intrauterine system (mirena) to treat complex atypical hyperplasia and grade 1 endometrioid endometrial cancer. *Gynecol Oncol.* 2016;125:S9. doi: 10.1016/j.ygyno.2011.12.016

56. Gunderson CC, Fader AN, Carson KA, et al. Oncologic and reproductive outcomes with progestin therapy in women with endometrial hyperplasia and grade 1 adenocarcinoma: a systematic review. *Gynecol Oncol.* 2012;125(2):477–482. doi: 10.1016/j.ygyno.2012.01.003

57. Hubbs JL, Saig RM, Abaid LN, et al. Systemic and local hormone therapy for endometrial hyperplasia and early adenocarcinoma. *Obstet Gynecol.* 2013;121(6):1172–1180. doi: 10.1097/AOG.0b013e31828d6186

58. Gallos ID, Ganesan R, Gupta JK. Prediction of regression and relapse of endometrial hyperplasia with conservative therapy. *Obstet Gynecol.* 2013;121(6):1165–1171. doi: 10.1097/AOG.0b013e31828cb563

59. Vetter MH, Smith B, Benedict J, et al. Preoperative predictors of endometrial cancer at time of hysterectomy for EIN or CAH. *Am J Obstet Gynecol.* 2020;222(1):60e1–60e7. doi: 10.1016/j.ajog.2019.08.002

60. Benoit MF, Ward KK. Abstract SGO 2019 annual meeting. 2019.

61. Cowan R, Nobre SP, Pradhan N, et al. Outcomes of incidentally detected ovarian cancers diagnosed at time of risk-reducing salpingo-oophorectomy in brca mutation carriers. *Gynecol Oncol.* 2021;161(2):521–526. doi: 10.1016/j.ygyno.2021.02.006

62. Blok F, Dasgupta S, Dinjens WNM, et al. Retrospective study of a 16 year cohort of BRCA1 and BRCA2 carriers presenting for RRSO: prevalence of invasive and in-situ carcinoma, with follow-up. *Gynecol Oncol.* 2019;153(2):326–334. doi: 10.1016/j.ygyno.2019.03.003

63. Jacobs I, Oram D, Fairbanks J, et al. A risk of malignancy index incorporating ca 125, ultrasound and menopausal status for the accurate preoperative diagnosis of ovarian cancer. *Br J Obstet Gynaecol.* 1990;97(10):922–929. doi: 10.1111/j.1471-0528.1990.tb02448.x

64. Ueland FR, DePriest PD, Pavlik EJ, et al. Preoperative differentiation of malignant from benign ovarian tumors: the efficacy of morphology indexing and doppler flow sonography. *Gynecol Oncol.* 2003;91(1):46–50. doi: 10.1016/s0090-8258(03)00414-1

65. van Nagell JR, Miller RW, DeSimone CP, et al. Long-term survival of women with epithelial ovarian cancer detected by ultrasonographic screening. *Obstet Gynecol.* 2011;118(6):1212–1221. doi: 10.1097/AOG.0b013e318238d030

66. Karlsen MA, Høgdall EVS, Christensen IJ, et al. A novel diagnostic index combining HE4, CA125 and age may improve triage of women with suspected ovarian cancer - an international multicenter study in women with an ovarian mass. *Gynecol Oncol.* 2015;138(3):640–646. doi: 10.1016/j.ygyno.2015.06.021

67. Goff BA, Mandel LS, Drescher CW, et al. Development of an ovarian cancer symptom index: possibilities for earlier detection. *Cancer.* 2007;109(2):221–227. doi: 10.1002/cncr.22371

68. Andersen MR, Goff BA, Lowe KA, et al. Combining a symptoms index with CA 125 to improve detection of ovarian cancer. *Cancer.* 2008;113(3):484–489. doi: 10.1002/cncr.23577

69. Andersen MR, Goff BA, Lowe KA, et al. Use of a symptom index, CA125, and HE4 to predict ovarian cancer. *Gynecol Oncol.* 2010;116(3):378–383. doi: 10.1016/j.ygyno.2009.10.087

70. Menon U, Gentry-Maharaj A, Hallett R, et al. Sensitivity and specificity of multimodal and ultrasound screening for ovarian cancer, and stage distribution of detected cancers: results of the prevalence screen of the UK collaborative trial of ovarian cancer screening (UKCTOCS). *Lancet Oncol.* 2009;10(4):327–340. doi: 10.1016/S1470-2045(09)70026-9

71. Jacobs IJ, Menon U, Ryan A, et al. Ovarian cancer screening and mortality in the UK collaborative trial of ovarian cancer screening (UKCTOCS): a

randomised controlled trial. *Lancet.* 2016;387(10022):945–956. doi: 10.1016/S0140-6736(15)01224-6

72. Menon U, Gentry-Maharaj A, Burnell M, et al. Ovarian cancer population screening and mortality after long-term follow-up in the UK collaborative trial of ovarian cancer screening (UKCTOCS): a randomized controlled trial. *Lancet.* 2021;397(10290):2182–2193. doi: 10.1016/S0140-6736(21)00731-5

73. Buys SS, Partridge E, Black A, et al. Effect of screening on ovarian cancer mortality: the prostate, lung, colorectal and ovarian (PLCO) cancer screening randomized controlled trial. *JAMA.* 2011;305(22):2295–2303. doi: 10.1001/jama.2011.766

74. Pinsky PF, Yu K, Kramer BS, et al. Extended mortality results for ovarian cancer screening in the PLCO trial with median 15years follow-up. *Gynecol Oncol.* 2016;143(2):270–275. doi: 10.1016/j.ygyno.2016.08.334

75. Kobayashi H, Yamada Y, Sado T, et al. A randomized study of screening for ovarian cancer: A multicenter study in japan. *Int J Gynecol Cancer.* 2008;18(3):414–420. doi: 10.1111/j.1525-1438.2007.01035.x

76. Pavlik EJ, Ueland FR, Miller RW, et al. Frequency and disposition of ovarian abnormalities followed with serial transvaginal ultrasonography. *Obstet Gynecol.* 2013;122(2 Pt 1):210–217. doi: 10.1097/AOG.0b013e318298def5

77. van Nagell JR, Burgess BT, Miller RW, et al. Survival of women with type I and II epithelial ovarian cancer detected by ultrasound screening. *Obstet Gynecol.* 2018;132(5):1091–1100. doi: 10.1097/AOG.0000000000002921

78. Greene MH, Piedmonte M, Alberts D, et al. A prospective study of risk-reducing salpingo-oophorectomy and longitudinal CA-125 screening among women at increased genetic risk of ovarian cancer: design and baseline characteristics: A gynecologic oncology group study. *Cancer Epidemiol Biomarkers Prev.* 2008;17(3):594–604. doi: 10.1158/1055-9965.EPI-07-2703

79. Mai PL, Sherman ME, Piedmonte M, et al. Pathologic findings at risk-reducing salpingo-oophorectomy among women at increased ovarian cancer risk: results from GOG-199. *JCO.* 2012;30(15_suppl):1519–1519. doi: 10.1200/jco.2012.30.15_suppl.1519

80. Morelli M, Venturella R, Mocciaro R, et al. Prophylactic salpingectomy in premenopausal low-risk women for ovarian cancer: primum non nocere. *Gynecol Oncol.* 2013;129(3):448–451. doi: 10.1016/j.ygyno.2013.03.023

81. Falconer H, Yin L, Grönberg H, et al. Ovarian cancer risk after salpingectomy: a nationwide population-based study. *J Natl Cancer Inst.* 2015;107(2):dju410. doi: 10.1093/jnci/dju410

82. Madsen C, Baandrup L, Dehlendorff C, et al. Tubal ligation and salpingectomy and the risk of epithelial ovarian cancer and borderline ovarian tumors: a nationwide case-control study. *Acta Obstet Gynecol Scand.* 2015;94(1):86–94. doi: 10.1111/aogs.12516

83. Falconer H, Yin L, Grönberg H, et al. Ovarian cancer risk after salpingectomy: a nationwide population-based study. *J Natl Cancer Inst.* 2015;107(2):dju410. doi: 10.1093/jnci/dju410

84. Sopik V, Rosen B, Giannakeas V, et al. Why have ovarian cancer mortality rates declined? part III. prospects for the future. *Gynecol Oncol.* 2015;138(3):757–761. doi: 10.1016/j.ygyno.2015.06.019

85. Qaseem A, Humphrey LL, Harris R, et al. Screening pelvic examination in adult women: a clinical practice guideline from the american college of physicians. *Ann Intern Med.* 2014;161(1):67–72. doi: 10.7326/M14-0701

2 Gynecologic Cancers

CERVICAL CANCER

Characteristics

There are approximately 570,000 new cases of cervical cancer world-wide annually. In 2022 there were 14,100 anticipated new cases identified with approximately 4,280 deaths in the United States.

- The most common symptom of cervical cancer is abnormal vaginal bleeding—specifically, postcoital and intermenstrual bleeding, menorrhagia, and PMPB. Other symptoms include pelvic fullness/pain, unilateral leg swelling, bladder irritability, and tenesmus. Cervical cancer is also commonly asymptomatic, found only following an abnormal Pap smear, colposcopic exam, or cervical biopsy.
- Common signs of advanced cervical cancer are a fungating cervical mass, unilateral leg edema, and obstructive renal failure.
- Cervical cancer often results from persistent infection with high-risk HPV types (most commonly 16 and 18). Risk factors associated with cervical cancer are: prior history of STDs, early age of first coitus, multiple sexual partners, multiparity, nonbarrier methods of birth control, and smoking.
- Cervical cancer primarily spreads by direct extension from the cervix to the parametria, vagina, uterine corpus, and the pelvis. Other routes of spread include lymphatic and hematogenous dissemination, as well as direct peritoneal seeding.
- LN metastasis usually occurs in a sequential fashion, traveling first to the parametrial LNs, then to pelvic (obturator, internal, and external iliac), common iliac, PA, then scalene LN.

Pretreatment Workup

The pretreatment workup of cervical cancer begins with a history and physical exam. Laboratory studies to assess hematologic, renal, and liver functions should be performed. Imaging studies should also be performed to include pelvic imaging and a CXR (Figure 2.1).

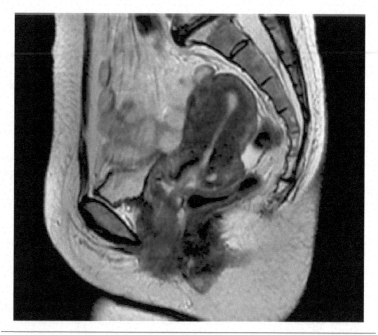

Figure 2.1 MRI of stage IIB squamous cell cervical cancer.

- FIGO-approved imaging studies previously only included barium enema, IVP, and CXR. Other modalities, such as CT (to assess LNs and evaluate for hydronephrosis), MRI (to assess integrity of tissue planes and extent of cervical disease), and PET/CT (to evaluate for distant metastasis), are also now FIGO- (2018) and AJCC-approved staging tests (2021), although they continue to have poor accessibility in medically underserved areas and countries.

- Cervical conization should be used to evaluate microscopic disease. Conization can differentiate between microinvasive versus invasive early-stage disease.

- For lesions that are macroscopic, an office examination with evaluation for hydronephrosis (CT/MRI/renal ultrasound) and CXR are indicated and cystoscopy/proctoscopy are only indicated if the patient is clinically symptomatic. Cystoscopy is also recommended when there is a barrel-shaped tumor.

- If patients cannot tolerate an office exam, or if there is ambiguity about the staging in an office setting, an EUA should be performed. There is data to suggest that EUA can significantly change clinical staging: 23% were upstaged, most to IIA or IIB disease. Patients were downstaged less often (9%) to IB2 and IIB. Proctoscopy was not found to be helpful, but cystoscopy identified 8% of patients with stage IVA disease, and a CXR was abnormal in 4% of patients.[1]

- Multiple studies have supported the use of PET scans. An analysis of 15 published (FDG)-PET studies on cervical cancer showed that the pooled sensitivity and specificity of FDG-PET for detecting pelvic LN metastasis were 79% (95% CI: 65%–90%) and 99% (95% CI: 96%–99%), compared with 72% (95% CI: 53%–87%) and 96% (95% CI: 92%–98%) for MRI, and 47% (95% CI: 21%–73%) for CT (specificity not available). The pooled sensitivity and specificity of FDG-PET for detecting PALNs were 84% (95% CI: 68%–94%) and 95% (95% CI: 89%–98%).[2] A study from Israel[3] revealed a sensitivity of 60%, a specificity of 94%, a PPV of 90%, and a NPV of 74%. PET–CT may not pick up lesions smaller than 1.5 cm. There is data to suggest that treatment modification can occur in 25% of patients based on PET–CT results.

Histology

There are several different histologic types of cervical cancer, the most common being squamous (85%). Other types include adenocarcinoma (15%–20%), verrucous carcinoma, adenosquamous carcinoma, clear cell carcinoma (CC), neuroendocrine carcinomas, and undifferentiated types. Ten percent of these are not HPV related.

- Adenocarcinoma: About 15% have no visible lesion because the lesion arises from the endocervical canal, forming a "barrel-shaped" lesion. Cells frequently stain CEA+. Variants are the more common mucinous endocervical, mucinous intestinal type, signet ring type, and colloid variants. Adenoma malignum/minimal deviation variant has an infiltrative pattern distinct from those listed elsewhere with cytologically benign-appearing cells on low power but moderate nuclear atypia seen on higher power and are seen in patients with PJS. There is a three-tiered system developed to classify risk of LN metastasis in invasive adenocarcinoma developed by Silva et al.[4]
  - Pattern A: Well-demarcated glands frequently form clusters or groups with lobular architecture and lack destructive stromal invasion or LVI. LN metastasis risk: 0%.
  - Pattern B: Localized destructive invasion with small clusters or individual tumor cells within desmoplastic stroma often arising from pattern A glands. Often well to moderately differentiated. LVI ±. LN metastasis risk: 4.4%.
  - Pattern C: Glands are diffusely infiltrated with an associated desmoplastic response. Confluent growth filling a 4 × field (5 mm) or mucin lakes present, solid poorly differentiated component with LVI. LN metastasis risk: 23.8%.[5]
- Verrucous carcinoma: This is a well-differentiated squamous cell carcinoma. It is known to recur locally, but does not metastasize. Historically, these tumors should not be treated with XRT because radiation can cause anaplastic transformation; however, recent evidence does not support this. It is associated with HPV6.

- Adenosquamous carcinoma: This is a mixed glandular and squamous carcinoma. It behaves similarly to adenocarcinoma.
- Glassy cell carcinoma: This is a poorly differentiated type of adenosquamous carcinoma.
- Clear cell carcinoma: This is a poorly differentiated carcinoma. It is nodular and reddish in gross appearance. It has a hobnail cell shape microscopically. It can be associated with intrauterine DES exposure.
- Neuroendocrine carcinoma: This includes the small-cell, large-cell, and carcinoid (typical and atypical) carcinomas. Small cell is the most common neuroendocrine tumor in the cervix. It contains adenoid basal cells with scarce myoepithelial differentiation. Small cell is often HPV 18, 16 related. CD56, NSE, chromogranin, synaptophysin, TTF-1, ACTH, somatostatin, and serotonin staining can all be positive.
- Papillary squamous cell: This is a variant of squamous cell carcinoma. It appears as transitional or cuboidal cells on microscopy.
- Mesonephric adenocarcinoma: Remnants of the mesonephric ducts are occasionally seen in the lateral aspects of the cervix, are PAS+, and do not contain intracytoplasmic mucin (Tables 2.1A–D, and 2.2).

Staging[6,7]

Staging was modified in 2018 to allow the option of clinical, pathologic, or radiological findings to assign stage. Positive LN are included into stage IIIC.

Treatment

The treatment of cervical cancer may involve the use of surgery, chemotherapy, XRT, systemic targeted therapy or a combination of therapies. About 70% of newly diagnosed patients with invasive carcinoma

Table 2.1A AJCC 9th Edition and FIGO 2018: T Category

T	FIGO	T Criteria
TX		Primary tumor cannot be assessed
T0		No evidence of primary tumor
T1	I	Cervical carcinoma confined to the uterus (extension to the corpus should be disregarded)
T1a	IA	Invasive carcinoma diagnosed only by microscopy; stromal invasion with a maximum depth of ≤5.0 mm measured from the base of the epithelium; vascular space involvement, venous or lymphatic, does not affect classification
T1a1	IA1	Measured stromal invasion of 3.0 mm or less in depth

(continued)

Table 2.1A AJCC 9th Edition and FIGO 2018: T Category *(continued)*

T	FIGO	T Criteria
T1a2	IA2	Measured stromal invasion of more than 3.0 mm and ≤5.0 mm in depth
T1b	IB	Clinically visible lesion confined to the cervix or microscopic lesion greater than 5mm of stromal invasion; includes all macroscopically visible lesions, even with superficial invasion
T1b1	IB1	Clinically visible or invasive lesion >5 mm in depth and ≤2 cm in dimension
T1b2	IB2	Clinically visible invasive lesion >2 cm and ≤4 cm in greatest dimension
T1b3	IB3	Clinically visible invasive lesion >4 cm in greatest dimension
T2	II	Cervical carcinoma invading beyond the uterus such as the vagina, but not the pelvic wall or to the lower third of the vagina
T2a	IIA	Tumor without parametrial invasion and confined to the upper 2/3 of the vagina
T2a1	IIA1	Invasive lesion ≤4 cm in greatest dimension
T2a2	IIA2	Invasive lesion >4 cm in greatest dimension
T2b	IIB	Tumor has spread to the parametrial area but not pelvic sidewall
T3	III	Tumor extending to the pelvic sidewall and/ or involving the lower third of the vagina and/ or causing hydronephrosis or nonfunctioning kidney
T3a	IIIA	Tumor involving the lower third of the vagina but not extending to the pelvic sidewall
T3b	IIIB	Tumor extending to the pelvic sidewall and/ or causing hydronephrosis or nonfunctioning kidney
T3c	IIIC	Involvement of pelvic and/or PALNs irrespective of tumor size and extent
T3c1	IIIC1	Pelvic LN metastasis only
T3c2	IIIC2	PALN metastasis
T4	IVA	Tumor invading the mucosa of the bladder or rectum and/ or extending beyond the true pelvis (bullous edema is not sufficient to classify a tumor as T4)

Table 2.1B AJCC 9th Edition and FIGO 2018: N Category

N	FIGO	N Criteria
NX		Regional LNs cannot be assessed
N0		No regional LN metastasis
N1		Pelvic LN metastasis N1mi: regional LN metastasis >0.2mm but ≤2mm N1a: regional LN metastasis >2 mm
N2		PALN metastasis: with or without positive pelvic LN N2mi: regional LN metastasis >0.2mm but ≤2mm N2a: regional LN metastasis >2 mm

(r) is imaging; (p) is pathology
suffix (f) added when FNA
suffix (sn) is added with SLN biopsy
ITCs have no impact on staging at this time.

Table 2.1C AJCC 9th Edition and FIGO 2018: M Category

M	FIGO	M Criteria
M0		No distant metastasis
M1	IVB	Distant metastasis (including peritoneal spread or involvement of the inguinal, supraclavicular, mediastinal, or distant LNs; lung; liver; or bone)

Table 2.1D AJCC 9th Edition and FIGO 2018: Stage Grouping

I	
IA	T1aN0M0
IA1	T1a1N0M0
IA2	T1a2N0M0
IB	T1bN0M0
IB1	T1b1N0M0
IB2	T1b2N0M0
IB3	T1b3N0M0

(continued)

Table 2.1D AJCC 9th Edition and FIGO 2018: Stage Grouping (*continued*)

II	
IIA	T2aN0M0
IIA1	T2a1N0M0
IIA2	T2a2N0M0
IIB	T2bN0M0
III	
IIIA	T3aN0M0
IIIB	T3bN0M0
IIIC	(TX, T0, T1-3)N1M0
IIIC1	(TX, T0, T1-3)N1M0
IIIC2	(TX, T0, T1-3)N2M0
IV	
IVA	T4(Any N)M0
IVB	(Any T)(Any N)M1

of the cervix have disease limited to the uterine cervix and are, there-fore, potential operative candidates. Of these, 54% to 84% of patients will need adjuvant therapies for intermediate or high-risk factors; so thorough investigation of the full extent of disease should be per-formed. NCI statements support treatment with the fewest number of interventions; thus, if high-risk factors are found on conization or in preoperative planning that predict a high probability for the need of adjuvant therapy, it may be prudent not to perform radical hys-terectomy and move towards definitive chemoradiation instead. The

Table 2.2 Cervical Cancer OS by Stage

Stage	5YS (%)
IA	97
IB	90
IIA	83
IIB	80
IIIA	50
IIIB	50
IIIC	60
IVA	50
IVB	28

LACC trial demonstrated that patients undergoing minimally invasive approaches to radical hysterectomy have worse OS than those who had an open/abdominal approach.[8]

Tumor testing: Testing can be ordered on specimens when staged as metastatic IVB or recurrent and includes:

- TMB
- PD-L1
- MSI genes
- NTRK gene fusion testing

Treatment Options by Stage
- Stage IA1:
  - No LVSI: A simple (type I/extrafascial) hysterectomy or CKC with 3-mm negative margins (if fertility-sparing treatment is desired) are adequate therapies. If margins on the CKC are positive, repeat CKC or simple trachelectomy should be performed. Extrafascial hysterectomy +/- LND or SLND are alternative options. Intracavitary XRT can be used alone if the patient is not a surgical candidate.
  - LVSI: A CKC with LND/SLND can be performed. If margins are positive, a repeat CKC or trachelectomy can be performed for fertility-sparing management. A radical trachelectomy with LND/SLND can also be performed. Non–fertility-sparing procedures include a type II (modified) radical hysterectomy with LND/SLND or WP EBXRT and brachytherapy.
- Stage IA2:
  - A type II radical hysterectomy with LND/SLND. Similar outcomes have been seen between types II and III radical hysterectomy[9] or
  - Pelvic EBXRT with brachytherapy. Fertility-sparing procedures include a CKC with LND/SLND or radical trachelectomy with LND/SLND.
- Stages IB1, IB2:
  - A radical hysterectomy and pelvic LND/SLND: PALND is recommended for all patients staged IB and higher. Surgical candidates are those with lesions that are not bulky or barrel shaped. A radical trachelectomy with LND/SLND can be considered for tumors not greater than 2 cm if fertility preservation is desired.
  - Definitive treatment can also be primary EBXRT and brachytherapy with concurrent cisplatin chemotherapy. Total dosing for XRT should be 80 to 85 Gy. Similar cure rates are seen with either radical surgery or XRT.[10]
- Stage IIA1: Radical hysterectomy with LND/SLND can be offered for small volume disease. Otherwise EBXRT and brachytherapy with platinum-based chemotherapy are recommended.

- Stages IB3-IVA (locally advanced):
  - A combination of EBXRT and brachytherapy with concurrent platinum-based chemotherapy is the standard of care. Patients with cervical lesions 4 cm or larger in size have a high rate of needing adjuvant therapies after a surgical approach and *primum non nocere* states the least injurious approach be the standard of care. Total dosing with XRT should be ≥85 Gy to the primary tumor with extended field radiation based on imaging, +/-FNA, or surgical LN staging.
  - A radical hysterectomy with P-LND with PALND or SLND can be offered in select stage IB3 and IIA2 patients unable to receive radiation.
  - Surgical LN staging can be considered via extraperitoneal or transperitoneal laparoscopic LND. If negative, tailored field EBXRT and brachytherapy with concurrent platinum-based chemotherapy can be administered. If positive, then the need arises for EBXRT to cover the PA and involved LN basins.
  - Surgery can be considered as adjuvant therapy in certain situations; for example, if there is residual tumor after definitive chemotherapy–XRT or uterine anatomy precludes adequate brachytherapy. Total dose with this approach is 75 to 80 Gy.
- Stage IB2, IB3, IIA2, IIB, IIIA, IIIB, IVA: CT of chest, abdomen, and pelvis should be obtained:
  - If imaging shows adenopathy:
    - Positive pelvic adenopathy but negative PA adenopathy: Consider laparoscopic LND of pelvic and PA basins or FNA of suspicious LN:
      - If positive PALN: WP EBXRT and brachytherapy with extended-field XRT concurrent with platinum-based chemotherapy.
      - If negative PALN: Then WP EBXRT with brachytherapy concurrent with platinum based chemotherapy (tailored fields is needed).
    - Positive pelvic and PA adenopathy on imaging: Consider laparoscopic LND followed by WP and PA EBXRT to affected LN basins with brachytherapy, concurrent with platinum based chemotherapy.
    - If distant metastases are seen: Administer systemic chemotherapy with individualized palliative XRT.
- Stage IVB: Chemotherapy should be used for disseminated disease and XRT can be considered for pelvic tumor control or palliation of symptoms, including bleeding.

- If cancer is incidentally found on a postoperative hysterectomy specimen:
  - Stage IA1 with LVSI or > stage IA2: Imaging should be obtained with pathologic review:
    - Negative margins and negative imaging:
      - WP EBXRT and brachytherapy with concurrent cisplatin chemotherapy should be offered, or
      - A parametrectomy with upper vaginectomy and P-LND with/without PA-LND can be performed
    - Positive margins or gross residual disease:
      - If imaging is negative for adenopathy: WP EBXRT with concurrent platinum-based chemotherapy with/without brachytherapy based on vaginal margins.
      - If imaging is positive for adenopathy: Consider debulking of grossly enlarged LN followed by WP and PA EBXRT with concurrent platinum-based chemotherapy with/without brachytherapy based on vaginal margins.
- Most randomized trials included 5% to 8% of patients with adenocarcinoma, so they are applicable to cite in treating adenocarcinoma of the cervix.
- Margin status is important in conization. In one study evaluating AIS,[11] 33% of patients with negative margins had residual disease at the time of hysterectomy and 14% had invasive cancer; 53% of those with positive margins had residual disease and 26% were found to have invasive cancers. In another study, which reviewed patients with invasive squamous cell cancer on conization,[12] 24% of patients had residual disease if they had negative margins and 60% were found to have residual disease if they had positive margins.
- The incidence of positive LNs with squamous cell and adenocarcinomas is 5% for stage IA2, 15% for stage IB1, 30% for stage IB2, 45% for stage IIB, and 60% for stage IIIB (by default is now 3C).
- The incidence of adnexal metastasis with adenocarcinoma is 1.7% compared to 0.5% for squamous cell lesions. According to GOG 49,[13] this is a nonsignificant difference, and all patients with ovarian metastasis had evidence of other extra-cervical disease.
- The rate of an aborted radical hysterectomy for grossly positive LNs is approximately 7% to 8%.[14] Per GOG 49, the rate of aborted radical hysterectomy was 8.3%.
- If a positive LN is found at the time of radical hysterectomy, there are two management options: completion of, or abortion of, radical hysterectomy.

- ○ Some proceed and complete the radical hysterectomy. The rationale is that removal of bulky LNs leaves less residual tumor for XRT to sterilize.

- ○ Another study showed that the local recurrence and distant recurrence rates were not significantly different for LN-positive aborted versus completed radical hysterectomy patients. The PFS was 74.9 months versus 46.8 months (p = .106) and the OS was 91.8 months versus 69.4 months (p = .886).[15] Potter[16] found similar outcomes and the trend favored definitive XRT. Leaving the uterus in situ can help with treatment planning and can move the small bowel out of the treatment field. Debulking of LN greater than 2 cm prior to abortion of hysterectomy may be beneficial additionally.

- ○ The number of positive LN affects OS. The 5YS decreases for each additional positive LN: one node (79%), two to three nodes (63%), four + nodes (40%).[17]

- Surgical staging in locally advanced cervical cancer may be beneficial. In one study, surgical staging of women with locally advanced cervical cancer was suggested to improve overall clinical outcome, as those with positive LNs had a modification in standard XRT fields in up to 43% of patients.[18]

- LN debulking can potentially improve the 5YS in patients with locally advanced cervical cancer.[19] One study showed that if grossly metastatic LNs were resected, the survival of women in that group approached the level of those women who had microscopic LN involvement only (50%, 5YS), which was significantly higher than the women with unresectable LNs (0%).[19] There was a 10.5% incidence of severe XRT-related morbidity and a 1% incidence of treatment-related deaths due to combined therapies.

- A *cut-through hysterectomy* refers to a cancer either found incidentally on final pathology or resected without radical surgery. Treatment of a "cut through" can include adjuvant EBXRT +/-brachytherapy with platinum-based chemotherapy or a radical parametrectomy. Indications for EBXRT and brachytherapy +/-cisplatin are positive margins, gross residual disease, positive imaging, or primary tumor characteristics meeting Sedlis criteria. There are data to suggest that the 5YS is better with adjuvant XRT versus radical parametrectomy with a 68.7% versus a 49% 5YS. This is stage and margin dependent. The 5YS for women staged IA2 and IIA was 96%,[20] but was much lower for women stage IIB or higher, who had a 5YS of 28%.

- Hydronephrosis found on imaging predicts a worse OS and PFS. Relief of ureteral obstruction has been associated with improved survival. Management with stenting via cystoscopy from below, or antegrade from above, is beneficial for preservation of renal function and enables full dosing of radiosensitizing chemotherapy.[21]

Surgical Treatment

- Hysterectomy types: Piver classification I–V is based on the degree of resection of vagina, parametria, cardinal ligaments, and uterosacral ligaments.[22]
  - Class I radical hysterectomy is the same as a simple hysterectomy. It is indicated for stage IA1 cervical cancers without LVSI.
  - Class II radical hysterectomy is a modified radical hysterectomy. It involves resection of the medial half of the cardinal and uterosacral ligaments. The uterine artery is taken at its junction with the ureter. The upper one fourth (or 1–2 cm) of the vagina is also removed. This results in a wider local treatment margin than a simple hysterectomy.
  - Class III radical hysterectomy is also called a *Wertheim/Meigs–Okabayashi hysterectomy*. Originally, Wertheim did not include lymphadenectomy, whereas Meigs and Okabayashi did. In this procedure, the cardinal and uterosacral ligaments are completely transected and one third to one half of the vagina is removed. The uterine artery is taken at its origin. The autonomic nerves for bladder and rectal function are also resected, which can result in a high incidence of prolonged or permanent bladder dysfunction.
  - Class IV radical hysterectomy is reserved for larger bulky lesions. This procedure involves completely transecting the cardinal and uterosacral ligaments at their origin. One half of the vagina is removed; therefore, sexual dysfunction occurs from the shortened vagina. The superior vesical artery is sacrificed and all periureteral tissue is removed.
  - Class V radical hysterectomy is reserved for tumors that invade to the lower urinary tract. It involves the removal of involved portions of the bladder as well as the distal ureters.
- There are data to suggest that for early-stage (IB–IIA) cervical cancer that there is no difference in recurrence rate or survival rate between class II or III radical hysterectomy. Surgeries took longer for the type III hysterectomies (Figure 2.2).[9]
- A scalene LND is done if there is a question about distant metastasis. There are data to suggest that 10.7% of patients with positive PALNs have positive scalene nodes. PET scanning may be a reasonable alternative to a scalene LND.[23]
  - The boundaries of the neck are the anterior and posterior triangles.
    - The anterior triangle is bordered by the sternocleidomastoid, the mandible, and the midline of the neck.
    - The posterior triangle is bordered by the sternocleidomastoid, the clavicle, and the trapezius. This is the larger triangle of the neck in which the scalene triangle lies.

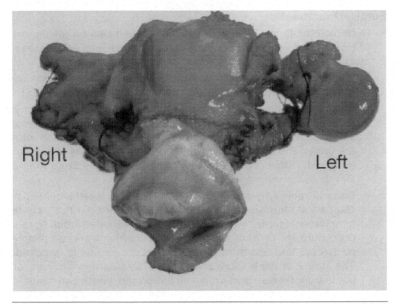

Figure 2.2 Type III radical hysterectomy.

- The boundaries of the scalene triangle are the inferior belly of the omohyoid muscle, the sternocleidomastoid, and the subclavian vein. The scalenus anterior muscle lines the floor of the triangle. The phrenic nerve runs through the scalene triangle, as does the thoracic duct. If the duct is transected, it must be ligated at both ends to prevent a fistula.
- Other surgical techniques and indications:
  - Radical vaginal hysterectomy (Schauta–Amreich procedure) is performed in two stages. The first stage involves a retroperitoneal pelvic LND, most often via laparoscopy. The second step is to perform a vaginal radical hysterectomy. This is recommended for tumors less than 2 cm in size.
  - Laparoscopic radical hysterectomy: This can also be approached with robotic assistance (please review LACC trial and tumor size considerations).
  - Radical trachelectomy:
    - This procedure is indicated in patients who desire fertility with tumors that are stage IB1 or lower, low-grade histology, and with a negative frozen section ECC. There are some feasibility data for tumors up to 4 cm. Of note, 60.7% of these patients had adjuvant therapies based on high pathologic risk factors to include XRT, chemotherapy, or both.[24] Care should be taken with the larger and more aggressive histologic types.

Neuroendocrine and adenoma malignum histologies fall into this category. Please refer to Chapter 6 for further fertility discussion.

- A radical trachelectomy involves the radical dissection and removal of the uterine cervix. This can be performed by either an abdominal, laparoscopic (with robotic assistance) or (Schauta–Amreich) vaginal approach. The cervix is amputated from the uterine corpus about 1 cm below the isthmus. An ECC is performed and sent for frozen pathology. If the ECC is positive, the radical hysterectomy is performed. If it is negative, a McDonald's or Shirodkar cerclage is usually placed at the time of surgery due to the risk of preterm labor from creating a shortened cervix. A Saling procedure, which advances the vaginal mucosa to cover the external os, can be performed at 14 weeks IUP to reduce the risk of ascending infection. A separate LND can be accomplished via extraperitoneal laparoscopic or transperitoneal laparoscopic approaches. Only the parametrial nodes can be removed during the vaginal portion of the surgery.

- Specific indications for surgical therapy and not XRT include a current pelvic abscess, the presence of a pelvic kidney, or a history of prior XRT for other indications.

- Ovarian transposition can be considered in some patients who wish to preserve their fertility or preserve their ovarian function. Studies have shown 41% to 71% of patients maintained their ovarian function after XRT with ovarian transposition.[25] Ovaries can migrate down and contraceptive therapy should still be encouraged if a salpingectomy is not performed.

XRT

- Total dosing is prescribed to defined anatomical points. Please refer to Chapter 5 for an involved discussion. The point A total dose should be at least 80 to 90 Gy. The point B dose is at least 50 to 60 Gy. WP EBXRT is usually dosed at 45 to 50.4 Gy. Dosing for grossly involved LN is 54–63 Gy with an additional boost of 10–15 Gy (using highly conformal EBXRT), microscopic involvement of LN is dosed at 40–45 Gy. A parametrial boost can be administered of 5 to 10 Gy. A sufficient vaginal margin is 3 cm. For patients with lower ⅓ vaginal disease, the bilateral inguinal regions should be covered. Brachytherapy provides a dose with LDR of 70–80 Gy, or with HDR of 30–40 Gy (small vs. large volume primary tumor size). The HDR rates are 0.6 × the LDR rate and converted using the linear-quadratic model equation. This is usually delivered in 5 fractions of 6 Gy HDR dose, equivalent to 40 Gy LDR.

- The duration of treatment with XRT affects outcomes in cervical cancer. As treatment time lengthens, the OS decreases. The goal is completion of treatment within 56 days. There is a 1% per day decrease in survival if treatment goes beyond 56 days (Table 2.3).

Table 2.3 XRT Outcomes for Cervical Cancer and Treatment Time Delay

Stage	Treatment Time (wk)	10-Y Pelvic Failure (%)	10-Y DSS (%)
IB	≤7	5	86
	7.1–9	22	78
	>9	36	55
IIA	≤7	14	73
	7.1–9	27	41
	>9	36	43
IIB	≤7	20	72
	7.1–9	28	60
	>9	34	65

- Chemotherapy is usually given concurrently with XRT. It can be given as cisplatin monotherapy dosed weekly at 40 or 50 mg/m² with a maximum of 70 mg, or as combination chemotherapy with cisplatin dosed at 40 or 50 mg/m² on day 1 and 5-FU dosed at 1,000 mg/m²/day as a continuous infusion for 4 days every 3 weeks. Carboplatin AUC 2 has also been used. For neuroendocrine tumors, etoposide should be added to cisplatin: cisplatin dosed at 25 mg/m² IV days 1 to 3 and etoposide 100 mg/m² IV days 1 to 3 of a 21-day cycle.

- There is a 25% chance of needing adjuvant XRT following radical hysterectomy for intermediate risk factors in patients with stage IB1 disease. For stages IB2, IB3 and IIA disease, this can increase to about 80%. There is data to suggest that 54% of patients with a tumor less than 4 cm will need adjuvant XRT.[10] For those with lesions greater than 4 cm in size, approximately 84% will need adjuvant XRT. Adjuvant XRT recommendations were based on pathological data to include positive LNs, positive parametria, close margins, and less than 3 mm uninvolved stroma.

- The rate of XRT complications increases in dual-therapy patients. In GOG 92, there was a 7% incidence of G 3 to 4 hematologic, GI, or GU complications in patients who had pelvic XRT after radical hysterectomy versus 2% who received NFT after radical hysterectomy.[26] In the Landoni study, there was a 28% complication rate after radical hysterectomy with adjuvant XRT compared to 12% for definitive XRT alone.

Adjuvant Posthysterectomy Treatment

Adjuvant therapies should be initiated by 6 weeks, postoperatively. Risk factors are based on observational data from GOG 49.[27]

Table 2.4 Intermediate Risk Factors for Cervical Cancer Treatment Stratification

LSVI	Stromal Invasion	Tumor Size
Positive	Deep one third	Any
Positive	Middle one third	≥2 cm
Negative	Deep or middle one third	≥4 cm
Positive	Superficial one third	≥5 cm

Source: Adapted from Ref. (26). Sedlis A. A randomized trial of pelvic radiation therapy vs. no further therapy in selected patients with stage IB carcinoma of the cervix after radical hysterectomy and pelvic lymphadenectomy: A Gynecologic Oncology Group study. *Gynecol Oncol.* 1999;73(2):177–183.

- **Intermediate risk factors** GOG 92:[26] EBXRT +/- brachytherapy is recommended for intermediate risk factor patients. Many providers add platinum-based chemotherapy to treatment for radiosensitization. Please refer to Table 2.4 for risk factor combinations that would lead to adjuvant therapies.
- **High-risk factors** GOG 109:[28] Combination chemotherapy (every-3-weeks cisplatin and 5-FU, or weekly cisplatin alone) and EBXRT with brachytherapy are indicated for patients following primary surgical treatment with HiR factors to include one or more of the following risk factors: LN metastasis, positive (or close, 0.5 cm) margins, or positive parametria.
- A Hg goal of at least 9.4 g/dL has been shown to increase the 5 YS by 9% for patients undergoing XRT[29] but the use of red cell stimulants has been associated with a 2 times higher risk of DVT. Use of transfusion can increase the Hg but this can be associated with immunosuppression, in addition to the TACO or TRALI reactions. In head, neck, and breast cancers, the aggressive use of transfusion and growth factors has been associated with poorer survival. GOG 191[30] randomized patients to aggressive transfusion or red cell stimulation for patients undergoing concurrent chemotherapy and XRT to maintain Hg at or above 12 g/dL compared to the standard level of 10 g/dL. This study was closed early due to higher DVT/VTE complications.

Differences between adenocarcinoma and squamous cell carcinoma:

- Adenocarcinoma has a higher rate of LN metastasis at 32%, compared to 15% for squamous cell carcinoma.[31]
- GOG 92: Those with adenocarcinoma had a better response to the addition of XRT treatment shown by recurrence rates of 44% in the observation group, compared to 9% in the XRT arm, compared to a 28% recurrence rate in the observation group versus 20% in the XRT arm for those with squamous cell carcinoma.

- GOG 109: For those patients with adenocarcinoma who received cisplatin/XRT, the recurrent rate was 83% compared to 50% with XRT alone, compared to those with squamous cell carcinoma who received cisplatin/XRT and had a recurrence rate of 80% compared to 68% for XRT alone.
- GOG 240: Those with adenocarcinoma did not have any survival benefit with the addition of bevacizumab.

Advanced Disease

Treatment options for stage IVB cervical cancer are limited. Chemotherapy alone or chemotherapy with palliative pelvic XRT and site-directed XRT are the two main options. Chemotherapy can include cisplatin in combination with a taxane, topotecan, gemcitabine, or vinorelbine. Combination antiangiogenic therapy with bevacizumab is beneficial (GOG 240) and immunotherapy/CPI has also been shown to improve OS.[69]

Recurrent Disease

A full metastatic workup should be performed if the disease reoccurs. If local recurrence alone is demonstrated, different surgical options exist. If there is extensive recurrent pelvic disease or distant metastasis, patients are often treated with systemic therapy and/or palliative XRT. The Moore criteria can help triage patients to treatment options.

- Most recurrences are diagnosed within the first 2 Y: 50% in the first Y; 75% in the second Y; 95% of recurrences are diagnosed in the first 5 Y.
- "Triad of trouble": Signs of recurrence which indicate that a mass has reached the pelvic sidewall are:
  - Sciatica (compression/invasion of the sciatic nerve)
  - Lower extremity edema (compression of pelvic lymphatics)
  - cva tenderness (hydronephrosis from compression/invasion of the ureter)
- Management is based on location, prior therapies given, PD-L1, NTRK gene fusion, MMRd, and TMB-H biomarker status, and patient comorbidities.
  - Surgery:
    - Radical hysterectomy: Can be considered if the uterus is in situ and the recurrent tumor is less than 2 cm and limited to the cervix. The rate of complications is high, however, with fistula occurring at 50%, and patients having a 5 YS of 62%.
    - Pelvic exenteration with/without IOXRT: total, anterior, or posterior. The 5 YS with positive pelvic LNs is 15% to 20% and this must be weighed with the morbidity of the procedure. There are certain patient selection factors that are important when considering exenteration: Local extension, positive LNs,

peritoneal disease, or malignant ascites are adverse factors related to decreased survival. One study found the following three risk factors predicted survival at 18 months: time to recurrence, size, and preoperative pelvic sidewall fixation.

- Some protocols include consideration of resection of disease at site of failure in noncentral recurrent disease patients with/ without IOXRT. This should be followed by systemic or tumor-directed (or both) therapy in most cases.

○ Systemic therapy:

- Cytotoxic: Cisplatin and paclitaxel showed an improved response rate compared to cisplatin alone (GOG 169). Topotecan and cisplatin also showed an improvement in PFS but not OS over cisplatin alone (GOG 170).

- Antiangiogenic: The addition of bevacizumab to cisplatin and paclitaxel has shown further improvement in PFS and OS (GOG 240).[32]

- Targeted therapy: Entrectinib/larotrectinib for NTRK gene fusion positive tumors. Tisotumab vedotin-ttfv has also been used.

- Immunotherapy: Pembrolizumab[68,69]

  - Preferred regimens for recurrent or metastatic disease

  - First-line combination treatment: Cisplatin/paclitaxel/beva-cizumab adding pembrolizumab if PD-L1+ (can use carbo-platin alternatively if cisplatin toxicities are present).

  - Second-line or later treatments: PD-L1+/MMRd/TMB-H tumor: Administer nivolumab or pembrolizumab.

  - NTRK gene funsion positive: larotrectinib or entrectinib.

○ Radiation:

- For radiotherapeutic curative-intent retreatment, patients can be broken down into three categories: central disease, limited peripheral disease, and massive peripheral disease. The central and limited peripheral disease patients are good candidates for curative intent, having a 30% to 70% chance for extended survival.

- Patients who are candidates for salvage reirradiation include those who are medically inoperable, those who refuse surgery, or those in whom surgery is not feasible.

- External beam doses of 39 to 72 Gy, brachytherapy doses of 60 to 89 Gy, or combination XRT doses up to 90 Gy can be used. This yields 57% control for external beam, 67% for brachyther-apy, and 44% for combination therapy.[33] For recurrence in the PA region, EBXRT can be delivered, but success rates for ade-nopathy greater than 2 cm are low. Therefore, resection with combination chemotherapy and XRT can be considered.[34]

- Interstitial XRT implants placed via laparotomy guidance have been reported to yield a 71% rate of local control with 36% of patients having no evidence of disease at follow-up.
- In the palliative setting, RTOG protocols have given 3.7 Gy twice daily for 2 consecutive days at 3- to 6-week intervals repeated up to three times.
- For palliative intent retreatment, the response rates are low and of short duration. Combined modality retreatment with chemotherapy in addition to XRT can be considered. Platinum compounds, taxanes, and ifosfamide have a response rate of 20% with a median duration of 4 to 6 months.

- Moore Criteria: Evaluated prognostic factors from 428 patients from GOG's 110, 169, 179 in an effort to predict response to chemotherapy in recurrent and metastatic cervical cancer.[35] These factors included: PS > 0, pelvic disease, receipt of prior radiosensitizer, time interval from diagnosis to first recurrence < 1 Y, and African American race. Three categories were formed: low risk 0 to 1 risk factors; moderate risk: 2 to 3 risk factors; and high risk: of 4 to 5 factors. The median OS ranged from 11.93 months for low risk to 5.58 for those with high-risk factors, and the ORR to additional chemotherapy was only 14.3% with a PFS of 3.38 months for those with high-risk factors.
- Fertility-sparing approaches: see Chapter 6 for algorithms.

Survival

- 5YS by stage and histology:
  - Stage I: squamous 65% to 90%; adenocarcinoma 70% to 75%
  - Stage II: squamous 45% to 80%; adenocarcinoma 30% to 40%
  - Stage III: squamous 60%; adenocarcinoma 20% to 30%
  - Stage IV: squamous less than 15%; adenocarcinoma less than 15%

Prognostic Factors for Survival

- Stage I:
  - LVSI (predicts LN metastasis)
  - Size of tumor
  - DOI (greater than half the thickness of cervix)
  - Tumor volume (>500 mm^3)
  - Presence of LN metastasis (decreases survival by 50%)
- Stages II to IV:
  - Stage
  - LN metastasis (decreases survival by 50%)
  - Tumor volume
  - Age
  - Performance status

Follow-Up

- Every 3 months for the first 2 Y
- Every 6 months for Y 3 to 5
- Annually thereafter
- The follow-up visit should include:
  - A directed physical and pelvic examination
  - An annual Pap smear without HPV testing is considered adequate surveillance
  - A Pap smear is not performed within the first 3 months following XRT due to XRT-associated changes
  - Colposcopy is recommended only for HSIL
  - Consideration can be given to CT scan of the abdomen and pelvis every 6 to 12 months
  - PET scanning can be considered

Neuroendocrine Tumors

Treatment algorithm for neuroendocrine cervical cancer:

- Stage IB2 and less, IIA1: Open radical hysterectomy with pelvic/PA LND followed by either a) chemoradiation with brachytherapy with two cycles of EP followed by two to four additional cycles of EP or b) five or more cycles of EP or primary chemoradiation with brachytherapy with two cycles of EP followed by two to four additional cycles of EP.
- Stage 1B3, IIA2: Primary EBXRT and brachytherapy with two cycles of EP chemosensitization then an additional two to four cycles of EP chemotherapy.
- Stage IIB, III, IVA: Primary chemoradiation with brachytherapy with two cycles of EP followed by an additional two to four cycles of EP.
- Stage IVB: Chemotherapy with five or more cycles of EP containing regimen individualized with palliative radiation.[36]
- Nivolumab + ipilimumab is also an option for those with no prior exposure to CI with an ORR of 21.9% vs 11.6% for nivolumab alone.

Notable Trials in Cervical Cancer

- GOG 49: This was a prospective surgical pathological study of stage I squamous cell carcinoma of the cervix. 1,120 patients with stage IA2 or IB tumors were evaluated, 940 patients were eligible, 732 squamous cell tumors were investigated, and 645 patients underwent P PA-LND. Four risk factors were found on multivariate analysis as independently associated with a higher risk of pelvic LN metastasis: greater than one-third cervical stromal invasion, LVSI, tumor size greater than 4 cm, and age ≤50 Y. On univariate analysis, parametrial involvement and grade were also found to be significant.[37]

- GOG 71: This study showed that there is no improvement in survival with the addition of hysterectomy after XRT. This study evaluated 256 patients with exophytic or barrel-shaped tumors, measuring ≥4 cm, who were randomized to EBXRT and brachytherapy, or attenuated EBXRT followed by extrafascial hysterectomy. Of the patients, 25% had tumors greater than 7 cm. There was a 27% versus 14% decrease in the local recurrence rate, but there was no difference in the OS. The 5Y PFS was 53% for the XRT arm versus 62% for the XRT with adjuvant hysterectomy arm ($p = .09$). Disease progression occurred in 46% of patients in the XRT arm versus 37% for the XRT with adjuvant hysterectomy arm ($p = .07$). XRT dosing was 80 Gy to point A in the XRT arm, whereas the adjuvant hysterectomy arm received 75 Gy to point A. The primary criticism of this study was that the adjuvant hysterectomy arm was underdosed. The study was powered for OS, with PFS as a secondary endpoint. For the subgroup with cervical lesions of 4, 5, or 6 cm, there was a borderline significance for PFS and OS in the adjuvant hysterectomy arm. Paradoxically, cervical tumors of 7 cm or greater had a worse survival when treated with adjuvant hysterectomy.[38]

- GOG 92: With 12 Y of follow-up, researchers looked at 277 patients with at least two of the following intermediate risk factors: greater than one-third stromal invasion, positive LVSI, or large clinical tumor diameter. These were all stage IB patients who underwent radical hysterectomy with LND and who had negative LNs and negative margins. Seventy percent had tumors greater than 3 cm. 137 patients were randomized to adjuvant XRT (50.4 Gy) and 140 patients received no further therapy. Patients with any combination of two or more risk factors who were treated with XRT were found to have a decreased risk of recurrence. The recurrence rate was 15% with XRT versus 28% for those who were observed over 2 Y, yielding a 47% decrease in recurrence risk. At 12-Y follow-up, essentially the same decrease in recurrence was seen except for those patients with adenocarcinoma, who had a significantly different recurrence of 9% versus 44%. There was no significant difference in OS (Table 2.4).[26,39]

- GOG 123: Evaluated 369 bulky stage IB (at least 4 cm) patients who were randomized to XRT followed by hysterectomy versus XRT and concurrent chemotherapy followed by hysterectomy. XRT dosing was 45 Gy EBXRT followed by brachytherapy to a total dose of 75 Gy to point A for both groups. An extrafascial hysterectomy was performed 3 to 6 weeks after XRT. Chemotherapy was dosed with cisplatin at 40 mg/m^2 weekly for a maximum of six doses. With a median follow-up of 36 months, the 3YS was 79% versus 83% with concurrent chemotherapy. The OS was 74% versus 83% with concurrent chemotherapy. The relative risk of death was 0.54. The recurrence rate was 37% versus 21% for the concurrent chemotherapy arm with an relative risk of recurrence of 0.51, favoring chemoradiation. Fewer patients in the concurrent chemotherapy arm had residual disease in the uterus.[40]

- GOG 85: Evaluated 388 patients with stages IIB to IVA disease. Patients were randomized to either XRT with hydroxyurea at 80 mg/kg twice weekly during XRT, or XRT with cisplatin at 50 mg/m^2 and 5-FU at 1,000 mg/m^2 × 96-hour infusion every 28 days. All had negative PA-LNDs. The relative risk of progression or death was 0.79 (95% CI: 0.62–0.99) in the cisplatin/5-FU (CF) group. There was also a decreased incidence of lung metastasis from 9% to 6% when platinum therapy was given. Survival was significantly better for the patients randomized to platinum-based therapy (p = .018).[41]

- GOG 120: Evaluated 526 patients with stages IIB to IVA with negative PALNs who were randomized to three arms. XRT was administered concurrently with either hydroxyurea alone, hydroxyurea–5-FU–cisplatin, or cisplatin alone. The dose of hydroxyurea was 2 g/m^2 twice weekly when in combination and 3 g/m^2 twice weekly when given alone. The dose of cisplatin when used alone was 40 mg/m^2 weekly, and the dose of cisplatin with 5-FU was 50 mg/m^2 days 1 and 29. 5-FU was dosed as a 96-hour infusion of 1,000 mg/m^2. The relative risk of PFS or death was 0.55 to 0.57 for the cisplatin-containing groups. There was also a lower rate of lung metastasis with a rate of 3% to 4% versus 10% favoring the cisplatin-containing arms. The OS rate was significantly higher in the cisplatin groups than in the hydroxyurea alone group with relative risk of death of 0.61 and 0.58, respectively.[42]

- GOG 109: Evaluated 243 patients staged as IA2 or IB. All were status-post radical hysterectomy and had high-risk factors to include positive nodes (85%) and/or positive margins (15%), and/or or positive parametria (15%). Patients were randomized to pelvic EBXRT dosed at 49.3 Gy or pelvic EBXRT with concurrent chemotherapy consisting of cisplatin at 70 mg/m^2 and 5-FU of 1,000 mg/m^2/day for 4 days every 3 weeks for four cycles, two cycles of which were given after completion of XRT. The 4Y PFS was 80% versus 63% favoring concurrent chemotherapy, yielding a HR of 2.01 for PFS and 1.96 for OS. The projected OS rate at 4Y was 71% with XRT alone and 81% with chemoradiation. The toxicity was higher (22% vs. 4%) in the concurrent chemotherapy arm. A reappraisal of the data suggested that concurrent chemotherapy was beneficial specifically for cervical lesions ≥2 cm and for patients with two or more positive LNs. The absolute improvement in 5YS for adjuvant chemoradiation in patients with tumors ≤2 cm was only 5% (77% vs. 82%), whereas for those with tumors greater than 2 cm it was 19% (58% vs. 77%). Similarly, the absolute 5YS benefit was less evident among patients with one nodal metastasis (79% vs. 83%) than when at least two nodes were positive (55% vs. 75%). Furthermore, this study also found that there was a significant difference with respect to histologies. AC subtypes had a better PFS when treated with combination chemotherapy and XRT.[28,43]

- GOG 136: Evaluated 86 patients with confirmed PALN metastases clinically staged I to IVA. Radiation doses were WP-XRT 39.6 to 48.6 Gy, point A intracavitary doses of 30 to 40 Gy, and point B doses 60 Gy combined with a parametrial boost. Extended-field XRT was dosed at 45 Gy given with concomitant chemotherapy consisting of 5-FU 1,000 mg/m²/day for 96 hours and cisplatin 50 mg/m² weeks 1 and 5. The 3Y OS was 39% and the 3Y PFI was 34%. Extended field RT with concomitant chemotherapy is feasible with a 3Y PFI of 33%. Ninety percent of the patients completed the study.[44]

- GOG 165: Evaluated clinically staged IIB, IIIB, and IVA cervical cancer patients who were treated with 45 Gy WP-XRT with a parametrial boost of 5.4 to 9 Gy using HDR or LDR. Standard therapy was weekly cisplatin 40 mg/m², and experimental therapy was PVI-FU at 225 mg/m²/day for 5 d/wk for six cycles concurrent with XRT. The study was closed prematurely when an analysis indicated that PVI-FU/XRT had a higher treatment failure rate (35% higher) (RR unadjusted, 1.29) and a higher mortality rate (RR unadjusted, 1.37). There was an increase in the failure rate at distant sites in the PVI-FU arm. The 4Y PFS for the cisplatin group was 57% compared to 50% with the PVI-FU group (NS). The 4Y pelvic failure rate was 16% and 14% in the cisplatin and PVI-FU arms. The distant failure rate (including abdominal, PA region, bone, liver, and lung) was higher in the PVI-FU group (29% vs. 18%). The PVI-FU group had a higher failure rate for lung metastases (9% vs. 5%) and abdominal failures (11% vs. 3%). PA failure occurred in only 7% and 5% of patients in the PVI-FU and cisplatin arms, respectively, despite the fact that only 18% of patients were surgically staged in the PA region.[45]

- RTOG-79–20: Evaluated 337 patients with stages IB, IIA, and IIB disease without clinically or radiologically involved PALN who were randomized to external beam WP-XRT dosed at 45 Gy or WP-XRT at 45 Gy plus extended field XRT dosed at 45 Gy. Patients who received WP-XRT alone had a 44% 10Y OS compared to a 55% 10Y OS for patients who had pelvic and PA-XRT. Though NS the difference between the DSS for the pelvic-only XRT arm versus the pelvic and PA-XRT arm were 40% and 42%, respectively. Ten-Y locoregional failure rate was similar (35% for pelvic only and 31% for pelvic and PA). Ten-Y incidence of G 4/5 toxicity in the WP-XRT-only arm versus the pelvic and PA arm was 4% and 8%, respectively.[46]

- RTOG-90–01: This study evaluated 380 surgically staged patients (IIB–IVA or IB–IIA >5 cm in size, or those with positive LN) and randomized them to WP and PA-XRT with brachytherapy versus WP-XRT and brachytherapy with concurrent cisplatin and 5-FU (75 mg/m²/day 1 and 1,000 mg/m²/day on days 2–5, every 21 days for two cycles). The RR was 0.48 for recurrence favoring cisplatin-based chemoradiotherapy. Total dosing was 85 Gy to point A. The patients in the chemotherapy arm had an improved 8Y OS of 67% versus 41%, and a DFS rate of 61% versus 46%. The chemotherapy arm had a decreased locoregional recurrence rate of 18% versus 35% and distant metastasis of 2% versus 35%. The chemotherapy arm had a nonsignificant increase in PA-LN failures at 7% versus 4%.[47,48]

- NCIC cervical cancer trial: This is the only trial to show no difference in survival with concurrent chemotherapy and XRT. It included 253 patients staged IB > 5 cm to IVA. This trial evaluated XRT versus weekly concurrent XRT and cisplatin (40 mg/m²) for 4 to 6 weeks. Criticisms of this study were that patients had a lower Hg level and longer treatment times. WP-XRT was dosed at 45 Gy with LDR at 35 Gy ×1 or HDR at 8 Gy 3 × versus the same XRT doses with weekly cisplatin at 40 mg/m² × 6. The 5YS was 62% versus 58% NS.[49]

- GOG 169: This was a randomized phase III clinical trial with 264 eligible patients. It compared single-agent cisplatin at 50 mg/m² in patients with stage IVB, persistent, or recurrent cervical cancer to combination cisplatin and paclitaxel dosed at 50 mg/m² and 135 mg/m² every 21 days. The addition of paclitaxel improved the respone rate (36% vs. 19%, p = .002) and PFS (4.8 months vs. 2.8 months, p = .001), but did not impact the median OS (9.7 vs. 8.8 months, p = NS).[50]

- GOG 179: Randomized patients with stage IVB, persistent, or recurrent cervical cancer to cisplatin 50 mg/m² q21d versus doublet therapy with topotecan 0.75 mg/m² days 1, 2, 3 and cisplatin 50 mg/m² on day 1, q21d. The PFS was 2.9 versus 4.6 months, favoring the topotecan–cisplatin combination. The OS was 6.5 versus 9.4 months (p = .017), favoring the platinum doublet. The respone rate was 13% for cisplatin alone versus 27% for the combination. Febrile neutropenia occurred more often with the topotecan–cisplatin arm with 17% versus 8% of patients having complications. G 3/4 neutropenia occurred in 70% of patients on the topotecan–cisplatin arm. QOL measures were not significantly different between the two arms. The platinum/paclitaxel regimens were less toxic and easier to administer so these regimens are favored instead.[51]

- GOG 204: Evaluated 513 patients with stage IVB or recurrent cervical cancer. Four platinum doublets were evaluated. The control arm was cisplatin–paclitaxel. The experimental-to-cisplatin-paclitaxel HRs of death were 1.15 (95% CI: 0.79–1.67) for vinorelbine–cisplatin (VC), 1.32 (95% CI: 0.91–1.92) for GC, and 1.26 (95% CI: 0.86–1.82) for TC. The HRs for PFS were 1.36 (95% CI: 0.97–1.90) for VC, 1.39 (95% CI: 0.99–1.96) for GC, and 1.27 (95% CI: 0.90–1.78) for TC. Response rates for PC, VC, GC, and TC were 29.1%, 25.9%, 22.3%, and 23.4%, respectively. The trends for RR, PFS, and OS (12.9 vs. 10 months) led to cisplatin/paclitaxel as the standard/preference with less anemia and thrombocytopenia.[52]

- GC concurrent chemotherapy for locally advanced cervical cancer. In this study, 515 patients with stage IIB to IVA disease were randomly assigned to arm A (cisplatin 40 mg/m² and gemcitabine 125 mg/m² weekly for 6 weeks with concurrent EBXRT dosed to 50.4

Gy in 28 fractions, followed by brachytherapy dosed 30 to 35 Gy and then two additional 21-day cycles of cisplatin, 50 mg/m^2 on day 1, plus gemcitabine, 1,000 mg/m^2 on days 1 and 8) or to arm B (cisplatin at 40 mg/m^2 weekly and concurrent EBXRT followed by brachytherapy). The PFS at 3 Y was 74.4% in arm A versus 65% in arm B. The OS (log-rank p = .0224; HR, 0.68; 95% CI: 0.49–0.95) and time to PD (log-rank p = .0012; HR, 0.54; 95% CI: 0.37–0.79) were both better for arm A. G 3/4 toxicities were 86.5% in arm A versus 46.3% in arm B. Problems with this study: The primary endpoint was changed midstudy to PFS; the sample size of approximately 500 evaluable patients was based on the original OS primary endpoint of 436 deaths out of 500 patients at an 80% power.[53]

- A second study evaluating cisplatin versus cisplatin–gemcitabine was performed in Asia. Seventy-four patients with II to IVA cervical cancer or stage I to II with positive pelvic/PALN were included. Of these, 37 were randomized to weekly cisplatin at 40 mg/m^2 and 37 were randomized to weekly cisplatin at 40 mg/m^2 with gemcitabine at 125 mg/m^2 for six cycles. The 3Y PFS was 65.1% for cisplatin alone versus 71% for cisplatin-gemcitabine (p = .71). The 3Y OS was 74.1% for cisplatin versus 85.9% for double therapy but crossed over at 5 Y (p = .89).[54]

- GOG 191: This studied 109 eligible patients with stage IIB to IVA cervical cancer with an Hg level less than 14 g/dL. Patients were assigned to concurrent weekly cisplatin and XRT with or without recombinant human erythropoietin (40,000 units SC weekly) to keep the Hg level at standard levels of 10 g/dL versus ≥12 g/dL. VTE occurred in four of 52 patients receiving chemotherapy and XRT compared to 11 of 57 patients treated with chemotherapy and XRT and erythropoietin, not all considered treatment related. No deaths occurred from VTE. The study closed prematurely, with less than 25% of the planned accrual, due to potential concerns for VTE events with erythropoietin.[30]

- GOG 240: A total of 452 evaluable patients with advanced or recurrent cervical cancer were randomly assigned in a 2 × 2 factorial design to cisplatin 50 mg/m^2 and paclitaxel 135 to 175 mg/m^2 or topotecan 0.75 mg/m^2 days 1 to 3, plus paclitaxel 175 mg/m^2 on day 1. Patients were also randomized to bevacizumab 15 mg/kg. Cycles were repeated every 21 days until DP or toxicity. The primary endpoint was OS. The topotecan–paclitaxel doublet was not superior to the cisplatin–paclitaxel doublet. The HR for death was 1.20. The addition of bevacizumab to chemotherapy was associated with an increased OS of 3.7 months (17 vs. 13.3 months; HR for death 0.71; 95% CI 0.54–0.95; p = .004). and higher RR (48% vs. 36%; p = .008). The addition of bevacizumab was associated with HTN G 2 or higher: 25 versus 2%, VTE: 8 versus 1%, and GI fistula G 3 or higher: 3 versus 0%. As a supplement, a QOL assessment was performed. FACT-Cx TOI scores did not differ significantly between patients who received bevacizumab versus those who did not, $p = .27.28$[32,55]

- GOG 263/RTOG-1171: adjuvant XRT versus adjuvant chemoradiation in intermediate risk, stage I–IIA cervical cancer after primary radical hysterectomy and pelvic LND: comparator study is GOG 92. The primary objective was the effect of treatment on RFS with a secondary objective of OS. An estimated 534 patients were randomized to one of two treatment arms after radical hysterectomy and pelvic LND. Arm I: Patients underwent pelvic EBXRT or IMRT 5 days a week for 5.5 weeks. Arm II: patients received cisplatin IV over 1 to 2 hours on day 1 and XRT as in Arm I. Treatment with cisplatin was once every 7 days at 40 mg/m^2 for up to six courses in the absence of DP or unacceptable toxicity. Inclusion criteria: Pathologically proven primary cervical cancer I to IIA with squamous cell carcinoma, adenosquamous carcinoma, or AC initially treated with a standard radical hysterectomy with pelvic lymphadenectomy and the following pathological characteristics: Positive capillary–LSVI and one of the following: deep third penetration; middle third penetration, clinical tumor ≥2 cm; superficial third penetration, clinical tumor ≥5 cm; negative capillary–lymphatic space involvement; middle or deep third penetration, clinical tumor ≥4 cm. Results pending.[56]

- GOG 265: ADXS 11–001 Lovaxin C: Advaxis consists of a recombinant strain of *Listeria monocytogenes* that secretes HPV 16 E7 protein, which has been attenuated by partial complementation of prfA, the transcriptional factor needed for expression of *Listeria* virulence. ADXS 11–001 (axalimogene filolisbac) uses a multicopy episomal expression system to secrete a 76kDa fusion protein consisting of the first 417 amino acids of *Listeria* protein LLO followed by the HPV 16 E7 protein. This induces an immune response that promotes a potent antitumor response targeting the E7 protein. The final results of 50 reviewed patients showed a 38% 12-month survival, which is a 52% improvement over the expected survival rate. The mean CR was 18.5 months ranging from 12.2 to 40.6 months.[57]

- JCOG0505: A phase III trial of 253 women with recurrent or metastatic cervical cancer showed that carboplatin/paclitaxel was not inferior to cisplatin/paclitaxel. The OS was 18.3 months for the cisplatin arm versus 17.5 months for the carboplatin doublet (HR = 0.994; 90% CI 0.79–1.25; $p = .32$). For patients who had not received cisplatin previously, the OS for the carboplatin doublet compared to the cisplatin doublet was 13 versus 23.2 months (HR 1.57; 95% CI 1.06–2.32). Thus, carboplatin may be used in place of cisplatin as an equally effective alternative.[58]

- GOG 127v: Phase II trial of nab-paclitaxel (Abraxane) in the treatment of recurrent or persistent advanced cervical cancer. Nanoparticle, albumin-bound paclitaxel (nab-paclitaxel) was administered at 125 mg/m^2 IV over 30 minutes on days 1, 8, and 15 of each 28-day cycle to 37 women with metastatic or recurrent cervical cancer that had progressed or relapsed following first-line cytotoxic drug treatment. Thirty-five eligible patients were enrolled, all patients had one prior chemotherapy regimen and 27 had prior XRT with concomitant cisplatin. The median number of nab-paclitaxel cycles was four (range 1–15). Ten (28.6%; CI 14.6%–46.3%) of the 35 patients had a PR and 15 patients (42.9%) had SD. The median PFS and OS were 5.0 and 9.4 months, respectively. The only NCI CTCAE G 4 event was neutropenia in two patients (5.7%). G 3 neurotoxicity was reported in one (2.9%) patient. Nab-paclitaxel has considerable activity and moderate toxicity in the treatment of drug-resistant, metastatic, and recurrent cervix cancer.[59]

- GOG 263: Evaluates 534 patients with stage I to IIA cervical cancer were reviewed. All had ≥2 intermediate risk adverse pathologic factors (Sedlis criteria from GOG 92) after radical hysterectomy and pelvic LND. Patients were randomized to WP-XRT vs WP-XRT with cisplatin at 40 mg/m^2 weekly; Outcomes pending.[60]

- Senticol 1: In this prospective feasibility study, 133 patients with FIGO stage IA–IB1 cervical cancer were evaluated between 2005 and 2007. All underwent laparoscopic radical hysterectomy and SLN identification. If the frozen section on the SLN was negative they were randomized to complete full pelvic and PA-LND or no further dissection. SLN identification was via combined technetium and patent blue injections. Histology included squamous, adeno, and adenosquamous carcinoma. Of patients, 14.7% had nodal micrometastasis and 5.2% had parametrial involvement. Of patients, 9% had adjuvant chemoradiation due to adverse prognostic factors. Five-Y results include: 8% recurred, 5% died of DP, there was no difference in PFS or OS, there were no FNs.[61]

- Senticol 2: In this study, 206 were patients randomized to radical hysterectomy with SLND with or without completion LND: 105 patients were in the SLN-alone group and 101 were in the complete pelvic LND group. No FNs were identified in the complete LND arm. Three-Y follow-up reviewed surgical morbidity and showed a 51.5% rate of morbidity compared to a 31.4% rate with SLND alone (morbidities not specified).[61] Combined results from SENTICOL I and II showed a correlation of parametrial involvement only if primary tumor size was >2cm and SLN was +.[62]

- SENTIREC trial: In this study, 245 patients were dispositioned to SLN mapping at time of radical hysterectomy. Patients were stratified by tumor size of 2cm. LND detection rate was 96.3% and 82% had bilateral detection; 15.5% overall had LN metastasis. For the 103 women with tumors >2 cm, 26.2% had LN metastasis, LND mapping sensitivity was 96.3% and NPV was 98.7%. PET concordant imaging sensitivity was 14.8% and specificity 85.5% with NPV of 73.9% and PPV of 26.7%. The conclusion was that for tumors <2cm, SLN mapping was safe and accurate, but for tumors >2 cm a complete PLND should be performed.[63]

- LACC trial: This is a randomized phase III noninferiority trial that compared outcomes of radical hysterectomy patients stage IA1 with LVSI, 1A2, IB1, cervical cancer via laparotomy versus laparoscopy. In it, 319 patients were randomized to MIS (84.4% laparoscopic and 15.6% robotic) with a 3.5% conversion rate and 312 to open surgery. Of participants, 91.9% had stage 1B1 disease. The rate of adjuvant postoperative chemo or radiotherapy was similar in 28.85 of the MIS versus 27.6% of the open group. The primary outcome was DFS at 4.5 Y. For patients with early-stage 1A1 with LVSI-1B2, the HR for DFS was 3.91 (95% CI, 2.02–7.58) favoring open surgery. In the ITT group, the DFS at 4.5 Y was 96.3% in the open group vs 84.3% in the MIS group. There was a higher rate of locoregional recurrence in the MIS group (HR 4.25 p = .002 CI 1.73–10.4) and between MIS approaches there was no difference. The trial reached an 84% power to declare noninferiority even after the safety stop was enacted. Outcomes for tumors less than 2 cm are unknown due to 91.9% of patients having tumors >2 cm. Those patients without prior cone and MIS had an HR 5.85 (p < .001, CI 2.47–13.9) for progression and death. The rate of carcinomatosis was 24% at recurrence for those with MIS.[8] QOL did not differ statistically between groups.[64]

- Melamed et al: This was a cohort study of 2,461 women who had a radical hysterectomy for stage IA2 or IB1 cervical cancer from 2010 to 2013. Of these, 1,225 women (49.8%) had MIS. Of the MIS women compared to open, they were more often White, privately insured, had higher socioeconomic status (SES) with smaller sized tumors. The median follow-up was 4 months and the 4-Y mortality was 9.1% among women who had MIS compared to 5.3% for those who had open surgery (HR, 1.65; 95% CI, 1.22–2.22; p = .002). As MIS was more common in later Y of the study, it coincided with a decline in the 4 Y relative survival rate of 0.8%/Y after 2006 (95% CI, 0.3–1.4, p = .01).[65]

- SHAPE Trial GOG 278: A randomized trial comparing radical hysterectomy and pelvic node dissection versus simple hysterectomy and pelvic LND in patients with LoR early stage cervical cancer. It attempted to demonstrate that simple hysterectomy and LND are not inferior to radical hysterectomy and LND in terms of pelvic relapse rate and are associated with better QOL/sexual health. Results pending.

- TAKO trial: A RCT of weekly cisplatin at 40 mg/m² versus every-3-week cisplatin at 75 mg/m² in combination with XRT in locally advanced-stage IIB to IVA cervical cancer. Results pending.

- TACO trial: This an RCT of tri-weekly cisplatin at 75 mg/m² for three cycles with concurrent XRT in locally advanced cervical cancer compared to weekly cisplatin at 40 mg/m² for 6 cycles with XRT in patients staged IB2, IIB-IVA. Results pending.

- INTERLACE Trial: INduction ChemoThERapy in Locally Advanced CErvical Cancer. This is an RCT of carboplatin AUC 2 and paclitaxel 80 mg/m² weekly for 6 weeks followed by standard concurrent cisplatin-based chemotherapy at 40 mg/m² weekly during XRT weeks 7 to 13, versus standard concurrent cisplatin-based chemotherapy with XRT. Results pending.[66]

- GOG 274/RTOG-1174: the OUTBACK Trial: This was a randomized phase III trial of 919 women that evaluated radiosensitizing cisplatin therapy with or without adjuvant carboplatin and paclitaxel chemotherapy after definitive XRT in patients with locally advanced cervical cancer. The primary objective was 5YOS with secondary endpoints of PFS, toxicities, and recurrence patterns. Of participants, 456 were in the control arm and 463 were assigned to the adjuvant chemotherapy arm. For arm I: Cisplatin was administered days 1, 8, 15, 22, and 29 concurrent with EBXRT followed by intracavitary brachytherapy. Arm II: Patients received concurrent cisplatin and EBXRT and brachytherapy as in arm I, followed 4 weeks later with adjuvant chemotherapy consisting of 3-hour paclitaxel 155 mg/m² and carboplatin AUC 5 on day 1 × four cycles every 3 weeks for four cycles. Eligible patients were diagnosed with FIGO 2009 stage IB1 node positive, IB2, II, IIIB, or IVA disease suitable for primary treatment with chemoradiation with curative intent. The median follow-up was 60 months and the 5YOS was comparable in the adjuvant arm versus the control (72% vs 71%, difference <1%, 95% CI -6 to +7; $p = .91$). The HR for OS was 0.91, (95% CI 0.70 to 1.18). The 5Y PFS was also insignificant for those assigned adjuvant arm versus control (63% vs 61%, difference 2%, 95% CI -5 to +9; $p = .61$). The HR for PFS was 0.87, (95% CI 0.70 to 1.08). Adjuvant therapy was started in 361 (78%) women assigned to receive it. AE of G 3 to 5 within a Y of randomization occurred in 81% who were assigned and received ACT versus 62% assigned control. Disease recurrence sites were similar between the treatment groups. Findings were adjuvant chemotherapy compared to standard cisplatin/XRT did not improve survival outcomes for women with locally advanced cervical cancer.[67]

- CONCERV, conservative surgery for women with LoR early-stage cervical cancer: Schmeler et al conducted a prospective trial of 100 women evaluating conization with LND and simple hysterectomy with LND to standard radical hysterectomy for early stage <2 cm cervical cancer patients. Of these, 44% underwent conization with negative margins and negative ECC, 40% had simple hysterectomy, and 16% enrolled after incidental findings of occult cancer after hysterectomy. Five percent of patients overall had +LN and one patient had residual disease in hysterectomy specimen. The recurrence rate was 4.3% with a pregnancy rate of 20%. GOG278 and SHAPE trials will provide additional information in this patient population.

- KEYNOTE-158 was a phase II basket study and a cohort of cervical cancer patients was reviewed. Pembrolizumab was administered to 98 metastatic or recurrent cervical cancer patients who had received prior treatment. Dosing was 200 mg IV every 3 weeks for 2 Y or until progression, toxicity, or physician/patient censoring. Eighty-two patients had PDL1-positive tumors. The primary endpoint was ORR. The median age was 46.0 Y (24–75 Y), the median follow-up was 10.2 m (range, 0.6 to 22.7 m). The ORR was 12.2% (95% CI, 6.5% to 20.4%). There were 3CR and 9 PR. All 12 responses were in patients with PD-L1–positive tumors, giving an ORR of 14.6% (95% CI, 7.8% to 24.2%); 14.3% (95% CI, 7.4% to 24.1%) of these responses were in those who had received one or more lines of chemotherapy for recurrent or metastatic disease. The median DOR was not reached (range, ≥3.7 to ≥18.6 months). Treatment-related AEs occurred in 65.3% of patients, hypothyroidism was the most common AE at 10.2%. G 3/4 treatment-related AE's occurred in 12.2% of patients.[68]

- Keynote-826: This study included 617 women with persistent, recurrent, or metastatic cervical cancer that was deemed not curable and were chemotherapy naive were randomly assigned 1:1 after stratification by PD-L1 CPS score and metastatic status. Of these, 308 women received 200mg pembrolizumab and 309 women received placebo Q3W up to 35 cycles in addition to both arms receiving paclitaxel chemotherapy with either cisplatin or carboplatin. Bevicuzimab was administered to 63.6% in the pembrolizumab group and 62.5% in the placebo group. A median PFS of 10.4 months was seen in all three groups with pembrolizumab and chemotherapy versus 8.2 months with placebo and chemotherapy for women who had a PD-L1 CPS score of 1 or greater (HR = 0.62; 95% CI, 0.5–0.77) and all women (HR = 0.65; 95% CI, 0.53–0.79) and 8.1 months for women with a PD-L1 CPS of 10 or greater (HR = 0.58; 95% CI, 0.44–0.77). OS rates at 24 months were 53% versus 41.7% for women with a PD-L1 CPS of ≥1, 50.4% versus 40.4% for all women, and 54.4% versus 44.6% for women with a PD-L1 CPS of ≥10. The 12-month PFS rate among all women was 44.7% with pembrolizumab versus 33.5% with placebo (HR = 0.65; 95% CI, 0.53–0.79), and was comparable between PD-L1 subgroups. The median OS for the entire population was 24.4 months with pembrolizumab versus 16.5 months with placebo (HR = 0.67; 95% CI, 0.54–0.84) ,and the median OS was not reached in either PD-L1 subgroup. A survival benefit was seen regardless of bevacizumab therapy.[69]

- EMPOWER: Cemiplimab for patients with recurrent or metastatic cervical cancer after prior cytotoxic chemotherapy. The phase III study included 608 patients: 304 were treated with cemiplimab and 304 had standard chemotherapy (n = 304). The median OS was longer in the cemiplimab group than in the chemotherapy group (12.0m vs. 8.5m; HR, 0.69; 95% CI, 0.56–0.84; p < .001). PFS was longer for the cemiplimab group in the overall population (HR, 0.75; 95% CI, 0.63–0.89; $p < .001$). There was a 31% reduction in the risk of death (HR: 0.69; 95% CI: 0.56–0.84; one-sided $p = .00011$). There was a 25% reduction in the risk of DP (HR: 0.75; 95% CI: 0.63–0.89; one-sided $p = .00048$). There was also a 16.4% ORR (50 patients; 95% CI: 12.5–21.1%; one-sided $p = .00004$), compared to 6.3% with chemotherapy (19 patients). The median DOR was 16 months with cemiplimab (95% CI: 12 months to not yet evaluable) and 7 months with chemotherapy (95% CI: 5–8 m). The OS benefit was consistent in both histologic subgroups (squamous-cell carcinoma and AC [including adenosquamous carcinoma]). Of patients, 78% had squamous cell carcinoma. In this patient subgroup, significant improvements were also seen with cemiplimab ($n = 239$), compared to chemotherapy ($n = 238$), including a 27% reduction in the risk of death (HR: 0.73; 95% CI: 0.58–0.91; one-sided $p = .00306$); a 29% reduction risk of PD (HR: 0.71; 95% CI: 0.58–0.86; one-sided $p = .00026$); an 18% ORR (42 patients; 95% CI: 13–23%), compared to 7% with chemotherapy (16 patients; 95% CI: 4–11%). A post-hoc analysis for the 22% of those with AC showed for cemiplimab-treated patients ($n = 65$) compared to chemotherapy ($n = 66$) a: 44% decrease in death risk (HR: 0.56; 95% CI: 0.36–0.85; $p < .005$), a 9% decrease for risk of PD (HR: 0.91; 95% CI: 0.62–1.34), and a 12% ORR (8 patients; 95% CI: 6–23%), versus 5% with chemotherapy (3 patients; 95% CI: 1–13%). Subgroup analysis by PD-L1 expression showed an ORR occurred in 18% (95% CI, 11–28) of the cemiplimab-treated group with expression $\geq$1% and in 11% (95% CI, 4-25) of those with expression <1%. AEs occurred in 88% vs 91% of cemiplimab versus chemotherapy patients: anemia at 25% versus 45%, nausea at 18% versus 33%, fatigue at 17% versus 16%, vomiting at 16% versus 23%, decreased appetite at 15% versus 16% and constipation at 15% versus for 20% chemotherapy. G 3/4 AEs occurred in 45% of cemiplimab patients versus 53.4% of chemotherapy patients: asthenia (2% vs. 1%, pyrexia <1% vs. 0%); and immune-related AEs were observed in 16% of cemiplimab versus <1% chemotherapy).[70]

- Innova TV 204: Tisotumab vedotin (Tivdak) was evaluated in a phase-II trial in 101 women with recurrent or metastatic cervical cancer with DP on or after doublet chemotherapy with bevacizumab. The antibody-drug conjugate administered at 2 mg/kg up to 200 mg q3w elicited an ORR of 24%, of whom 7% were CR with a median follow-up of 10 months.[71]

- Zalifrelimab and/or Balstilimab alone (NCT03495882) were evaluated in 125 patients with recurrent or progressive cervical cancer after platinum-based chemotherapy. The combination treatment provided an ORR of 25.6% with an 8.8% CR. Among the 67 patients with a positive PD-L1 status, the ORR was 32.8% compared with 9.1% in the PD-L1-negative subgroup ($n = 33$). The median DOR was not reached (9.3 months–not reached). The 6-month DOR was 86.4% and the 12-month rate was 66.7%.[72]

- RaPiDS trial (GOG 3028): This is a randomized, blinded, two-arm phase-II study evaluating balstilimab alone (monotherapy) or with zalifrelimab (combination therapy) in patients with recurrent/metastatic cervical cancer with progression or relapse after front-line, platinum-based chemotherapy. Results pending.

- The anti–PD-1/CTLA-4 inhibitor combination of balstilimab plus zalifrelimab (AGEN1884) elicited durable responses and notable OS in previously treated recurrent/metastatic cervical cancer patients.

- "Less radical surgery for early-stage cervical cancer: A systematic review."[73] A retrospective review of women with stage 1A2 to 1B1 diseases treated with simple hysterectomy was undertaken in 2,662 women. Data were abstracted to include tumor characteristics, other treatment modalities, adjuvant therapy, recurrence, and survival outcomes. A subgroup analysis compared studies with simple versus radical hysterectomy outcomes. Twenty-one studies were reviewed, of which three were RCTs, 14 retrospective studies, two prospective studies, and two population-level data sets. Of women studied, 36.1% had stage IA2 disease and 61.0% stage IB1 disease and 96.8% had tumors ≤2 cm in size, 15.4% had LVSI. About 71.8% of women who had a simple hysterectomy also had LN dissection, and 30.7% of women had adjuvant chemotherapy or radiation. The total death rate was 5.5%. Evaluation by stage, showed a 2.7% mortality rate for those with IA2 disease and a 7.3% mortality rate for those with IB1 disease. Of note, 18 studies reported outcomes for both simple and radical hysterectomy, with a 4.5% death rate in the radical hysterectomy group and a 5.8% death rate in the simple hysterectomy group. Estimated and reported HR showed no significant association for death between radical and simple hysterectomies for stage IA2 but increased risk of death for stage IB1.

- RetroEMBRACE study: RetroEMBRACE (Image-guided intensity modulated External beam radiochemotherapy and MRI-based adaptive BRAchytherapy in locally advanced Cervical cancer) was a multi-institutional database of image-guided adaptive brachytherapy (IGABT) reviewing 731 patients at 12 sites.[74] It demonstrated that combined IGABT with EBXRT/cisplatin chemotherapy leads to a local control rate of 91%, partial control of 87%, an OS of 74%, and CSS of 79% with limited G ¾ morbidity. IGABT showed a trend for improved OS compared 2D brachytherapy.[74] Local control was achieved with a 3-Y local failure of 7% for stage 2B. The target volume at the time of IGBT (CTVHRVolume) and dose to 90% of the target volume CTV HR D90 are predictors for outcome. A dose of ≥85 Gy (D90) delivered over 7 weeks provided a 3-Y local control rate of 94% in limited size CTVHR (20 cm³), 93% in intermediate size (30 cm³) and 86% in large size (70 cm³) CTVHR. CTVIR and GTVres dose of ≥60Gy and ≥95Gy (D98) led to similar local control.[75] Effect of tumor dose, volume, and overall treatment time on local control after radiochemotherapy, including MRI-guided brachytherapy of locally advanced cervical cancer. The addition of interstitial needles to IC applications allowed dose escalation to CTVHR D90, yielding superior local control in larger tumor volumes (=30 cm³) at the time of IGBT, without difference in late morbidities.[76]

TUBO-OVARIAN CANCERS: OVARIAN, FALLOPIAN TUBE, AND PRIMARY PERITONEAL CANCERS

Characteristics

- Upon review of pathogenesis for high-grade serous adnexal cancers and reflecting standard clinical practice, ovarian, fallopian tube, and primary peritoneal cancers (PPCs) have now been classified uniformly as HGSTOC. Sex cord stromal and germ cell tumors (GCT) are classified separately and considered to originate from the ovary itself. The more uncommon epithelial subtype origin is undetermined. One in 70 women will develop TOC in her lifetime. In 2022, 19,880 new cases are approximated with 12,810 deaths. As awareness has increased regarding the possible origin of HGSTOC, close histopathologic review can identify the transition within the fallopian tubes from benign to serous carcinoma (Figure 2.3).

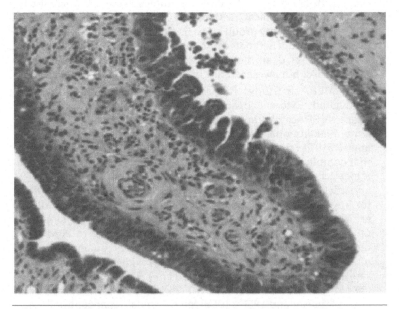

Figure 2.3 STIC identified in a patient surgically staged as IIIC HGSTOC.

- Serous tubo-ovarian cancer is most commonly found in advanced stages: 84% of women present with stage IIIC and 12% to 21% present with stage IV disease. Most women die from bowel complications/obstruction.
  - Symptoms include abdominal fullness, dyspepsia, constipation, tenesmus, pelvic fullness or pressure, bloating, and anorexia. Many of these make up the OCSI.
  - The route of spread for TOC is primarily transcoelomic. Cancer cells flake off the ovarian/fallopian tube surface and implant throughout the abdomen and pelvis. Other routes of spread are lymphatic and hematogenous.

Pretreatment Workup

- The pretreatment workup includes a history and physical examination, LN survey, and laboratory tests, including a CBC, CMP, coagulation profile, CA-125, and other indicated tumor markers. A CXR is recommended in addition to abdominal/pelvic imaging (CT/MRI). Colonoscopy and EGD can be considered based on symptoms. Specific attention should be given to pain elicited during the pelvic exam, the presence of a mass that is fixed or solid, the presence of nodularity, and the overall mobility of the rectosigmoid colon and parametrium (Figures 2.4 and 2.5).

Treatment

- Primary treatment can be surgical, via primary debulking surgery (PDS) or with NACT.
- Surgery usually consists of an exploratory laparotomy, abdominal cytology, hysterectomy, BSO, omentectomy, and cytoreduction.
- Patients with evidence of up to stage IIIB cancer should be surgically staged to include peritoneal biopsies and a pelvic and PA-LND. Three-fourths of advanced-stage cancers will have positive retroperitoneal LN. LN drainage tends to follow the ovarian vessels. Dissection around the high precaval and PA regions is important.
- The definition of debulking:
  - R0: Complete debulking is removal of all gross tumor to no residual visible disease (microscopic status).
  - R1. Optimal debulking is removal of all gross tumor to less than 1 cm of visible macroscopic disease.
  - R2. Suboptimal resection is defined as a remaining visible tumor with a diameter greater than 1 cm.
- Surgical staging is often inadequate when performed by general surgeons (68%) or general gynecologists (48%), compared to gynecologic oncologists (3%).
- If NACT is chosen as the primary treatment, surgical debulking typically follows after two to three cycles of chemotherapy.

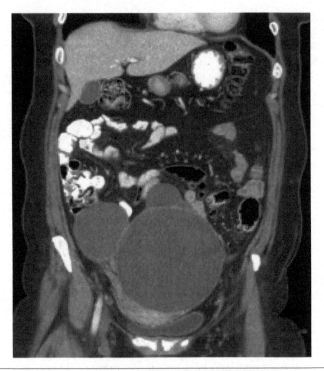

Figure 2.4 OC/pelvic mass CT.

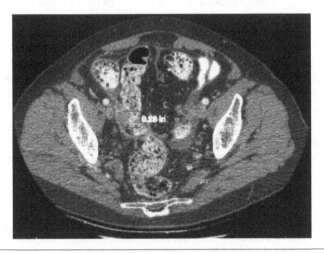

Figure 2.5 Partial LBO from HGSTOC.

Histology[77]

The following is a list of the WHO 2020 classification of tubo-ovarian tumors:

- Epithelial tumors
  - Serous tumors
    - Serous cystadenoma, adenofibroma and surface papilloma
    - Serous borderline tumor
      - Serous borderline tumor, micropapillary variant
    - Low grade serous carcinoma (LGSC)
    - High grade serous carcinoma (HGSC)
  - Mucinous tumors
    - Mucinous cystadenoma and adenofibroma
    - Mucinous borderline tumor
    - Mucinous carcinoma
  - Endometrioid tumors
    - Endometrioid cystadenoma and adenofibroma
    - Endometrioid borderline tumor
    - Endometrioid carcinoma
  - Clear cell tumors
    - CC cystadenoma and adenofibroma
    - CC borderline tumor
    - Clear cell carcinoma (CCC)
  - Seromucinous tumors
    - Seromucinous cystadenoma and adenofibroma
    - Seromucinous borderline tumor
  - Brenner tumors
    - Benign Brenner tumor
    - Borderline Brenner tumor
    - Malignant Brenner tumor
- Other carcinomas
    - Mesonephric-like AC
    - Undifferentiated and dedifferentiated carcinoma
    - Carcinosarcoma
    - Mixed carcinoma
    - Mesenchymal tumors
- Endometrioid stromal sarcoma
  - Low Grade
  - High Grade
- Smooth muscle tumors
  - Leiomyoma

- o Smooth muscle tumor of uncertain malignant potential
- o Leiomyosarcoma (LMS)
- Ovarian myxoma
- Mixed epithelial and mesenchymal tumors
  - o Adenosarcoma
- Sex cord stromal tumors
  - o Pure stromal tumors
    - Fibroma, NOS
    - Cellular fibroma
    - Thecoma
    - Luteinized thecoma associated with sclerosing peritonitis
    - Sclerosing stromal tumor
    - Microcystic stromal tumor
    - Signet ring stromal tumor
    - Leydig cell tumor
    - Steroid cell tumor, NOS
    - Malignant steroid cell tumor
    - Fibrosarcoma
  - o Pure sex cord tumors
    - Adult granulosa cell tumor
    - Juvenile granulosa cell tumor
    - Sertoli cell tumor, NOS
    - Sex cord tumor with annular tubules
  - o Mixed sex cord stromal tumors
    - Sertoli–Leydig cell tumor
      - □ Well differentiated
      - □ Moderately differentiated
      - □ Poorly differentiated
      - □ Retiform
    - Sex cord stromal tumor, NOS
    - Gynandroblastoma
- Germ Cell Tumors
  - o Teratoma, benign
  - o Immature teratoma (IT), NOS
  - o Dysgerminoma
  - o Yolk sac tumor
  - o Embryonal carcinoma
  - o Choriocarcinoma, NOS
  - o Mixed GCT

- ○ Monodermal teratomas and somatic type tumors arising from a dermoid cyst
  - Struma ovarii, NOS
  - Struma ovarii, malignant
  - Strumal carcinoid
  - Teratoma with malignant transformation
  - Cystic teratoma, NOS
- Germ cell sex cord stromal tumors
  - ○ Gonadoblastoma
    - Dissecting gonadoblastoma
    - Undifferentiated gonadal tissue
  - ○ Mixed germ cell–sex cord stromal tumor, unclassified
- Miscellaneous tumors
  - ○ Small cell carcinoma of the ovary, hypercalcemic type
  - ○ Carcinoid: insular/trabecular/stromal/mucinous (G1 only)
  - ○ Neuroendocrine (G3 only, determined by Ki-67 IHC, necrosis, and mitotic count)
    - Small cell (nonhypercalcemic)
    - Large cell
    - Mixed
  - ○ Unclassified
  - ○ Metastatic secondary tumors: 5% to 6% of adnexal masses are metastases from the breast, GI tract, or urinary tract

Staging

FIGO staging was last amended in 2014. Staging is surgical (Tables 2.5A–D).

Epithelial Tubo-Ovarian Cancer

Characteristics

- Risk factors for EOC include age (median age of 61 Y), low or nulli-parity, infertility, and genetic risk.
- Genetic mutations: the *BRCA 1* and *2* genes are located on chromosome 17q21 and 13q12-13, respectively. Mutations in these genes can cause autosomal dominant inherited forms of familial cancer and yield a combined 80% overall risk of TOC; 11% to 25% of patients of serous TOCs harbor one of these mutations: Rad50/51C/51D, BRIP1, BARD1, CHEK2, MRE11A, MSH2, MLH1, MSH6, PMS2, PPM1Df, POLE, POL-D1, PALB2, 17SNPs, NBN, PALB2, TP53. HNPCC yields a 10% risk of TOC and can present with other cancers such as endometrial cancer (60% risk), colon cancer (60% risk), and urothelial cancers.

Table 2.5A AJCC 8th Edition: T Category

T	FIGO	T Criteria
TX		Primary tumor cannot be assessed
T0		No evidence of primary tumor
T1	I	Tumor limited to ovaries (one or both) or fallopian tube(s)
T1a	IA	Tumor limited to one ovary (capsule intact) or fallopian tube surface; no malignant cells in ascites or peritoneal washings
T1b	IB	Tumor limited to one or both ovaries (capsules intact) or fallopian tubes; no tumor on ovarian or fallopian tube surface; no malignant cells in ascites or peritoneal washings
T1c	IC	Tumor limited to one or both ovaries or fallopian tubes, with any of the following
T1c1	IC1	Surgical spill
T1c2	IC2	Capsule ruptured before surgery or tumor on ovarian or fallopian tube surface
T1c3	IC3	Malignant cells in ascites or peritoneal washings
T2	II	Tumor involves one or both ovaries or fallopian tubes or PPC with pelvic extension below the pelvic brim
T2a	IIA	Extension and/or implants on the uterus and/or fallopian tube(s) and/or ovaries
T2b	IIB	Extension to and/or implants on other pelvic tissues
T3	III	Tumor involves one or both ovaries or fallopian tubes, or PPC, with microscopically confirmed peritoneal metastasis outside the pelvis, and/or metastasis to the retroperitoneal (pelvic and/or PA) LNs
T3a	IIIA2	Microscopic extrapelvic (above the pelvic brim) peritoneal involvement, with or without positive retroperitoneal LNs
T3b	IIIB	Macroscopic peritoneal metastasis beyond the pelvis, 2 cm or less in greatest dimension, with or without metastasis to the retroperitoneal LNs
T3c	IIIC	Macroscopic peritoneal metastasis beyond the pelvis, more than 2 cm in greatest dimension, with or without metastasis to the retroperitoneal LNs (includes extension of tumor to capsule of liver and spleen without parenchymal involvement of either organ)

Table 2.5B AJCC 8th Edition: N Category

N	FIGO	N Criteria
NX		Regional LNs cannot be assessed
N0		No regional LN metastasis
N0(i+)		ITCs in regional LN(s) not greater than 0.2 mm
N1	IIIA1	Positive retroperitoneal LN only (histologically confirmed)
N1a	IIIA1i	Metastasis up to 10 mm in greatest dimension
N1b	IIIA1ii	Metastasis more than 10 mm in greatest dimension

Table 2.5C AJCC 8th Edition: M Category

M	FIGO	M Criteria
M0		No distant metastasis
M1	IV	Distant metastasis, including pleural effusion with positive cytology; liver or splenic parenchymal metastasis; metastasis to extra-abdominal organs (including inguinal LNs and LNs outside the abdominal cavity); and transmural involvement of intestine
M1a	IVA	Pleural effusion with positive cytology
M1b	IVB	Liver or splenic parenchymal metastases: metastases to extra- abdominal organs (including inguinal LNs and LNs outside the abdominal cavity); transmural involvement of intestine

Table 2.5D AJCC 8th Edition: Stage Grouping

FIGO	AJCC
I	
IA	T1aN0M0
IB	T1bN0M0
IC	T1c(c1-c3)N0M0
II	
IIA	T2aN0M0
IIB	T2bN0M0

(continued)

Table 2.5D AJCC 8th Edition: Stage Grouping (*continued*)

FIGO	AJCC
III	
IIIA1	T3a1(T1/T2)N1M0
IIIA2	T3a2(N0/N1)M0
IIIB	T3b(N0/N1)M0
IIIC	T3c(N0/N1)M0
IV	
IVA	(AnyT)(Any N)M1a
IVB	(AnyT)(Any N)M1b

- The use of OCP and pregnancy reduce the overall risk (RR = 0.66). OCPs also reduce risk for HGSTOC in carriers of genetic mutations.
- Ten to 14% of apparent early-stage OCs are staged IIIA1i/ii (based exclusively on retroperitoneal LN involvement).
- The ovaries can be "fertile soil" for metastatic disease. Metastatic disease can be distinguished from a primary ovarian tumor by the following: Metastatic tumors to the ovaries are bilateral in 77% of cases, have multifocal and nodular implants, and often smaller in size. Primary tumors are commonly larger and usually unilateral (bilateral only in 13%).
- Terminology has been suggested to distinguish between low-grade and high-grade TOCs. It is not universally adopted.
  - Type I tumors are the low-grade serous tumors. This is distinct from LMP/borderline tumors.
    - The annual incidence is 3.8%, with an OS of 99 months. Diagnosis is with low mitotic activity (< 12 mitosis/10 HPF). Of cases, 99% are found at stage III. Even with six cycles of chemotherapy, 88% of patients had stable disease (a 5% ORR). Nine percent respond to hormonal treatment. Bevacizumab has been shown to provide a sustained CR in recurrent disease.[78]
    - Type I tumors respond to chemotherapy, although not as vigorously as type II because chemoresistance is due to the low growth fraction. In an in vitro chemoresponse profile: 86% of tumors demonstrated a sensitive chemoresponse assay result to at least one agent, 35.7% were pan-sensitive to all seven standard cytotoxic agents: carboplatin, cisplatin, docetaxel, doxorubicin, gemcitabine, paclitaxel, topotecan.[79] Twenty-three percent of low grade serous tumors responded in an AGO database.[80]
    - Those with MAPK mutations can have a better PFS and OS.[81]

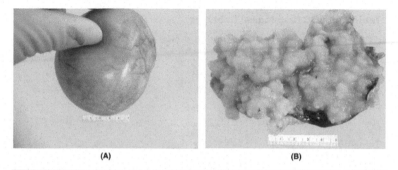

(A)   (B)

Figure 2.6 (A) Exterior of pelvic mass. (B) Gross bivalve of the same pelvic mass demonstrating papillary projections of HGSTOC.

- Type II tumors are the most common type of tubo-ovarian cancers, namely, high-grade serous. Eighty to 90% of HGSTOCs respond to standard chemotherapies (Figure 2.6A and B).

Pretreatment Workup

Workup follows the general preoperative/staging workup as described earlier.

Histology (Table 2.6)

- Serous carcinoma is the most common type of EOC. Serous cancers are graded in a two-tiered fashion: low and high-grade. IHC profiling includes: p53+, WT-1 positive, PAX-8 positive, ER/PR indeterminate, CK7+ (see Figure 2.6A and B).

- Endometrioid carcinoma: This represents about 10% of EOCs. This includes variable cystic and solid components with tubular glands commonly confluent. It resembles endometrial glands. Grading is consistent with uterine endometrioid cancer. Squamous differentiation can be present in one third of cases. When present in the ovary, synchronous versus metastatic uterine cancer should be considered.

- CCC: These tumors are difficult to treat; 63% are refractory to primary platinum chemotherapy. There is an increased risk of DVT: 42% versus 18% when compared to serous histologies in one study.[82] There is a 15% rate of VTE during primary treatment, and 9% occurrence at the time of recurrence in another study.[83] The OS is approximately 12 months for patients with advanced-stage disease.

- Mucinous carcinoma: Tumors are often large and serum CEA can be positive. They have a higher rate of discordance between frozen and final pathology at 34%: 11% were downgraded and 23% were upgraded. This is due in part to their larger size. LN metastases are rare in apparent stage I cancers and an LND can potentially be omitted in these cases without adverse effect on PFS or

Table 2.6 EOC Histological Subtypes

Histologic Subtypes	Malignant Epithelial Ovarian Tumors (%)	Bilaterality (%)
Serous	46	73
Mucinous	36	47
Endometrioid	8	33
CC	3	13
Transitional	2	
Mixed	3	
Undifferentiated	2	
Unclassified	1	
Brenner	1.5	

OS.[84] Appendectomy can be performed to ensure primary tumor site identification but is not mandatory. There is a high frequency of KRAS mutations. Chemotherapy can be carbo/taxol, 5FU/leucovorin/oxaliplatin, or capecitabine/oxaliplatin regimens.

- Brenner tumors: Brenner tumors of the ovary are relatively uncommon neoplasms, constituting 1.4% to 2.5% of all ovarian tumors. Histologically, a Brenner tumor is characterized by varying numbers of rounded nests of transitional or squamous-like epithelium and glandular structures of cylindrical cells within abundant fibrous nonepithelial tissue. Most Brenner tumors are benign, only 2% to 5% are malignant. Malignant components of the tumor show heterogeneous epithelial growth and atypia with intervening stroma, consisting of transitional cells, squamous or undifferentiated carcinoma, or a mixture of these types. The criteria proposed by Hull and Campbell in 1973 are as follows: (a) frankly malignant histologic features must be present, (b) there must be intimate association between the malignant element and a benign Brenner tumor, (c) mucinous cystadenomas should preferably be absent or must be well separated from both the benign and the malignant Brenner tumor, (d) stromal invasion by epithelial elements of the malignant Brenner tumor must be demonstrated.

Staging

Staging follows FIGO 2021 and AJCC surgical staging protocols.

- Upstaging based on LN metastasis has been reviewed in 14 studies. The mean incidence of LN metastases in clinical stages I to II EOC was 14.2% (range 6.1%–29.6%) of which 7.1% were only in the PA region, 2.9% only in the pelvic region, and 4.3% in both the PA and pelvic regions.[85] G 1 tumors had a mean incidence of LN metastases of 4.0%, G 2 tumors = 16.8%, and G 3 tumors = 20.0%. According to histologic subtype, the highest incidence of LN metastases was found in the serous subtype (23.3%), the lowest in the mucinous subtype (2.6%). Patterns of LN metastases were largely independent of laterality: Among those with unilateral lesions and positive nodes, 50% had ipsilateral LN involvement, 40% had bilateral involvement, and 7% to 13% had isolated contralateral positive LN.[86]

Treatment

Treatment can be primary surgical staging with debulking if indicated, followed by adjuvant chemotherapy for all tumors staged greater than IA G 1. NACT followed by surgery can be considered for patients who are poor surgical candidates (large pleural effusions with poor ventilation capacity, severe CHF, recent myocardial infarction, cardiac stent, recent laparotomy in the last 6 months, or recent PE) or who have extensive disease that is potentially unresectable (based on operative skill, patient comorbidities, or risk scoring). Optimal debulking to no visible residual disease is the primary goal. Adjuvant chemotherapy treatment should start within 25 days of surgery. Each additional 10% cytoreduction of disease yields a 5.5% increase in median survival.[87]

Treatment by Stage

- Stage IA G 1 tumors: Comprehensive staging surgery; with hysterectomy, BSO, LND, staging biopsies, omentectomy. If fertility preservation is desired, consider leaving the uterus and contralateral tube and ovary.
- Stage IA, G 2 or 3, and stage IB and IC, any G: Primary treatment is comprehensive staging surgery as indicated previously. If fertility is desired, consider leaving the uterus and contralateral tube and ovary. Adjuvant chemotherapy is platinum based with a taxane for three to six cycles.
- Stages II, III, IV: Either NACT or PDS may be offered. NACT has been shown to offer lower peri- and postoperative morbidity but PDS may offer superior survival.
  - ○ Primary treatment is surgery to include hysterectomy BSO omentectomy and cytoreduction. Adjuvant chemotherapy is platinum based with a taxane for six cycles. This can be administered IV or IP/IV. The addition of PARP-inhibitors as frontline maintenance therapy can be considered.
  - ○ Consideration can be given to NACT for:
    - ▪ The medically unfit or high perioperative risk patient (recent VTE, MI, Frailty score)
    - ▪ Per surgical risk assessment score (Fagotti) or Mayo algorithms

- If response is seen with NACT after two to three cycles, then perform interval debulking surgery (IDS)
  - Ensure pretreatment biopsy confirms histology.
  - If SD during NACT: Continue NACT up to 6 cycles and reevaluate.

The Mayo triage algorithm is relative but can help when deciding to proceed with PDS or NACT if primary cytoreduction is deemed feasible. Patients are considered high risk if any one of the following criteria are met. If high risk the patient should receive NACT:[88]
  - Albumin <3.5 g/dL
  - Age
    - ≥80
    - 75–79 with one of the following:
      - ECOG PS 1 (ASA score 3–4)
      - Stage IV disease in the liver or lung parenchyma
  - Complex surgery likely to involve more than a hysterectomy/BSO/omentectomy
- Cytoreductive surgery for stage IV TOC can be attempted with 30% achieving optimal cytoreduction; 30% of patients can be expected to have complications (mostly infectious or wound). The preoperative performance status should be two or lower. Bristow et al.[89] demonstrated that survival depended on location of the stage IV disease: The median survival for patients with a pleural effusion was 19 months, lung metastasis was 12 months, parenchymal liver metastasis was 18 months, and other extraperitoneal sites were 26 months. If patients had liver metastasis and had optimal intra- and extrahepatic cytoreduction to less than 1 cm, the median OS was 50 months; if there was optimal extrahepatic and suboptimal hepatic resection, the median OS was 27 months; and if there was suboptimal resection at all sites, there was an OS of 8 months.
- Removal of LNs for advanced-stage disease has been studied[90] via the LIONS trial;[91] 427 patients with stage IIB, IIIC, or IV all underwent surgery, including removal of bulky LNs greater than 1 cm in diameter. Intraoperative randomization was performed and the control arm completed PDS surgery, whereas the treatment arm underwent additional retroperitoneal lymphadenectomy to remove pelvic (at least 25 nodes) and PA (at least 15 nodes) LNs. After surgery, all patients received platinum-based chemotherapy. The 5Y PFI was 31.2% for the LND group compared to 21.6% for those in the control arm. The LND group was more likely to require blood transfusions, had a longer surgery, and had more postoperative complications. At 68.4 months, 202 of the 427 patients had died. There was no difference in the risk of death: 48.5% of the LND group and 47% of the control group were alive 68.4 months after surgery.

Predictive Models for Optimal Surgical Cytoreduction

- Different presurgical models have attempted to stratify predictive values of various findings for optimal debulking versus candidacy for neoadjuvant therapy (ascites, carcinomatosis, tumor size, CA-125 level) but the proposed models usually fail with validation sets. False positive criteria range from 10% to 68% for laboratory, clinical, or radiologic criteria. If there is PD (refractory disease) while on NACT, a change in chemotherapy regimen should be considered. If the tumor has regressed, it is appropriate to surgically assess the patient and attempt surgical debulking, typically after two to three cycles of chemotherapy.

- A surgical assessment algorithm has been proposed with the potential to categorize patients by location and bulk of disease into theoretically optimally resectable versus not resectable, called: *scope and score* based on the Fagotti criteria. Care should be taken with this approach as surgeons are passionate about their surgical skill but can vary differently in their opinions and skill sets.[92]

  o Fagotti scoring considers seven parameters and is a laparoscopic evaluation for feasibility of PDS versus unresectable to optimal disease status. If patients are deemed not optimally resectable (score ≥10), they are thus dispositioned to NACT. It was externally validated and modified by Brun[93] (Table 2.7).

  o If TOC is diagnosed incidentally after a TH-BSO without staging, surgical staging should be considered within 3 weeks. The risk of undiagnosed higher stage disease is 22% to 29%[84]; 4% to 25% of unstaged clinical stage I OCs have positive LNs, and the incidence of isolated contralateral positive LNs ranges from 7% to 13%.

  o The timing of ovarian cyst rupture can make a difference. According to one study,[95] preoperative cyst rupture had a larger influence on PFS than intraoperative cyst rupture. For preoperative cyst rupture, the HR for OS was 2.65 versus 1.64 for intraoperative cyst rupture.[96] Recent data on intraoperative rupture from a retrospective database review showed an HR for worse PFS of 1.92 95% CI, 1.34–2.76, $p < .003$) for those with capsule rupture. A worse OS was also present for those with capsule rupture (HR 1.48, 95% CI 1.15–1.91).[97]

  o Tumor biology: The impact of disease distribution in stage III OC patients was evaluated.[98] In this evaluation, 417 patients from three randomized GOG trials who were microscopically cytoreduced and given adjuvant IV platinum/paclitaxel were reviewed. Patients were divided into three groups based on preoperative disease burden: minimal disease was defined by pelvic tumor and retroperitoneal metastasis; APD was considered disease limited to the pelvis, retroperitoneum, lower abdomen, and omentum; and UAD

Table 2.7 Fagotti Scoring System for HGSTOC

Laparoscopic Feature	Score 0	Score 2
Peritoneal carcinomatosis	Carcinomatosis involving a limited area (along the paracolic gutter or the pelvic peritoneum) and surgically removable by peritonectomy	Unresectable massive peritoneal involvement as well as with a military pattern of distribution
Diaphragmatic disease	No infiltrating carcinomatosis and nodules confluent with most of the diaphragmatic surface	Widespread infiltrating carcinomatosis or nodules confluent with most of the diaphragmatic surface
Mesenteric disease	No large infiltrating nodules and no involvement of the root of the mesentery (indicated by limited movement of various intestinal segments)	Large infiltrating nodules or involvement of the root of the mesentery (indicated by limited movement of various intestinal segments)
Omental disease	No tumor diffusion observed along the omentum up to the large stomach curvature	Tumor diffusion observed along the omentum up to the large stomach curvature
Bowel infiltration	No bowel resection assumed and no miliary carcinomatosis observed	Bowel resection assumed or miliary carcinomatosis observed
Stomach infiltration	No obvious neoplastic involvement of the gastric wall	Obvious neoplastic involvement of the gastric wall
Liver metastasis	No surface lesions	Any surface lesion

was considered disease affecting the diaphragm, spleen, liver, or pancreas. The median OS was not reached in MD patients, survival was 80 months in the APD group, and 56 months in the UAD group ($p < .05$). The 5YS was 67% for he MD group, 63% for APD. and 45% for UAD. In multivariate analysis, the UAD group had a significantly worse prognosis than MD and APD both individually and combined (PFS HR 1.44; $p = .008$ and OS HR 1.77; $p = .0004$). Thus, it is suggested that there is a biological difference in OC patients proportional to the amount of disease at presentation.

○ 4 subtypes of HGSTOC were identified from the TCGA Network: "immunoreactive," "differentiated," "proliferative," and "mesenchymal".[99] The longest survival was seen for the immunoreactive subtype. Patients whose tumor samples expressed the proliferative signature (unadjusted HR = 1.50, 95% CI = 0.96 to 2.34, *p* = .08; adjusted HR = 1.52, 95% CI = 0.96 to 2.42, *p* = .07) or the mesenchymal signature (unadjusted HR = 2.12, 95% CI = 1.35 to 3.34, *p* = .001; adjusted HR = 1.84, 95% CI = 1.15 to 2.94, *p* = .01) had shorter survival compared to the immunoreactive subtype. Molecular classification of HGSTOC using transcriptional profiling then identified a de novo classification. Survival differed statistically significantly between de novo subtypes (log rank, *p* = .006) and was again the best for the immunoreactive-like subtype, and worst for the proliferative- or mesenchymal-like subtypes (HR = 1.89, 95% CI = 1.18–3.02, *p* = .008, HR = 2.45, 95% CI = 1.43–4.18, *p* = .001). Better prognostic information was provided by the de novo classification than that of the TCGA classification (likelihood ratio tests, *p* = .003 and *p* = .04, respectively). Single-driver molecular events specific to these subtypes haven't been clearly identified, but miR-508 has been found to regulate a cascade of genes in the mesenchymal subtype, including core genes in the epithelial–mesenchymal transition sequence: downregulation of miR-508 due to promoter hypermethylation has been seen to correlate with metastatic behavior and has been cited as a master regulator. These molecular subtypes that have the potential to guide therapy decisions.[100] Thus, miR-508-3p has been identified as the determinant for the mesenchymal trait and marks it as a strong prognostic biomarker for OC.[101]

○ A mechanism of resistance to platinum-based chemotherapies and PARP inhibitors in *BRCA*-mutant cancers is acquisition of *BRCA* reversion mutations. These mutations restore protein function. cfDNA extracted from pretreatment and postprogression plasma in patients known somatic or germline *BRCA* mutations after treatment with rucaparib were analyzed and *BRCA* reversion mutations were found in pretreatment cfDNA at 18% (2/11) of platinum-refractory and 13% (5/38) of PI-R cancers, compared to 2% (1/48) of platinum-sensitive cancers (*p* = .049). Patients with no reversion mutations in pretreatment cfDNA had longer rucaparib PFS than those with reversion mutations (median, 9.0 vs. 1.8 months; HR, 0.12; *p*<.0001). Sequencing of cfDNA can detect multiple *BRCA* reversion mutations.[102]

Genetic Testing

Panel testing is recommended for most epithelial TOCs for germline *BRCA* mutations and HRd status as well as somatic tumor mutations, NRTK gene fusion protein, and tumor mutation burden. Patients tested for *BRCA* mutations before 2014 and negative on that query are recommended to have repeat and full-panel testing. Genetic testing is not recommended for neuroendocrine tumors.

Chemotherapy for Epithelial Tubo-OC

- **First-line/frontline chemotherapy** involves platinum-based chemotherapy regimens with a taxane. Single-agent platinum regimens can be considered in older or compromised patients.
- **Second-line agents** are used when cancer recurs after first-line therapy has been given.
  - ○ **Platinum-sensitive and platinum-resistant (Pl-R) disease**. These are defined based on disease recurrence in relation to the 6-month time period following completion of first-line platinum-based chemotherapy.
    - ▪ Platinum-sensitive disease: Tumor has recurred but more than 6 months has elapsed since primary treatment with platinum-containing regimens. Second-line chemotherapy with platinum-based regimens should be used.
    - ▪ *Platinum resistance* is defined as disease recurrence occurring less than 6 months after completion of primary platinum-based treatment. If recurrence occurs at less than 6 months, non–platinum-based salvage therapies should be used.
    - ▪ *Platinum refractory* is defined as patients who have PD while on chemotherapy.
    - ▪ Recurrence rates for second-line chemotherapy depend on the time to recurrence after primary chemotherapy. The longer the interval from primary therapy, the better the RR: 6 to 12 months, 27%; 13 to 24 months, 33%; greater than 24 months, 59%.
- **Neoadjuvant chemotherapy** is chemotherapy given prior to surgery. Surgery is usually attempted after two to three cycles of chemotherapy. This has been shown to reduce the radical nature of surgery with a decreased risk of colostomy and hemorrhage.
- **Consolidation chemotherapy** is used after primary or adjuvant chemotherapy to decrease the chance of cancer recurrence in patients with CCR. This is usually a short duration of treatment.
- **Maintenance chemotherapy** is used after primary or adjuvant chemotherapy, or after second-line therapies, to decrease the chance of cancer recurrence in patients with CCR. This is usually of a longer duration than consolidation therapy.
- **Intraperitoneal chemotherapy** administered directly into the abdominal cavity. IP chemotherapy using platinum and taxane regimens is indicated for optimally debulked patients stage II or higher.
- **Intraoperative hyperthermic intraperitoneal chemotherapy** involves heated cytotoxic regimens administered at the time of primary or recurrent debulking surgery and circulated intraperitoneally for a specific amount of time.

- ○ Benefits:
  - A high volume of chemotherapy can be delivered, and a homogeneous distribution can be achieved. This is often not practical in conventional IP therapy because of abdominal distension and pain, but it is feasible in HIPEC, since the patient is under anesthesia.
  - There is no interval between cytoreduction and chemotherapy. The cytotoxic therapy is applied at the time of R0-R1 disease, and there are no adhesions that might alter the distribution of the drug.
  - Hyperthermia (>41°C) has a pharmacokinetic benefit. Several studies have convincingly shown that hyperthermia can increase both the tumor penetration of cisplatin as well as DNA crosslinking.
  - High concentrations of chemotherapy can be achieved in the IP compartment with low systemic exposure—in a single intraoperative treatment.
  - There is a continuous mechanical flow of perfusion solution.
- ○ Many combinations of cytotoxic agents have been used for HIPEC:
  - Single agents to include carboplatin 800 mg/m^2 for 60 to 120 minutes at 41°C to 43°C, oxaliplatin 460 mg/m^2 for 30 minutes; cisplatin 100 mg/m^2 for 90 minutes at 41°C to 43°C.
  - Cisplatin 350 mg/m^2 and alpha-interferon 5 million IU/m^2 and for 90 minutes at 43°C to 44°C, cisplatin 100 mg/m^2 and mitomycin C 15 mg/m^2 for 60 minutes at 41°C to 43°C, paclitaxel 60 to 75 mg/m^2 and cisplatin 100 mg/m^2 or doxorubicin 0.1 mg/kg (if PI-R) for 120 minutes at 40°C to 43°C.
  - At IDS: Van Driel protocol HIPEC regimen: Cisplatin 100mg/m^2 infused at completion of cytoreduction at 42°C; perfusion speed 1L/min over 90 minutes. Fifty percent of the dose administered at start, 25% at 30 min, 25% at 60 min. At the start of HIPEC: Sodium thiosulfate: 9g/m^2 in 200 mL distilled water followed by 12 g/m^2 thiosulfate IV continuous infusion over 6 hours (the 12 g/m^2 should be dissolved in 1L of distilled water and infused at 167 mL/hr. After 90 minutes, the inflow is stopped, the abdomen is drained, and surgery moves toward closure.
- ○ However, NCCN states the absence of sufficient levels of scientific evidence to support the use of HIPEC in patients with TOC with peritoneal dissemination at primary surgical treatment does not allow a general recommendation. HIPEC at IDS is now a level 2A recommendation.[103]
- ○ Carcinoid: Treatment should commence if the patient is symptomatic. Treatment is with octreotide or lanreotide, an mTOR inhibitor (everolimus), a combination of everolimus and octreotide or

a combination of Lu-177 dotatate (lutetium) with octreotide. The NETTER-1 trial showed a higher ORR compared to octreotide alone at 18%, versus 3% in somatostatin receptor-/+imaging.[36]

After Completion of Adjuvant Therapy: Maintenance therapy based on Genetic Profile should be considered.

- If no bevacizumab was used and the patient's genetic profile is BRCA 1/2 WT or unknown:
  - CR/PR: observe or niraparib
  - SD/PD:
    - Platinum sensitive: platinum combination chemotherapy, or clinical trial
      - Consider waiting to start until symptoms present if only CA-125 is elevated
    - Platinum resistant: clinical trial or second-line therapies (cytotoxic, targeted, hormonal, or immunotherapy)
- If no bevacizumab was used and the patient's genetic profile is BRCA 1/2 mutated:
  - CR/PR: olaparib or niraparib or observation if stage II or higher
  - SD/PD: depends whether patient is platinum sensitive or resistant
- If bevacizumab was used and the patient is:
  - BRCA 1/2 WT/HRp/unknown:
    - CR/PR: Continue bevacizumab.
  - BRCA 1/2 WT/HRd:
    - CR/PR: Continue bevacizumab and add olaparib.
  - BRCA 1/2 mutated:
    - CR/PR: Continue bevacizumab and add olaparib or niraparib.
    - SD/PD: Treatment depends on whether the patient is platinum sensitive or resistant (Figure 2.7).

Duration of PARP-I Therapy

- Olaparib and bevacizumab: 15 months of bevacizumab and 24 months of olaparib
  - Niraparib: 36 months
  - Olaparib: 25 months
  - Rucaparib: not determined
- Immunotherapy:
  - Pembrolizumab: for MMRp/MMRd or TMB-H tumors
  - Dostarlimab-gxly: for MMRd/MMRp tumors
- Targeted therapy:
  - NRTK gene fusion positive tumors: entrectinib or larotrectinib

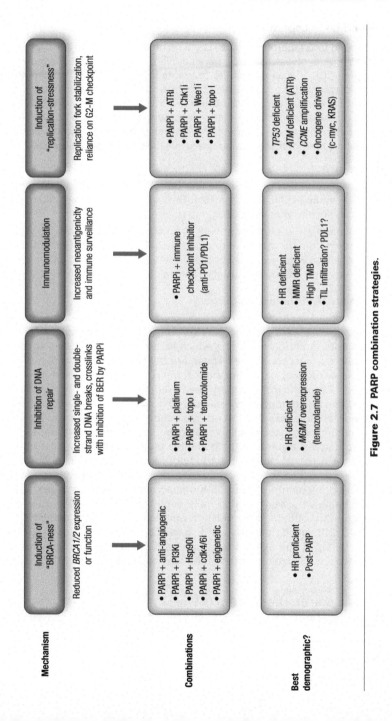

Figure 2.7 PARP combination strategies.

Second Look Laparotomy

- Second look laparotomy (SLL) is the pathological surgical assessment for residual disease after primary adjuvant chemotherapy in a patient with a CCR. It is used to guide decisions for either continuing chemotherapy, changing chemotherapy, or discontinuing chemotherapy. It can also be used to guide treatment in patients who were suboptimally debulked, or who were primarily unstaged. Routine SLL is not the current standard of care; 40% of second-look patients are pathologically positive, and of those who are negative, 50% will recur (Table 2.8).[104]

Recurrence

- Most recurrences occur within the first 2 Y. The risk of recurrence for a G 1, stage I OC is less than 10%. The risk of recurrence for stage III OC is much higher, over 50%.
  - ○ Treatment is commonly with chemotherapy based on duration from primary response to recurrence. Once secondary CR or PR has occurred, maintenance therapy with a PARP-I or other biologic/anti angiogenesis agent can be considered.

Secondary Cytoreduction Surgery

- Secondary cytoreduction surgery (SCS) is the removal of gross recurrent disease after primary or secondary chemotherapy. There are criteria attributed to Chi, which help stratify patients as appropriate surgical candidates. These are based on time, location, and number of recurrent tumor sites. If the recurrence occurs at greater than 30 months from primary chemotherapy, secondary cytoreduction can be attempted regardless of the number of involved sites. If the interval is less than 30 months, and there are one to two sites of recurrence, cytoreduction can again be attempted. If there is carcinomatosis, ascites, or the patient is platinum resistant, it is often not wise to attempt secondary cytoreduction. For those who had less than 0.5 cm of residual disease after secondary cytoreduction, an improvement in OS to 56 months was seen versus 27 months for those who were suboptimally debulked. The overall success at secondary optimal cytoreduction ranges between 24% and 84%.[105] GOG 213 results dissuade SCS based on generalized criteria but DESKTOP III and SOC-1 trials support PFS and OS improvements if specific qualifications are met. Review of Chi and GOG 213 criteria

Table 2.8 SLL for HGSTOC 5YS Outcomes

SLL Disease Status	5YS (%)
No evidence of disease	50
Microscopic	35
Macroscopic	5

can be compared to more contemporary iMODEL criteria (SOC-1) and DESKTOP III in select patients regarding secondary debulking.

PARP Inhibitors and AML/MDS

- PARP inhibitors used as maintenance monotherapy reduce the hazard of cancer progression or death in *BRCA* mutant patients by 60% to 70%, in BRCAWT/HRd patients up to 50%, and about 32% in HR-proficient patients. Secondary leukemias also known as treatment-related myelodysplastic syndromes *MDS* and/or acute myeloid leukemia *AML*. The average time to development is 18 months.

- In a meta analysis of RCTs of ovarian/breast/pancreas/prostate cancers, 5,739 patients were reviewed and an IRR of 5.43 was found in those using PARPi's but not in comparative patients without a history of PARPi use (IRR 1.01). Duration of exposure to PARPi was not related to MDS development. A rate of 2.77 cases of MDS/1,000 personY was identified for PARPi use. Attention to cytopenias during therapy may be an early signal of MDS development and quick referral to medical oncology for further evaluation is warranted.[106,107]

Cerebellar Degeneration

- Cerebellar degeneration can occur from antibodies to OC. This is called *paraneoplastic cerebellar degeneration.* The incidence is 2:1,000 patients with gynecologic cancers. There are two main antibodies: The anti-Yo antibody reacts against the Purkinje cells and the anti-Hu antibody reacts against all neurons.

Survival

- Relative survival
- 2YS: 65%, 5YS: 44%, 10YS: 36%[108] (Tables 2.9 and 2.10)
- 10YS: Thirty-one percent of women survive more than 10Y. Younger age, early stage, low G, and nonserous histology are significant predictors of long-term survival. One third of those who survived to 10Y had stages III or IV per 1989 staging, 16% of patients with late-stage serous cancer survived more than 10Y.[109]

Survival Care

- Follow-up:
  - Every 3 months for 2Y
  - Every 6 months up to 5Y
  - Annually for subsequent visits
- At each visit:
  - Physical and pelvic examination
  - Symptom review
  - Consider CA-125: Discussion should be held with the patient regarding surveillance with tumor markers. Rustin et al demonstrated no improvement in survival when tumor markers were

Table 2.9 HGSTOC 5YS by Stage

Stage	Relative 5YS (%)
I	90
IA	94
IB	92
IC	85
II	70
IIA	78
IIB	73
III	39
IIIA	59
IIIB	52
IIIC	39
IV	17

followed. Patients had a poorer QOL with additional unsuccessful cycles of chemotherapy given based on laboratory data. Assessment of symptoms, along with physical examination, can guide the clinician regarding when to order lab tests, imaging, and when to initiate second-line chemotherapy.[110]

- CT imaging: CT cannot often detect subcentimeter disease.
- PET is not recommended.

Epithelial TOC Notable Trials

- **Surgical-Approach Trials**
  - LION Trial: A total of 647 patients stages IIb to IV underwent intraoperative randomization after macroscopic complete resection and assessment of normal-sized LND from December 2008 through January 2012 and were assigned to undergo LND (323 patients) or not (324).[91] The primary endpoint was OS. For women who had LND, the median number of LNs removed was 57 (35 pelvic and 22 PA LN). The median OS was 69.2 months in the

Table 2.10 5YS by Residual Disease

Residual disease	5YS (%)
Microscopic	40–75
Optimal	30–40
Suboptimal	5

no-LND group and 65.5 months in the LND group (HR for death in the LND group, 1.06; 95% CI, 0.83–1.34; p = .65), and median PFS was 25.5 months in both groups (HR for progression or death in the LND group, 1.11; 95% CI, 0.92–1.34; p = .29). Serious postoperative complications occurred more frequently in the LND group (e.g., incidence of repeat laparotomy, 12.4% vs. 6.5% [p = .01]; mortality within 60 days after surgery, 3.1% vs. 0.9% [p = .049]). Systematic pelvic and paraaortic LND in patients with stage 2B–4 OC who had optimal intraabdominal macroscopic complete resection with normal LN both before and during surgery was not associated with longer OS or PFS than the no LND group, and was associated with a higher incidence of postoperative complications. The LION trial differed from the Panici trial by three components: Patients were included only if they achieved R0, patients were excluded if they had clinically enlarged LN, and there was meticulous quality control.

- ○ Minimally invasive surgery for cytoreduction results in ~50% conversion rate to laparotomy at IDS after NACT to achieve R1 or less disease.[111] This was a multi-institutional review of 282 women with staged III/IV OC of whom 80.5% had HGSTOC. 78 patients (27.7%) had diagnostic laparoscopy and 72 were scored per Fagotti protocol prior to NACT. Twenty-three percent were optimally cytoreduced to R1 status and 61% to R0, giving an overall optimal cytoreduction rate of 84%. In multivariate analyses, age 75+ (p ≤ .001), residual disease (>1 cm; p = .03), and SCS ≥3 (p = .04) were significantly predictive of worse DSS when morbidity and ASA score were also in the model. Of the 51 patients (18.8% of the total study group) who underwent MIS IDS attempts, 24 (47%) were converted to laparotomy to achieve optimal debulking, whereas 25 were able to have laparoscopic optimal cytoreduction.

- **Primary Adjuvant Chemotherapy Trials**
  - ○ ICON 1: This trial evaluated 477 patients who had early OC "staged" with hysterectomy, BSO, and recommended omentectomy. Patients were eligible if the treating physician was uncertain whether the patient required chemotherapy. Ninety-three percent of patients were "stage I." Patients were randomized between NFT and single-agent carboplatin (AUC 5); CAP; or another platinum regimen. Histology was 32% serous, 15% CC, 23% mucinous. Most patients were apparent stage I; however, there were 7% of patients with stage II or III disease; 70% were G 2 or 3. At 51 months, the OS was 79% in the chemotherapy arm versus 70% in the NFT arm. The 5Y PFS was 73% in the chemotherapy group versus 62% in the NFT group. For clinical stage I disease that did not get staged, there was a 38% recurrence rate without further treatment and a 30% death rate. Chemotherapy had an HR of 0.66 for survival.[112]

○ ACTION: This trial ran concurrently with ICON 1. Of 448 patients 30% were comprehensively staged. Patients were randomized to observation or to chemotherapy. Chemotherapy consisted of four to six cycles of single-agent platinum or a platinum-containing regimen. Forty percent of patients were stage IA or IB and 60% had G 1 or G 2 disease. The 5 YS in the observation and adjuvant chemotherapy arms were 75% and 85%. Patients who received chemotherapy had a better RFS (HR 0.63). In non-optimally staged patients, the adjuvant chemotherapy group had an improved OS and RFS (HR 1.75 and HR 1.78, respectively). Among patients in the observation arm, optimal staging provided an improvement in OS and RFS (HR 2.31 and HR 1.82, respectively). There was no benefit seen from adjuvant chemotherapy in the optimally staged patients. This suggests that in the suboptimally staged group, there were undiagnosed higher-staged patients who benefited when given chemotherapy. A 10Y follow-up found support for most of the original conclusions, except that OS after optimal surgical staging was improved among patients who received adjuvant chemotherapy (HR of death 1.89).[113,114]

○ ICON 2: This trial evaluated 1,526 eligible surgically staged patients who needed primary adjuvant chemotherapy. Patients were staged I to IV and were randomized to single-agent platinum-based chemotherapy or CAP. This trial was stopped early due to the availability of taxanes. These patients were then grouped into the control arm of ICON 3 as their outcomes were statistically nonsignificant with an OS HR of 1.0. The median survival in both groups was 33 months and the 2 YS was 60% for both arms. CAP was more toxic.[115]

○ ICON 3: This trial evaluated 274 eligible surgically staged patients stages I to IV, 20% of whom were stages I and II. Patients were randomized between a paclitaxel–carboplatin doublet versus the ICON 2 group of single-agent carboplatin or CAP. The OS was 36 months for carboplatin–paclitaxel and 35 months for the control groups of single-agent carboplatin and CAP. The PFS was 17 months versus 16 months for the control arm. There were a lot of confounding factors in this study: A large number of patients were deemed to have recurrent disease based on elevated CA-125 levels prior to showing clinical recurrence. In addition, 30% of those who did not get paclitaxel as primary treatment received paclitaxel as second-line treatment.[116]

○ ICON 4: This trial evaluated 802 eligible patients with recurrent platinum-sensitive OC; 75% recurred more than 12 months following initial therapy. Patients were randomized to paclitaxel 175 to 185 mg/m^2 and cisplatin 50 mg/m^2 or carboplatin AUC 5 versus single-agent cisplatin 75 mg/m^2 or carboplatin AUC 5. The doublet therapy showed a statistically significant improvement over the single-agent group with a median PFS of 13 months versus 10 months (HR 0.76; p = .0004). The doublet therapy showed an improvement in median survival by 5 months (29 months versus 24 months; HR of 0.82, p = .02). This translated to a 2 YS of 57% versus 50% and a 1Y PFS of 50% versus 40%. Criticisms of this trial were that 75% of patients were in a good prognosis group. This is essentially a trial of platinum-sensitive disease.[116]

○ ICON 5/GOG 182 EORTC 55012: This trial evaluated 4,312 surgically staged stage III and IV patients for primary adjuvant therapy. The control arm was the doublet of carboplatin AUC 6 and paclitaxel 175 mg/m^2, administered for eight cycles. The experimental arms consisted of carboplatin–paclitaxel–gemcitabine as sequential doublets or in triplicate, for a total of eight cycles, or carboplatin–paclitaxel–topotecan as sequential doublets for a total of eight cycles, and carboplatin–paclitaxel–liposomal doxorubicin as a triplicate regimen for eight cycles. There was no difference in median PFS or OS with the PFS in the control arm being 16 months and the OS being 44 months, both in the optimally and suboptimally debulked patients. The median PFS for patients with suboptimal, gross optimal (<1 cm residual), and microscopic residual disease were 13, 16, and 29 months, respectively, and the median OS rates were 33, 40, and 68 months, respectively.[117]

○ ICON 7/AGO-OVAR 11: This trial evaluated 1,528 eligible patients in stages I to IV, of whom 26% were suboptimally debulked. The control arm was carboplatin AUC 5 or 6 and paclitaxel 175 mg/m^2 IV every 3 weeks for six cycles. The experimental arm consisted of carboplatin and paclitaxel at the same doses with the addition of bevacizumab at 7.5 mg/kg IV every 3 weeks for six cycles, with maintenance bevacizumab continued for an additional 12 cycles or until progression of disease. Median follow-up was 48.9 months. At 42 months, PFS was 22.4 months without bevacizumab versus 24.1 months with bevacizumab (p = .04 log rank). In HiR patients, the PFS was 14.5 months versus 18.1 months with bevacizumab and median OS was 28.8 versus 36.6 months with bevacizumab. At 48.9 months though, no difference in PFS was seen. For the entire population at 48.9 months, the RMST (OS) demonstrated an improvement of only 0.9 months from 44.6 to 45.5 months (95% CI, log rank p = .85, pH test p = .02) with bevacizumab—not significant (NS). In a subgroup analysis, RMST for the poor prognosis group (stage IV, inoperable stage III [6%], and suboptimally debulked >1 cm stage III) demonstrated a 4.8-month RMST improvement from 34.5 to 39.3 months (log rank p = .03 PH test = 0.007). In the average prognosis group, the RMST was 49.7 months versus 48.4 months (p = .2) in the bevacizumab group. No benefit from bevacizumab was seen in low-grade serous tumors, CC tumors, or low-stage high-risk patients (stage I–IIA CC or G3). HTN attributed to bevacizumab was seen in 18% of patients who received bevacizumab versus 2% of patients in the control arm. Bowel perforation was seen in 10 patients in the bevacizumab group versus three patients in the control arm.[118,119]

○ GOG 1: Eighty-six evaluable surgical stage I patients were randomized to observation, WP-XRT, or melphalan chemotherapy. Recurrence was 17% in the observation group, 30% in those irradiated, and 6% in those who received chemotherapy. Recurrence was related to grade: G 1, 11%; G 2, 22%; G 3, 27%.[120]

○ GOG 111: This trial evaluated 386 eligible suboptimally debulked stage III and IV patients. Patients with greater than 1-cm residual disease were randomly assigned to receive cisplatin 75 mg/m^2 and cyclophosphamide 750 mg/m^2 or cisplatin 75 mg/m^2 and 24-hour paclitaxel 135 mg/m^2. ORR in the first arm was 73% compared to 60%. PFS was longer in the paclitaxel-containing arm at 17.9 months versus 12.9 months. OS was longer in the paclitaxel arm at 37.5 months compared to 24.4 months.[121]

○ OV-10: This trial evaluated cyclophosphamide and cisplatin versus 3-hour paclitaxel and cisplatin in 680 eligible patients with stage IIB, IIC, III, or IV disease, who were optimally and suboptimally debulked. The ORR was 58.6% in the cisplatin and paclitaxel arm versus 44.7% in the cyclophosphamide and cisplatin arm. The PFS was 15.5 months versus 11.5 months favoring the paclitaxel arm and the OS was 35.6 months versus 25.8 months, again, all favoring paclitaxel.[122]

○ GOG 132: This trial evaluated 648 suboptimal stage III and any stage IV patients. There were three arms: a doublet of cisplatin and paclitaxel dosed at 75 and 135 mg/kg, single-agent paclitaxel dosed at 200 mg/kg, and single-agent cisplatin dosed at 100 mg/kg. The PFS, respectively, were 14 months, 11 months, and 16 months. The OS, respectively, were 26 months, 26 months, and 30 months. The response rates were, respectively, 67%, 67%, and 47%.[123]

○ GOG 157: This trial evaluated three versus six cycles of paclitaxel and carboplatin in 427 eligible patients staged IAG3, IBG3, IC, and II. The primary endpoint was recurrence rate. There were 457 patients registered, 213 in each arm. Of these, 70% were stage I, 30% were stage II, and 30% were CC cancers in each arm. The recurrence rate was 27.4% for three cycles versus 19% for six cycles (95% CI: 0.53–1.13). The probability of surviving 5 Y was 81% for three cycles versus 83% for six cycles (95% CI: 0.66–1.57). The HR for recurrence was 0.74, p = .18 (NS). Criticisms of the study were insufficient power to detect a difference, and only 29% (126) of patients were staged appropriately. Chan updated the data in 2006 and found a benefit to six cycles of chemotherapy specifically for serous tumors with a 5Y RFS of 83% compared to 60% in those who received six versus three cycles of chemotherapy, respectively (p = .007). Those with serous tumors had a significantly lower risk of recurrence after six versus three cycles of chemotherapy (HR 0.33; 95% CI: 0.14–0.77; p = .04) in contrast to nonserous tumors (HR 0.94; 95% CI: 0.60–1.49).[124,125]

o GOG 158: This trial compared 792 optimally cytoreduced stage III OC patients to 24-hour paclitaxel and cisplatin versus 3-hour paclitaxel and carboplatin. This was designed as a noninferiority study and there was a provision for SLL, which about 50% chose to do (Greer et al subset analysis proved that SLL was not beneficial). 85% were able to receive all six cycles. The PFS was 19 months for paclitaxel and cisplatin and 20 months for paclitaxel and carboplatin. The OS was 48 months for paclitaxel cisplatin and 57 months for paclitaxel carboplatin. The relative risk of recurrence was 0.88 (95% CI: 0.75–1.03), and the RR for OS was 0.84 (95% CI: 0.7–1.02) favoring carboplatin and paclitaxel. The carboplatin arm had less myelotoxicity and electrolyte problems, with similar neurotoxicity.[104,126]

o GOG 218: This randomized trial evaluated 1,873 staged III or IV suboptimally debulked patients with a control arm of carboplatin and paclitaxel. The investigational arms consisted of carboplatin and paclitaxel with either bevacizumab for 5 months during primary therapy or an extended dosing of bevacizumab after six initial cycles of carboplatin, paclitaxel, and bevacizumab for a total of 18 cycles. The PFS was, respectively, 10.3, 11.2, and 14.1 months; the PFS HR was 0.91/0.72. The OS, respectively, was 39.9, 38.7, and 39.7 months; OS HR was 1.036/0.92. Maximum separation of the PFS occurred at 15 months and the curves merged 9 months later. The degree of neutropenia was associated with a greater PFS and OS (HR 0.76 and 0.73, respectively).[127]

o SCOTROC 1: This trial evaluated 1,077 patients with stage IC to IV disease and randomized them to docetaxel 75 mg/m^2 versus paclitaxel at 175 mg/m^2 each with carboplatin at an AUC of 5 for six cycles. The PFS was 15 months versus 14.8 months. Docetaxel was found not to be inferior. The OS was 64.2% versus 68.9%, respectively.[128]

o OCTAVIA: This single-arm study evaluated 189 patients treated with primary adjuvant bevacizumab plus weekly paclitaxel and carboplatin every 21 days. For patients with stage IIB to IV or G 3/CC stage I/IIA, bevacizumab was dosed at 7.5 mg/kg on day 1; paclitaxel at 80 mg/m^2 on days 1, 8, 15; and carboplatin at an AUC 6 on day 1 IV every 21 days for six to eight cycles, followed by single-agent maintenance bevacizumab to total 1 Y. Seventy-four percent of the patients had stage IIIC/IV disease. The primary objective was PFS. Patients received a median of six chemotherapy and 17 bevacizumab cycles. At the predefined cut-off of 24 months after last patient enrollment, 99 patients (52%) had progressed and 19 (10%) had died, all from OC. The median PFS was 23.7 months (95% CI: 19.8–26.4 months), 1Y PFS rate was 85.6%, RECIST RR was 84.6%, and median response duration was 14.7 months. Most patients (≥90%) completed at least six chemotherapy cycles. G ≥3 peripheral sensory neuropathy occurred in 5% and febrile neutropenia in 0.5%. There was one case of GI perforation (0.5%) and no treatment-related deaths.[129]

o AGO-OVAR 9: This was a randomized phase III frontline chemotherapy trial by the GCIG for previously untreated patients with stages I to IV EOC. There were 1,742 patients randomly allocated to receive a combination of TCG or TC. TC was given day 1 every 21 days for a planned minimum of six courses. Gemcitabine was given on days 1 and 8 of each cycle in the TCG arm. The median PFS for the TCG arm versus TC arm was 17.8 months and 19.3 months, respectively (HR 1.18; 95% CI: 1.06–1.32; p = .0044). The median OS for he TCG and TC arm was 49.5 months and 51.5 months, respectively. Patients on the TCG arm experienced more G 3 to 4 hematologic toxicity and fatigue compared to patients treated on the TC arm. QOL analysis showed a disadvantage in the TCG arm.[130]

o AGO-OVAR 10/MIMOSA study: Abagovomab is an anti-idiotypic antibody produced by mouse hybridoma and generated against OCA-125. Abagovomab maintenance therapy or placebo was administered as a 2 mg/1 mL suspension once every 2 weeks for 6 weeks then once every 4 weeks until recurrence for up to 21 months after primary surgery with adjuvant platinum–taxane chemotherapy in 888 EOC patients randomized in a 2:1 ratio. A robust immune response was seen but the HR for RFS and OS were 1.099 (95% CI: 0.919–1.315; p = .301) and 1.15 (95% CI: 0.872–1.518; p = .322), respectively. A prior phase I/II trial of 119 patients showed prolonged survival in those who demonstrated an immune response to vaccination (23.5 vs. 4.9 months) contrary to this phase III trial.[131]

o AGO-OVCAR 12/LUME-Ovar1: (Nintedanib) 1,366 women with stage IIB to IV with EOC underwent PDS to R1/R0 status. Patients were randomly assigned (2:1) to receive six cycles of carboplatin (AUC 5 mg/mL/min or 6 mg/mL/min) and paclitaxel (175 mg/m²) in addition to either 200 mg of nintedanib (nintedanib group) or placebo (placebo group) twice daily on days 2 to 21 of every 3-week cycle for up to 120 weeks. The primary endpoint was PFS. Addition of antiangiogenic to standard chemotherapy increased median PFS in the nintedanib group versus the placebo group (17.2 months [95% CI: 16.6–19.9] vs. 16.6 months [95% CI: 13.9–19.1]; HR 0.84 [95% CI: 0.72–0.98]; p = .024). The most common AEs were: diarrhea in the nintedanib group at 22% versus in the placebo group at 3%, and neutropenia in the nintedanib group (42%) versus placebo (36%). Serious AEs were reported in 42% of the nintedanib group and 34% of the placebo group; 2% of patients in the nintedanib group experienced serious AEs associated with death compared with 3% in the placebo group. Nintedanib in combination with carboplatin and paclitaxel prolonged the PFS in first-line treatment of OC patients with a higher impact in patients with low postoperative tumor burden.[132]

o AGO-OVAR 15: This randomized phase II study compared carboplatin, paclitaxel, and lonafarnib to carboplatin and paclitaxel alone as front-line treatment in 105 EOC patients, FIGO stages IIB to IV. Lonafarnib was dosed at 100 mg PO BID during chemotherapy and increased to 200 mg for up to 6 months after chemotherapy for maintenance therapy. PFS was 11.5 months in the lonafarnib, carboplatin, and paclitaxel taxol (LTC) arm versus 16.4 months in the TC arm (p = .0141); the median OS was 20.6 months versus 43.4 months in the TC arm (p = .012). For those with R1 to R2 disease, lonafarnib was inferior treatment, thus, further investigation was not recommended.[133]

o AGO-OVAR-17 BOOST Trial: This was a prospective randomized phase III trial evaluating the optimal treatment duration of first-line bevacizumab in combination with carboplatin and paclitaxel. Nine-hundred-twenty-seven patients with FIGO stages IIB to IV EOC were randomized 1:1 to paclitaxel 175 mg/m^2 and carboplatin AUC 5 q21 days with bevacizumab 15 mg/kg q21 days with an additional 22 cycles (15m) of bevacizumab versus the same dosing of C/P and bevacizumab, but maintenance bevacizumab was continued for an additional 44 cycles (30 months). Patients were stratified by FIGO stage/residual tumor. The primary endpoint was PFS. The trial ran from 2011 to 2013, with a good distribution of characteristics between arms: The median age was 61 Y, 58% were R0, and 77% had HGSTOC. AE happened in 11% of the patients on bevacizumab for 15 months compared to 14% receiving bevacizumab for 30 months. The median PFS was 24.2 months in the 15-month arm compared to 26.0 months for the 30-month group with an HR of 0.99 95% CI 0.85–1.15 p = .90. BEV treatment duration of 15 months remains standard of care. The median OS was 54.3 months compared to 60 months with an HR of 1.04 95% CI 0.87–1.23, p = .68. Thus, the standard duration of maintenance bevicumizab as established by GOG 218 continues to be 15 months.[134]

o GOG 252: In this study, 1,560 patients were randomly assigned to six cycles of IV paclitaxel at 80 mg/m^2 once weekly with IV carboplatin AUC 6 versus IV paclitaxel at 80 mg/m^2 once weekly with IP carboplatin AUC 6 versus once every 3 weeks IV paclitaxel at 135 mg/m^2 over 3 hours day 1, IP cisplatin 75 mg/m^2 day 2, and IP paclitaxel 60 mg/m^2 day 8 (IP cisplatin)—followed by bevacizumab at 15 mg/kg IV every 3 weeks in cycles 2 to 22 for all patients.[135] At month 84.8 of follow-up, the median PFS duration was 24.9 months in the IV carboplatin arm, 27.4 months in the IP carboplatin arm, and 26.2 months in the IP cisplatin arm. On subgroup analysis of 1,380 patients with stage II/III and R1, the median PFS was 26.9 (IV-carboplatin), 28.7 (IP-carboplatin), and 27.8 months (IP cisplatin), respectively. The median PFS for patients with stage II/III and R0 disease was 35.9, 38.8, and 35.5 months, respectively. Median OS for all enrolled was 75.5, 78.9, and 72.9 months, respectively, and median OS for stage II/III with no gross residual disease was 108.6, 114.2, and 107.9 months at 10 Y. Neurotoxicity scores were comparable between arms, but mean TOIFACT-ovary scores were worse for those in the IP cisplatin arm during treatment. Thus, the PFS was not significant for a meaningful difference for either IP arm with the addition of bevacizumab. There was no difference in OS between IV/IP. Bevacizumab may have masked results compared to GOG 172 as well as lower doses of cisplatin in the IP cohort, acknowledging higher doses had more toxicity in GOG 172.

○ Carboplatin monotherapy versus standard doublet frontline therapy in older patients: This was an international, open-label, phase III trial of 120 OC patients who scored 3 or higher on the Geriatric Vulnerability Score undergoing frontline therapy. Patients were stratified by country and surgical outcome between 2013 and 2017.[137] Patients received 6 cycles of (a) carboplatin, AUC 5 with paclitaxel at 175 mg/m² IV every 3 weeks; (b) single-agent carboplatin, AUC 5 or 6 IV every 3 weeks; or (c) weekly carboplatin, AUC 2 with paclitaxel at 60 mg/m², on days 1, 8, and 15 every 4 weeks. The primary outcome was treatment feasibility and DFS. The mean and median age was 80 Y; 43 patients (36%) were scored at 4 and 13 (11%) had a score of 5; 40 (33%) had stage IV disease. The trial was terminated early because single-agent carboplatin showed a worse OS. Six cycles were completed in 26 of 40 (65%), 19 of 40 (48%), and 24 of 40 (60%) patients in the groups described, respectively. Treatment-related AEs were less common with the standard every-3-weeks combination (17 of 40 [43%]) than single-agent carboplatin or weekly combination therapy (both 23 of 40 [58%]). Treatment-related deaths occurred in four patients (2 of 40 [5%] in each combination group).

• **Dose-Density Trials**

○ GOG 97: This study investigated four cycles versus eight cycles of cyclophosphamide and cisplatin in 458 eligible patients. The four-cycle regimen dosed the chemotherapy doublets at 1,000/100 mg/m², whereas the eight-cycle doublet dosed the chemotherapy at 500/50 mg/m² given every 3 weeks. This provided no difference in OS, and the total dosing was the same.[138]

- Fruscio weekly cisplatin: This trial evaluated 285 eligible patients and randomized them to weekly cisplatin at 50 mg/m² for 9 weeks versus cisplatin at 75 mg/m² for six cycles every 3 weeks. At 16.8 Y follow-up, no difference in PFS was seen (17.2 months vs. 18.1 months, HR 1.08) and no difference in OS was seen (35 months vs. 32 months, HR 0.97) for the dose-dense weekly cisplatin versus standard treatment.[139]

- The Scottish Dose Dense Trial: this Trial evaluated six cycles of cyclophosphamide at 750 mg/m² and cisplatin at doses of either 50 or 100 mg/m² q21 days in 159 patients. The OS for the 100 and 50 mg/m² patients was 32.4% and 26.6%, and the overall relative death rate was 0.68 ($p = .043$). From this trial, the standard 75 mg/m² dose was chosen for its modest toxicity.[140]

- The Dutch/Danish Study: This trial randomized 222 patients between different doublet doses of carboplatin and cyclophosphamide. Carboplatin was dosed at an AUC of either 4 or 8 q28 days for six cycles in combination with cyclophosphamide at a constant dose of 500 mg/m². There was no difference in OS (2 YS 45%) or CPR (32% and 30%).[141]

- Gore et al randomized 227 patients to single-agent carboplatin at either an AUC of 6 for six courses or an AUC of 12 for four courses every 4 weeks. There was no difference in PFS or OS at 5 Y at 31% and 34%, respectively. There was more toxicity in the AUC 12 arm.[142]

- GOG 134: This trial included 271 eligible patients with persistent, recurrent, or PD who were evaluated with paclitaxel dosed at 135 mg/m²/24 hr, paclitaxel at 175 mg/m²/24 hr, or paclitaxel at 250 mg/m²/24 hr. The 135 mg/m² arm was closed early. The partial and CR to paclitaxel at 250 mg/m² (36%) was higher than those receiving 175 mg/m² (27%, $p = .027$). The median duration for OS was 13.1 months and 12.3 months for paclitaxel 175 and 250 mg/m², respectively. Thus, paclitaxel exhibited a dose effect with regard to RR, but there was no survival benefit.[143]

- European–Canadian randomized trial of paclitaxel in relapsed OC: This trial evaluated infusion length of paclitaxel in recurrent OC in 391 eligible patients. This was a 2 × 2 study design of 3-hour versus 24-hour infusion and 135 mg/m² versus 175 mg/m². The high-dose group had a longer PFS at 19 weeks versus 14 weeks ($p = .02$). The 175 mg/m² dose was found to have a better RR at 19% versus the 135 mg/m² dose with a RR of 16% (NS). There was no difference in survival.[144]

- NOVEL Trial JGOG 3016: This phase III trial evaluated 631 patients with stages II, III, and IV EOC, stratified by residual disease less than 1 cm or greater than 1 cm as well as by histology (CC/mucinous vs. serous/others) to carboplatin AUC 6 q21 days for six to nine cycles versus dose-dense weekly paclitaxel 80 mg/m^2 on days 1, 8, 15 with carboplatin AUC 6 day 1 q21 days for six to nine cycles. Carboplatin was dosed at an AUC 6 and given every 3 weeks with either: weekly paclitaxel at 80 mg/m^2 or standard 3-week dosing at 180 mg/m^2. The median follow-up was 76.8 months. The median PFS was 28.2 months (95% CI: 22.3–33.8) versus 17.5 months ([15.7–21.7]; HR 0.76; 95% CI: 0.62–0.91; p = .0037). The median OS was 100.5 months (95% CI: 65.2–∞) in the dose-dense treatment group and 62.2 months (95% CI: 52.1–82.6) in the conventional treatment group (HR 0.79; 95% CI: 0.63–0.99; p = .039). The HR for progression was 0.71 (95% CI: 0.58–0.88; p = .0015). The 3Y OS was 72% versus 65% (p = .03), respectively. The 5Y OS was 58.6% versus 51.0%, respectively, with an HR of 0.79.[145,146]

o GOG 262: 692 patients were enrolled in a phase III randomized trial in which 84% elected to receive bevacizumab in addition to either paclitaxel 175 mg/m^2 every 3 weeks with carboplatin AUC 6 for six cycles, or paclitaxel dosed weekly 80 mg/m^2 plus carboplatin AUC 6 for six cycles. In the ITT analysis, weekly paclitaxel was not associated with longer PFS than paclitaxel administered every 3 weeks (14.7 months and 14.0 months, respectively; HR for progression or death = 0.89; 95% CI: 0.74–1.06; p = .18). For those patients who did not receive bevacizumab, weekly paclitaxel was associated with PFS that was 3.9 months longer than that observed with paclitaxel administered every 3 weeks (14.2 vs. 10.3 months; HR 0.62; 95% CI: 0.40–0.95; p = .03 This is similar to JGOG 3016 outcomes). However, among patients who received bevacizumab, weekly paclitaxel did not significantly prolong PFS, as compared with paclitaxel administered every 3 weeks (14.9 months and 14.7 months, respectively; HR 0.99; 95% CI: 0.83–1.20; p = .60). A test for interaction that assessed homogeneity of the treatment effect showed a significant difference between treatment with bevacizumab and without bevacizumab (p = .047). Patients who received weekly paclitaxel had a higher rate of G 3 or 4 anemia than did those who received paclitaxel every 3 weeks (36% vs. 16%), as well as a higher G 2 to 4 sensory neuropathy (26% vs. 18%); although lower rates of G 3 or 4 neutropenia (72% vs. 83%) were observed. Weekly paclitaxel, compared to every-21-day paclitaxel did not prolong PFS.[147]

o MITO-7 (dose intense): In this study, 810 patients with stages IC to IV EOC were randomized in a 1:1 fashion to carboplatin AUC 6 and Taxol 175 mg/m^2 every 3 weeks for six cycles versus carboplatin AUC 2 and paclitaxel 60 mg/m^2 every week for 18 weeks. Primary endpoints were PFS and QOL. The median follow-up was 22.3 months. The median PFS was 17.3 months for every-3-weeks treatment versus 18.3 months for weekly treatment; HR 0.96; 95% CI: 0.8–1.16; p = .66. The weekly group had less neutropenia and neuropathy. 25% of the total population had NACT, 24% were not operated on, 23% were suboptimally debulked, 25% were stage IV, and 67% had serous histology. The 2 YS was 79% with every-3-weeks treatment and 77% with weekly treatment. This was not a dose-dense study so is not a parallel to the JGOG study.[148]

○ ICON 8: This was a phase III randomized trial of 1,566 women randomized to three different frontline chemotherapy arms after undergoing primary cytoreductive surgery or before NACT that compared the efficacy and safety of two dose-dense weekly regimens to standard 3-weekly chemotherapy in women with stage Ic to IV HGSTOC. The study ran between 2011 and 2014.[149] The groups were (a) carboplatin AUC5 or AUC6 and 175 mg/m^2 paclitaxel every 3 weeks, (b) carboplatin AUC5 or AUC6 every 3 weeks and 80 mg/m^2 paclitaxel weekly, or (c) carboplatin AUC2 and 80 mg/m^2 paclitaxel both administered weekly. The primary outcomes were PFS and OS. Total paclitaxel dose was reviewed per group and median total paclitaxel dose for group a was 1010 mg/m^2, group b was 1233 mg/m^2, and group c was 1274 mg/m^2. Of participants, 1,018 (65%) experienced DP by 2017. Seventy-two percent (365), completed six treatment cycles in group a, 60% (305) in group b, and 63% (322) in group c, although 90% (454), 89% (454), and 85% (437) completed six PBC cycles, respectively. No significant PFS increase was observed with either weekly regimen (RMST 24.4 months [97.5% CI, 23.0–26.0] for group a, 24.9m [24.0-25.9] for group b, and 25.3m [23.9-26.9] for group c; the median PFS was 17.7 months [IQR 10.6—not reached] in group a, 20.8 months [11.9-59.0] in group b, 21.0 months [12.0-54.0] in group c; LR p = .35 for group b vs. group a; group c vs. a p = .51). Although G 3/4 toxic effects increased with weekly treatment, they were overall uncomplicated. Febrile neutropenia and sensory neuropathy rates were comparable among groups.

- **IP Trials**
   ○ GOG 104: This trial evaluated 546 patients for primary adjuvant chemotherapy after "optimal" debulking to a size of less than 2 cm. IV cyclophosphamide was given at 600 mg/m^2 for six cycles every 3 weeks with either IP cisplatin or IV cisplatin (both dosed at 100 mg/m^2). The median OS was significant favoring the IP arm at 49 months versus the IV group at 41 months. The HR for death was lower in the IP group, 0.76; 95% CI: 0.61 to 0.96; p = .02.[150]

   ○ GOG 114: This trial evaluated 462 stage III patients who were optimally debulked to less than 1 cm. Patients were randomized to IV cisplatin at 75 mg/m^2 and IV paclitaxel 135 mg/m^2 over 24 hours every 3 weeks for six cycles versus IV carboplatin at an AUC 9 for two cycles q28 days followed by IP cisplatin at 100 mg/m^2 with IV paclitaxel 135 mg/m^2 over 24 hours every 3 weeks for six cycles.

SLL was optional. The PFS was 27.6 months versus 22.5 months with $p = .01$, the OS was 63.2 months versus 52.5 months with a $p = .05$, all favoring IP therapy.[151]

o GOG 172: This trial evaluated 415 stage III patients who were optimally debulked to less than 1 cm residual. Patients were randomized to either IV paclitaxel at 135 mg/m² over 24 hours, with cisplatin dosed at 75 mg/m² or to IP cisplatin on day 1 dosed at 100 mg/m² with IV paclitaxel at 135 mg/m² over 24 hours on day 2, and paclitaxel again on day 8 dosed at 60 mg/m² IP. Sixty-four percent had gross residual disease after primary surgery and 50% of patients chose a second-look surgery. Of participants, 41% of the IV group versus 57% of the IP group had a CPR at SLL. Only 42% of the IP group completed all IP cycles, whereas 83% of the IV group received all six cycles. The PFS was 18.3 months for the IV arm versus 23.8 months for the IP arm ($p = .05$). The OS was 49.7 months for the IV arm versus 65.6 months for the IP arm with a 16-month survival advantage favoring IP therapy ($p = .03$). A 5.5-month PFS was seen. Patients with no visible residual disease did well with a 78-month median survival for those on the IV arm and the median survival has not been reached for the IP arm.[152] In a subgroup analysis of *BRCA* expression, the IP group had a better OS of 84.1 (mut) versus 47.7 months (WT).[153]

o A 10Y follow-up of GOG 114 and 172: This was a combined review of two IP studies that included 876 patients that showed the median PFS for IP therapy was 25 months compared to 20 months for IV therapy. The OS was 61.8 versus 51.4 months, respectively. The risk of death decreased by 12% for each cycle of IP chemotherapy completed. The DFS for those who received IP therapy with R0 disease (complete cytoreduction) was 60.4 months, with an OS of 127.6 months.[154]

o Prognostic factors for stage III EOC treated with IP chemotherapy: This was a combined review of surgically debulked patients from GOG IP studies 114 and 172: a second 10Y follow-up of GOGs 114 and 172. IP versus IV OS was 61.8 months versus 51.4 months with risk reduction of death 23%. Those patients with R0 disease who received IP therapy had a PFS of 38 months with a median OS not yet reached and a median follow-up of 53 months. An OS of 127 months with R0 disease after PDS was seen in this subgroup. The OS for those treated on the IV arm with R0 disease was 78 months. The difference in the median OS between the IV and IP arms was 16 months, the difference between RD1 versus RD0 exceeded 39 months. Considering all patients in GOGs 114 and 172, the difference in OS between the IV and IP arms was 11 months, whereas the difference between RD1 and RD0 for those receiving IP was over 60 months. This then concludes there is high value in resecting all gross disease with acceptable morbidity. Twenty-nine percent of patients underwent bowel resection, which is a surrogate for surgical effort.[155]

- ○ On GOG 172, 205 patients were randomized to IP therapy. Of these, 58% did not complete treatment, 13% did not receive IP treatment, 57% completed one to two cycles, 29% received three to five cycles. Of participants, 34% were not able to complete treatment because of catheter-related issues, 38% due to poor tolerance to the treatment; 29% did not have IP treatment because of DP of other complications.[156]

- ○ GOG 9921: This was a phase I feasibility study evaluating dose modification of GOG 172. It evaluated 23 patients. IP cisplatin was dosed at 75 mg/m² with IV paclitaxel at 135 mg/m² over 3 hours on day 1, with IP paclitaxel 60 mg/m² administered on day 8 of a 21-day cycle with a 95% rate of adherence for an outpatient regimen.[157]

- **IP Catheter Outcomes**
  - ○ GOG 172: Of the 58% of patients not completing six IP cycles, one third were catheter related (catheter infection in 20 of 41 cases, blocked catheter in 10 of 41 cases). One third were related to IP treatment (pain, bowel complications, patient refusal, other non-catheter infection). One third of discontinuations were probably unrelated to the catheter (nausea, renal, metabolic). Left colon resection or colostomy was related to a decreased ability to tolerate IP chemotherapy. Appendectomy, small bowel resection, or right colon surgery did not appear to affect IP tolerance. Optimal placement is the use of a 9.6-F catheter through a separate incision (not the laparotomy incision), and tunneled at least 10 cm, with 10 cm length left in the peritoneal cavity. A waiting time of 24 hours postinsertion before use was recommended to avoid leakage.[158]

  - ○ GOG 252: This was a phase III trial of patients with stage II to IV epithelial TOC to include suboptimally debulked patients. 1,560 were randomized to one of three arms: Arm 1 (control arm similar to GOG 262): IV paclitaxel at 80 mg/m² weekly with IV carboplatin AUC 6 every 3 weeks and IV bevacizumab 15 mg/kg every 3 weeks continuing with maintenance bevacizumab ×22 weeks. Arm 2: IV paclitaxel 80 mg/m² weekly with IP carboplatin AUC 6 every 3 weeks and IV bevacizumab 15 mg/kg every 3 weeks with maintenance bevacizumab ×22 weeks. Arm 3: IV paclitaxel at 135 mg/m² on day 1 followed by IP cisplatin at 75 mg/m² on day 2, then IP paclitaxel at 60 mg/m² on day 8, and bevacizumab at 15 mg/kg every 3 weeks with maintenance bevacizumab for 22 weeks. The median age was 58, 34% were stage III, 10% stage II, 72% were G3 serous, 57% achieved R0 debulking, 90% in arm 1 completed platinum therapy, 90% in arm 2, and 84% in arm 3. PFS was the primary outcome. Median PFS for the 461 patients in arm 1 was 26.8 months, for the 464 patients in arm 2 it was 28.7 months (log rank p = .661), and for the 456 patients in arm 3 it was 27.8 months (log rank p = .122). Of note: This was not a platinum dose intense trial similar to GOG 172, and bevacizumab was added as primary therapy and maintenance, similar to GOG 218.[159]

○ iPocc Trial (GOTIC-001/JGOG-3019): This was a superiority trial evaluating 655 patients with dose-dense weekly IV paclitaxel at 80 mg/m² administered in combination with carboplatin AUC 6 every 3 weeks either IV or IP. No bevacizumab or maintenance therapy was allowed. Eligible patients had EOC stages II to IV; 299 received IV, whereas 303 received IP. The PFS was 20.7 versus 23.5 months for IV versus IP. The OS was 67 versus 64.9 months IV versus IP (p = .041 CI .77–1.17). For those with R2 disease, the OR for response was better for the IP group at .89 CI .55–1.42. OS was not improved by IP therapy.[159,160]

○ OV-21/PETROC: This was a two-stage, phase II trial of 275 women with EOC staged IIB to IVA treated with IV platinum-based NACT followed by optimal (<1 cm) debulking surgery then randomized to one of the three treatment arms: (a) IV carboplatin/paclitaxel, (b) IP cisplatin with IV/IP paclitaxel, or (c) IP carboplatin plus IV/IP paclitaxel. The primary endpoint was a 9-month PD rate. The trial ran between 2009 to 2015. The IP cisplatin arm failed to progress beyond first-stage accrual due to not meeting preset superiority rules. The final analysis compared IV carboplatin/paclitaxel (n = 101) with IP carboplatin, IV/IP paclitaxel (n = 102). The ITT PD rate at 9 months was lower in the IP carboplatin arm compared to the IV carboplatin arm: 24.5% (95% CI 16.2%–32.9%) versus 38.6% (95% CI 29.1%–48.1%), p = .065. The study was underpowered to detect differences in PFS: HR PFS 0.82 (95% CI 0.57–1.17); p = .27 and OS HR 0.80 (95% CI 0.47–1.35, p = .40). The IP carboplatin regimen was well tolerated. Thus, for R0 women with stage IIIC or IVA EOC treated with NACT, IP carboplatin-based chemotherapy is well tolerated and associated with an improved 9-month PD rate compared to IV carboplatin-based chemotherapy.[161]

• **Maintenance/Consolidation Trials**

○ GOG 178: This trial evaluated consolidation therapy in 222 eligible stage III and IV patients and randomized patients to 12 versus three cycles of paclitaxel at 175 mg/m² after completion of six cycles of platinum/paclitaxel with a clinical CR. At 50% enrollment, the protocol dictated interim analysis. This showed an improvement in PFS favoring 12 cycles with an HR of 2.31 demonstrating a 28-month versus 21-month PFS (p = .002, 99% CI: 1.08 to 4.94). The study was closed at this point. Patients were allowed to crossover so all those on the three-cycle arm could complete up to 12 cycles of therapy.[162]

○ Follow-up study to GOG 178: Criticisms cited from this study were the crossover may have masked a difference between study arms, there was insufficient power within the study, and treatment at relapse equalized outcomes. The PFS was 22 versus 14 months favoring the 12-month paclitaxel. OS was 53 versus 48 months (*p* = .34, NS).[163]

○ Initiation of salvage chemotherapy: This was a retrospective institutional evaluation of maintenance therapy versus expectant management in patients with recurrent disease that reviewed 59 eligible patients with a median follow-up of 51 months. The median time from CCR to start of second-line chemotherapy was 21 months; the median time to the start of third-line agents was 43 months. Twelve months elapsed between completion of first-line therapy and recurrence in 50% of patients. Thus, a similar time frame of 40 months between clinical CR and the start of third-line therapies exists, which is comparable to results in GOG 178.[164]

○ GOG 175: This trial evaluated 542 eligible patients who were staged IA or IB G 3 or CC, all stage IC and all stage II OC. They were all given IV carboplatin AUC 6 and paclitaxel 175 mg/m^2 for three cycles followed by randomization to either observation or weekly paclitaxel for 24 weeks. The 5Y recurrence probability rate was 23% for those observed, and 20% for those who received maintenance paclitaxel, HR 0.8. The 5 YS was 85.4% versus 86.2% (NS).[165]

○ Study 19: Olaparib maintenance therapy. In this study, 256 patients with platinum-sensitive, relapsed, HGSTOC who had received two or more platinum-based regimens and had had a partial or CR to their most recent platinum-based regimen were included in this double-blind phase II randomized study. BRCA1/2 mutation status was not required but was known in 36.6% of patients at study entry. Olaparib was dosed at 400 mg twice daily. The primary endpoint was PFS. A total of 136 were assigned to the olaparib group and 129 to the placebo group. The PFS was significantly longer with olaparib than with placebo (median, 8.4 months vs. 4.8 months from randomization on completion of chemotherapy; HR for progression or death, 0.35; 95% CI: 0.25–0.49; *p* <.001). Subgroup analyses of PFS showed that, regardless of subgroup, patients in the olaparib group had a lower risk of progression. AEs reported in the olaparib group versus the placebo group were nausea (68% vs. 35%), fatigue (49% vs. 38%), vomiting (32% vs. 14%), and anemia (17% vs. 5%); the majority of AEs were G 1 or 2. An interim analysis of OS (38% maturity, meaning that 38% of the patients had died) showed no significant difference between groups (HR with olaparib, 0.94; 95% CI: 0.63–1.39; *p* = .75). A subset analysis showed patients with mutations were most likely to benefit.

There was an 82% reduction in risk of DP or death in muta-tion patients, translating to a median PFS of 11.2 months with drug compared to 4.3 months on placebo. OS data for mutation patients were 34.9 versus 31.9 months (NS). The highest bene-fit was seen in BRCA-mutation carriers with platinum-sensitive disease.[167]

○ Solo-1: Solo 1 was a phase III double-blind trial that evaluated the efficacy of olaparib as maintenance therapy in 391 patients with advanced (stage 3/4) newly diagnosed HGSTOC or endometri-oid cancer identified to have a *BRCA1*, *BRCA2*, mutation, or both (*BRCA1/2*) after a CCR or partial clinical response to frontline platinum-based chemotherapy.[168] Olaparib was dosed at 300mg PO BID or placebo. The primary endpoint was PFS.260 patients were assigned to olaparib and 131 to placebo in a 2:1 ratio. Of patients, 388 had a germline *BRCA1/2* mutation, and two patients had a somatic *BRCA1/2* mutation. At median follow-up of 41 months, the risk of DP or death was 70% lower with olaparib than with placebo (Kaplan–Meier estimate of the rate of freedom from DP and from death at 3Y, 60% vs. 27%; HR for DP or death, 0.30; 95% CI, 0.23–0.41; *p* <.001). At 5Y from trial enrollment clo-sure, maintenance olaparib doubled the 5YDFS with 48.3% of the olaparib group not experiencing DP versus 20.5% of the placebo arm with the median DFS of 56.0 months versuss 13.8 months, respectively (HR: 0.33). There was no statistical difference in QOL between treatment regimens.[169] There was an improvement in PFS in the BRCA-mutated cohort on olaparib for 3Y and also an improvement in PFS2 overall.

○ AGO-OVAR 16: A phase III study evaluated the efficacy and safety of pazopanib monotherapy versus placebo in women who have not progressed after first-line chemotherapy for epithelial ovar-ian, fallopian tube, or PPC. In it, 940 patients were randomized 1:1 to receive either 800 mg of pazopanib once daily or placebo for up to 24 months. The median follow-up was 24.3 months. The median PFS was 17.9 months in the pazopanib arm and 12.3 months in the placebo arm (HR − 0.77; *p* = .0021). The interim survival analysis did not show any significant difference between the two study arms after events in 36.5% of the study population. In an exploratory analysis of ethnicity, pazopanib appeared to have superior benefit in the 78% of patients who were not of East Asian descent (HR − 0.69; median PFS benefit, 5.9 months), com-pared to 22% of patients of East Asian descent who had an HR of 1.16. Toxicity was high and treatment discontinuation occurred more often in the pazopanib arm: 33% of patients discontinued treatment compared with 5.6% of patients in the placebo arm. The incidence of G 3 or 4 AEs was higher in the pazopanib arm: HTN in 30.8%, neutropenia in 9.9%, liver-related toxicity in 9.4%, diarrhea in 8.2%, thrombocytopenia in 2.5%, and palmar–plantar erythrodysesthesia in 1.9%. Three patients in the pazopanib arm had a fatal AE—a myocardial infarction, pneumonia, and posterior reversible encephalopathy syndrome.[468] One patient in the placebo arm had fatal acute leukemia. The third OS interim analysis showed futility with HR of 0.96 CI 0.805-1.145 between arms with median OS of 59.1 months in the pazopanib group compared to 64 months in the placebo group.[166]

o MANGO-2/ILIAD: This was a phase IV trial using biomarker data for OC patients treated on study 55041 with bevacizumab and carboplatin followed by erlotinib maintenance versus observation in patients with no evidence of DP after first-line platinum-based chemotherapy. Somatic mutations in KRAS, BRAF, NRAS, PIK3CA, EGFR, and PTEN were determined in 318 (38%) and expression of EGFR, pAkt, pMAPK, E-cadherin and Vimentin, and EGFR and HER2 gene copy numbers in 218 (26%) of a total of 835 randomized patients. Biomarker data were correlated with PFS and OS. Only 28 mutations were observed among KRAS, BRAF, NRAS, PIK3CA, EGFR, and PTEN (in 7.5% of patients), of which the most frequent were in KRAS and PIK3CA. EGFR mutations occurred in only three patients. When all mutations were pooled, patients with at least one mutation in KRAS, NRAS, BRAF, PIK3CA, or EGFR had longer PFS (33.1 vs. 12.3 months; HR 0.57; 95% CI: 0.33–0.99; p = .042) compared to those with wild-type tumors. EGFR overexpression was detected in 93 of 218 patients (42.7%), and 66 of 180 patients (36.7%) had EGFR gene amplification or high levels of copy number gain. Fifty-eight of 128 patients had positive pMAPK expression (45.3%), which was associated with inferior OS (38.9 vs. 67.0 months; HR 1.81; 95% CI: 1.11–2.97; p = .016). Patients with positive EGFR fluorescence in situ hybridization (FISH) status had worse OS (46.1 months) than those with negative status (67.0 months; HR 1.56; 95% CI: 1.01–2.40; p = .044) and shorter PFS (9.6 vs. 16.1 months; HR 1.57; 95% CI: 1.11–2.22; p = .010). None of the investigated biomarkers correlated with responsiveness to erlotinib. Conclusion: Increased EGFR gene copy number was associated with worse OS and PFS in patients with OC.[170]

o PAOLA-1: This was a randomized, double-blind phase III trial of 806 patients with newly diagnosed, advanced-stage HGSTOC who responded to frontline platinum-taxane chemotherapy plus bevacizumab. Patients were eligible regardless of surgical resection status or BRCA mutation status.[171] Assigned in a 2:1 ratio to olaparib at 300 mg PO BID, or placebo up to 24 months, all patients received bevacizumab dosed at 15mg/kg every 3 weeks for up to 15 months in total. The primary endpoint was the time from randomization until DP or death. Of participants,

537 received olaparib and 269 received placebo. At a median follow-up of 22.9 months, the median PFS was 22.1 months with olaparib plus bevacizumab, and 16.6 months with placebo plus bevacizumab (HR for DP or death, 0.59; 95% CI, 0.49 to 0.72; p <.001). Subgroup analysis for patients that were HRd deficient showed an HR (olaparib vs. placebo group) for DP or death was 0.33 (95% CI, 0.25 to 0.45), including tumors that were BRCA mutation + (median PFS, 37.2 vs. 17.7m), and 0.43 (95% CI, 0.28–0.66) in patients who were HRd +/– but BRCA– (median PFS, 28.1 vs. 16.6 months).

o PRIMA/ENGOT-OV26/GOG-3012: Niraparib was evaluated in a phase III double blind trial that assigned 733 advanced OC patients in a 2:1 ratio to niraparib or placebo once daily after response to frontline platinum-based chemotherapy.[172] The primary endpoint was PFS, both in patients who were HRd, and the overall population. Of patients, 373 (50.9%) had tumors that were HRd. For the HRd group, the median PFS was longer in the niraparib group at 21.9 months than in the placebo group at 10.4 months (HR, 0.43; 95% CI: 0.31–0.59; p <.001). For the overall population, the PFS was 13.8 months and 8.2 months (HR 0.62; 95% CI, 0.50–0.76; p <.001). At 24 months, the OS was 84% in the niraparib group and 77% in the placebo group (HR 0.70; 95% CI, 0.44–1.11). G 3 and higher AEs were anemia (31.0%), thrombocytopenia (28.7%), and neutropenia (12.8%). No treatment-related deaths occurred.

o JAVELIN Ovarian 100: This was an open-label, three-arm, parallel, randomized, phase III trial in women with stage III to IV epithelial ovarian, fallopian tube, or peritoneal cancer (following debulking surgery, or candidates for NACT). Patients were randomly assigned (1:1:1) to receive (a) six cycles of carboplatin AUC 5/6 IV every 3 weeks with paclitaxel 175 mg/m^2 every 3 weeks or weekly at 80 mg/m^2 [investigators' choice] followed by avelumab maintenance at 10 mg/kg IV q 2 weeks; (b) chemotherapy plus avelumab (10 mg/kg IV q 3 weeks) followed by avelumab maintenance; (c) chemotherapy followed by observation. The primary endpoint was PFS and the study ran between 2016 to 2018. A total of 998 patients were assigned (a) n = 332, (b) n = 331, and (c) n = 335). At interim analysis prespecified futility boundaries were crossed and the trial was closed. The median follow-up was 10.8 months (IQR 7.1–14.9); 11.1 months (7.0–15.3) for group a, 11.0 months (7.4–14.5) for group b, and 10.2 months (6.7–14.0) for group c. The median PFS was 16.8 months (95% CI 13.5–NE) group for a, 18.1 months (14.8–NE) for group b, and NE (18.2 months–NE) for group c. The stratified HR for PFS was 1.43 (95% CI 1.05–1.95; one-sided p = .99) for group a and 1.14 (0.83–1.56; one-sided p = .79) for group b compared to group c. The most common AE were G 3 to 4 anemia at 21% for group a and 19% in group a b compared to 16% in group

c. Thus, there is minimal data to support the use of avelumab as primary treatment.[173]

o ATHENA-NONO/GOG-3020/ENGOT-ov45: This was a phase III randomized study of high grade ovarian cancer patients staged III-IV who were randomized 4:1 after primary debulking surgery and 4–8 cycles of frontline platinum/taxane double chemotherapy to rucaparib 600 mg PO BOD or placebo. 538 total patients were enrolled and stratified by HRd status. For the HRd group, the median PFS was 28.7 months for rucaparib vs. 11.3 months for placebo. For the HRp group the PFS was 12.1 months vs. 9.1 months. and for the ITT group the PFS was 20.2 vs. 9.2 months for rucaparib vs. placebo (HR 0.47, 0.65, and 0.52 respectively. AE's were anemia and neutropenia at 28.7 and 14.6 vs. 0 and 0.9% for rucaparib or placebo groups respectively. Rucaparib monotherapy maintenance regardless of primary surgical postoperative residual disease or genetic mutation status extended the PFS for ovarian cancer patients.[469]

o PRIME: This was a phase 3 study of 384 patients followed for 27.5 months comparing niraparib maintenance at 200 mg daily for 36 months to placebo for stage IIII/IV OC patients after frontline platinum-based chemotherapy. In the study, 255 patients received the study drug and 129 placebo. The PFS was 24.8 months versus 8.3 months. The OS data is immature. For BRCAm the PFS was 222.3 versus 10.8 months and BRCAWT 19.3 versus 8.3 months.[174]

o VELIA/GOG-3005: This was a phase III, placebo-controlled trial that evaluated the efficacy of veliparib added to frontline chemotherapy with carboplatin and paclitaxel and continued as maintenance monotherapy in patients with stage III/IV HGSTOC.[136] In the study, 1,140 patients were assigned in a 1:1:1 ratio to receive (a) chemotherapy plus placebo followed by placebo maintenance (control), (b) chemotherapy plus veliparib followed by placebo maintenance, or (c) chemotherapy plus veliparib followed by veliparib maintenance. Surgical cytoreduction could be primary or neoadjuvant after three cycles of trial treatment. Combination chemotherapy was for six cycles, with maintenance therapy for an additional 30. The primary endpoint was PFS in group c compared with group a. Stratification was by *BRCA*-mutation, HRd (which included the *BRCA*-mutation cohort), and in the ITT population. For the *BRCA*-mutation cohort, the median PFS was 34.7 months in group c and 22.0 months in control group (HR for progression or death, 0.44; 95% CI, 0.28-0.68; $p < .001$); in the HRd cohort it was 31.9 months and 20.5 months, respectively (HR, 0.57; 95 CI, 0.43-0.76; $p < .001$); and in the ITT population, it was 23.5 months and 17.3 months (HR, 0.68; 95% CI, 0.56-0.83; $p < .001$). Veliparib led to a higher incidence of anemia and thrombocytopenia when combined with chemotherapy as well as nausea and fatigue overall. Among all cohorts, the regimen of carboplatin, paclitaxel, and veliparib induction therapy followed by veliparib maintenance therapy led to significantly longer PFS than carboplatin plus paclitaxel induction therapy alone. Synergy was suggested with veliparib and platinum chemotherapy in the frontline setting before the addition of maintenance therapy. The HR for reduction in recurrence or DP was 56% in patients with *BRCA* mutations, 43% in patients with HRd, and 32% in the ITT population. The benefit of veliparib combined with carboplatin and paclitaxel and continued as maintenance was seen across each of the primary endpoint patient populations (HR = 0.68; $p < .001$). Assessment of ORR from patients with measurable disease after primary surgery ($n = 290$, 25% of the ITT population) and along with baseline CA-125 levels and during treatment cycles showed that veliparib provided an incremental antitumor activity when combined with frontline platinum chemotherapy prior to maintenance. During the first six cycles, the veliparib-containing arms yielded the following: a higher percentage of patients with ORR and CR per RECIST, version 1.1; a higher percentage of patients with at least a 90% reduction in CA-125 levels; a higher CA-125 response prior to surgery in patients undergoing IDS; and an increased CA-125 response in both HRd and non-HRd patient populations—thus, there may be an extended window of benefit for PARP inhibition versus a maintenance-alone method. A difference in study design is that patients with SD at the end of chemotherapy were eligible for maintenance therapy and this population represented 28% of the control arm at the end of chemotherapy.

- **Recurrent Disease Trials**
  - EORTC 55005: GC versus carboplatin: This trial evaluated platinum-sensitive relapsed EOC in 356 eligible patients. Single-agent carboplatin AUC 5 was compared to carboplatin AUC 4 with gemcitabine dosed at 1,000 mg/m^2 given on days 1 and 8, every 21 days. The PFS was improved with the addition of gemcitabine (8.6 months vs. 5.8 months HR 0.72 (95% CI: 0.58–0.90; $p = .0031$)). The study was not powered to detect a difference in OS. The ORR was 47% with the addition of gemcitabine versus 30% with single-agent carboplatin (HR 0.96; 95% CI: 0.75–1.23; $p = .7349$). In 60% of patients illness recurred at greater than 12 months and in 40% recurred between 6 months and 12 months.[175]
  - A randomized phase III study of PLD versus topotecan in recurrent EOC: This trial evaluated 474 patients with recurrent disease in response to single-agent therapy. Liposomal doxorubicin was dosed at 50 mg/m^2 every 4 weeks, and topotecan was dosed at 1.5 mg/m^2/day for 5 days every 3 weeks. The median survival for

patients was 63 weeks for PLD versus 60 weeks for topotecan (HR 1.216; 95% CI: 1–1.478; p = .05). For those patients who had platinum-sensitive disease there was a significant difference in time until progression: 108 weeks versus 70 weeks, favoring PLD (HR 1.432; 95% CI: 1.066–1.923; p = .017). For patients with PI-R disease, OS was similar.[176]

o OCEANS: This trial evaluated 484 eligible patients who received carboplatin AUC 4 and gemcitabine 1,000 mg/m² on days 1 and 8 with or without the addition of bevacizumab at 15 mg/kg IV every 3 weeks in recurrent platinum-sensitive disease. Six to 10 cycles were given with a median follow-up of 58.2 months in the bevacizumab arm and 56.4 months in the placebo arm. An ORR of 78.5% versus 57.4% was seen. Duration of response was 10.4 months versus 7.4 months (HR 0.534; 95% CI: 0.408–0.698), favoring the bevacizumab arm. The median OS was comparable between arms, with 33.6 months in the bevacizumab arm versus 32.9 months in the placebo arm (HR 0.95 log rank p = .65), thus no difference between arms. The PFS demonstrated an HR of 0.48, favoring the bevacizumab arm, with months until progression of 12.4 versus 8.4. G 3 HTN occurred in 17.4% of the experimental arm versus 1% with placebo. OS results were possibly confounded by extensive use of subsequent anticancer therapies.[177,178]

o CALYPSO EORTC 55051: In this international noninferiority trial, 976 patients with recurrent late relapsing (>6 months after first- or second-line platinum- and paclitaxel-based therapies) platinum-sensitive OC were treated with the doublets of carboplatin AUC 5 and liposomal doxorubicin (CD) dosed at 30 mg/m² every 4 weeks (CD) versus the standard of carboplatin AUC 5 and paclitaxel 175 mg/m² for at least six cycles every 3 weeks (CP). Forty percent of patients had received two prior regimens before entering the study. A maximum of nine cycles were administered. The ORR was 63%, including 38% of patients who achieved a CR. Patients in the CD arm had a better PFS of 11.3 months compared to the CP arm with 9.4 months (HR 0.82 (95% CI: 0.72, 0.94; p = .005)). The median survival times were 30.7 months and 33 months for the CD arm versus the CP arm (NS). CD led to delayed progression but similar OS compared to CP in platinum-sensitive OC. In a subset analysis, patients with a tumor-free interval >24 months were analyzed separately. A total of 259 very platinum-sensitive patients were included (n = 131, CD; n = 128, CP). The median PFS was 12.0 months for the CD arm and 12.3 months for CP (HR 1.05; 95% CI: 0.79–1.40; p = .73 for superiority) and median OS was 40.2 months for CD and 43.9 for CP (HR 1.18; 95% CI: 0.85–1.63; p = .33 for superiority). ORRs were 42% and 38%, respectively (p = .46). This subset analysis found that CP and CD were equally effective treatment regimens for patients with very platinum-sensitive recurrent ovarian cancer but the favorable risk-benefit profile suggested that carboplatin-PLD should be the treatment of choice for these patients due to better toxicity profiles.[179,180]

o AURELIA trial AGO-OVAR 2.15: In this study, 361 patients with platinum resistant disease following frontline platinum chemotherapy randomly allocated to single non-platinum chemotherapy agent alone or with bevacizumab (10 mg/kg every 2 weeks or 15 mg/kg every 3 weeks). The non-platinum agents were investigator chosen from either: PLD 40 mg/m^2 q28 days, weekly paclitaxel at 80 mg/m^2, topotecan 1.25 mg/ m^2 on days 1 to 5 q3 weeks, or topotecan 4 mg/m^2 on days 1, 8, 15 q28 days. Cross over to bevacizumab alone was allowed and occurred in 40% of patients. The primary endpoint was PFS. Patients in the chemotherapy-alone arm had a median PFS of 3.4 months versus 6.7 months with bevacizumab (HR 0.48, 95% CI: 0.38–0.60; p <.001). The RECIST ORR was 11.8% in the chemotherapy-alone arm versus 27.3% in the group with bevacizumab added (p = .001). The HR for OS was 0.85 (95% CI: 0.66–1.08; p <.174). There was no difference in OS between chemotherapy regimens (HR 0.85; 95% CI: 0.66–1.08 unstratified log-rank p <.174). The median OS was 13.3 months for chemotherapy versus 16.6 months for chemotherapy plus bevacizumab (95% CI: 13.7–19). GI perforation occurred in 2.2% of bevacizumab-treated patients. The QOL arm showed a greater than 15% improvement in abdominal/GI symptoms at weeks 8/9 with the addition of bevacizumab; 21.9% versus 9.3% difference. The PFS HRs were 0.57 (95% CI: 0.39–0.83) for PLD (median 5.4 vs. 3.5 months, favoring the addition of bevacizumab), 0.46 (95% CI: 0.30–0.71) in the paclitaxel cohort (median 10.4 vs. 3.9m), and 0.32 (95% CI: 0.21–0.49) for the topotecan cohort (median 5.8 vs. 2.1m). The ORR evaluable by RECIST criteria was greater in regimens that included bevacizumab compared to chemotherapy alone for all cohorts: PLD cohort 13.7% versus 7.8% (95% CI: −7.2% to 19.0%), paclitaxel cohort 53.3% versus 30.2% (95% CI: 1.7%–44.5%), and topotecan cohort 17.0% versus 0.0% (95% CI: 5.1%–28.9%). The unadjusted HRs for bevacizumab-containing chemotherapy versus chemotherapy alone were: HR 0.91 (95% CI: 0.62–1.36) for the PLD cohort (median 13.7 vs. 14.1 months), HR 0.65 for the paclitaxel cohort (95% CI: 0.42–1.02; median 22.4 vs. 13.2 months), and HR 1.09 (95% CI: 0.72–1.67) for the topotecan cohort (median 13.8 vs. 13.3 months). In the chemotherapy-alone arms, progression, median PFS, and ORR varied among groups. Topotecan was usually given weekly and seemed less active than weekly paclitaxel, whereas PLD had intermediate results. There was no difference in OS between treatment arms in the PLD and topotecan cohorts, but Kaplan–Meier curves for OS were clearly separated in the paclitaxel cohort; thus, a combination of paclitaxel and bevacizumab may enhance both of their antiangiogenic effects and potentially account for their better HRs in AURELIA.[181,182]

o MITO-8: This was an unmasked, prospective, randomized, superiority trial to evaluate the effect of prolongation of PFI with monotherapy non-platinum based chemotherapy (NPBC) in 215 patients with relapsed OC who experienced DP 6 to 12 months after their last platinum treatment.[183] Patients were assigned 1:1 to NPBC followed by PBC at subsequent relapse or the standard reverse treatment sequence. OS was the primary endpoint. There were 108 patients enrolled in the standard arm and 107 in the experimental arm. The trial ended early due to slow enrollment. PFI was prolonged in the experimental arm (median, 7.8 vs. 0.01 months) but there was no OS benefit in the experimental arm (median, 21.8 vs. 24.5 months; HR, 1.38; 95% CI, 0.99–1.94; $p = .06$). PFS after the sequence was shorter in the experimental arm (median, 12.8 vs. 16.4 months; HR, 1.41; 95% CI, 1.04–1.92; $p = .025$). Global QOL change after three cycles was worse in the experimental arm. Thus, PBC should not be delayed in favor of an NPBC in patients with platinum-sensitive OC.

o JAVELIN 200 Trial: In this open-label, parallel-group, three-arm, phase III trial, 566 recurrent HGSTOC patients were randomized.[184] Each patient had to have a maximum of three lines of previous therapy for platinum-sensitive disease, none for PI-R disease. Assignment was 1:1:1 to (a) avelumab at 10 mg/kg IV q2 weeks, (b) avelumab plus PLD at 40 mg/m² IV q4 weeks, and (c) PLD. All were stratified by disease platinum status, number of prior chemotherapy regimens, and bulky disease. Primary endpoints were PFS by and OS in this superiority study to PLD. The trial ran between 2016–2017. In it, 188 patients were randomized to the combination group, 190 to the PLD group, and 188 to the avelumab group. Median PFS was 3.7 months (95% CI 3.3–5.1) in the combination group, 3.5 months (2.1–4.0) in the PLD group, and 1.9 months (1.8–1.9) in the avelumab group (combination vs. PLD: stratified HR 0.78 [repeated 93.1% CI 0.59–1.24], one-sided $p = .030$; avelumab vs. PLD: 1.68 [1.32–2.60], one-sided $p > .99$). Median OS was 15.7 months (95% CI 12.7–18.7) in the combination group, 13.1 months (11.8–15.5) in the PLD group, and 11.8 months (8.9–14.1) in the avelumab group (combination vs. PLD: stratified HR 0.89 [repeated 88.85% CI 0.74–1.24], one-sided $p = .21$; avelumab vs. PLD: 1.14 [0.95–1.58], one-sided $p = .83$]). The most common G 3 AE was PPE syndrome. Serious AEs occurred in 32 (18%) patients in the combination group, 19 (11%) in the PLD group, and 14 (7%) in the avelumab group. Thus, neither combination nor monotherapy improved PFS or OS significantly for these PI-R refractory OC patients.

○ TRINOVA-1: This was a randomized, double-blind international phase III study in women with recurrent EOC evaluating trebananib in antiangiogenesis. The study enrolled 919 women. Patient eligibility criteria included having been treated with three or fewer previous regimens, and a platinum-free interval of less than 12 months. Patients were randomly assigned to weekly IV paclitaxel (80 mg/m^2) plus either weekly masked IV placebo or trebananib (15 mg/kg). Patients were stratified on the basis of platinum-free interval (≥ 0 and ≤ 6 months vs. >6 and ≤ 12 months), presence or absence of measurable disease, and region. The primary endpoint was PFS. The median PFS in the trebananib arm was 7.4 months (95% CI: 7.0–7.8) versus 5.4 months (95% CI: 4.7–5.5) in the placebo arm (HR 0.70; 95% CI: 0.61–0.80; $p < .001$). The ORR was 29.8% vs. 38.4% ($p = .0071$). The median OS was 19.3 months in the trebananib arm versus 18.3 months in the control arm (NS); (HR 0.95; 95% CI: 0.81–1.11; $p = .52$). In a subgroup analysis, trebananib improved the median OS compared with placebo (14.5 vs. 12.3 months; HR 0.72; 95% CI: 0.55–0.93; $p = .011$) in patients with ascites at baseline ($n = 295$). In the intent-to-treat population, trebananib significantly improved median PFS-2 compared with placebo (12.5 vs. 10.9 months; HR 0.85; 95% CI: 0.74–0.98; $p = .024$). PFS-2 confirmed that the PFS benefit associated with trebananib was maintained through the second DP, independent of the choice of subsequent therapy.[185,186]

○ TRINOVA-2 AGO-OVAR 2.19/ENGOT-OV-6: This was a randomized phase III trial evaluating PLD plus trebananib or placebo in patients with recurrent partially platinum-sensitive or -resistant disease that enrolled 223 patients. No subgroup of patients showed a favorable PFS with experimental treatment but those with baseline ascites treated with trebananib showed a trend toward improved PFS (HR 0.6; 95% CI: 0.35–1.04). Trebananib use was associated with an improved RR but no improvement in OS.[187]

○ ICON6: This was a three-arm, double-blind, placebo-controlled randomized trial using the oral VEGFR-1,2,3 inhibitor, cediranib, in relapsed platinum-sensitive OC. The study enrolled 456 patients, with a median age of 62 Y. Previous treatment interval greater than 12 months (67%) was balanced between arms. The primary endpoint was PFS. Patients were randomized 2:3:3 for up to six cycles of platinum-based chemotherapy with either placebo, cediranib 20 mg/day during chemotherapy (paclitaxel/carboplatin, gemcitabine/carboplatin, or single-agent carboplatin) followed by placebo for up to 18 months (concurrent) or cediranib 20 mg/day followed by maintenance cediranib (concurrent +maintenance). Cediranib plus platinum-based chemotherapy followed by maintenance cediranib provided a benefit compared to chemotherapy alone, with an improved PFS from 9.4 to 12.5 months and an improved OS by 2.7 months (17.6–20.3 months HR 0.7; log-rank test p = .0419). PFS comparing reference and concurrent plus maintenance using a log-rank test gave a p-value of .00001 with an associated HR of 0.57 (95% CI: 0.45–0.74). However, because of nonproportional hazards (p = .0237 for PFS and p = .0042 for OS) the HR can be difficult to interpret, and instead survival time was estimated using restricted means (RM) and HRs were given for completeness. The RM estimates an increased time to progression of 3.2 months from 9.4 to 12.6, during 2 Y. Similarly using RM, OS increased by 2.7 months from 17.6 to 20.3 (HR 0.70; log-rank test p = .0419). PFS using RM for the reference versus concurrent arms saw an increase of 2.0 months from 9.4 to 11.4 months (HR 0.68; log-rank test p = .0022). AEs significantly more common in the cediranib-maintenance arm were HTN, diarrhea, hypothyroidism, hoarseness, hemorrhage, proteinuria, and fatigue.[188]

○ NOVA trial: Niraparib OVArian trial (MK-4827): This was a double-blind, placebo-controlled phase III trial of niraparib. In this study, 490 patients with high-grade serous, platinum-sensitive, relapsed OC were enrolled into one of two independent cohorts based on germline BRCA mutation status. Cohort 1 were germline BRCA mutation carriers (gBRCAmut), and cohort 2 comprised those who were not germline BRCA mutation carriers (non-gBRCAmut). The non-gBRCAmut cohort included patients with HRd-positive tumors, including those with somatic BRCA mutations and other HR defects, and patients with HRd-negative tumors. Within each cohort, patients were randomized 2:1 to receive niraparib or placebo and were treated continuously with placebo or 300 mg of niraparib until progression. Among BRCAm patients, the niraparib arm showed a HR of 0.27 for PFS compared to control. The median PFS for patients treated with niraparib was 21.0 months, vs. 5.5 months for control (p <.0001). For patients who were HRd positive the niraparib arm PFS, had an HR of 0.38. The median PFS for HRd-positive patients treated with niraparib was 12.9 months, compared to 3.8 months for control (p < .0001). A statistical significance in the overall nongermline BRCA mutant cohort was also seen for niraparib, which included patients with both HRd-positive and HRd-negative tumors. The niraparib arm had an HR of 0.45. The median PFS for patients treated with niraparib was 9.3 months, compared to 3.9 months for control (p <.0001). The most common G 3/4 AEs were thrombocytopenia (28.3%), anemia (24.8%), and neutropenia (11.2%). The discontinuation rate was 14.7% for niraparib-treated patients and 2.2% for control. The rates of AML in the niraparib (1.3%) and control (1.2%) arms were similar. There were no deaths among patients during study treatment.[189] Second line maintenance for patients with recurrent EOC was restricted to HRd+ and BRCAm patients due to final OS analysis that showed an HR of 1.06 seen in those who were HR proficient and BRCA Wt between treatment and control arms.

○ QUADRA: QUADRA was a phase II, open-label, single-arm, phase II study that assessed the safety and activity of niraparib in 464 women with relapsed HGSTOC.[190] This was a heavily pretreated cohort with a median number of four prior regimens (IQR 3-5). Niraparib was dosed PO at 300 mg once daily continuously, beginning on day 1 and every 28 days for a cycle, until DP. The primary objective was investigator-assessed confirmed OR in patients with HRd-positive tumors (including patients with BRCA and without BRCA mutations) sensitive to their last platinum-based therapy who had received three or four previous chemotherapy regimens. The median follow-up for OS was 12.2 months (IQR 3.7-22.1). Of participants, 151 (33%) were resistant and 161 (35%) were refractory to their last platinum therapy. Thirteen (28%) of 47 patients obtained OR according to RECIST (95% CI 15.6–42.6; one-sided p = .00053). The most common G 3> AEs were anemia in 113 (24%) and thrombocytopenia in 95 (21%). The most common AEs were SBO in 34 (7%), thrombocytopenia in 34 (7%), and vomiting in 27 (6%) of patients. One patient died due to treatment-related GI bleed. Patients with early dose reduction did not have efficacy compromised if their baseline body weight was <77 kg or platelets <150,000/uL.

○ Niraparib Maintenance Therapy in Platinum-Sensitive, Recurrent OC.[189] This randomized, double-blind phase III trial evaluated the efficacy of niraparib versus placebo as maintenance treatment for 553 patients with platinum-sensitive, recurrent OC. Patients were categorized by germline BRCA mutation (gBRCA cohort and non-gBRCA cohort) and the type of non-gBRCA mutation. Assignment was a 2:1 ratio for niraparib at 300 mg or placebo once daily. The primary endpoint was PFS. The 203 patients in the gBRCA cohort (138 assigned to niraparib and 65 to placebo), and 350 patients in the non-gBRCA cohort (234 assigned to niraparib and 116 to placebo) had a median duration of PFS of 21.0 versus 5.5 months in the gBRCA cohort (HR, 0.27; 95% CI, 0.17–0.41), compared with 12.9ths versus 3.8 months in the non-gBRCA cohort for patients who had tumors with HRd (HR, 0.38; 95% CI, 0.24–0.59) and 9.3 months versus 3.9 months in the overall non-gBRCA cohort (HR, 0.45; 95% CI, 0.34–0.61; p <.001 for all three comparisons). Common G 3/4 AEs reported in the niraparib group were thrombocytopenia (33.8%), anemia (25.3%), and neutropenia (19.6%); all managed dose reductions. The median PFS was significantly longer among those receiving niraparib than among those receiving placebo, regardless of the presence or absence of gBRCA mutations or HRd status.

- ○ NORA: This was a phase III, double-blind, placebo-controlled study in 265 women with platinum-sensitive recurrent OC with response to their penultimate platinum-containing regimen who were randomized in a 2:1 fashion to maintenance niraparib dosed at 300 mg/day PO or matched placebo until DP or toxicity.[191] Patients with a body weight <77 kg or a platelet count <150 × 103/μL received 200 mg/day PO as an individualized starting dose (ISD). BRCA status was documented. The primary endpoint was PFS and the study ran from 2017 to 2019. Of participants, 177 patients received niraparib and 88 placebo; 249 patients received an ISD (300 mg, n = 14; 200 mg, n = 235). The median PFS was longer for those randomized to niraparib vs. placebo: 18.3m (95% CI, 10.9—not evaluable) versus 5.4 (95% CI, 3.7–5.7) (HR = 0.32; 95% CI, 0.23–0.45; p <.0001). There was a similar benefit seen in PFS for patients dosed at ISD, regardless of BRCA mutation status. G ≥3AEs occurred in 50.8% and 19.3% of patients who received niraparib and placebo, respectively; the most common events were neutrophil count decreased (20.3% versus 8.0%) and anemia (14.7% versus 2.3%). Thus, niraparib maintenance therapy reduced the risk of DP or death by 68% and ISD is effective and safe.

- ○ Fuzuloparib maintenance therapy: This was a phase III, double-blind trial of fuzuloparib as maintenance therapy in patients with platinum-sensitive, recurrent HGSTOC or G2 endometrioid histology. Patients had to have at least two prior platinum-based chemotherapies and achieved CR or PR on their last regimen with ECOG 0-1. Patients were randomized 2:1 to fuzuloparib at 150mg (n = 167) or placebo (n = 85) in 4-week cycles. It demonstrated a 7.4-month improvement in median PFS at median follow-up of 8.5 months (12.9 vs 5.5m; p <.0001) at an interim assessment and a 75.5% reduced risk of DP or death versus placebo (HR = 0.25) regardless of BRCA mutation status, and had a manageable safety profile. The primary endpoint was PFS, secondary endpoints included chemotherapy-free interval, OS, ORR, and safety. BRCA mutations were confirmed in 40% of patients. About 25% of patients had received two or more prior platinum-based regimens, and greater than half achieved CR. Treatment discontinuation happened in 40.1% of patients on fuzuloparib versus 4.8% of patients on placebo, and 24.6% required dose reduction versus none on placebo. The most common AEs were nausea, anemia, and other hematologic toxicities. G 3 + AEs in the fuzuloparib group were hematologic, including anemia (25.1%), thrombocytopenia (16.8%), and neutropenia (12.6%).[192]

- ○ OVA-301: In a phase III, randomized trial, trabectedin plus PLD in recurrent OC resulted in a 35% risk reduction of DP or death (HR 0.65, 95% CI: 0.45–0.92; p = .0152). In the study, 337 patients were randomized to the combination trabectedin/PLD arm versus 335 patients randomized to the PLD arm. The median PFS was 7.4 versus 5.5 months. There was a 41% decrease in the risk of death (HR 0.59; 95% CI: 0.43–0.82; p = .0015). The median survival was 23.0 versus 17.1 months favoring the trabectedin arm. Similar proportions of patients received subsequent therapy in each arm (76% vs. 77%), although patients in the trabectedin/PLD arm had a slightly lower proportion of further platinum (49% vs. 55%). It is important to note that, patients in the trabectedin/PLD arm survived significantly longer after subsequent platinum (HR 0.63; p = .0357; median 13.3 vs. 9.8 months). This hypothesis-generating analysis demonstrates that superior benefits with trabectedin/ PLD in terms of PFS and survival in the overall population appear particularly enhanced in patients with partially sensitive disease (PFI 6–12 months).[193]

o MITO-11: This was an open-label, randomized, phase II trial addressing the effect of adding pazopanib to paclitaxel for patients with PI-R or platinum-refractory advanced OC. Patients previously treated with a maximum of two lines of chemotherapy, ECOG PS 0–1, who had no residual peripheral neurotoxicity were randomly assigned (1:1) to receive weekly paclitaxel 80 mg/m² with or without pazopanib 800 mg daily, and stratified by center, number of previous lines of chemotherapy, and platinum-free interval status. The primary endpoint was PFS, assessed in the modified intention-to-treat population. The study enrolled 74 patients: 37 were assigned to receive paclitaxel and pazopanib and 37 assigned to paclitaxel only. The median follow-up was 16.1 months (IQR 12.5–20.8). The PFS was significantly longer in the pazopanib plus paclitaxel group than in the paclitaxel-only group (median 6.35 months [95% CI: 5.36–11.02] vs. 3.49 months [2.01–5.66]; HR 0.42 [95% CI: 0.25–0.69]; p = .0002). No unexpected toxic effects or deaths were recorded. AEs were more common in the pazopanib and paclitaxel group to include neutropenia (30% vs. 3%], fatigue (11% vs. 6%), leucopenia (11% vs. 3%), and HTN (8% vs. 0%). One patient in the pazopanib group had a small bowel perforation. The PFS was 6.3 versus 3.5 months (HR 0.42, 95% CI: 0.25–0.69). The RR was 50% versus 21% (p = .03).[194]

o GOG 26FF: This phase II study evaluated single-agent paclitaxel at 170 mg/m² IV over 24 hours every 3 weeks in 43 refractory or PI-R OC patients. The ORR was 37%. The median PFI was 4.2 months, the median survival was 16 months. PFS was 4 months.[195]

o GOG-186F: This was a phase II study that estimated the activity of docetaxel 60 mg/m² IV over 1 hour followed by trabectedin 1.1 mg/ m² over 3 hours with filgrastim, pegfilgrastim, or sargramostim every 3 weeks. Seventy-one patients with recurrent and measurable disease, PS ≤2, and no more than three prior regimens were eligible. A historical GOG taxane control study was used for direct comparison. The goal of this study was to determine whether the trabectedin regimen had an RR of ≥36% with 90% power. The median number of cycles given was six (438 total cycles, range 1–22). The number of patients responding was 21 (30%; 90% CI: 21%–40%). The OR for responding was 2.2 (90% one-sided CI: 1.07–∞). The median PFS and OS were 4.5 months and 16.9 months, respectively. The median duration of response was 6.2 months.[196]

○ GOG 186i: In this study, 107 women with recurrent platinum-sensitive or resistant EOC treated with one to three prior chemotherapy lines were randomized to bevacizumab or bevacizumab with fosbretabulin (a vascular disrupting agent). PFS was improved to 7.3 versus 4.8 months (HR 0.69; 95% CI: 0.47–1 at 90%). RRs were 36% versus 28%. Although not a statistically significant result, patients receiving the combination had an ORR of 35.7% (n = 42) compared to 28.2% for patients on bevacizumab alone (n = 39). The study achieved its primary endpoint and demonstrated a statistically significant increase in PFS for the combination as compared to bevacizumab alone (p = .049; HR 0.685). In a posthoc subgroup analysis, data showed that in patients who were PI-R, the addition of fosbretabulin to bevacizumab increased the ORR to 40% (n = 10) compared to 12.5% (n = 8) for bevacizumab. Among those patients, the median PFS was 6.7 months for those on bevacizumab and fosbretabulin compared to 3.4 months for those receiving bevacizumab alone (p = .01; HR0.57). Patients in the combination arm experienced an increased incidence of G3 HTN compared to the control arm.[197]

○ GOG186j: This phase II trial evaluated weekly paclitaxel with or without pazopanib in women with recurrent EOC and one to three lines of prior chemotherapy. In the study 100 women were analyzed and PFS was the primary endpoint. Compared to weekly paclitaxel there was no significant difference in PFS: The median was 7.5 versus 6.2 months (HR 0.84; 90% CI: 0.57–1.22) in the combination versus single-agent group. The RR was 32% versus 23%, respectively. HTN was more common in the combination arm and led to treatment discontinuation in 37% versus 10% of the paclitaxel-only arm. More patients progressed on the control arm at 65% versus 32%.[198]

○ AGO-OVAR 2.20: PENELOPE trial: This was a two-part, randomized, phase III, double-blind trial evaluating pertuzumab in combination with standard chemotherapy in women with recurrent PI-R EOC and low HER3 mRNA expression. In this study, 156 patients were randomized to pertuzumab or placebo. Pertuzumab was administered at 840 mg IV loading dose followed by q21 day dosing at 420 mg IV in combination with either paclitaxel at 80 mg/m^2 on days 1, 8, 15 every 3 weeks or gemcitabine 1,000 mg/m^2 on days 1, 8 every 3 weeks, or topotecan 1.25 mg/m^2 on days 1 to 5 every 3 weeks. PFS was 4.3 months for pertuzumab plus chemotherapy versus 2.6 months for placebo for chemotherapy.

PFS was extended in the paclitaxel (most pronounced) and gemcitabine cohorts specifically and further exploration of this agent in combination regimens can be explored. A longer PFS was also seen in those with no prior antiangiogenic therapy.[199]

○ Combination cediranib and olaparib versus olaparib alone: This was a randomized, phase II study of women with recurrent platinum-sensitive OC. In the study, 46 women received olaparib at 400 mg PO BID and 44 received combination therapy with olaparib dosed at 200 mg PO BID with cediranib 30 mg PO daily. The median PFS was significantly longer with cediranib/olaparib compared with olaparib alone (17.7 vs. 9.2 months; HR 0.42; p = .005). In a subset analysis of gBRCA mutation status, a significant improvement in PFS in gBRCA WT or unknown patients receiving cediranib–olaparib compared with olaparib alone (16.5 vs. 5.7 months; p = .008) with no significant improvement in PFS observed in the gBRCAm patients (19.4 vs. 16.5 months; p = .16).[200,201]

○ Cediranib in recurrent or persistent ovarian, peritoneal, or fallopian tube cancer: This was a phase II trial of cediranib dosed at 30 mg daily. It evaluated 74 patients: 39 were platinum sensitive (Pl-S) and 35 were Pl-R. For those who were Pl-S, 26% had a PR and 51% had SD. In the Pl-R arm there were no PR, but 66% had SD. The median PFS for all patients, was 4.9 months, for the Pl-S patients the PFS was 7.2 months and for the platinum-resistant patients, the PFS was 3.7 months. The median OS was 18.9 months, 27.7 for the platinum-sensitive, and 11.9 for the Pl-R patients.[202]

○ Combination olaparib/cediranib: In this study, 90 patients were randomized 1:1 to cediranib with olaparib versus olaraib in platinum-sensitive recurrent EOC. The median PFS overall was 16.5 versus 8.2 months (HR 0.5, 95% CI: 0.3–0.83, p = .006); in the BRCA germline mutant group it was 16.4 versus 16.5 months (HR 0.76, 95% CI: 0.38–1.49, p = .42); and in the BRCAwt/unknown group it was 23.7 versus 5.7 months (HR 0.31, 95% CI: 0.15–0.66, p = .0013). The median overall OS was 44.2 versus 33.3 months (HR 0.64, 95% CI: 0.36–1.11, p = .11), for the BRCA germline mutant group it was 44.2 versus 40.1 (HR 0.86, 95% CI: 0.41–1.82; p = .7), and for the BRCAwt/unk group it was 37.8 versus 23 months (HR 0.44, 95% CI: 0.19–1.01; p = .047).[200]

○ SORAYA trial: This was a phase III trial of Mirvetuximab soravtansine-gynx (Elahere) was evaluated in 106 HGSTOC patients who were platinum resistant and folate receptor alpha 2+ positive and had 1-3 prior systemic treatment regimens including bevacizumab and 47% had received a PARP inhibitor. Dosing was 6 mg/kg every 3 weeks. The ORR was 32.4% with a CR of 4.8%, a PR of 26.9% and median duration of response of 6.9 months. A reduction in tumor size was seen at 71.4%. The antibody drug conjugate targets teh FR-alpha linked to DM4 which is an anti-tubulin drug.[470]

o ICON-9: Results pending: This is a randomized open-label trial in 618 patients with platinum-sensitive recurrent EOC evaluating maintenance olaparib and cediranib versus maintenance olaparib.

o SOLO-2: This study evaluated 295 germline BRCA 1/2 mutant patients with platinum-sensitive (two or more prior platinum therapies in PR or CR) relapsed EOC who were randomized 2:1 in a phase III trial to treatment with olaparib 300 mg BID compared to placebo maintenance therapy. The olaparib arm had a 19-month DFS compared to the placebo arm at 5.5 months (HR 0.3, 95% CI: 0.22–0.41, p <.0001). PFS in the olaparib arm was 30.2 months compared to 5.5 months in the placebo arm (HR 0.25, 95% CI: 0.18–0.35, p <.0001). A benefit in time to second progression or death was also seen (HR 0.50 95%, CI: 0.34–0.72, p = .0002) with the median not reached compared to 18.4 months. G 3 AEs were identified in 36.9% of patients on the olaparib arm compared to 18.2% in the placebo arm. Of participants, 75.6% had nausea compared to 2.6% in the placebo arm. There was no difference in QOL for patients on olaparib versus placebo. Other than for anemia, toxicities were low G and manageable.[203]

o SOLO-3: This was a randomized, open-label, phase III study of 266 germline BRCA-mutated platinum-sensitive relapsed OC who had seen at least two prior lines of platinum-based chemotherapy.[204] Patients were randomly assigned 2:1 to olaparib 300 mg BID or physician's choice single-agent nonplatinum chemotherapy (PLD, paclitaxel, gemcitabine, or topotecan). The primary endpoint was ORR with the secondary endpoint being PFS in the intent-to-treat population. In the study, 178 patients were assigned to olaparib and 88 to chemotherapy. In patients with measurable disease (olaparib, n = 151; chemotherapy, n = 72), the ORR was 72.2% with olaparib compared to 51.4% with chemotherapy (OR 2.53, 95% CI: 1.40–4.58; p = .002). In the subgroup that had received two prior lines of treatment, the ORR was 84.6% compared to 61.5%, respectively (OR 3.44, 95% CI: 1.42–8.54). PFS showed Olaparib patients had a median of 13.4 months versus placebo of 9.2 months (HR 0.62, 95% CI: 0.43–0.91; p = .013). PFS2 was 23.6 versus 19.6 months (HR 0.8, p = .229, CI: .56–1.15) and the OS was 34.9 versus 32.9 (HR 1.07, p = .714, CI: .76–1.49).

o ARIEL2 (Assessment of Rucaparib In OC Trial): This phase II study for patients with relapsed, high-grade, platinum-sensitive OC evaluated the clinical activity of rucaparib dosed at 600 mg BID in three predetermined HRd subgroups: BRCA mutated (germline or somatic), BRCA WT/LOH high, and BRCA WT/LOH low. The primary endpoint for the study was PFS. Median PFS was 12.8 months (95% CI: 9.0–14.7) in the BRCA mutated group, 5.7 months

(5.3–7.6) in the BRCA WT/LOH high group, and 5.2 months (3.6-5.5) in the BRCA WT/LOH low subgroup. BRCA mutated (HR 0.27, 95% CI: 0.16–0.44, p < .0001) and BRCA WT/LOH high (HR 0.62, 0.42–0.90, p = .011) groups had a significantly longer PFS than the BRCA WT/LOH low subgroup. Anemia (22% patients) and elevated liver enzymes (12%) were the two most common G 3 side effects. Interim results identified robust activity with a 65% ORR in patients with a germline BRCA mutation and improved RR of 36% in BRCA WT patients with HRd measured by high LOH in tumors.[205]

o ARIEL-3: This was a phase III, double-blind, placebo-controlled trial of rucaparib maintenance therapy in platinum-sensitive HGSTOC or endometrioid histology who had received at least two previous platinum-based chemotherapy regimens with response to the last platinum-based regimen.[206] In the study, 564 patients were assigned in a 2:1 fashion to rucaparib 600mg POD BID or placebo in 28-day cycles with stratification on HRd mutation status, PFI following the last platinum therapy, and CR versus PR. The primary endpoint was PFS. Three nested cohorts were evaluated: those with BRCA mutations, patients with HRd, and ITT. The study ran between 2014 and 2016 with 375 patients assigned to rucaparib and 189 to placebo. Median follow-up was 28.1 months (IQR 22.0-33.6). In the ITT population, the median chemotherapy-free interval (CFI) was 14.3 months (95% CI: 13.0–17.4) for the rucaparib group versus 8.8 months (8.0-10.3) for the placebo group (HR 0.43, 95% CI: 0.35–0.53]; p < .0001), median time to first subsequent therapy was 12.4 months (11.1-15.2) versus 7.2 months (6.4-8.6; HR 0.43 [0.35-0.52]; p < .0001), median PFS2 was 21.0 months (18.9-23.6) versus 16.5 months (15.2-18.4; HR 0.66 [0.53-0.82]; p = .0002), and median time to first subsequent therapy was 22.4 months (19.1-24.5) versus 17.3 months (14.9-19.4; HR 0.68 [0.54-0.85]; p = .0007). CFI, TFST, PFS2, and TSST were longer with rucaparib than placebo in the BRCA-mutant and HRd groups. The most frequent AE greater than G 3 was anemia (22% for the rucaparib group vs. 1% for the placebo group). Serious AEs were reported in 22% versus 11% of patients, respectively. Rates of dose modification were higher in patients older than 65 Y.

o ARIEL4 Trial: In this study, 349 HGSTOC patients with BRCA germline or somatic mutations and at least two prior chemotherapy regimens, including at least one platinum-based regimen, but no prior PARP inhibitor were enrolled to receive rucaparib (n = 233) or standard chemotherapy (n = 116).[207] For those randomized to chemotherapy, investigator's choice consisted of platinum monotherapy or carboplatin/paclitaxel, carboplatin/gemcitabine, or cisplatin/gemcitabine for patients who were platinum sensitive, and patients who were platinum resistant received paclitaxel monotherapy. Crossover was allowed for chemotherapy patients at DP. The median PFS for the rucaparib group was 7.4 months and 5.7 months with chemotherapy (HR, 0.64; 95% CI, 0.49–0.84; p = .001). Patients with a *BRCA* reversion mutation had a worse PFS if receiving rucaparib than with chemotherapy. The median PFS was 2.9 months and 5.5 months, respectively (HR, 2.77; 95% CI, 0.99–7.76). The ORR was 40.3% with rucaparib and 32.3% with chemotherapy (p = .13). The CR rate was 4.7% and 2.1%, respectively. The median DOR was 9.4 months and 7.2 months, respectively (HR, 0.59; 95% CI, 0.36–0.98). Third-line treatment was withdrawn after lower OS for rucaparib vs standard chemotherapy was observed of 19.4 months compared to 25.4 months with a HR of 1.31. The rucaparib arm had higher rates of treatment AEs, including anemia, nausea, asthenia/fatigue, elevated liver enzymes, vomiting, abdominal pain, and thrombocytopenia. Rates of neutropenia, diarrhea, and alopecia were higher in the chemotherapy arm. Treatment discontinuation due to AEs occurred in 8.2% of patients in the rucaparib arm and 12.4% of those in the chemotherapy arm. There were five cases of MDS/AML, all in the rucaparib arm.

○ DESKTOP I: In this study, 267 platinum-sensitive recurrent OC patients were retrospectively reviewed for predictability of secondary cytoreduction. Complete secondary resection was associated with longer survival compared to any residual postoperative disease (45.2 vs. 19.7 months). Variables associated with complete resection were performance status, early-stage FIGO disease (I/II), residual disease after primary surgery (none vs. any), absence of ascites, and less than 500 mL of ascites. A combination of good PS, early FIGO stage, no residual disease, and absent ascites predicted complete resection in 79% of patients.[208]

○ DESKTOP II AGO-OVAR OP.2: This trial evaluated 516 recurrent platinum-sensitive OC patients. Patients were screened with the DESKTOP I prediction factors for operability for recurrent disease: (a) complete resection at first surgery, (b) ECOG performance status 0/1, and (c) absence of ascites. The DESKTOP II trial was intended to verify the DESKTOP I trial. In the study, 51% were classified as score positive; of these 261 patients, 129 were operated on. The rate of complete resection was 76%, confirming score validity and; 11% had second operations for complications.[209]

○ GOG 254: Sunitinib evaluation in the treatment of persistent or recurrent CC OC: In this study, 30 patients were treated in this phase II trial of sunitinib 50 mg per day for 4 weeks administered in repeated 6-week cycles until DP or toxicity. Of these, 6.7% had a PR or CR. The median PFS was 2.7 months. The median OS was 12.8 months. There was minimal activity in second- and third-line treatment in recurrent CC OC.[210]

○ KEYNOTE-100: This was a phase II trial of 376 patients with recurrent OC divided into two groups evaluating monotherapy with pembrolizumab.[211] Cohort A had received one to three prior regimens of chemotherapy with a PFI or TFI between 3 to 12 months, whereas cohort B had received four to six prior treatments with a PFI/TFI of ≥3 months. A dose of 200 mg IV q3 weeks of pembrolizumab was given until progression, toxicity, or 2 Y on study treatment. Primary endpoints were ORR and PD-L1 expression whereas secondary endpoints were DOR, disease control rate, PFS, OS, and safety. There were 285 patients were in cohort A and 91 in cohort B. The ORR was 7.4% for cohort A and 9.9% for cohort B, the median DOR was 8.2 months and not reached, and the DCR was 37.2% and 37.4%, respectively. The ORR was 4.1% for CPS <1, 5.7% CPS ≥1, and 10.0% for CPS ≥10. PFS was 2.1 months for both cohorts. Median OS was not reached for cohort A and was 17.6 months for cohort B. Thus, there was an ORR of 8% and a PD-L1 CPS was predictive of response and all patients who had a CR had CPS of >10.

○ Paragon trial: This trial was a prospective basket protocol examining the activity of anastrozole in 49 patients with hormone receptor (ER and/or PR) positive recurrent gynecological cancers.[212] Those patients with PI-R or refractory recurrent EOC evaluated by RECIST or GCIG CA-125 criteria were reviewed. Anastrozole was dosed at 1 mg daily until progression or toxicity. Clinical benefit was observed in 13 (27%; 95% CI: 16%–40%). No CR or PR responses were observed. Median PFS was 2.7 months (95% CI, 2.0–2.8 months), median time of benefit was 2.8 months (95% CI, 2.6–5.7 months), and most patients (83%) progressed in 6 months. Seven patients continued treatment for more than 6 months.

○ Volasertib in platinum resistant or refractory OC: In this study, 109 patients were randomized to single-agent, investigator-chosen nonplatinum chemotherapy (PLD, topotecan, paclitaxel, or gemcitabine) or volasertib (an inhibitor of Polo-like kinases) at 300 mg IV q21 days until DP or toxicity. The primary endpoint was 24-week disease control rates. The disease control rate for volasertib was 30.6% versus 43.1% for chemotherapy. Median PFS was 13.1 versus 20.6 weeks favoring chemotherapy. Eleven percent of patients receiving volasertib had a durable RR with PFS of more than 1 Y, and none had that RR with chemotherapy. Thus, single-agent volasertib has shown antitumor activity in this OC patient population.[213]

○ FANG vaccine: This was a phase II trial consisting of 331 women who achieved a CCR with standard adjuvant chemotherapy. Patients were randomized 2:1 to receive an autologous tumor-based vaccine product incorporating a plasmid encoding GMCSF and a novel bi-shRNAi targeting furin convertase, thereby down-regulating endogenous immunosuppressive TGF β1 and β2. Patients with advanced cancer received up to 12 monthly intra-dermal injections of FANG vaccine (1 × 107 or 2.5 × 107 cells/mL injection). GMCSF, TGFβ1, TGFβ2, and furin proteins were quantified by ELISA. PFS was 19.3 in the vaccine group versus 12.4 months in the observation group and saw an improved 3Y recurrence rate of 90% versus 60%. The researchers harvested cells from the tumor removed during the initial surgery to develop the personalized immunotherapy. Patients assigned the vaccine then received 1 × 107 cells/intradermal injection monthly for up to 12 doses. Researchers evaluated T-cell activation per interferon-gamma ELISPOT. A greater proportion of patients who were chemotherapynaive achieved interferon-gamma ELISPOT response in the current analysis compared with the previous phase I trial (92% vs. 50%).[214]

- **Interval Debulking Trials**
  - EORTC 44865: This trial randomized 319 patients with stage III and IV after suboptimal surgery to chemotherapy with cyclo-phosphamide and cisplatin for six cycles or to chemotherapy with cyclophosphamide and cisplatin for three cycles with inter-val debulking followed by three more cycles. The interval debulk-ing group had a significantly better median PFS of 18 months versus 13 months. The median OS was 26 months versus 20 months, favoring the interval debulking group. The risk of death decreased by 33%, $p = .008$.[215]
  - GOG 152: This trial randomized 424 eligible patients stage III and IV after suboptimal surgery to chemotherapy with cisplatin and paclitaxel for six cycles or to chemotherapy for three cycles with interval debulking, followed by three more cycles of chemo-therapy. The median PFS was 10.5 months versus 10.7 months (HR 1.07; 95% CI: 0.869 to 1.31; $p = .54$). The OS was 33.7 in the chemotherapy alone group compared to 33.9 months in the IDS group. The relative risk for death was 0.99 (95% CI: 0.786–1.24; $p = .92$).[216]

There were differences between the two preceding interval debulking studies. Namely, there was a more effective second-line therapy (pacl-itaxel) in the GOG study, the chemotherapy regimens were different, residual disease was 5 cm or less for fewer than two thirds of patients in GOG 152 versus one third of patients in the EORTC study, and gen-eralists did a majority of the primary surgery in the EORTC study. Furthermore, residual disease after three cycles of chemotherapy was greater than 1 cm in 65% of patients in the EORTC study, thus there was an increased chance of optimal cytoreduction in the EORTC study, compared to only 45% who were converted to optimal debulking in the GOG study.

- SOCQER 1: SOCQER 1 was a single institution prospective evaluation of QOL following primary PDS or IDS in 93 women, 24 of whom had extensive OC surgery, 32 who had standard OC surgery (based on Aletti Surgical Complexity Score of 3 or lower) compared to 32 patients who had surgery for benign indications. These were reviewed at sequential time points. The cohort undergoing extensive surgery had deterioration in the immediate and short term QOL measures. But by 9 months scores in all three cohorts were equal.[217]
- Timing of surgery in patients with a PR or SD after NACT in advanced OC.[218] 265 patients were reviewed with 57% having stage IV disease, of whom 87% were HGSTOC. There was an overall R0 rate of 81% at surgical completion. Analysis showed that more than 4 cycles of NACT was not associated with a worse PFS or OS than 3-4 cycles (HR 1.02, 95% CI: 0.74–1.42 and HR 1.12, 95% CI, 0.73–1.72). Any amount of RD had worse PFS and OS irrespective of the number of NACT cycles. Thus, the ability to obtain R0 should guide decision making for timing of surgery.

HIPEC/IDS Studies

- Vergote commented in a review of HIPEC at IDS that the standard of care continues to be surgery and IV chemotherapy as HIPEC does not improve survival in advanced OC.[219]
- OVHIPEC: This trial showed an improvement in RFS and OS compared to surgery alone in a phase III randomized trial of 245 patients. Patients who had at least SD after three cycles of carboplatin AUC 5/6 with paclitaxel 175 mg/m^2 to IDS with or without HIPEC with cisplatin at 100mg/m^2. Randomization occurred at the time of surgery and was stratified by feasibility of R0 versus R1 debulking. Three adjuvant cycles of carboplatin/paclitaxel were then given. The HR for disease recurrence or death was 0.66; 95% CI: 0.50–0.87; p = .003). The median FRS was 10.7 months for the surgery-alone cohort and 14.2 months for the surgery-HIPEC group. At 4.7 Y for median follow-up, 76 patients (62%) in the surgery group and 61 patients (50%) in the surgery-HIPEC group died (HR, 0.67; 95% CI, 0.48–0.94; p = .02). The median OS was 33.9 months for the surgery group and 45.7 months for the surgery-HIPEC group. The percentage of patients who had AEs of G 3 or 4 was similar in the two groups at 25% in the surgery versus 27% surgery-HIPEC. Criticisms of this trial include a lower number of patients randomized because of slow accrual; a lower than anticipated PFS and OS in both arms compared to the original power and an amended statistical plan; the study was of small size, there were imbalances between the two arms with more low-grade tumors in the HIPEC arm; the timing of randomization before the start of IDS; the lack of clear inclusion criteria for NACT; and heterogeneous results, with largest effects seen at the smaller centers, and there was concern that AEs were incompletely reported.[103]

- Lim et al. randomized 184 patients stage III/IV patients after PDS or IDS with R1/R0 disease to IV paclitaxel and carboplatin as a control vs HIPEC at IDS. The HIPEC consisted of cisplatin at 75 mg/m^2 over 90 minutes. The cohorts were well balanced for demographics and tumor characteristics. The 5Y PFS was similar at 20.9% in the HIPEC group versus 16.0% for those in the control arm; NS. The 5Y OS was similar with 51.0% in the HIPEC group versus 49.4% in the control. In the NAC group (similar to the OVHIPEC trial), PFS and OS were similar (PFS, 20 months in the HIPEC arm vs. 19 months in the control arm; OS, 54 months in the HIPEC arm vs. 51 months in the control arm).[220,221]

- Jou et al. showed that HIPEC after neoadjuvant chemotherapy and interval debulking is associated with development of platinum-refractory or -resistant disease. This was a prospective study of patients who received NACT and IDS with or without HIPEC as part of frontline therapy in 68 HGSTOC patients. The study ran from 2010-19 and included 20 patients who had HIPEC compared to 48 who did not. Results showed that HIPEC patients had higher rates of R0 disease (95% vs 50%), longer mean length of surgery (530 vs. 216 min), more G 3/4 postoperative morbidity (65% vs. 4%), and longer LOS (8 vs. 5 days). HIPEC patients were found to be at higher risk for platinum-refractory progression or platinum-resistance recurrence (50% vs. 23%; RR = 2.18; 95% CI: 1.11, 4.30, p = .024). The median PFS was 11.5 versus 12 months and all-cause mortality was 19.1 versus 30.5 months, respectively.

- Zivanovic et al. showed in an open-label phase II trial of 98 recurrent platinum-sensitive EOC patients enrolled between 2014 to 2019 who were intraoperatively randomized to HIPEC with carboplatin at 800 mg/m^2 (n = 49) or no HIPEC (n = 49), followed by five (HIPEC group) or six cycles (no HIPEC group) of carboplatin-based doublet chemotherapy (+paclitaxel, or +gemcitabine, or +liposomal doxorubicin). PFS was the primary endpoint. R0 status was obtained 82% of patients in the HIPEC group and 94% of the non-HIPEC group (p = .12). Bowel resection was performed in 37% versus 65% of patients (p = .008). No perioperative deaths occurred. There were no intergroup differences for ostomies, LOS (6 vs. 5 days, p = .05). The 2Y PFS or death showed no statistical difference in the eight patients (16.3%, 1-sided 90% CI = 0.099–1.0) who were without DP or death in the HIPEC group versus 12 (24.5%, 1-sided 90% CI = 16.5%–100%) in the non-HIPEC group. The median PFS was 12.3 months versus 15.7 months, respectively (HR = 1.54, 95% CI = 1.00–2.37, p = .05). The median OS was 52.5 versus 59.7 months (HR = 1.39, 95% CI = 0.73–2.67, p = .31).[222]

Secondary Cytoreduction Studies

- GOG 213 (bevacizumab): This was a phase III randomized study with two primary objectives: (a) to examine the role of bevacizumab at 15 mg/kg in combination with paclitaxel at 175 mg/m^2 and carboplatin

AUC 5 followed by bevacizumab maintenance, and (b) to examine the role of secondary cytoreduction before initiation of chemotherapy in recurrent patients. The primary endpoint was OS. Secondary endpoints were safety toxicity, allergy, PFS, and QOL. In the study, 674 patients were randomized. Prior bevacizumab was received in 67/606 patients. The median age was 60. For the chemotherapy arm: CTB combination chemotherapy improved the HR of death by 18.6% (HR 0.827; 95% CI: 0.683–1.005; $p = .056$) with a median OS of 42.2 versus 37.3 months. The PFS was improved with CTB with an HR 0.614 (95% CI: 0.522–0.722; $p < .0001$) with median PFS 13.8 versus 10.4 months. It extended the OS to 42.2 months versus 37.3 months but the p-value was NS at 0.056. Estimated completion for the surgical debulking arm is March 2019.[223]

- GOG 213 (secondary cytoreduction): This study examined 485 patients with platinum-sensitive recurrent OC and deemed surgically resectable to R0 were randomly assigned to secondary cytoreduction followed by platinum based chemotherapy (PBC), or PBC without surgery in this superiority trial.[224] Patients had to have received one previous therapy, and have a PFI of 6 months or more. Second-line chemotherapy included paclitaxel–carboplatin or GC; +the use of bevacizumab was at the investigator's discretion. The primary endpoint was OS. In the study, 240 patients underwent secondary cytoreduction and 245 proceeded to chemotherapy alone. The median follow-up was 48.1 months. R0 was achieved in 67% of patients who received surgery in the cytoreduction group. PBC with bevacizumab followed by bevacizumab maintenance was given to 84% of patients overall, and not different between groups. The HR for death (surgery vs. no surgery) was 1.29 (95% CI [CI], 0.97–1.72; $p = .08$), corresponding to a median OS of 50.6 months and 64.7 months, respectively. Adjustment for PFI and choice of chemotherapy did not change the results. The HR was 0.82 for DP or death (surgery vs. no surgery) 82 (95% CI, 0.66–1.01; median PFS, 18.9 months [21.4 months confirmed] and 16.2 months). Thirty-day surgical morbidity was 9%; and one patient died in the surgery group. Patient-reported QOL was lower for the immediate 6 weeks after surgery, but was not different between groups after recovery.

- DESKTOP III AGO-OVAR OP.4: This was a randomized superiority trial in 407 patients comparing secondary cytoreduction followed by chemotherapy to chemotherapy alone in recurrent platinum-sensitive OC. The AGO score was used to select patients with a less than 30% risk of R1 disease. The primary endpoint was the difference in OS between groups. AGO score + was ECOG PS 0, ascites ≤500 mL, and R0 at initial surgery). Patients were prospectively randomized between 2010 to 2014. The TFIp (pathologic) exceeded 12 months in 75% of patients. In the study, 206 patients were allocated to the surgery arm of whom 187 (91%) ultimately had surgery. R0 was obtained in 75.5%; 90% of patients in both arms received platinum-containing second-line chemotherapy. Results showed a median OS of 53.7 months with SCS and 46.2 months with chemotherapy alone (HR 0.76, 95% CI: 0.59–0.97, p = .03); the median PFS was 18.4 and 14 months (HR: 0.66, 95% CI: 0.54–0.82, p < .001), the median time to start next chemotherapy was 17.9 versus 13.7 months, favoring the SCS arm (HR 0.65, 95% CI: 0.52–0.81, p < .001). An OS benefit >12 months was seen for patients with R0 surgery compared to patients without surgery (median 61.9 months vs. 46.2 months); patients with surgery and incomplete resection had a median of 28.8 months OS. The 2-month mortality rate was 0 and 0.5% in the SCS versus chemotherapy-only arms. Repeat surgery for complications was performed in 3.7% of SCS patients. Other G 3/4 AEs did not differ significantly between arms. The benefit of SCS was exclusively seen in patients with R0 status indicating the importance of both the optimal selection of patients by AGO score and for expert surgeons.[225,226]

- SOC-1 trial: This multicenter randomized trial for women with first recurrence of FIGO stage IC to IV platinum-sensitive EOCran between 2012 to 2019. First-line treatment must have consisted of optimal (≤1 cm) cytoreductive surgery and (neoadjuvant) platinum/taxol-based chemotherapy. Inclusion criteria were ascites < 500 mL (pocket < 8 cm), potential for R0 resection status, and a ECOG PS 0–1 based on the iMODEL score (compilation of FIGO stage, residual disease at primary debulking, length of platinum-free interval, ECOG performance status, CA-125 level at recurrence, presence of ascites, and a PET-CT). In the study, 357 women were randomized between the standard of at least six cycles of IV platinum-based chemotherapy only (175 patients) or secondary cytoreductive surgery followed by at least six cycles of IV platinum-based chemotherapy (182 patients). The median PFS was 11.9 months versus 17.4 months for no-surgery versus secondary surgery groups (HR 0.58, 95% CI 0.45–0.74; p < .0001). The median OS was 53.9 months versus 58.1 months for the no-surgery versus surgery groups (HR 0.82, 95%CI: 0.57–1.19). Crossover occurred in 11 patients for the no-surgery group.[227]

- **Neoadjuvant Therapy Trials**
  - EORTC 55971: This trial evaluated 632 eligible patients who were staged IIIC or IV. They were randomized to upfront debulking surgery versus three cycles of neoadjuvant platinum-based chemotherapy followed by interval surgery and subsequent chemotherapy. Inclusion criteria were biopsy-proven EOC, in combination with a pelvic mass, the presence of metastases of ≥2 cm outside the pelvis, and a CA-125:CEA ratio ≥25. The median follow-up was 4.8 Y. Baseline characteristics for arms A and B were, respectively: median largest metastasis, 80/80 mm; FIGO stage IIIC, 76%/76%. The largest residual tumor was ≤1 cm in 48% after PDS (arm A) and 83% after IDS (arm B). Complications of

PDS and IDS were postoperative mortality 2.7%/0.6%; sepsis 8%/2%; G 3/4 and hemorrhage 7%/4%. The PFS was 11 months in both arms (HR 0.99; 95% CI: 0.87–1.13). An OS of 29 and 30 months was seen for arms A and B (HR 0.98; 95% CI: 0.85–1.14).[201]

- Some critics suggest that this OS is still less than the 36 months seen in the carboplatin/paclitaxel arm of GOG 111 evaluating sub-optimally debulked OC. Regarding neoadjuvant therapy versus PDS, the overall PFS was similar for both arms, approximately 12 months. OS was 30 versus 29 months overall. For those with R0 disease, OS was 38 versus 45 months, R1 disease 27 versus 32 months, R2 disease 25 versus 26 months.

- MRC CHORUS trial: This study attempted to confirm the results of EORTC 55971. In this study, 550 patients with clinical FIGO stages III to IV OC were randomized to surgery followed by six cycles of chemotherapy or NACT. The median age was 65, the median tumor size was 8 cm, 25% were stage IV, and 19% had a WHO PS of 2. There was a well-balanced randomization. In the ITT analysis, a median OS of 22.8 months for PDS was observed versus 24.5 months for NACT (HR 0.87; 95% CI: 0.76–0.98) favoring NACT. The median PFS was 10.2 versus 11.7 months (HR 0.91; 95% CI: 0.81–1.02).[228]

- Exploratory analysis of EORTC 55971: Which patients benefit most from primary surgery or NACT in stage IIIC or IV EOC? In this study, 670 patients from EROTC 55971 were reviewed. These patients had been randomly assigned to PDS or NACT. Clinical factors were reviewed for those who could benefit more from the differing primary approaches. The size of the largest metastatic tumor and clinical stage were significantly associated with the magnitude of the benefit from treatment in terms of 5 YS. Stage IIIC patients with tumors less than 4.5 cm benefited more from PDS whereas stage IV patients with metastatic tumors greater than 4.5 cm benefited more from NACT. Primary outcome was OS. The potential 5YS in the population of treated patients would be 27.3%, 7.8% higher than if all were treated with primary surgery, and 5.6% higher than if all were treated with NACT.[229]

- A meta-analysis suggests that for each extra cycle of NACT, there is a 4.1-month decrease in survival. Within this meta-analysis, each 10% increase in cytoreduction yielded a 5.5% median increase in survival time, which equates to 3 months.[89]

- SCORPION trial: This was a phase III trial evaluating 110 patients randomized to either PDS followed by adjuvant chemotherapy or NACT followed by IDS. Patients were triaged preoperatively to laparoscopic staging to assess tumor load. Tumor load was documented as a Fagotti score. 45.5% of the PDS patients had R0 status postoperatively compared to 57.7% of those who received NACT; p = .206. Of the patients in the PDS arm , 52.7% had G 3–4 complications compared to 5.7% in the IDS arm, p = .0001.[230–232]

○ NACT has also been found not to improve the rate of complete resection or affect the morbidity of IDS in another study. This retrospective study reviewed 200 patients in separate cohorts based on Y of diagnosis. Cohort 1 was those diagnosed from 2009 to 2011 with PDS; cohort 2 was those diagnosed after 2011 to 2013 (at publication of EORTC Vergote) and they underwent visceral-peritoneal debulking after three cycles of NACT. Patients with CR or PD never underwent surgical resection. Patients had diagnostic laparoscopy before debulking to evaluate for small bowel serosal disease or porta hepatic encasement. If no small bowel or porta hepatic involvement, conversion to laparotomy and debulking was attempted. Debulking was completed in 90% of patients in both groups. There was no difference in operating room times, EBL, hospital stay, or postoperative complications between cohorts.[233]

○ Yet another study shows that PDS should be the primary management approach for advanced EOC. Those who had NACT were more likely to have no residual disease (50.1% vs. 41.5%). The 7 YS for PDS was found to be 41% versus 8.6% if NACT was used. For those who obtained R0 at PDS, the 7YS was 73.6% versus 21%. Those who had PDS with R0 status and had IP chemotherapy had a 7YS of 90%.[234]

○ TRUST Study (Trial of Radical Upfront Surgical Therapy in advanced ovarian cancer) (ENGOT ov33/AGO-OVAR OP7): Pending 2024.

○ SUNNY Trial (Study of upfront surgery vs NACT followed by IDS for patients with stage IIIC and IV OC, SGOG SUNNY [SOC-2] trial): Pending 2023.

○ Summation of OS and PFS in seminal NACT, IP, and PDS trials.
  ▪ JGOG Dose-dense* paclitaxel vs conventional q21 days dosing:
    □ OS 100.5 vs 62.2 months
    □ PFS 28.2 months vs 17.5 months
  ▪ GOG 172 IP* vs IV dosing
    □ OS 65.5 vs 49.7 months
    □ PFS 23.8 months versus 18.3 months
  ▪ Landrum's review on GOG 114/172 data on R1/R0 patients IP* versus IV
    □ OS 43.2 months versus 20.1 months
    □ PFS 100 months versus 50.9 months
  ▪ Chan's GOG 262 dose-dense paclitaxel versus q21 day with bevacizumab

- □ PFS 14.7 months vs 14 months overall. But subgroup analysis:
  - − 14.2 months vs 10.3 months dose-dense* no bevacizumab
  - − 14.9 months vs 14.7 months dose-dense plus bevacizumab
- Vergote's EORTC neoadjuvant vs PDS* both using q21 day dosing
  - □ PFS similar: both around 12 months
  - □ OS is similar at 30 months neoadjuvant vs 29 months PDS, but see the following for subgroup analysis by R status
  - □ R0: 38 months vs 45 months favoring PDS
  - □ R1: 27 months vs 32 months favoring PDS
  - □ R2: 25 months vs 26 months
- EORTC 55971 (Vergote) stages 3c-IV 670 patients median OR time 180 versus 165 minutes, noninferior
  - □ R1 80.6 versus 41.6 NACT versus PDS
  - □ CGR 51.2 versus 19.4
  - □ PFS 12, 12
  - □ OS 30 versus 29m
- CHORUS (Kehoe) stages II to IV 550 patients, OR time 180 versus 165 minutes
  - □ R1 73% versus 41%
  - □ R0 39% versus 17%
  - □ PFS 12 versus 10.7 months
  - □ OS 24.1 versus 22.6 months
- JCOG 0602 (Onda) stages III to IV, 301 patients, OR time 273 versus 341 minutes
  - □ R1 82% versus 37%
  - □ R0 64% versus 12%
  - □ PFS 16.4 versus 15.1 months
  - □ OS 44.3 versus 49 months
- SCORPION (Fagotti) stages IIIC to IV, 171 patients surgical quality controlled, OR time 275 vs 451 minutes
  - □ R1 100% versus 92.8%
  - □ R0 57.7 versus 45.5
  - □ PFS 14 versus 15 months
  - □ OS NR versus 41 months

Low-Grade Serous Studies
- FRAME trial. This is a phase I/II trial of 24 patients with recurrent LGSTOC.[235] This trial administered VS-6766 (dual RAF/MEK inhibitor) and defactinib (a FAK inhibitor) regardless of KRAS mutation status. At least one prior line of platinum-based chemotherapy was

necessary for inclusion. Of 24 patients, a 52% ORR was seen (11 of 21 response evaluable patients), with KRAS mutant ORR at 70% (seven of 10 response-evaluable patients), KRAS wt ORR at 44% (four of nine response-evaluable patients) and KRAS status undetermined ORR at 0% (0 of 2 response evaluable patients). Side effects were G 1/2 rash, creatine kinase elevation, nausea, hyperbilirubinemia, and diarrhea, and all were reversible.[236]

- RAMP 201 Trial (Raf And Mek Program) ENGOTov60/GOG3052: This is a phase II study of VS-6766 alone and in combination with defactinib in recurrent LGSOC.[237] Part A will determine the optimal regimen based on confirmed ORR (independent radiology review) in KRAS-mutated LGSOC. Part B will determine the efficacy of the optimal regimen identified in part A in KRAS-mutated and KRAS wild-type LGSOC. The minimum expected enrollment is 52 subjects with KRAS-mutated tumors (32 subjects in part A and 20 in part B) and 36 with KRAS wt tumors in part B. Patients will be randomized to receive VS-6766 (4.0 mg PO, twice weekly 3 weeks on, 1 week off) or VS6766 with defactinib (VS-6766 3.2 mg PO, twice weekly +defactinib 200 mg PO BID 3 weeks on, 1 week off) until progression. Results pending.

- MILO/ENGOT-ov11 (Biminetinib): 303 patients with recurrent LGSTOC were randomized to binimetinib at 45 mg PO BID versus physician choice of cytotoxic chemotherapy after at least one prior platinum-based regimen. Median PFS in the study group was 9.1 months versus 10.6 months with a median DOR of 8.1 months versus 6.7 months and median OS of 25.3 versus 20.8 months. This MEK inhibitor did not meet its primary end point but it did show activity across other efficacy evaluation points.[238]

- GOG 281/LOGS: This was a phase II/III study of 260 patients assigned either to trametinib (n = 130) or standard-of-care group (SOC) (n = 130). Trametinib was dosed 2 mg PO QD. SOC chemotherapy options included IV paclitaxel 80 mg/m^2 weekly x 3 weeks of a 4-week cycle, IV liposomal doxorubicin 40–50 mg/m^2 once every 4 weeks, IV topotecan 4 mg/m^2 weekly x 3 weeks of a 4-week cycle; PO letrozole 2.5 mg qd; or PO tamoxifen 20 mg BID. The primary endpoint was PFS: Median PFS for the trametinib group was 13 months (95% CI: 9.9–15.0) versus 7.2 months (5.6–9.9) for the SOC (HR 0.48 [95% CI: 0.36–0.64]; p <.0001). G 3/4 AEs were skin rash (13%), anemia (13%), HTN (12%), diarrhea (10%), nausea (9%), and fatigue (8%) in the study arm.[239]

- **Translational Studies**
  - OVCAD study: "Ovarian Cancer—Diagnosis of a Silent Killer" is a study aimed to investigate new predictors for early detection of minimal residual disease in EOC. In this study, 275 consecutive patients with EOC were included and their clinical outcomes with regard to pathology, surgery, and chemotherapy

were reviewed. Evaluable patients had stage II to IV cancer who underwent cytoreductive surgery, adjuvant platinum-based chemotherapy, and had tissue specimens collected. Characteristics of the patients included the following: Median age of diagnosis was 58 Y, 94.5% stage III/IV, 96% G 2/3, 86% with serous histology, 67.6% with peritoneal implants, 76% with ascites, and 52% with positive lymph nodes. The majority of patients underwent a BSO (90.9%) and omentectomy (92.4%); 77.3% underwent hysterectomy. Of patients, 37.7% had a resection of the large bowel, whereas 13.4% of patients had a small bowel resection. Of patients, 69.5% had a P-LND and 66.9% underwent PA-LND. "Macroscopic" cytoreduction was achieved in 68.4%. Platinum-based chemotherapy was used in 98.2% of the patients. At the time of median follow-up (37 months), 70 patients (25.5%) had PI-R recurrent disease. Results from this trial are being used in a myriad of other reviews.[240]

○ VITAL study: Gemogenovatucel-T (Vigil) immunotherapy demonstrates clinical benefit in HRp OC.[241,242] Vigil (gemogenovatucel-T) is an autologous tumor cell vaccine developed for OC maintenance therapy. It is constructed from individual patient-harvested malignant tissue during PDS. The vaccine incorporates a multigenic plasmid encoding the GMCSF gene and a bi-short-hairpin RNA construct, which is a furin inhibitor, the proprotein convertase that targets downstream TGF-beta1/2. The plasmid is transfected into the host T cells and introduces the individual tumor-specific neoantigen repertoire to dendritic and CD8 cells, enhancing major histocompatibility complex presentation via colony-stimulating factors, and inhibiting immunosuppressive cytokines. In a 1:1 randomized, double-blind, placebo-controlled phase II study, 91 patients with stage IIIb/IV HRp (BRCA/WT) molecular profile OC were given four to 12 doses after frontline surgery followed by platinum/taxane chemotherapy in CCR. Dosing was 1 × 107 cell/mL intradermally (n = 47 median age 63 Y, 81% stage III) or placebo (n = 44, median age 62.5, 88.6% stage III) given once monthly x 12 or until progression. Myriad myChoice CDx assay with scores of less than 42 were deemed proficient. RFS was the primary endpoint. Of the 62 women with BRCA/WT disease who underwent HRd testing, 45 were HRp. The overall RFS was better with HR 0.386; 90% CI 0.199–0.750, p = .007 and OS HR 0.342; 90% CI 0.141–0.832; p = .019 There was a longer median RFS among women with HRp tumors who were assigned to the vaccine group (n = 25) compared with those assigned placebo (n = 20; 10.6m vs. 5.7m; HR = 0.386; 90% CI, 0.199–0.75). There was improved OS among women with HRp tumors in the vaccine group versus the placebo group (median, not reached vs.

26.9 months; HR = 0.342; 90% CI, 0.14–0.83). There was a statistically significant benefit in both RFS with a doubling from 10 months to 20 months, with an OS benefit from 28 months to 38 months. At median follow-up of 58 months, the OS benefit was maintained in the Vigil group, with an HR of 0.417 (p = .02) and a 2YOS (92% vs. 55%), and 3YOS (70% vs. 40%) for those who received the vaccine.

Low Malignant Potential Ovarian Tumors: Borderline Tumors

Characteristics

- Low malignant potential (LMP) tumors represent 5% to 15% of ovarian malignancies. The median age at diagnosis ranges from 39 to 45 Y old. Twenty percent of these tumors are diagnosed at stage III or IV. There are no known risk factors.
- Clinical features include a mass, abdominal pain, bloating, abdominal distension, early satiety, dyspepsia, and an elevated CA-125.
- The route of spread is often transcoelomic, and can be lymphatic.
- Prognostic factors are stage, residual tumor, the presence of invasive implants, and micropapillary histology.

Histology

- Pathologically, there is the absence of stromal invasion and the tumors have at least two of the following: nuclear atypia, mitotic activity, pseudostratification, and epithelial budding. There are two main histologic types: serous and mucinous. If foci are found of stromal invasion measuring 3 to 5 mm or 10 mm^2, the tumor is considered microinvasive. Outcomes for microinvasive tumors are usually favorable and parallel LMP tumors. If a mucinous borderline tumor is found to have three or more layers of epithelial cell stratification, it is considered a carcinoma. There is guidance from WHO that LMP tumors may represent the early part of the disease spectrum for invasive TOCs.
- Frozen-section diagnosis of borderline tumors can be difficult. In one study of patients with a final diagnosis of LMP tumor, 10% were diagnosed as having invasive cancer and 25% were reported to have benign cystadenomas on intraoperative frozen section. Therefore, the sensitivity of the frozen section analysis for LMP's was 65% (95% CI: 55%, 75%).[243] Size greater than 8 cm, micropapillary, endometrioid, or CCC histologies can contribute to this difficulty.
- The micropapillary subtype is a distinct entity and carries an adverse prognosis. BRAF mutations are commonly found in this subtype. The distinguishing architecture is a height-to-width ratio of 5:1. It is often associated with invasive implants. Micropapillary histology has a higher rate of recurrence at 26%.

- Serous LMP tumors represent 62% of all LMP tumors; 30% are diagnosed as stage I, and they are often bilateral; 10% to 20% have invasive implants.
- Mucinous LMP tumors represent about 38% of LMP tumors and 80% to 90% are found as stage I; 5% are bilateral. There is a greater malignant potential with these tumors than with the serous LMP tumors.
- Invasive implants are a major factor in determining whether to treat with adjuvant therapies or not. The 7YOS for patients with noninvasive implants is 96%, and for those with invasive implants, 66%. The risk of invasive implants accompanies histology: for serous borderline tumors the risk is 6%, but increases to 49% with micropapillary tumors.

Pretreatment Workup
- Workup is the same as for TOC.

Staging
- Staging is the same as for TOC. Contralateral tubo-ovarian and uterine conservation may be considered in patients considering future fertility with completion surgery after childbearing.

Treatment
- Treatment is primarily surgical and follows the same directives as those for malignant OC: complete surgical staging with full cytoreduction to microscopic disease status.
- Fertility-sparing treatment is a reasonable option if desired. A cystectomy or USO can be performed with additional staging LND, biopsies, and omentectomy. The recurrence rate overall is 12%. If a cystectomy is performed, the recurrence rate is 23%, compared to 8% with a USO. The median time to recurrence is 2.6 Y after a cystectomy and 4.7 Y after a USO.
- If surgical staging was not performed or this was an incidental pathologic finding, there is data to suggest that repeat staging is not beneficial in this patient population, given that no micropapillary histology is present. One series[243] compared early-stage LMP tumors in 31 staged patients to 42 unstaged patients ($p = .01$). Of these, 17% of patients had their stage upgraded based on surgical staging, but 5YOS was 93% for all stages. The OS was similar in both groups. LN positivity made no difference in OS. Often, endosalpingiosis is seen in the LN.
- Adjuvant chemotherapy should be considered if there are invasive implants. Treatment usually includes adjuvant chemotherapy that is platinum based. There is an average 25% recurrence rate for LMP tumors to chemotherapy. At second look, the response to

chemotherapy was 15% if noninvasive implants were present, versus 57% if invasive implants were present, thus borderline tumors are not completely chemoresistant.[244]

Recurrence

- Recurrence in a spared contralateral ovary can occur in 16% to 23% of patients, but is treated by resection of the tube and ovary. There were no deaths in those managed conservatively.
- Recurrent disease is often indolent. Recommended treatment is repeat cytoreduction. Overall, 5% to 10% of tumors recur. There are data to suggest that 73% recur as low-grade invasive cancers.[245]

Survival

Survival Care

- Follows the same pattern as that of EOC (Table 2.11).

Fallopian Tube Cancer

Characteristics

- The origin of primary HGST OC, based on advancing genetic investigations and correlation with histopathologic evidence is most likely metastatic PFTC. Thus, fallopian tube, ovarian, and PPCs are now grouped under the same umbrella for diagnosis, treatment, and management as TOCs. The incidence of PFTC was stated to be 0.41/100,000 women.[246] Bilateral involvement is found in 5% to 30% of patients, and one third of patients have LN metastasis at the time of staging. Route of spread is transcoelomic, lymphatic, and hematogenous.
- Hu's criteria were established to assist in the definitive diagnosis of PFTC.[247] This was further modified by Sedlis in 1978[248] and the criteria are: (a) the main tumor is in the tube and arises from the endosalpinx, (b) the pattern histologically reproduces the epithelium of fallopian tube mucosa and shows a papillary pattern, (c) the transition between benign and malignant tubal epithelium should be demonstrable, and (d) and the ovaries and endometrium are normal or contain less tumor than the tube.

Table 2.11 LMP OC 10-YS by Stage

Stage	Relative 10-YS (%)
I	99
II	98
III	96
IV	77

- There is often a triad of symptoms: pelvic pain, a pelvic mass, and watery vaginal discharge (hydrops tubae profluens). This occurs in 11% of patients. A pelvic mass is diagnosed in 12% to 66% of patients.

Pretreatment Workup

- Workup includes a history and physical examination with lab tests. Tumor markers including a CA-125 are drawn. An abnormal Pap smear has been found to be positive in 18% to 60% of patients. Imaging with US, CT, or MRI can be helpful.

Histology

- Ninety percent of tumors are serous, but other subtypes are found, including endometrioid, transitional, and mixed mesodermal Müllerian tumor.

Staging

- Staging follows the same criteria as that for EOC.

Treatment

- Primary treatment is usually surgical to follow the general EOC protocols.
- Surgery includes full staging with a TH-BSO, LND (if less than stage IIIC), omentectomy, peritoneal biopsies, and debulking to microscopic residual disease.
- Chemotherapy follows the same principles as that of EOC with first-line platinum- and paclitaxel-based combination regimens.
- Treatment by stage and G:
  - Stage I G 1: definitive surgery
  - Stage I G 2 or 3: surgery and adjuvant chemotherapy
  - Stage II to IV: surgery and (neo) adjuvant chemotherapy

Survival

Survival Care

- Follows the same principles as that of EOC (Table 2.12).

Table 2.12 Fallopian Tube Cancer 5YS by Stage

Stage	Relative 5YS (%)
I	87
II	86
III	52
IV	40

Primary Peritoneal Cancer

- Differentiation between primary peritoneal cancer (PPC) and primary tubo-ovarian carcinomas can be difficult. PPC may be unrecognized metastatic STIC or PFTC. Pathologic criteria previously established to determine a primary peritoneal site are: the bulk of tumor is on the peritoneum rather than on the ovaries, normal-sized ovaries are present or the ovaries are enlarged by a benign process, tumor involves the ovaries to a depth that is less than 5 mm and a width that is less than 5 mm, and the tumor is serous by nature. Again, peritoneal, tubal, and OCs are now grouped under one heading for diagnosis, treatment, and management.
- PPC can be considered an expression of HBOC syndromes. There is a 2% to 4.3% risk of PPC after prophylactic oophorectomy in hereditary cancer mutation carriers.
- Workup, staging, treatment, survival, and survival care follow the same principles as that of EOC.

Germ Cell Tumors

Characteristics

- Germ cell tumors (GCTs) are hypothesized to arise from an unfertilized ovum. They represent 15% to 20% of ovarian cancers, and 70% of ovarian tumors in women less than 30 Y of age. The median age at diagnosis is 19 Y, 30% are malignant, 60% to 75% are stage I at diagnosis, and 25% to 30% are stage III at diagnosis.
- Clinical symptoms include a mass, abdominal distension, bloating, pelvic pressure, or pain. Pain can occur from mass effect, torsion, and/or hemorrhage.
- Paraneoplastic syndromes are common: Hyperthyroidism can occur from teratomatous thyroid tissue, HTN from renin-producing teratomas, hypoglycemia from insulin production, as well as autoimmune hemolytic anemia from teratomas.
- See Table 2.13 for 5YS rates.

Table 2.13 Germ Cell OC 5YS by Stage	
Stage	Relative 5YS (%)
I	98
II	94
III	87
IV	69

Pretreatment Workup

- The pretreatment workup includes a physical examination; CXR; abdominal pelvic imaging to include pelvic US, CT, or MRI; serum tumor markers; and a karyotype in short or premenarchal females.
- Serum tumor markers specific to histology include:
  - Dysgerminoma: hCG, LDH
  - Endodermal sinus tumor: AFP, LDH
  - Immature Teratoma (IT): AFP, LDH
  - Embryonal carcinoma: hCG, AFP, LDH
  - Choriocarcinoma: hCG
  - Polyembryoma: hCG, AFP, LDH
  - Mixed: hCG, AFP, LDH

Staging

- Staging for GCT is per TOC FIGO and AJCC protocols.
- Inadequately staged patients can be managed in two ways: with surgical re-exploration and staging; or chemotherapy without re-exploration, especially if the histologic subtype demands chemotherapy regardless of stage.

Treatment

- Surgical exploration is advised if a mass greater than 2 cm is found in premenarchal girls, or a mass greater than 6 to 8 cm is found in adolescents or postmenopausal females. If tumor markers, such as AFP or hCG, are found elevated, and pregnancy is ruled out, exploration should also be considered. Surgical treatment includes washings, a USO if fertility is desired, along with staging biopsies, omentectomy, LND, and debulking of disease. If fertility is not desired, a hysterectomy with BSO is indicated in addition to the preceding staging procedures.
- The role of optimal cytoreduction is also important with these tumors. In a study of 76 patients, a 28% recurrence rate was seen if they were completely resected, versus a 68% recurrence rate if there was residual disease.[249] In another study of patients treated with PVB, those with measurable disease had a 34% DFS versus 65% if optimally debulked.[250]
- Adjuvant chemotherapy is recommended for all tumors except for stage IA dysgerminomas and stage IAG1 ITs. Chemotherapy is recommended to be platinum based and consists of BEP or EP for three to four cycles. Total bleomycin dose should be evaluated to ensure it does not surpass 450 mg/m^2, which is the toxicity level.
- The appropriate number of BEP cycles is debated. Three cycles are recommended for optimally debulked stages I to III disease. Four cycles are given for suboptimally debulked disease or stage IV disease. If tumor markers are still elevated, chemotherapy should continue for two cycles past normalization of these markers.

Recurrence

- Recurrence is documented by physical examination, a rise in serum tumor markers, or imaging. Ninety percent of relapses occur within 2 Y.

- GCTs are classified as platinum resistant if there is recurrence within 4 to 6 weeks. Patients with elevated tumor markers at presentation who do not achieve a negative marker status at four cycles are considered to have a failed response. Salvage chemotherapy should be implemented.

- Some clinicians have recommended salvage cytoreduction showing a 61% 5YS if optimally salvaged versus 14% 5YS in those not secondarily optimally cytoreduced.[251]

- TIP (paclitaxel, cisplatin, ifosfamide, or high-dose chemotherapy with bone-marrow transplant can be considered).

Follow-Up

- For nondysgerminomatous tumors, follow-up should occur every 3 months for the first 2 Y, then every 6 months up to 5 Y.

- For dysgerminomas, a 10 Y follow-up is recommended. Serum hCG and AFP should be measured for all patients, even if not initially elevated. The tumor relapse rate is 10% to 20%.

Histologic Subtypes and Directed Therapies

- **Dysgerminomas** represent 40% of GCT; 95% are found in stage I. There is greater malignant potential if the tumor is larger than 10 cm, there is an elevated LDH, a high mitotic index, and necrosis. Five percent of tumors produce hCG and PLAP, due to the presence of syncytiotrophoblastic tissue.

  o Adjuvant therapy is indicated for patients staged IB or greater. BEP for three to four cycles is the recommended regimen; alternatively XRT can be considered.

  o It is important to check a karyotype because 15% of patients are intersex with XY gonadal dysgenesis. If this is found, a prophylactic bilateral gonadectomy should be considered because of the high risk for contralateral dysgerminoma. Gonadectomy should be performed before puberty except in females with testicular feminization. The gonads should be removed after puberty in these cases.

  o If a dysgerminoma is found incidentally after primary surgery, restaging can be considered but is not always indicated, if there is no bulky disease.

  o For stage IA patients, there is a 20% recurrence rate. If patients were unstaged, consider surveillance and salvage therapies initiated at recurrence. If there is recurrent disease, XRT or chemotherapy can be administered.

- Gonadoblastomas are rare benign GCTs. These tumors have up to a 10% chance of malignant transformation. The gonads should be removed if a gonadoblastoma is found in a dysgenic gonad.
- Endodermal sinus tumors represent 22% of GCT.
  - The histologic pearl is the presence of Schiller–Duval bodies. These are hyaline bodies that resemble the glomerulus in the kidney.
  - All patients require adjuvant postoperative chemotherapy, which should begin within 7 to 10 days of surgery due to rapid growth of disease. Recommended therapy is BEP for three to four cycles, or POMB-ACE every 3 weeks for four cycles. Survival is 2% to 10% without chemotherapy. This is the most virulent of the GCTs.
- Embryonal carcinoma is a rare tumor that occurs in younger patients. There are no trophoblastic tissues in this tumor. Adjuvant treatment should consist of BEP chemotherapy regardless of stage.
- Choriocarcinoma is a rare tumor, especially the nongestational type. Adjuvant treatment should consist of BEP chemotherapy regardless of stage.
- Polyembryoma is an extremely rare GCT with fewer than 40 cases reported in the literature. Embryoid bodies are seen at pathology. Adjuvant treatment consists of BEP chemotherapy regardless of stage.
- Mixed GCT constitutes 1% to 15% of all GCTs. They most commonly consist of dysgerminomatous and endodermal sinus tumor components. Adjuvant treatment should consist of BEP chemotherapy regardless of stage.
- Mature cystic teratoma (MCT), also known as a *dermoid*, represents 95% of ovarian teratomas. All three germ cell layers are represented. This tumor does not constitute a malignancy. It can present as a mass, and it can cause pain via torsion or rupture (Figure 2.8).
  - The tubercle of Rokitansky is a mural density seen on radiologic imaging.
  - Treatment is surgical with a cystectomy or USO.
  - Malignant degeneration can occur in 1% to 2% of MCTs. This is usually found in a focus of squamous cell carcinoma from skin lining the cyst. Intraoperative spill of sebaceous contents can cause a chemical peritonitis.
  - Gliomatosis peritonei is the presence of benign peritoneal implants of mature neuroglia. These implants usually undergo remission upon resection of the primary tumor.
- **Immature cystic teratoma (ITs)** constitute 20% of GCTs. An IT is defined as the presence of any immature neural tissue. Immature neural tissue is seen as rosettes or neurotubules within the tumor.

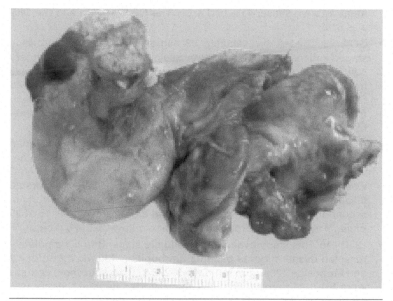

Figure 2.8 Dermoid tumor with teeth.

- The amount of immature tissue on one low-power slide determines the grade. The grading system for IT is grade (G) 1, one LPF (10x) of neural elements in any slide; G2, no greater than a total of three LPFs of neural elements in any slide; G3, greater than three LPFs full of neural elements on at least one slide.
- Chemotherapy is indicated for all patients except stage IA G 1. Recommended therapy is BEP every 3 weeks for three to four cycles.
- A SLL is recommended if there is residual tumor seen on imaging after completion of chemotherapy. This can remove chemoresistant disease or determine whether there was conversion to mature teratoma.

GCT Trials
- GOG 10: In this study, 76 patients with malignant GCTs received VAC postoperatively; 54 patients were optimally debulked; 28% of these failed compared to 68% of those who were incompletely resected and failed. Therefore, PVB was trialed for those who were suboptimally resected.[249]
- GOG 45: In this trial, 97 eligible patients with stage II to IV or recurrent disease were treated with three to four cycles of PVB. Of 35 patients with tumors other than dysgerminoma who had clinically

measurable disease, 43% had a CR. The OS was 71% and the DFS was 51%.[250]

- GOG 78: This study evaluated 93 eligible patients with surgically staged and resected GCTs. Three cycles of BEP were given as primary adjuvant therapy; 89 of the 93 patients were continuously disease free. At SLL, two patients were found to have foci of IT but remained CCR. Final conclusions were that 91 of 93 patients were progression free after surgery and three cycles of BEP. Patients with IT may benefit from secondary debulking if residual disease is identified.[252]

- GOG 90: Twenty patients with incompletely resected ovarian dysgerminoma were treated with cisplatin, bleomycin, and either vinblastine or etoposide. Consolidation chemotherapy with VAC was included for some. Eleven patients had clinically measurable disease postoperatively, and 10 responded completely. Fourteen second-look procedures were done, and all were negative; 19 of 20 patients were disease free with a median follow-up of 26 months.[253]

- GOG 116: This study evaluated 39 eligible stage IB to III completely resected dysgerminoma patients. Carboplatin 400 mg/m^2 on day 1 and etoposide 120 mg/m^2 on days 1, 2, 3 q28 days for three courses were used as primary adjuvant therapy. This doublet therapy was found to be well tolerated for those who needed to reduce chemotoxicity. There were no recurrences. Critics suggest the lack of bleomycin can contribute to an inferior outcome such as that seen in testes cancer (pharmacologic sanctuary), so the doublet should not be used without bleomycin in ovarian GCTs.[254]

- A GOG assessment of SLL in GCT evaluated 117 patients from GOG studies 45, 78, and 90. Of the 45 patients treated with BEP after optimal debulking, 38 had a negative SLL. They concluded there was no need for SLL. A subgroup analysis suggested that SLL may be of value in approximately 33% of patients with suboptimal debulking for GCT with teratomatous elements. Of the 24 patients with teratoma in the primary tumor, 16 patients had bulky residual disease; 14 of 16 patients were disease free after secondary debulking.[255]

Sex Cord Stromal Tumors

Characteristics

- Sex cord stromal tumors represent 5% to 8% ovarian malignancies and 5% of childhood tumors. They are bilateral in 2% of patients. Of these tumors, 85% produce steroid hormones. The route of spread is transcoelomic, lymphatic, and hematogenous.

- See Table 2.14 for 5YS rates.

Pretreatment Workup

- The pretreatment workup includes serum hormonal evaluation (free testosterone, estradiol, 17-hydroxy-progesterone, serum cortisol, DHEAS, DHEA, AFP, LDH, inhibin A, inhibin B, and hCG), and imaging, including CXR and US, CT, or MRI.

Table 2.14 Sex Cord Stromal Ovarian Cancer 5YS by Stage

Stage	5YS (%)
I	95
II	78
III	65
IV	35

Staging

- Staging is the same as for other OC. There are data to suggest a primary LND does not often yield positive results.[256]

Treatment

- Surgical treatment is with washings, a USO if fertility is desired, along with staging biopsies, omentectomy, +/-LND, and debulking of disease. A D&C should be considered if fertility preservation is undertaken especially for granulosa cell tumors. If fertility is not desired, a hysterectomy with BSO is indicated.
  - Stage 1 low risk: observation
  - Stage 1 high risk: (ruptured 1C or G3 or heterologous elements)
    - Observation or platinum-based chemotherapy (carbo/taxol or BEP)
  - Stage II-IV: platinum-based chemotherapy or XRT
  - Recurrent disease: can treat with carbo/taxol, BEP, an AI, or Leupron

Histology

- **Stromal tumors (Table 2.15)**
  - **Granulosa cell tumors**
    - Granulosa cell tumors represent 1% to 2% of ovarian tumors.
    - These tumors tend to produce high levels of estrogen that can cause the refeminization of postmenopausal patients, and isosexual-precious puberty in prepubertal girls. Patients may experience associated vaginal bleeding, with up to 50% of patients having endometrial hyperplasia and up to 5% with a concordant uterine cancer.
    - The histologic pearls are the presence of Call–Exner bodies and coffee bean nuclei.
    - Most granulosa tumors are of the adult type (95%) and the rest are of the juvenile type.
    - The juvenile type is relatively benign in early stages but can be aggressive in advanced stages. Associated syndromes are Ollier's disease (enchondromatosis) and Maffucci's syndrome

Table 2.15 Ovarian Stromal Tumor WHO Classification Overview and Risk of Malignancy

Granulosa cell tumors	
Adult	Malignant
Juvenile	Malignant
Thecoma	
Thecomas, typical	Benign
Thecomas, luteinized	Malignant potential
Thecoma with increased mitotic figures	Malignant potential
Fibroma	
Cellular fibroma	Malignant potential
Cellular fibroma with increased mitotic figures	Malignant potential
Fibrosarcoma	Malignant
Stromal tumor with minor sex cord elements	Benign
Sclerosing stromal tumor	Benign
Signet ring stromal tumors	Benign
Unclassified	Malignant potential
Sertoli–Leydig cell tumors	
Well differentiated	Malignant potential
Intermediate differentiation	Malignant
Poorly differentiated	Malignant
Sertoli–Leydig tumors with heterologous elements	Malignant
Sertoli cell tumors	Malignant potential
Leydig cell tumors	Benign
Stromal–Leydig cell tumors	Benign
SCTAT	Malignant
Microscopic SCTAT associated with PJS	Benign
Gynandroblastoma	Malignant/malignant potential
Unclassified sex cord stromal tumors	Malignant potential
Steroid cell tumors	Malignant

Source: Tavassoeli FA, Devilee P, eds. *WHO Classification of Tumours, Pathology and Genetics: Tumours of the Breast and Female Genital Organs.* Lyon: IARC; 2003.[257]

(hemangiomas and sarcomas). The OS for stage I juvenile tumors is 97% versus 23% for stage III/IV. There are no Call–Exner bodies in the juvenile type.

- It is important to check a serum estradiol (>30 pg/mL in a postmenopausal woman is abnormal) and both the α and β inhibin levels.
- Treatment is surgical with comprehensive staging.
- Adjuvant chemotherapy is considered for stage IC and higher. Recurrence is often indolent at 5 to 20 Y. See MITO-9 study.
- Prognostic factors for adverse outcomes are size greater than 10 cm, rupture, greater than 2 mitosis/10 HPF, LVSI, and nuclear atypia.
- For recurrent or metastatic disease, patients can be retreated with BEP or other regimens to possibly include platinum with paclitaxel, high-dose progestins, GnRH agonists, or XRT. One study demonstrated a 43% CCR with XRT in patients with measurable disease.[258] Another study has shown an 86% RR for granulosa cell tumors treated with XRT.[259]

○ **Thecomas**
- Thecomas represent 1% of ovarian tumors and are bilateral in 3%. They are benign tumors that can produce estrogen.

○ **Fibroma**
- Fibromas are the most common sex cord stromal tumor and 10% are bilateral. They are benign tumors. They occasionally secrete estrogen. They have an association with **Meigs syndrome**, which is the presence of an adnexal fibroma, ascites, and a pleural effusion.

○ **Androblastoma**
- This tumor is diagnosed at a median age of 30 Y. This tumor can cause virilization. It is important to follow the serum AFP and testosterone. Adjuvant chemotherapy is recommended if the tumor contains heterologous elements or is poorly differentiated. Recurrence is usually within the first 2 Y.

○ **Sertoli cell tumor**
- Sertoli cell tumor is also called a *Pick's adenoma*.
- It produces estrogen in 65% of patients and can also produce androgens. It rarely produces hyperaldosteronism with associated hyperkalemia and HTN.
- The histologic pearl is the Pick's body.
- There is an increased risk of malignancy if hemorrhage, necrosis, a high mitotic count, or poor differentiation are present.

○ **Leydig cell tumors**
- Leydig cell tumors produce androgens in 80% and estrogen in 10% of patients; 2.5% are malignant. They usually present after the age of 50 Y and are associated with thyroid disease.

- ○ **Sertoli–Leydig cell tumor**
  - Sertoli–Leydig cell tumors can cause virilization in one half to two thirds of patients. Most tumors produce testosterone and this can cause menstrual irregularities.
  - The histologic pearl is the Crystals of Reinke.
  - Ninety percent are found at stage I, and less than 20% are malignant.
  - For those that are malignant: 10% are G 2 and 60% are G 3. Malignant tumors tend to have more necrosis, are larger, and hemorrhage more frequently.
  - Adjuvant chemotherapy should consist of BEP if malignant.
- **Gynandroblastoma**
  - ○ Gynandroblastoma tumors can produce androgens and estrogens. These tumors can have both granulosa and Sertoli–Leydig components.
- **SCTAT**
  - ○ SCTAT can produce estrogen. Two thirds are bilateral.
    - These tumors can be associated with Peutz–Jeghers syndrome and are benign when they have this association. PJ syndrome has an associated 15% risk of cervical adenocarcinoma (adenoma malignum) and hysterectomy should be considered after fertility is concluded.
    - If patients are not diagnosed with PJ syndrome, these tumors are considered malignant. Treatment for non-PJ syndrome patients is surgical with a USO, LND, and staging. A D&C, ECC, and colposcopy should be performed if fertility is desired; otherwise, a TH-BSO is needed.
- **Unclassified**
  - ○ **Lipid cell tumors**
    - Lipid cell tumors can be virilizing and produce Cushing's syndrome. They produce estrogen, progesterone, and testosterone.
    - These are malignant in 20% of cases. Indications of malignancy are pleomorphism, necrosis, a high mitotic count, and a size greater than 8 cm.
    - Adjuvant BEP chemotherapy is recommended if found to be malignant.
  - ○ **Sex cord tumors NOS**
    - Sex cord tumors NOS produce a variety of hormones; up to 17% of patients have Cushing's disease.
    - Forty-three percent of these tumors are malignant. Malignant tumors contain fibrothecomatous areas and/or granulosa cell-like proliferation as well as areas of tubular differentiation.
    - Adjuvant BEP chemotherapy is recommended if malignant.

5YS

- Dysgerminoma
  - Stage I: 90% to 95%
  - All stages: 60% to 90%
- Endodermal sinus tumor
  - Stage I and II: 90%
  - Stage III and IV: 50%
- Immature teratoma
  - Stage I: 90% to 95%
  - All stages: 70% to 80%
  - G 1: 82%
  - G 2: 62%
  - G 3: 30%
- Embryonal carcinoma
  - All stages: 39%
- Choriocarcinoma: poor
- Polyembryoma: poor
- Mixed: depends on tumor composition
- Granulosa cell:
  - Stages I, II: 85% to 95%
  - Stages III, IV: 55% to 60%
- Sertoli–Leydig:
  - G 3: poor survival

Sex Cord Stromal Tumor Trials

- GOG 115: This study evaluated 57 eligible patients who had incompletely resected stages II to IV ovarian stromal malignancies. BEP was used as first-line therapy every 3 weeks for four cycles. The endpoint was negative SLL: 37% had negative findings. Patients with measurable disease had the highest risk of progression and death. BEP was found to be active in stromal tumors.[260]
- GOG 264: This was a randomized phase II trial of paclitaxel and carboplatin versus bleomycin etoposide and cisplatin for newly diagnosed advanced-stage and recurrent chemo-naive sex cord stromal tumors of the ovary. Results pending with estimated completion date of 2022.
- MITO-9: Forty patients with stage 1C granulosa cell tumor were retrospectively reviewed. 35% had fertility-sparing treatment, 22.5% received adjuvant BEP or carboplatin/taxol, 35% relapsed, and there was no difference in DFS between those who received and those who did not receive adjuvant chemotherapy. The 5Y DFS was 27% compared to 50%, p = .4. Adjuvant chemotherapy was

not predictive for recurrence although incomplete surgical staging was. This study was limited by being a retrospective review and by its low power.[261]

- Surveillance options after initial surgery for pediatric and adolescent girls with stage I ovarian GCTs are debatable. High risk histologies or stage IB and higher should be, in our opinion, considered for adjuvant chemotherapy.

  ○ A report from the Children's Oncology Group states that some girls can be watched rather than treated upfront due to high salvage rates. Careful discussion should be held with patient and family due to this being a small study, 48% recurrent with surveillance, and one death was observed. Twenty-five girls were reviewed with a median age of 12 Y. Of these, 23 patients had an elevated AFP at diagnosis. The predominant histology was yolk sac tumor (YST), with embryonal, or choriocarcinoma also represented. The median follow-up was 42 months. Surveillance involved measurement of serum tumor markers and radiologic imaging at defined intervals, AFP and b-HCG every 3 weeks through week 9, monthly from 2 to 6 months, and every 3 months from 6 to 24 months. LND was not required, sparing of fallopian tubes was allowed, and no staging biopsies were needed. In those with residual or recurrent disease, a compressed BEP regimen was initiated every 3 weeks for three cycles. Twelve patients had evidence of persistent or recurrent disease. The 4Y EFS was 52%, the median time to recurrence was 2 months. All patients had elevated AFP at recurrence. Eleven of 12 patients received successful salvage chemotherapy with a 4Y OS of 96%. There was one death. The compressed regimen of BEP was cisplatin 33 mg/m^2 on days 1 to 3, etoposide 167 mg/m^2 on days 1 to 3, bleomycin 15 mg/m^2 on day 1 for three cycles.[262]

UTERINE CANCER

Characteristics

- Uterine corpus cancer is the most common female gynecologic cancer in the United States with an estimated 65,950 cases and 12,550 deaths in the United States in 2022. Currently, endometrial adenocarcinoma is the most common malignancy of the female genital tract and ranks as the fourth most common cancer in females.

- **Risk factors** for endometrial cancer include the triad of obesity, diabetes, and HTN. Other risk factors are a prolonged exposure to estrogens, nulliparity, early menarche, late menopause, and unopposed estrogen hormone therapy. Fifty-seven percent of cancers are attributable to obesity. The lifetime risk of uterine cancer with a normal BMI is 3%, but with each five-unit increase in BMI, the risk of uterine cancer increases 50%.[263]

Table 2.16 Uterine Hyperplasia and Risk of Progression to Cancer

Type of Hyperplasia	Total Cases	Persisted (%)	Progressed (%)	Mean Y Follow-Up
Simple	93	19	1	15.2
Complex	29	17	3	13.5
Atypical simple	23	23	8	11.4
Atypical complex	45	14	29	11.4

- Most women present with abnormal uterine bleeding. Of those postmenopausal women who do present with bleeding, 10% result in a diagnosis of uterine cancer.
- Other presenting signs and symptoms can be menorrhagia, intermenstrual bleeding, pain, pyometria, hematometria, and an abnormal Pap smear.
- EIN (atypical hyperplasia +/- glandular complexity) has known rates for progression to uterine cancer (Table 2.16).[264]
  - According to one collaborative study, a diagnosis of complex atypical hyperplasia was associated with a 43% chance of concurrent endometrial cancer. Of these specimens, 31% had myometrial invasion and 10% had greater than 50% DOI.[265]

Prognostic Factors

Stage is the most important prognostic factor. Other factors include DOI, LVSI, G, histology, tumor size, patient age, and hormone receptor status.

Pretreatment Workup

- Workup for abnormal bleeding begins with a history and physical examination. Evaluation involves EMB with ECC or D&C. Pelvic US and Pap smear may also be performed, but are insufficient modalities used alone for persistent abnormal bleeding.
- An EMS thickness that is 5 mm or greater in a postmenopausal patient is abnormal and biopsy should be performed. The accuracy of EMB and D&C are relatively the same, between 91% and 99%, when compared with final pathology.[265]
- Women with the following should be ruled out for cancer via EMB: postmenopausal women with bleeding; postmenopausal patients with pyometria; asymptomatic postmenopausal women with endometrial cells on Pap smear (especially if atypical); perimenopausal patients with intermenstrual bleeding or increasingly heavy periods; and premenopausal patients with abnormal uterine bleeding, particularly if there is a history of anovulation.
- EMB should be performed for AUB in patients over 45, or in women younger than 45 with history of unopposed estrogen, failed medical management, and persistent AUB. Twenty-five percent of cancers

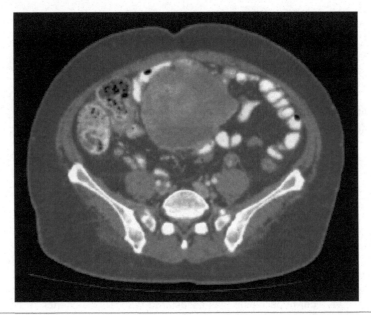

Figure 2.9 Uterine cancer on CT.

occur in premenopausal women and 5% occur in women younger than 40 Y of age.

- The pretreatment workup for uterine cancer includes a CXR and abdominal pelvic imaging. This can be with a pelvic US CT, or MRI. Chest CT can be added to CT abdomen/pelvic for high-grade malignancies. Lab tests include a CBC, CMP, and CA-125 (which can predict LN metastasis; Figure 2.9).

Categorical Divisions

- **TCGA/Genetic groupings (2014) and ESGO/ESTRO/ESP risk groups 2021:** Guidelines for risk group determination are now a hybrid: integrating molecular diagnostics and clinicopathologic variables. Adjuvant recommendations are to be determined by genetic grouping in addition to pathologic risk factors.[266–269]
- Tumor should be assessed for tumor size, DOI, grade histologic type, LVSI, and extent of disease. Then IHC staining should be performed using IHC for MLH1, MSH2, MSH6, PMS2 markers, as well as p53. HER2 IHC should be considered in TP53 aberrant carcinoma regardless of histotyping. Sanger sequencing should follow to include evaluation of POLE mutation. Hypermethylation of MLH1 should also be investigated either by sodium bisulfite conversion and sequencing, differential enzymatic cleavage of DNA, or affinity capture of methylated DNA if MLH1 IHC is absent.

○ If POLE mutated = hotspot mutation
○ If MMRd: MSI-H
○ if p53 IHC intact = CN low = NSMP
○ if p53 IHC deficient = CN high

PRoMisE is a molecular classification system that uses three IHC stains as surrogate markers of the TCGA molecular subtypes.[270,271]

- MMRd includes MSI-H: Genomic and somatic mutations present or epigenetic changes (hypermethylated), have intermediate prognosis; deficiency highlights possible future PDL1 immunotherapy use.

- P53 abnormal: considered high risk previously known as *copy number high*) is consistent with missense or null mutations, tend to be serous/ CC/some G3 endometrialcarcinomas and often with poor outcomes.

- POLE EDM (POLE exonuclease domain mutated): Considered low have the better PFS, sequencing demonstrates a hotspot mutation in the in the exonuclease domain of DNA polymerase epsilon [POLE])

- NSMP: no specific molecular profile/p53wt, previously known as *copy number low*. Commonly G1/2 endometrioid adenocarcinomas with PTEN *PIK3CA, ARID1A, CTNNB1*, and *KRAS* as frequent mutations. Has intermediate prognosis.

Further subclassification by L1CAM IHC of the intermediate groups (NSMP and MSI) shows that L1CAM positive has a poor outcome and could triage toward adjuvant therapies.

The average percentage per molecular profile type is:

- MSI: 19%
- NSMP/p53 wt: 64%
- POLE: 13%
- p53: abnormal 4%

Tumors that are MMRd are often due to epigenetic change via hypermethylation in 75%, whereas somatic gene mutations occur in 15%, and germline or Lynch mutations occur in about 10%. Lynch cases have the best prognosis.[272]

MSI high tumors consist of low- and high- grade endometrial cancers and have MMR protein defects superimposed on the CN low tumors (Figure 2.10).

L1CAM further stratifies the endometrial carcinoma patients that have the NSMP no.[270,271,273]

For metastatic or recurrent tumors: tumor mutation burden (TMB) testing and NTRK gene fusion testing can be offered

- **Histologic grouping:** Epidemiological and clinical studies suggest that endometrial cancers be separated by histologic appearance and behavior into two groups: type I and II tumors. Genetic evaluation is moving toward categorizing tumors outside standard histological status into four separate molecular categories.

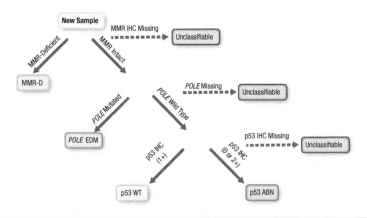

Figure 2.10 A simple, genomics-based clinical classifier for endometrial cancer.

Talhouk A, McConechy MK, Leung S, et al. Confirmation of ProMisE: A simple, genomics-based clinical classifier for endometrial cancer. *Cancer*. 2017;123: 802–813. https://doi.org/10.1002/cncr.30496

- ○ Type I tumors are the most common. The main risk factor in type I carcinomas is hyperestrogenism. These tend to be hormonally responsive and have an 83% all-stage 5YS. These cancers typically have a favorable prognosis with appropriate therapy (Figure 2.11).
  - The most common type I cancer is endometrioid adenocarcinoma, which occurs in 75% of cases.
  - Adenosquamous carcinoma is diagnosed in 18% to 25% of uterine cancers. The behavior is similar to that of endometrioid cancer.
  - Villoglandular carcinoma occurs in 6% of uterine cancers. This subtype is distinguished by delicate fibrovascular cores. It is usually of low grade and is more differentiated than endometrioid adenocarcinoma.
  - Secretory carcinoma occurs in 2% of uterine cancers and appears as a well-differentiated glandular pattern with intracytoplasmic vacuoles containing glycogen, similar to secretory endometrium. It is usually G 1.
  - Mucinous carcinoma is diagnosed in 5% of cases and mucin is present as the major cellular component. There are columnar cells that are basally oriented or pseudostratified. It is necessary to rule out other cancers such as colon, mucinous ovarian, and primary endocervical cancers. It has the same prognosis as endometrioid cancer.
  - Squamous carcinoma is associated with cervical stenosis, pyometria, and chronic inflammation. It is important to rule out a primary cervical cancer origin. It has a poorer prognosis.

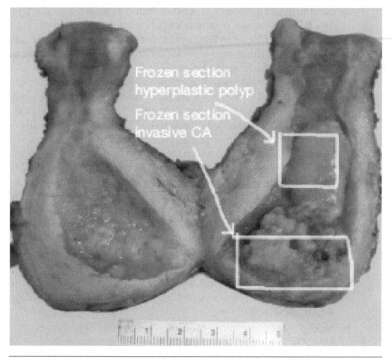

Figure 2.11 Endometrioid uterine cancer.

- Uterine tumors resembling ovarian sex cord tumors: A panel of four IHC markers, including calretinin, inhibin, CD99, and Melan A, has emerged that seems to indicate the most characteristic sex cord markers. Positivity for calretinin and at least one of the other named markers may thus confirm the diagnosis of UTROSCT.[274]
- IHC can be used to differentiate type I from type II tumors. Type I tend to be ER/progesterone receptor (PR)+, p53–, and WT-1 negative.
- Type II cancers are poorly differentiated tumors and are histologically represented by the serous, CC, and MMMT histologies. Type II tumors are more biologically aggressive and have a 53% 5YS for all stages. Type II tumors account for 15% of uterine carcinomas, but represent 50% of all relapses. These type II tumors are classified as high risk high grade and are unresponsive to hormonal therapy.
  - **Serous** uterine carcinoma is diagnosed in 10% to 15% of endometrial cancers. If there is a serous component of at least 10%, it is called a *mixed tumor*. This subtype resembles serous

carcinoma of the ovary. It is often found at an advanced stage. The DOI is often not predictive of LN metastasis, and extrauterine disease is found in 60% of tumors. If the cancer is identified in a polyp without other evidence of uterine disease, 38% of patients will be found to have extrauterine spread. IP spread is common even when DOI is minimal. When comprehensively staged, 70% of patients are found to have advanced-stage disease: 25% of apparent stage I cancers[275] have omental metastasis and 25% of patients have UAD.[276] Microscopically, there are fibrous papillary fronds, picket fencing of the terminal cells, LVSI is common, and psammoma bodies are often present. It is high grade by definition. There is a 2% rate of *BRCA1* mutations in uterine serous cancer patients. Nine percent of women with a history of breast cancer followed by uterine serous cancer have a *BRCA 1/2* mutation.[277] IHC for serous cancers is ER/PR variable, WT-1 negative, p53+, and Her2 IHC should be performed.

- Clear cell carcinoma (CCC) is diagnosed in 5% of uterine cancers. It also is an aggressive tumor. The cells contain a large amount of glycogen and when processed for histology, the glycogen in the cells gives an appearance of cellular clearing and nuclear hobnailing.

- Mixed Mesodermal Mullerian Tumors/Carcinosarcomas MMMTs (CS) are now thought to be metaplastic epithelial (or carcinomatous) cancers. These tumors tend to occur in older women with a median age of 65 to 75 Y. Other characteristics include obesity, nulliparity, and diabetes. Tumor can be seen via speculum examination in 50% of women. Pathologically, there is a mixture of carcinomatous and sarcomatous tissues. The carcinomatous component is most commonly endometrioid, but can be of serous or CC histology. Prognosis is mainly dependent on the epithelioid histology. The sarcomatous/nonepithelial component is commonly an ESS, but can be LMS, rhabdosarcoma, or chondrosarcoma. The presence or absence of heterologous elements is not predictive of outcome. Studies have shown similar allelic losses present in both the carcinomatous and sarcomatous areas of MMMTs in multiple patients. This suggests a late divergence in phenotype and a common abnormal clone for the entire cancer. Prior tamoxifen use has been implicated in this tumor's development. The median time of exposure to diagnosis of MMMT was 9 Y and ranges to a relative risk of 15.9.[278] Prior pelvic XRT has also been noted to have a causal effect: in 23 patients with prior pelvic XRT, 35% had an MMMT uterine cancer. Surgical management is critical for staging and optimization of treatment. Twenty percent of patients with clinical stage I and II are upstaged by LND. Cytoreduction in advanced-stage

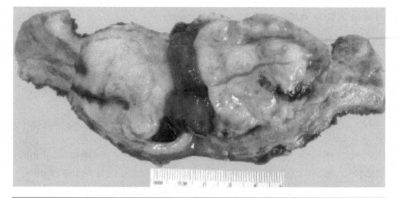

Figure 2.12 MMMT uterine cancer.

disease (III and IV) with optimal resection was associated with improved survival of 52.3 months versus 8.6 months (*p* < .0001). (Figure 2.12).[279]

- Dedifferentiated/undifferentiated: These are high risk type II tumors.

Staging

- Staging is **surgical**. In 1988, the staging was changed from clinical to surgical. Surgical staging was further revised in 2021 (Table 2.17A–D). Tumors that are staged clinically (patients that are not surgical candidates) should be stage by FIGO 1971 criteria.
- **Grade** is specified as a three-tiered system: G 1 tumors are highly differentiated, with less than 5% of the tumor containing solid areas; G 2 tumors are moderately differentiated with 6% to 50% solid areas; G 3 tumors are poorly differentiated carcinomas with greater than 50% of the tumor containing solid components. If nuclear atypia is present at a higher degree than the stated histological grade the overall grade is increased by one level.

Treatment

- Treatment is primarily surgical staging to include pelvic washings, total hysterectomy, BSO, assessment of lymph nodes, omentectomy and peritoneal biopsies (especially for type II tumors), and surgical debulking of extrauterine/metastatic disease.
  - Treatment approaches:
    - Laparotomy
    - Minimally invasive (preferred)
      - Laparoscopic assisted (total or vaginal)
      - Robotic assisted

Table 2.17A AJCC 8th Edition: T Category

T	FIGO	T Criteria
TX		Primary tumor cannot be assessed.
T0		No evidence of primary tumor.
T1	I	Tumor confined to the corpus uteri, including endocervical glandular involvement.
T1a	IA	Tumor limited to the endometrium or invading less than half the myometrium.
T1b	IB	Tumor invades one half or more of the myometrium.
T2	II	Tumor invades the stromal connective tissue of the cervix but does not extend beyond the uterus.
T3	III	Tumor involves the serosa, adnexa, vagina, or parametrium.
T3a	IIIA	Tumor involves the serosa and/or adnexa (direct extension or metastasis).
T3b	IIIB	Vaginal involvement (direct extension or metastasis) or parametrial involvement is present.
T4	IVA	Tumor invades the bladder mucosa and/or bowel mucosa (bullous edema is not sufficient to classify a tumor as T4).

Table 2.17B N Category

N	FIGO	N Criteria
NX		Regional LNs cannot be assessed
N0		No regional LN metastasis
N0(i+)		ITCs in regional LN(s) not > 0.2 mm
N1	IIIC1	Regional LN metastasis to pelvic LNs
N2	IIIC	Regional LN metastasis to PALNs, with or without positive pelvic LNs

Table 2.17C M Category

M	FIGO	M Criteria
M0		No distant metastasis
M1	IVB	Distant metastasis (includes metastasis to inguinal LNs, IP disease, lung, liver, or bone)

Table 2.17D Stage Grouping

I	
IA	T1aN0M0
IB	T1bN0M0
II	T2N0M0
III	
IIIA	T3aN0M0
IIIB	T3bN0M0
IIIC1	(T1-T3)(N1)M0
IIIC2	(T1-T3)(N2)M0
IV	
IVA	T4(Any N)M0
IVB	(Any T)(Any N)M1

- ○ Treatment modifications:
  - Conversion to laparotomy from laparoscopy: In one study this occurred in 17.5% of patients with a BMI of 25, 26.5% with a BMI of 34 to 35, and 57% of patients with BMI greater than 40. Port site metastasis occurred in 1%.[280]
  - The ability of infrarenal/PALND was 81% in one study when the BMI was greater than 35 kg/m², compared to 95% when the BMI was less than 35.[281]
  - Ovarian conservation in young women with uterine cancer: Only 18% of women less than 45 Y old have stage IAG1 disease. The risk of a synchronous ovarian malignancy can be as high as 19% to 25% in younger women. BSO should be considered for all women with uterine cancer. If ovarian conservation is desired, patients should be stage IA and G1.
    - □ A retrospective review showed that conservation was not independently associated with survival (HR 0.94; 95% CI: 0.65–1.37).[282]
    - □ Younger women have a higher risk of genetic mutations. The risk of HNPCC syndrome and ovarian malignancy is up to 10% if women harbor this genetic mutation. MRI is the best mode to evaluate for DOI and cervical involvement when considering preoperative radiologic evaluation for possible uterine or ovarian preservation.[283,284]
    - □ A two-step proposal for women diagnosed with endometrial cancer ≤45 Y and clinical stage 1 G 1 disease with

endometrioid histology and a surgical hysterectomy candidate were reviewed: 1) Preoperative assessment should consist of no family history of ovarian, endometrial, or colon cancer (syndromic); menopausal status (check FSH, if high and in menopause little benefit to ovarian conservation); no secondary primary cancer; CA-125 ≤35; no abnormal imaging results suggestive of metastasis; and MMR analysis on EMB is normal. If all of these results are normal, advancement to surgery with hysterectomy, with ovarian conservation can be considered. 2) Intraoperative assessment should then be incorporated into the management protocol and includes evaluation for the following: extrauterine metastasis, frozen section review for possible upgrade to moderate or high grade (G2/3), deep DOI cervical invasion, abnormal ovary/endometriosis on ovary, or secondary primary cancer identified.

- Morcellation: The risk of a fibroid harboring a LMS is 0.3% to 0.49%. Regardless, morcellation is not recommended for uterine cancer cases to avoid tumor spill and spread, or alter pathologic evaluation. Alternatives to morcellation for laparoscopic approaches to surgery are minilaparotomy or morcellation within an endoscopic bag to facilitate vaginal delivery of the specimen.[285,286] The FDA 2020 recommendation is that laparoscopic power morcellation for myomectomy or hysterectomy be performed only with a tissue containment system and preoperative use of MRI. EMB before hysterectomy can help rule out occult adenocarcinoma but is not reliable for diagnosing sarcomas.

- Sentinel LND: Memorial Sloan Kettering SLND algorithm: A colored dye (ICG, methylene blue, patent blue, isosulfan blue) with or without radiolabeled albumin (technetium-99m) is injected into the cervix, then laparoscopic evaluation proceeds with: (a) peritoneal and serosal visual evaluation and washings; (b) retroperitoneal evaluation, including excision of all mapped SLNs and all suspicious nodes regardless of mapping; (c) if mapping fails on a hemi-pelvis, a side-specific pelvic, common iliac, and interiliac LND is performed. PA-LND is then performed at the attendings' discretion.[287] Protocols for ICG SLN identification 4cc of ICG is injected superficially or deep into the cervical stroma and imaging with the near infrared camera can identify SLN.

- When performed, surgeon experience, adherence to a sentinel LND algorithm or clinical study, and the use of pathologic "ultrastaging" are key factors for successful SLN mapping. Serous/CC/MMMT histologies have a FN rate of 4.3%.[288]

- It is important to classify the size of the SLN metastasis when using SLN mapping as ITC $\leq$ 2 mm, micrometastasis >0.2mm to 2 mm, or a marcometastasis >2 mm.

- **Lymph node dissection**
  - The boundaries for Pelvic-LND are as follows: the distal half of the common iliac vessels, the anterior and medial aspect of the external iliac vessels, the ureter or (superior vesicle artery below the common iliacs) medially, the circumflex iliac vein distally, and the obturator nerve inferiorly.
    - Para-aortic LN boundaries are the fat pads over and lateral to the great vessels, the IMA superiorly, and the mid common iliac vessels inferiorly. For a high PA dissection, the LNs up to the renal vessels are removed medial to the ureters and anterior to the great vessels.
  - There is much controversy regarding the benefit and/or extent of an LND. LND has been shown not to increase the duration of surgery significantly. Some practitioners perform an LND based on tumor risk factors. Others recommend a comprehensive LND for all surgical candidates. Others have provided data that show that an LND is not therapeutic but can provide staging information to guide adjuvant therapies.
  - For those providers who choose a selective LND, the Mayo criteria are often employed to determine whether a patient is low risk for LN metastasis. The Mayo criteria are G 1 or 2 disease, tumor size that is 2 cm or less, and ≤50% DOI. If all these criteria are met, patients have a less than 5% chance of positive LNs.[289] Frozen section should be employed for this decision analysis. The accuracy of frozen section decreases with grade: 87% accurate with G 1, 65% with G 2, only 31% with G 3.[290] Doering et al correlated visual inspection for DOI with frozen section and found 91% accuracy,[291] and Franchi et al supported this data with 85% accuracy and 72% sensitivity.[292]
  - For those who perform comprehensive LND, the following benefits are cited: There may be a therapeutic benefit with removal of micrometastasis, there is a 22% chance of extrauterine disease found with surgical staging, and 20% of tumors are upgraded at final pathology. Data have shown that removing nodes provides a survival benefit.[293,294] An improvement in survival from 72% to 88% has been reported for patients undergoing lymphadenectomy with more than 11 LNs removed.[295] Using SEER data, Chan et al showed that in patients staged IB G 3 and above, more than 20 LNs removed was found to provide the best OS.[296] In low-risk patients, there was no association with LN count and survival. The PORTEC 1 trial subset of stage IC G 3 (unstaged) patients who were treated with pelvic XRT had a 5YS of only 58%. Most

recurrences were distant.[297] In contrast, stage IIIC patients staged and treated have a 5 YS of 57% to 72%.[298,299]

○ In some instances, LND is not performed. This can occur when cancer is found incidentally after hysterectomy. Postoperative pathological review can risk-stratify patients for possible post hoc staging. There can be intraoperative complications that prevent full staging, or the patient may be medically intolerant of the procedure. Body habitus may also prohibit adequate staging: In the Lap-2 data, 50% of patients with a BMI greater than 40 were not able to have a PALND performed.[280] For those who support no LND, data from the following two randomized studies are commonly used.

- The Panici study evaluated 514 eligible clinical stage I uterine cancer patients. Patients were randomly assigned to systematic PLND versus no LND. Researchers found that early and late postoperative complications were higher in the systematic LND group. LND improved staging as more patients were found to have advanced-stage disease with LN involvement (13.3% vs. 3.2%). However, the 5Y DFS and OS were similar (81% vs. 85.9% in the lymphadenectomy arm and 81.7% vs. 90% in the nonlymphadenectomy arm).[300]

- The ASTEC: (A Study in the Treatment of Endometrial Cancer) study[301,302] evaluated 1,408 women with clinical stage I endometrial cancer and randomized them to standard surgery (hysterectomy, BSO, washings with PALN palpation) or standard surgery plus lymphadenectomy. The primary outcome for this study was OS. The HR for death was higher in those who underwent comprehensive staging with LND, 1.16 ($p = .3$; 95% CI: 0.87–1.54). The absolute difference in 5Y OS was 1%.

- Based on a surgical/pathological review of patients thought to have disease confined to the uterus, extrauterine disease has been found in 22% of patients, LN metastasis has been found to occur in 9% to 13% of patients, and isolated PA LNs have been found in 2% of patients. The rate of positive PA LNs is approximately half the rate of positive pelvic LNs (Figure 2.13). For those who were identified with positive PA LNs, 47 of 48 patients had one or more of the following: grossly positive pelvic LN, grossly positive adnexal metastasis, or outer one third DOI.[303] Omental metastasis has been found in up to 8% of patients (Table 2.18).

○ Cervical involvement

- If gross cervical involvement is seen at diagnosis: Cervical biopsy and pelvic MRI should be performed for confirmation. If negative, TH-BSO and staging can be considered. If cervical biopsy is positive, a radical hysterectomy with BSO and LND can be performed—but there is the high likelihood of needing

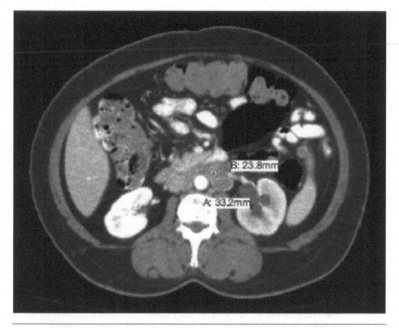

Figure 2.13 Uterine cancer on CT with PA lymphadenopathy.

Table 2.18 GOG 33 Risk Factors for LN Metastasis

Risk Factor	Pelvic*	PA
Grade		
Grade 1	3	2
Grade 2	9	5
Grade 3	18	11
DOI		
Superficial	5	3
Middle	6	1
Deep	25	17
Site of disease		
Fundus	8	4
Cervix	16	14
LVSI		
Negative	7	9
Positive	27	19

*Percentage who developed nodal metastasis.

adjuvant radiation regardless and given the higher morbidity of radical hysterectomy and similar treatment outcomes, this is not always recommended. No survival benefit was seen in one retrospective study comparing radical versus simple hysterectomy in patients with gross cervical involvement.[471] Preoperative XRT consisting of EBXRT and brachytherapy to a total dose of 75 to 80 Gy to point A can be alternative management. An adjuvant simple hysterectomy can then be considered. If not a surgical candidate, EBXRT and brachytherapy with consideration of systemic chemotherapy should be implemented. Reevaluation at a later date for surgical therapy should be performed. Systemic chemotherapy can also be an option alone for surgically inoperable patients.

- There are data to suggest that performing a radical hysterectomy, based on a positive ECC only, commonly shows no evidence of cancer on final pathology and may be overtreatment.[304] Pelvic MRI can help identify cervical stromal involvement preoperatively.

- If gross parametrial involvement is identified by physical examination or preoperative imaging, primary EBXRT with or without brachytherapy with dosing analogous to that for cervical cancer (75–80 Gy) can be considered, followed by a simple hysterectomy, with or without chemotherapy.

○ Sentinel LN:

- Management of positive SLN has not been decided: Completion LND, adjuvant EBXRT, or combination adjuvant chemo/EBXRT are all options.

- ITCs in SLN: otherwise stage I/II endometrioid endometrial cancer:[305] This study evaluated 175 patients in a retrospective study when SLN were identified to harbor ITCs (<200 cells and <0.2 mm) in patients with otherwise stage I/II endometrioid histology uterine cancer defined by HIR GOG249 criteria. Ninety underwent LND alone, and 85 had SLND f/b completion LND. By non-ITC stage, 39% were IB and 12% stage II. Of these, 76 (43%) received no additional therapy or vaginal brachytherapy only, 21 (12%) had EBXRT, and 78 (45%) received chemotherapy +/-radiation. Those who got chemotherapy frequently had deep myoinvasion, LVSI, and were higher grade. The median follow-up time was 31 months and nine (5.1%) patients recurred; of whom five were distant, three retroperitoneal (4.6%), and one vaginal. Extra-vaginal recurrences were similar in patients with or without chemotherapy (5.2% vs. 3.8%, p = .68). After controlling for stage, LVSI and grade, chemotherapy and EBRT were not associated with RFS (HR = 0.63, 95% CI: 0.11–3.52, and HR = 0.90, 95% CI: 0.22–3.61, respectively). Given the rate of 4.6% for recurrence in LN basins for patients with stage I/II endometrioid uterine cancer and ITCs in SLNs regardless of treatment, adjuvant therapy may not be significantly associated with RFS.

○ Positive cytology:

- Rethinking the old 3A uterine cancer (positive washings):[306] A retrospective review of 1,916 patients who had a hysterectomy for uterine cancer had peritoneal cytology (PC) reviewed. Subgroups were stratified by surgical stages (early/advanced stages), tumor types (types 1/2), and risk classifications (low, intermediate, high). Positive PC was identified as an adverse prognostic factor in analyses of all positive cases and in all subgroup analyses regardless of stratification methods. In survival curve comparisons, the PFS and DSS in early-stage patients with positive PC were distinctly demarcated between those stage II patients with negative PC and stage III patients. In subgroup analyses stratified by risk classification of the early-stage cancers, positive PC was related to lower PFS in the intermediate- and high risk groups but not in the low-risk group. Thus, **consideration of early stage** PC-positive cases, except for the low risk group, may be recommended for upstaging and careful deliberation of adjuvant therapy, compared with PC-negative cases.

- Positive washings for high-risk uterine subtypes (1A noninvasive serous, CC, CS) can change adjuvant therapy recommendations and escalate treatment recommendations to include chemotherapy.

- There are data to suggest that the incidence of omental metastasis is 6% to 8% and is associated with grade of disease, extrauterine involvement, LN metastasis, deep DOI and positive cytology.

○ Extrauterine disease:

- If there is **extrauterine disease** confirmed at presentation, NACT can be considered but most patients should proceed with total hysterectomy, BSO, and surgical staging with debulking. If tumor appears to be surgically unresectable at presentation, EBXRT with/without brachytherapy and consideration of chemotherapy should be offered. Systemic therapy alone is another option. If liver metastasis is present and biopsy confirmed, systemic therapy with or without EBXRT and/or hormonal therapy can be considered. Palliative TH-BSO can be considered—see notable studies.

- Nine percent of patients have metastatic disease at initial presentation. There is mounting evidence that definitive local therapies may increase survival for some types of metastatic cancers. In addition to systemic therapy, TAH with maximal cytoreduction has been shown to increase survival for patients with abdominal or pelvic metastases.[307]

- **Adjuvant treatment**
  - **Based on no molecular profiling and surgically staged cancers:**
    - High intermediate risk (HIR) early-stage disease is often treated with adjuvant XRT. HIR is classified by two different studies.
      - PORTEC 1: This study stratified patients into an intermediate HiR subgroup for which treatment was recommended: patient age older than 60 Y, DOI greater than half myometrial thickness, or G 2 or 3 tumor.
      - GOG 99 stratified patients by age and risk factors. If a patient fell into any of the following groups, they were considered HIR: patients age ≥70 Y with one risk factor, age 50 to 69 Y with two risk factors, and any age with all three. The risk factors are outer one-third MI, G 2 or 3 tumor, and LVSI.
      - Absent RF:
        - Stage IA G1,2,3: Vaginal brachytherapy (G1/2 with LVSI, G3) is recommended, observation for G1/2 and age <60 is an option.
        - Stage IB G1,2,3: Commonly, vaginal brachytherapy (G1/2) with/without WP EBXRT (G3) is recommended.
      - RF present:
        - Stage IA G1-2: Observation or brachytherapy can be offered.
        - Stage IAG3: Brachytherapy, WP EBXRT, or observation can be offered.
        - Stage IBG1-2: Brachytherapy, WP EBXRT, or observation can be offered.
        - Stage IBG3: Brachytherapy with/without WP EBXRT with/without chemotherapy can be recommended.
    - High-risk early-stage disease is defined variably. Stage I serous, CC, MMMT, dedifferentiated, and variably G 3 endometrioid cancers put patients into the high-risk early-stage disease category. Stage IA type II tumors are recommended to have adjuvant therapy: preferably a combination of XRT and chemotherapy (three cycles of chemotherapy with brachytherapy). Stage IB cancers are recommended to have chemotherapy (three to six cycles) with brachytherapy or EBXRT and brachytherapy. There are data to show that (FIGO 1988) stage 1CG3 type I tumors had a 58% 5YS. Some clinicians recommend chemotherapy and XRT for these high-risk patients.
    - Stage II disease: Adjuvant XRT is recommended and cumulative data support both WP EBXRT and brachytherapy treatment. Chemotherapy should be considered if a type II cancer is present and variably for G3 endometrioid cancer.

○ If cancer is found incidentally on post hysterectomy specimen and:

- Stage IA G1–2, <60 Y, no LVSI, observation is recommended.
- Stage IA G3, age <60 Y, no LVSI, and no myometrial invasion observation or brachytherapy.
- If stage IA G3, or stage 1B G1–2, ≥60 Y, no LVSI: Consider imaging; but brachytherapy is recommended.
- Stage 1A G1-3 with LVSI, stage 1B G1-2 with LSVI, stage IBG3 with LVSI, or stage II: Imaging and surgical staging should be considered, if imaging is negative. If imaging is positive or concerning, restaging should occur.
- If stage IIIA or higher: Adjuvant therapy recommendations should follow.

- **Adjuvant treatment**
  ○ **Based on molecular studies and surgically staged cancers**: Treatment is based on a combination of stage, pathologic, and molecular risk factors. Early-stage disease is defined as stages I and II. *Advanced stage* is defined as stages III and IV. A hybrid approach to adjuvant therapy recommendations for stage I/II disease is now accepted. When stratifying by molecular risk: Stages III/IV do not at this time qualify for stratification by molecular classifications and molecular renderings should not influence adjuvant therapy decisions.
    - Stage IA MMMRd/NSMP low grade with negative or focal LVSI are classified as low risk.
    - Stage IB MMMd/NSMP with negative or focal LVSI are intermediate or HIR based on tumor grade.
    - Stage I p53 mutant are intermediate/HIR based on DOI:
      □ No myometrial invasion +/-adjuvant therapy
      □ With myometrial invasion adjuvant treatment is recommended
    - Stage I-II POLE mutations are low risk regardless of DOI.

- **Advanced-stage endometrial cancer.** For advanced-stage disease (stages III/IV) treatment is primarily surgical with comprehensive staging and cytoreduction to microscopic status if possible. Adjuvant therapy is commonly multimodal, including both XRT and chemotherapy, and can include hormonal therapies. Maintenance therapy for advanced stages after cytotoxic chemotherapy has been suggested (SIENDO trial).
  ○ Stage IIIA: chemotherapy, EBXRT and/or brachytherapy, or both
  ○ Stage IIIB: chemotherapy and/or EBXRT, and brachytherapy
  ○ Stage IIIC: chemotherapy and/or EBXRT and/or brachytherapy
  ○ Stage IV: chemotherapy with/without EBXRT and/or brachytherapy

- There is literature to support cytoreduction in advanced metastatic uterine cancer.
  - Greer treated 31 patients with stage IVB disease with WAR. Those with residual disease less than 2 cm had a corrected 5YS of 80% and an absolute 5YS of 63%, whereas there were no survivors in the group with residual disease greater than 2 cm.[308]
  - Goff evaluated patients with stage IV disease. Those who were cytoreduced had a longer median survival of 18 months compared to an 8-month survival in those who were not able to be cytoreduced.[309]
  - Bristow reviewed 65 patients with stage IVB endometrial cancer who underwent cytoreduction. Optimal cytoreduction (residual tumor ≤1 cm in maximal diameter) was accomplished in 55%. The median survival rate of patients who underwent optimal surgery was 34 months versus 11 months for patients with greater than 1 cm residual disease. Furthermore, patients with microscopic residual tumor survived significantly longer (median survival 46 months) compared to patients optimally cytoreduced but with macroscopic disease.[310]
  - Shih also suggested optimal cytoreduction for stage IV uterine cancer patients. Median survival: The median PFS was 40.3 months for patients with microscopic disease, 11 months for patients with any residual disease, and 2.2 months for patients who did not have attempted cytoreduction. The median OS was 42.2 months for patients with microscopic disease, 19 months for patients with any residual disease, and 2.2 months for patients who did not have attempted cytoreduction.[311]
  - There are data to support that most stage IIIA patients (adnexal spread from primary uterine disease) adnexal tumors are clonally related metastatic tumors from the primary uterine tumor as demonstrated on genetic analysis.[312]

Overview

- Type II cancers to include p53 abnormal, and some MMRd/NSMP tumors
  - Early-stage type II cancers (serous, CC, or MMMT histology): There are data to support platinum-based chemotherapy in addition to XRT for patients staged IA or above. Of stage IB patients, 77% not treated with adjuvant chemotherapy recurred versus no recurrences in the treated group; 20% of stage (FIGO 1988) IC patients who received chemotherapy recurred versus 80% who did not. Recurrences tended to occur at the vaginal cuff in patients not treated with brachytherapy, thus brachytherapy in combination with chemotherapy was recommended for all patients staged IA (with residual) or higher.[313]

- ○ Maximal cytoreduction for stage IV serous uterine cancer can offer an improvement in survival. Bristow showed that patients with optimal cytoreduction had a median survival of 26.2 months versus 9.6 months in patients with suboptimal surgery. Patients with microscopic residual tumor had a significantly longer median survival of 30.4 months versus those with 0.1 to 1 cm residual disease, who had a median survival of 20.5 months. A 41-month, versus a 34-month, versus an 11-month OS was observed for those patients who were microscopically cytoreduced, optimally cytoreduced to less than 1 cm, or suboptimally cytoreduced, respectively.[310]
- Histologies and treatment
  - ○ Uterine clear cell cancer accounts for about 10% of endometrial cancers and is considered a type II cancer with an ORR to chemotherapy of about 32%.[314] The median 5YS is 20.9% Histologic patterns are solid, papillary, cystic, and tubular. IHC positivity includes CK7, CAM5.2, 34BetaE12, CEA, BCL02, p53, vimentin, leu-M1. PR and CK20 have often been negative. Frequent somatic mutations have been TP53 39%, PIK3CA 23.8%, PIK3R1 15.9%, ARID1A 15.9%, PP2R1A 15.9%, SPOP 14.3%, TAF1 9.5%, MSI 11.3%. with TAF1 being a candidate driver. Of patients, 40% to 50% have extrauterine spread at the time of diagnosis. The prevalence of LN metastasis is about 25% for pelvic and 15% for PA. Overall, SLND has been deemed appropriate. For stage IA/B cancers, chemotherapy can be advised, due to the high rate of recurrence. Brachytherapy is recommended for stages IA/IB following OS outcomes in the NCDB study. Only patients IA <1/2 DOI can discuss observation as an option. The FIRES trial had only 6 cases of CCC on their evaluation. GOG 249 enrolled 28 patients with CCC (5%). PORTEC-3 included only 62 (<10%) CCC. In the TCGA analysis, CCC tumors were not evaluated. For stages III/IV and recurrent CCC, chemotherapy is often recommended but response rates are often low: 25% for monotherapy with doxorubicin, up to 49% for adriamycin/cisplatin, 57% for TAP. GOG 209 only enrolled 46 patients with CCC demonstrating that cisplatin/paclitaxel was not inferior to TAP. In GOG 258, 22 (3%) patients had CCC. EBXRT can be recommended for LN +patients but not for peritoneal involvement. Standard regimens for recurrent CCC are platinum/paclitaxel adriamycin monotherapy, and consideration of immunotherapy or clinical trials, whereas secondary surgery or radiation has limited data and is not often recommended. Basket trials are reasonable options given that similar gene expression exists for CCC regardless of organ of origin.
    - ▪ Stage IA non-invasive negative washings: Observe.
    - ▪ Stage IA noninvasive positive washings: Brachytherapy and systemic therapy Are recommended.

- Stage IA invasive, IB, II: Systemic therapy with XRT (brachytherapy, external beam, or both) is recommended.
- Stage III, IV: Systemic therapy with XRT (brachytherapy, external beam, or both) is recommended.

- Serous uterine cancer: Serous uterine cancer accounts for about 10% of uterine cancers but is responsible for 40% of all uterine cancer-related deaths.[315] Histologically, it has a solid growth pattern with a high mitotic count, nuclear atypia, demonstrating papillae with/without a fibrovascular core, slit-like spaces, and psammoma bodies are present in 30% to 40% cases. By default, it is always high grade. IHC demonstrates positivity to p53, p16, PAX8, AE1/AE3, and CK7 and is negative for Ck20, ER/PR and WT-1. It is MMR proficient in 90% of cases and is considered copy number high on the TCGA nomenclature. Genetic changes include MYC, ERBB2, CCNE1, TP53, and LRP1B deletion (resistance to liposomal doxorubicin) with MMRd in 2% to 6% of cases and PTEN mutation in 11%. Upstaging at the time of surgery via omental biopsy/omentectomy demonstrates stage IV disease in 2% to 17% of cases. For those with bulky abdominal disease, comprehensive LND should not be performed in preference only for removal of bulky LN. Optimal cytoreduction following the premises of HGSTOC can be done, as can NACT principles. Adjuvant therapy with carboplatin and paclitaxel chemotherapy for early-stage disease is supported with or without brachytherapy.[316] Adjuvant chemotherapy for advanced-stage disease with the addition of trastuzumab for HER2+ patients at 8 mg/kg for the first dose and 6 mg/kg in the following cycles is recommended. The addition of radiotherapy in stages III/IV disease can be discussed as well.
  - Adjuvant chemotherapy for early-stage disease: as seen in GOG249 which randomized patients to EBXRT versus chemotherapy/brachytherapy. Fifteen percent of this study consisted of USC patients and showed similar outcomes for OS and RFS as compared with type I cancers, but there was a nonsignificant improvement in the chemotherapy/brachytherapy arm compared to XRT, perhaps due to the low power in the subset of USC patients. Adjuvant chemotherapy for advanced-stage disease is supported by the following: MaNGO ILIADE-III had 14% of patients with USC and combination chemo–XRT improved the PFS. PORTEC-3 had 15.3% of patients with USC and adjuvant chemo radiotherapy versus XRT alone showed an improved DFS and OS specific to USC, yielding a 5YS in 71.4% versus 52.8% with XRT alone, and 5Y FFS of 59.7% versus 47.9%. GOG 258 had 17.8% USC patients and compared XRT/chemo to chemo alone, demonstrating that RFS did not differ, but the numbers were too small to see a difference in the USC subgroup analysis. Treatment for recurrent/PD usually includes chemotherapy +/– immunotherapy, immunotherapy alone, or clinical trial. AntiPDL-1 monotherapy is usually

ineffective. Survival care reserves imaging for patients who are symptomatic or physical exam reveals concerns for recurrence with CT. PET or MRI can be considered selectively and monitoring of CA-125 levels is not supported by clinical trial data.

- Stage IA noninvasive negative washings: brachytherapy
- Stage IA noninvasive positive washings: systemic therapy and brachytherapy
- Stage IA invasive, stage IB, II: systemic therapy with XRT (either external beam, brachytherapy, or both), or EBXRT +/- brachytherapy
- Stage III, IV: systemic therapy with XRT (either external beam, brachytherapy, or both)

- MMMT (CS) used to be classified as a uterine sarcoma. Recent data have suggested an improvement in survival with surgical cytoreduction.[317,318] Uterine MMMT represents 3% to 9% of cases. Fifteen of uterine cancer deaths are due to the MMMT subtype. The mean age at diagnosis is 68Y. Regional or distant metastasis are present in 50% at the time of presentation and 10% to 15% of patients have LN involvement. The 5YS is 56%, 31%, 13%, 0% by stage. The predisposition for diagnosis is 2 to 3 time higher in African American women compared to Caucasian women. Mutational analysis identified TP53 and KRAS as frequent mutations, as well as chromatin remodeling pathways with histones H2A and B contributing to the sarcomatous component transformation. MMRd is rare in this tumor type, as are POLE mutations, which are found in 4.3%. Adjuvant treatment is highly recommended. For stages I and II: There is a 4 × higher death rate when there is no treatment compared to chemotherapy, and 50% of those managed with observation recurred within an average of 6 months from diagnosis to recurrence. An adjuvant XRT trial from the EORTC evaluated a subset of CS patients and found a trend toward improvement in local control with WP-XRT, but there was no improvement in survival.[319] Chemotherapy in combination with XRT has been shown to be effective in treatment of MMMTs. Ifosfamide and paclitaxel have been shown to produce a RR of 45%.[320] There have been no prospective phase III trials on chemotherapy with vaginal brachytherapy to assess superiority. For advanced stages 3/4: GOG trials 108/161/232b have investigated different treatment modalities. GOG 232b was a phase II trial of 46 patients who received paclitaxel/carboplatin that showed an ORR of 54%, a 13% CR, 41% PR, a PFS of 7.6 months and an OS 14.7 months, which was improved relative to GOG 161. GOG261 followed and was a phase III noninferiority study comparing PC to paclitaxel/ifosfamide: It showed the PFS was 16.3 months compared to 11.7 months with an OS of 37.3 months versus 29 months. Paclitaxel/carboplatin was noninferior to paclitaxel/ifosfamide with a trend toward improved OS with superior PFS for PC. A phase II trial of cabozantinib and nivolumab for recurrent uterine cancer included nine patients with MMMT: one patient had PR of 11.9 months and four patients had SD. MMMT checkpoint inhibitors should be considered in MMMT tumors as POLE mutations do not respond to immunotherapy. MEK inhibitors can address those tumors with KRAS mutations, and PI3K inhibitors/mTOR agents can target those with mutations in the PI3K/AKT/PTEN pathways.

○ Stage IA: systemic therapy and brachytherapy with consideration of EBXRT

○ Stage IB, II, III, IV: systemic therapy with XRT (either external beam, brachytherapy, or both)

Recurrence

Recurrent disease can be broken into local recurrence or distant recurrence. Local recurrence is divided into vaginal and pelvic. A full metastatic workup should be performed with a physical examination; imaging of the chest, abdomen, and pelvis; lab tests for baseline organ function; and possibly PET imaging. Patients who were previously radiated in the pelvis tend to fail distantly at 70%, only 16% recur vaginally, and 14% recur in the pelvis. Patients without prior pelvic XRT tend to fail vaginally at 50%, 21% fail in the pelvis, and 30% distantly.

- Molecular analysis:
  ○ If MMR testing has not been previously performed, testing should be ordered.
  ○ If MLH1 loss is identified, promoter methylation should be assessed.
  ○ NTRK gene fusion should be evaluated.
  ○ TMB should be evaluated.
  ○ Her2 status should be evaluated if aberrant TP53 identified.
- If the recurrence is vaginal, XRT can be administered. Prior XRT does affect response. In the PORTEC 1 trial, data on relapsed patients showed a 5YS of 65% if patients had no prior adjuvant XRT versus 19% if they had prior XRT. The treatment of recurrence is WP-XRT in combination with brachytherapy dosed to 75 to 80 Gy if no prior XRT. There are data to support surgical cytoreduction of vaginal lesions to less than 2 cm. This is associated with an improvement in OS to 43 months versus 10 months.[321]
  ○ If no prior XRT to the site of recurrence, then surgical cytoreduction to <2 cm should occur if possible with/without IOXRT, or EBXRT and brachytherapy dosed at 75 to 80 Gy.
  ○ If prior XRT given:
    ▪ And prior brachytherapy only, then EBXRT or surgical resection with/without IOXRT can be provided.
    ▪ If prior EBXRT, surgical resection with/without IOXRT or hormonal therapy, or chemotherapy can be offered.

- For pelvic recurrence, including pelvic LN involvement:
  - Surgical resection can be considered followed by tumor-directed EBXRT with/without chemotherapy.
  - EBXRT with/without chemotherapy
- For extrapelvic recurrences:
  - For isolated recurrence: Surgical resection with/without XRT or ablative therapy can be considered.
  - If upper abdominal recurrence is resectable it should be surgically reduced, chemotherapy should follow, and consideration of EBXRT can be offered.
  - If not resectable and low grade asymptomatic, or ER/PR positive, hormone therapy can be attempted and, if disease progresses, then systemic chemotherapy should be provided. If symptomatic, G 2/3, or there is large volume disease, then chemotherapy with/without palliative XRT should be provided.
  - For widely metastatic disease: If low grade asymptomatic, or ER/PR positive, hormone therapy can be attempted and, if disease progresses, then systemic chemotherapy should be administered. If symptomatic, G 2/3, or large volume disease, then chemotherapy with/without palliative XRT should be provided.
- Different chemotherapy regimens have been used. CAP: cyclophosphamide (500 mg/m^2), doxorubicin (40 mg/m^2), and cisplatin (70 mg/m^2), given every 4 weeks; single-agent paclitaxel at 250 mg/m^2 as 24-hour infusion (has shown a 36% RR); or a combination of paclitaxel (175 mg/m^2) and carboplatin AUC 6, has shown a 40% RR with an 8% CR.[322]
- Hormonal therapies, specifically progestins, have also been used. MPA at a dose of 200 mg/day had a better RR than 1,000 mg/day in the GOG 81 study. The ORR was 25%, and there was a higher response in ER- and PR-positive patients. The combination of megace and tamoxifen showed an ORR of 27%, with 53% of patients responding for longer than 20 months. Megace has also been used at a dose of 80 to 160 mg twice daily with an 18% to 34% RR.[323] For those patients who are ER positive, tamoxifen or an aromatase inhibitor can be considered.
- Targeted therapies:
  - If the patient is *Her-2/neu* positive (usually serous), trastuzumab was found to have a 13% RR in a phase II trial (GOG 181B).[324]
  - Cediranib monotherapy at 30 mg PO daily for a 28-day cycle was evaluated in 48 patients with recurrent or persistent endometrial cancer. The median age was 65.5 Y, 52% had prior XRT and 73% had one prior chemotherapy regimen. A PR was seen in 12.5%. Median PFS was 2.65 months and median OS was 12.5 months and was well tolerated.[325]

- For all tumors that are MMRd/MSI-H or TMB-H, the immune checkpoint inhibitors pembrolizumab or nivolumab can be used (Keynote 158 cohorts D and K).
- The TKI lenvatinib in combination with pembrolizumab can be used for tumors that are MMRp/MSS.
- The addition of bevacizumab to recurrent disease in addition to carboplatin and paclitaxel has not shown benefit.
- HNPCC/MMR-d-confirmed patients: Pertulimuzab has been shown to be an actionable mutation medication.
- Dostarlimab-gxly can be used for MMRd/MMRp.
- Avelumab can be used for MMRd/MMRp.
- Larotrectinib or entrectinib can be used for NTRK gene fusion and tumors.
- Cabozantinib can be used with nivolumab.[326]

Fertility-Sparing Options
- If the patient has fertility concerns, workup should include CT of the abdomen/pelvis; MRI of the pelvis, and pathology should be expertly reviewed. See Chapter 6 for more fertility-sparing options.
- For consideration of fertility preservation, metastatic disease must be absent on workup, no DOI seen on MRI, no contraindications (such as PE) should exist to medical therapy or desired pregnancy, grade must be well differentiated (G1), histology should be endometrioid subtype, and patients should undergo counseling with a reproductive endocrinologist as well as give full informed consent that medical management is not the standard of care.
- Treatment: Continuous progestin-based therapy with megace, medroxyprogesterone, or levonorgestrel IUD. Resampling of the uterus should occur with D&C/EMB every 3 to 6 months. If there is a CR by 6 months, conception can be encouraged. Completion hysterectomy should be offered at the end of desired fertility. If cancer is still present at 6 to 9 months, hysterectomy with BSO and staging is recommended.

Postoperative Hormone Replacement Therapy
Postoperative HRT namely, estrogen, has been studied for QOL and risk of recurrence. GOG 137[327] evaluated estrogen HRT given to women with a history of uterine cancer. There was no increased risk of recurrence identified. (RR was 1.27 80% CI: 0.916–1.77—the CI crossed 1.0, thus careful consideration of outcomes should be applied.)

Synchronous Ovarian Neoplasm
Five percent to 10% of women with uterine cancer may have a **synchronous ovarian neoplasm.** Up to 25% of women under 40 Y can have

this concurrent diagnosis. Concordant endometrioid histology in both the uterus and ovary are present 45% to 86% of the time. There is concordant grade in 69% of patients. Empirical criteria favoring metastatic uterine cancer over a synchronous ovarian tumor are multinodular ovarian involvement, deep myometrial invasion, LVSI, bilateral ovarian involvement, and visualization of intratubal transit. Surgical staging or adjuvant recommendations are based on the worst-case scenario; that is, if the ovarian tumor is G 3 and the uterine tumor is G 1, chemotherapy would commonly be recommended.

Survival
(Tables 2.19A–2.19C)

Follow-Up
- Every 3 months for the first 2 Y
- Every 6 months for the next 3 Y
- Annual examinations thereafter

Table 2.19A Endometrioid Uterine Cancer 5YS by Stage

Stage	5YS Endometrioid (%)
1A	88
1B	75
II	69
IIIA	58
IIIB	50
IIIC	47
IVA	17
IVB	15

Source: Lewin SN, Herzog TJ, Barrena Medel NI, et al. Comparative performance of the 2009 International Federation of Gynecology and Obstetrics' staging system for uterine corpus cancer. *Obstet Gynecol.* 2010;116(5):1141–1149.[407]

Table 2.19B Serous Uterine Cancer 5YS by Stage

Stage	5YS Serous Uterine Cancer (%)
I	66–90
II	50
III	20
IV	5–10

Table 2.19C MMMT/CS Uterine Cancer 5YS by Stage	
Stage	5YS CS (%)
I	70
II	45
III	30
IV	15

- Physical and pelvic examination should occur at each visit. Pap smears have not been found to increase the detection of recurrence, nor has annual CXR. CA-125 can be drawn if it was initially elevated.

Tamoxifen and Uterine Cancer

Adjuvant treatment of pre- and postmenopausal women with hormone receptor positive **breast cancer** has been **tamoxifen**. There are known gynecologic side effects from this medication. Aromatase inhibitors have been evaluated as crossover or primary therapy, replacing tamoxifen treatment. Gynecologic side effects of tamoxifen can be vaginal bleeding, growth of uterine polyps in 8% to 36% of women, endometrial hyperplasia in 2% to 20%, and endometrial cancer ranging from 0% to 8%. The overall risk of subsequent uterine corpus cancer was increased more than twofold (O/E 2.17; 95% CI: 1.95–2.41) relative to the general SEER population in one study. The relative risk was substantially higher for MMMTs (O/E 4.62, O 34; 95% CI: 3.20–6.46) than for endometrial adenocarcinomas (O/E 2.07, O 306; 95% CI: 1.85–2.32), although the excess absolute risk was smaller—an additional 1.4 versus 8.4 cancers per 10,000 women per Y, respectively.

US diagnoses revealed an EMS that is greater than 5 mm in 50% of patients on tamoxifen; but endometrial stripes up to 8 mm can be considered normal in these patients. A routine annual EMB is not recommended. EMB is recommended for women who are symptomatic with abnormal or PMPB or significant atypical vaginal discharge.[328]

Notable Studies in Uterine Cancer

High-Risk Early-Stage Disease Adjuvant Therapy Studies

- Aalders studied 540 patients with stage I endometrial cancer status post TAH BSO, but who were not surgically staged. All received brachytherapy and were randomized to WP-XRT or NFT. There was no improvement in OS. The 5YS was 89% in the EBXRT arm versus 91% in the NFT (NS). Vaginal and pelvic recurrences were 6.9% in the NFT arm versus 1.9% if given pelvic XRT. Distant metastasis occurred more often in the XRT arm. In the subset of patients with stage IC G 3 disease, there were fewer recurrences in the EBXRT arm, 18% versus 7%.[329]

- PORTEC 1: In this study, 715 eligible patients underwent TAH BSO without surgical staging or lymphadenectomy. Patients were included if they had either G 1 disease with greater than 50% invasion, G 2 with any invasion, or G 3 with less than 50% invasion. Less than 2% of histologies were other than endometrioid. Patients were randomized to no additional therapy versus WP-XRT to 46 Gy. The 5Y recurrence rate was 4% versus 14%, favoring XRT (p <.001) and the 5YS was 81% versus 85% (NS). Distant metastasis was similar at 7% and 8%. The 8 Y RFS was 68% for both groups. The 8Y OS was 71% in the XRT group and 77% in the control group (NS) due to salvage of relapse in the NFT arm (85% of vaginal recurrences were salvageable). An HIR subgroup was identified: patient age older than 60 Y, DOI greater than half myometrial thickness, or G 2 or 3 tumor. In this HIR group, the recurrence rate was 23% versus 5%, favoring XRT. Seventy-three percent of recurrences were in the vagina. Survival after recurrence was better for the control group than the XRT group. For the pelvic recurrence patients, 51% were salvaged if they had not received XRT versus 19% if they had received adjuvant XRT. Stage IB G 3 patients had higher rates of distant metastasis (15%). A subgroup of patients staged IC G 3 were not randomized but all received WP-XRT. These patients all had a 5 YS of 58%. A 15-Y follow-up report yielded a median follow-up of 13.3 Y, with a 5.8% locoregional recurrence in the XRT arm versus 15.5% in the NFT arm. Seventy-four percent of these recurrences were isolated vaginal recurrences.[330–332]
- ILIADE II Systemic pelvic lymphadenectomy randomized trial: In this study, 514 eligible patients underwent TH-BSO and were randomized to systemic P-LND or no LND. LND improved surgical staging with 13.3% versus 3.2% of patients identified with LN metastasis. At 49 months of follow-up, the 5Y DFS and OS were 81% and 85.9% in the LND arm and 81.7% and 90% in the no LND arm. There was no improvement in DFS or OS with LND. Researchers found the rate of recurrence in LN beds was 1.5% in each arm; therefore, LN basins were not where patients recurred.[301]
- GOG 99: In this study, 392 eligible patients with type I cancers staged IB, IC, IIA, and occult IIB were evaluated. All were surgically staged with TAH, BSO, pelvic and PALND. Of patients, 75% had endometrioid histology, 80% had G 1 or 2 tumors, 25% had LVSI, and 10% were stage II. Patients were randomized to WP-XRT to 50.4 Gy without brachytherapy, or NFT. Median follow-up was 68 months. The overall recurrence rate was 12% in the NFT group and decreased to 3% with XRT. The OS was 86% in the NFT group versus 92% in the XRT arm (NS). An HIR group was identified, which accounted for 132 patients (one third of those enrolled) and two thirds of the study-related deaths. This HIR group included patients of age ≥70 Y with one risk factor, age 50 to 69Y with two risk factors, and any age with all three. The risk factors were outer one-third DOI, G 2 or 3 tumor,

and LVSI. For this subgroup, the recurrence rate was reduced with adjuvant XRT from 26% to 6%. The major difference was the vaginal vault recurrences: 13 recurred vaginally in the NFT versus two that recurred in the XRT arm, and of these two, both had refused XRT. Five percent in each group had distant metastasis.[333]

- PORTEC 2: This study evaluated 427 patients with stage I or stage IIA endometrial carcinoma with HIR factors. Patients were randomized to pelvic XRT (46 Gy) or vaginal brachytherapy (21 Gy HDR or 30 Gy LDR). The 5-Y vaginal recurrence rate was 1.8% for vaginal brachytherapy versus 1.6% for pelvic XRT. The 5-Y rates of locoregional relapse were 5.1% for vaginal brachytherapy and 2.1% for pelvic XRT. There were no differences in overall or DFS. At 126 months, LVSI and unfavorable molecular alterations (TP53-mutation or >10% L1CAM expression; HR 8.53, 95% CI: 2.7–27.3) and EBXRT (HR 0.16, 95%, CI: 0.04–0.70) were independent prognostic factors for pelvic and locoregional recurrence (HR 0.37, 95% CI: 0.14–0.95 and HR 6.7, 95% CI: 2.5–17.9, respectively), but not for vaginal recurrence. EBXRT should be considered for patients with HIR cancers and tumor with LVSI.[334]

- PORTEC3: This was a randomized, phase III trial of 660 women with high-risk uterine cancer FIGO (2009) endometrioid histology stage IG 3 with deep MI or LVSI (or both), stage II, stage III, or CC or serous histology stages I to III (62UCC 10.6%; 15.3% 101 USC).[335] Assignment was (1:1) to receive WPXRT dosed at 48.6 Gy in 1.8 Gy fractions or WPXRT and chemotherapy starting with two cycles of cisplatin 50 at mg/m^2 given during WPXRT, followed by 4 cycles of carboplatin AUC5 and paclitaxel 175 mg/m^2. The two primary endpoints were OS and FFS; 330 women were assigned to chemo-WPXRT and 330 were assigned to WPXRT with a median follow-up of 60.2 m (IQR 48.1-73.1). 5YOS was 81.8% (95% CI 77.5–86.2) with chemo-WPXRT versus 76.7% (72.1-81.6) with WPXRT (HR 0.76, 95% CI 0.54–1.06; p = .11); 5R FFS was 75.5% (95% CI 70.3–79.9) versus 68.6% (63.1-73.4; HR 0.71, 95% CI 0.53–0.95; p = .022). G 3/4 AE occurred in 198 (60%) patients who received chemo-WPXRT versus 41 (12%) of patients who received WPXRT (p < .0001). Neuropathy (G 2 +) was persistent more after chemo-WPXRT than after WPXRT (20 [8%] women vs. one [1%] at 3 Y; p < .0001). Platinum-based chemotherapy added to WPXRT and followed with adjuvant combination chemotherapy for high-risk uterine cancer did not improve 5YOS, although it did increase failure-free survival. Thus, uterine cancer is not susceptible to chemo sensitization and combination therapy was better for advanced-stage disease (IIIC). It appears that uterine cancer cannot be sensitized with current therapies.[336]

- PORTEC-4: This is a three-arm study that will evaluate approximately 500 patients in a 2:1 fashion with HIR endometrial cancer. Patients are randomized to receive vaginal brachytherapy (either 21

Gy in three fractions vs. 15 Gy in three fractions to 5 mm depth vaginal cuff) versus observation vs. EBXRT stratified on biomarker status. Eligible patients had histologically confirmed endometrioid type endometrial carcinoma, via TH-BSO, FIGO 2009 stage I, with one of the following combinations of substage, age, and G: stage IA, any age and G 3 without LVSI; stage IB, age 60 Y or above and G 1 or 2; stage IB, any age, G 1 and 2 with documented LVSI. NTR3263. Results pending.[337]

- Taxane plus platinum regimens versus doxorubicin cisplatin for high risk uterine cancers.[338] This was a phase III RCT that enrolled patients with stage I/II patients deemed high risk (DOI >50% and G2/3 to include serous/CC/undifferentiated) or stages III/IV that did not extend beyond the abdomen. All patients had LND and residual tumor was 2 cm or less. Patients were assigned 1:1:1 to six cycles of doxorubicin 60 mg/m^2 plus cisplatin 50 mg/m^2 day 1; docetaxel 70 mg/m^2 plus cisplatin 60 mg/m2 day 1; or paclitaxel 180 mg/m^2 plus carboplatin AUC 6 day 1 — every 3 weeks for 6 cycles. The primary outcome was PFS; 788 were patients randomized with a median follow-up of 7 Y showing no difference between groups for PFS. The 5Y PFS was 73.3% for doxo/cis, 79% for docetaxel/cis, and 73.9% paclitaxel/carbo. The 5YOS was 82.7%, 88.1%, 86.1% respectively. The doxo/cis group had more hematologic adverse effects except for thrombocytopenia, which was higher in the paclitaxel/carbo group. GI symptoms were more common is the cisplatin regimens, myalgias and neurotoxicities were more common in the paclitaxel group. The PFS of patients who had LN metastasis was better in the docetaxel/cisplatin and paclitaxel/carbo groups, suggesting tropism for taxanes to LN. Neutropenia was reduced in the docetaxel cisplatin group, and docetaxel/cisplatin was better tolerated than other regimens.

- RTOG-9708: This was a phase II study in 46 patients with high-risk uterine cancer stages I to III cancer who underwent TAH, BSO, +/− LND. High-risk pathologic features were G 2/3, DOI greater than 1/2, and cervical stromal involvement, or pelvic confined extrauterine disease. Patients were given adjuvant pelvic XRT to 45 Gy with concurrent cisplatin 50 mg/m^2 on days 1 and 28. Vaginal brachytherapy was given after EBXRT. Four additional cycles of cisplatin 50 mg/m^2 and paclitaxel 175 mg/m^2 were given every 28 days after completion of XRT. The median follow-up was 4.3 Y. At 4 Y, the locoregional recurrence rate was 4% and distant recurrence rates 19%. OS and DFS rates at 4 Y were 85% and 81%, respectively. For stage III patients, 4Y rates for survival and DFS were 77% and 72%, respectively. There were no recurrences for patients with stage IC, IIA, or IIB.[339]

- JGOG-2033: This study evaluated 385 patients with stage IC to stage IIIC endometrial carcinoma who were randomized to WP-XRT versus cyclophosphamide (333 mg/m^2), doxorubicin (40 mg/m^2), and cisplatin (50 mg/m^2; CAP chemotherapy) every 4 weeks for three or more courses. The 5Y PFS was nearly the same at 83.5% in the pelvic XRT group and 81.8% in the CAP group. The 5YOS was 85% in the XRT group versus 87% in the chemotherapy group (NS). A subgroup of HIR patients—who were defined as having (a) stage IC disease in patients over 70Y of age or having G 3 tumor or (b) stage II or stage IIIA (positive cytology) with greater than 50% DOI—were found to have significantly better outcomes with chemotherapy: The PFS for the XRT arm was 66% versus 84% for the chemotherapy arm, and the OS was 74% in the XRT group versus 90% in the chemotherapy group.[340]

- SEPAL study: In this study, cohorts from two different gynecologic oncology teams totaling 671 patients were retrospectively analyzed with respect to the use of PA-LND. Routine PA-LND was standard practice at one facility and not at the other. Both facilities offered systemic P-LND. A median P-LND count was 34 in the P-LND group versus 59 in the combined PA and P-LND group. Patients at intermediate or high risk of recurrence were offered adjuvant chemotherapy and XRT. The OS was longer in the combination PA and P-LND group with a HR of 0.53. The risk of death was reduced independent of adjuvant therapies so it was recommended that a combined PA and P-LND be performed for all intermediate and high risk patients.[341]

- FIRES trial: This study was a prospective, cohort of clinically stage 1 endometrial cancer patients of all histologies and grades.[288] A robotic approach to MIS was used. ICG was the mapping agent used. The primary endpoint was sensitivity for detection of metastatic disease in the SLN. The study ran between 2012 to 2015, 340 patients underwent SLN mapping followed by complete PLND with PA LND performed in 196 (58%) of patients. 293 (86%) patients were successfully mapped with at least 1 LND. Forty-one (12%) patients had positive LN. Nodal metastases were identified in the SLNs of 35 (97%) of these 36 patients, yielding a sensitivity to detect node-positive disease of 97.2% (95% CI 85.0–100), and a NPV of 99.6% (97.9–100). The FN was 2.8% for endometrioid and 4.3% for G3/serous tumors of whom 89% were successfully mapped.

- GOG 249: In this study, 601 patients were randomized after TH BSO in a phase III trial of WP-XRT versus VCB/C in patients with high-risk, early-stage endometrial cancer. The primary outcome was RFS. All patients were required to undergo hysterectomy. Staging was encouraged, but not required. All patients had stage I endometrioid disease with GOG 33 based high-risk criteria (based on age, grade, DOI, and LVSI), stage II, or stage I and II serous or CC tumors. Patients assigned to WP-XRT were treated with standard four-field or IMRT techniques. Additional VCB was optional for patients with serous or CC tumors or stage II disease. Patients assigned to VCB/C received HDR or LDR brachytherapy followed by paclitaxel 175 mg/m^2 (3 hours) plus carboplatin AUC 6 q21 days for a total of three cycles.

Of the 601 patients, 289 received WP-XRT and 291 received VCB/C. The median age was 63 Y, 74% had stage I disease, and 89% underwent lymphadenectomy; 71% had endometrioid histology, 15% had serous, and 5%[303] had CC. Of patients, 91% completed WP-XRT and 87% completed VCB/C. Recurrence sites totaled 5 versus 3 vaginal, 2 versus 19 pelvic, and 32 versus 24 distant failures with WP-XRT versus VCB/C. The median follow-up was 53 months, the 5Y RFS was 0.76 (95% CI, 0.70 to 0.81) for WPXRT and 0.76 (95% CI, 0.70 to 0.81) for VCB/C (HR, 0.92; 90% CI, 0.69 to 1.23). The 5YOS was 0.87 (95% CI, 0.83 to 0.91) for WPXRT and 0.85 (95% CI, 0.81 to 0.90) for VCB/C (HR, 1.04; 90% CI, 0.71 to 1.52). Recurrence rates for regional and distant sites were similar between arms. Nodal recurrences (both pelvic and PA) were more common with VCB/C (9% vs. 4%). The superiority of VCB/C compared with pelvic XRT was not demonstrated. Acute toxicity was greater with VCB/C while late toxicities were similar[342,343]

- MaNGO ILIADE-III NSGO-EC-9501/EORTC-55991: This was a pooled study from two randomized trials evaluating 534 patients with FIGO 1988 staged I-IIIC (pelvic LN only involvement) endometrial cancer. The primary endpoint was PFS. Patients were randomly assigned to adjuvant XRT with or without sequential chemotherapy. Comprehensive surgical staging with LND was not mandatory and 30% did not have LND. Inclusion criteria were serous, CC or anaplastic tumors by definition. Serous and CC tumors were included in the NSGO/EORTC trial only. Optional vaginal brachytherapy was decided before randomization. Pelvic XRT was given before chemotherapy in the combination arm. Chemotherapy consisted of either four courses of doxorubicin/epirubicin 50 mg/m^2 and cisplatin 50 mg/m^2 every 4 weeks; paclitaxel 175 mg/m^2 and epirubicin 60 mg/m^2, or doxorubicin 40 mg/m^2 and carboplatin AUC 5; or paclitaxel 175 mg/m^2 and carboplatin AUC 5-6 every 21 days. The PFS difference in the NSGO/EORTC trial favored combination XRT and chemotherapy with HR 0.64 (95% CI: 0.41–99; p = .04.) In the MaNGO trial the HR was 0.61 but was NS. When the data was pooled, the HR was 0.63 (95% CI: 0.41–0.99; p = .009) favoring combination therapy. The pooled trial data showed significant differences in cancer specific survival with a HR of 0.55 (95% CI: 0.35–0.88; p = .01). This trial then showed the sequential use of chemotherapy after XRT was associated with a 36% decrease in the rate of relapse or death and a 49% decrease in the rate of relapse or death from endometrial cancer.

- RTOG-0921: This was a phase II study of postoperative IMRT with concurrent cisplatin and bevacizumab followed by carboplatin and paclitaxel for patients with endometrial cancer. Thirty eligible patients with TH-BSO LND and had ≥1 of the following high-risk factors: G 3 carcinoma with greater than 50% DOI, G 2 or 3 disease with any cervical stromal invasion, or known extrauterine extension confined to the pelvis. Treatment consisted of pelvic IMRT and concurrent 50 mg/m^2 cisplatin on days 1 and 29 of XRT and bevacizumab (at a dose of 5 mg/kg on days 1, 15, and 29 of XRT) followed by adjuvant carboplatin AUC 5 and paclitaxel 135 mg/m^2 for four cycles. Within 90 days, 23.3% patients developed G ≥3 treatment-related nonhematologic toxicities; an additional six patients experienced G ≥3 toxicities between 90 and 365 days after treatment. The 2YOS rate was 96.7% and the DFS rate was 79.1%. No patient developed a within-field pelvic failure and no stage IIIA and lower had recurrent disease with a median follow-up of 26 months.[344]

- Surgical–pathological findings in type 1 and 2 endometrial cancer: This NRG Oncology/GOG study was a surgical pathological study of uterine adenocarcinoma or MMMT cancer patients enrolled in GOG 210. In it, 5,866 patients with extra-uterine disease were evaluated and all uterine histologies were included, with 1,630 of the total being type II tumors. Molecular analysis using data from The Cancer Genome Analysis identified certain predictive proteins: 16% of patients were found to have somatic *BRCA* mutations. Tumors with mutations of either *PTEN* and *BRCA2* were associated with improved survival.[345]

Advanced and Recurrent Endometrial Cancer Studies

- GOG 28: This study evaluated melphalan, 5-FU, and megace versus doxorubicin, 5-FU and cyclophosphamide in 358 patients with FIGO stages III and IV or recurrent endometrial cancer. The ORR in those with measurable disease was 38% in both groups; 36% of each group had SD, and only 26.4% progressed on treatment. The OS was 10.6 versus 10.1 months, respectively (both NS).[346]

- GOG 48: This study evaluated 356 eligible patients and compared doxorubicin to the doublet of doxorubicin and cyclophosphamide. All patients had received prior therapy with progestins subsequent to progression of disease. A RR of 22% versus 32% was found and an OS of 6.8 versus 7.6 months was identified with a 17% reduction in the rate of death.[347]

- GOG 94: This trial evaluated 77 stage III/IV type I and 103 type II endometrial cancers. A subgroup (phase II study) of patients with stage I/II serous and CC uterine cancer patients were also evaluated. Treatment was WAR. The 3Y RFS was 29% and 27% for the type I and type II cancers, respectively. The OS were 31% and 35%, respectively. The 5Y PFS was 54%. The OS was 34%. This led to the development of GOG 122.[348,349]

- GOG 107: This study evaluated doxorubicin 60 mg/m^2 versus doxorubicin 60 mg/m^2 and cisplatin 50 mg/m^2 every 3 weeks in 281 eligible patients with stage III/IV or recurrent endometrial cancer. The ORR was 25% versus 42%. The median PFS was 3.8 versus 5.7 months, and the median OS was 9.2 versus 9 months for doxorubicin alone versus the doublet, respectively. The doublet improved response rate and PFS with little impact on OS.[350]

- GOG 122: This trial randomized 400 patients with stage III, IV, and recurrent disease to WAR versus doxorubicin 60 mg/m² and cisplatin 50 mg/m² (AP) for seven cycles plus an additional eighth cycle of cisplatin alone every 3 weeks. Of patients, 85% had a P-LND and 75% had a PA-LND. XRT was dosed at 45 Gy total (30 Gy WAR +15 Gy boost to the PALN and to the pelvis). Eighty-five percent had microscopic residual disease, 25% were stage IV, and 50% were stage IIIC. The PFS HR was 0.71 favoring AP demonstrating a 12% decrease in recurrence at 5 Y with chemotherapy. The OS HR was 0.68 favoring chemotherapy. A 13% increase in OS was seen at 5 Y in the chemotherapy arm. The 5 YS was 53% with chemotherapy versus 42% with XRT.[351]

- GOG 139: This trial evaluated a possible circadian difference in the administration of doxorubicin and cisplatin in 342 patients with stages III, IV, and recurrent disease. No benefit was found to timing the administration of chemotherapy based on increased GSH levels early in the morning. The RR was 46% versus 49%. The PFS was 6.5 months for the standard timed therapy and 5.9 months for the circadian timed therapy. The OS was 11.2 for standard versus 13.2 months for the circadian therapy (both NS).[352]

- GOG 163: This trial evaluated 328 chemotherapy-naïve uterine cancer patients FIGO stages III/IV, or recurrent (prior XRT and hormone therapy not excluded), were randomly assigned to doxorubicin 60 mg/m² followed by cisplatin 50 mg/m² (arm 1, n = 157) or doxorubicin 50 mg/m² followed 4 hours later by paclitaxel 150 mg/m² over 24 hours plus filgrastim 5 mcg/kg on days 3-12 (arm 2, n = 160). Both regimens were repeated every 3 weeks for a maximum of seven cycles. There was no significant difference in RR, PFS, or OS. The ORR in arm 2 relative to arm 1 stratified by PS was 1.12 [95% CI: 0.69–1.79; p = .36, one-tailed]. The median PFS was 7.2 months on arm 1 and 6 months on arm 2. The HR relative to arm 1 was 1.01 (95% CI: 0.80–1.28; p = .46, one-tailed). The median OS was 12.6 months on arm 1 and 13.6 months on arm 2. The death HR relative to arm 1 was 1.00 (95% CI: 0.78–1.27; p = .49, one-tailed) Toxicities were primarily hematological, with 54% (arm 1) and 50% (arm 2) of patients experiencing G 4 granulocytopenia. There was no difference in PFS or OS in either group. The RR was 40% versus 43%; the PFS was 7.2 versus 6 months; and the OS was 12.6 versus 13.6 months (NS).[353]

- GOG 177: This study looked at the combination of paclitaxel 160 mg/m², doxorubicin 45 mg/m², and cisplatin 50 mg/m² (TAP) with G-CSF support versus the doublet of doxorubicin 60 mg/m² and cisplatin 50 mg/m² (AP): 273 patients with stage III, IV, or recurrent disease were treated every 3 weeks for seven cycles or until progression; 50% of patients on both arms received all cycles of therapy. There was a 22% CR in the TAP arm versus a 7% CR on the AP arm and a PR of 36% versus 27%. The ORRs were 57% versus 34%, the PFS was 8.3 versus 5.3 months, and the median OS was 15.3 versus 12.1 months, all favoring TAP.[354]

- GOG 184: In this study, 552 eligible patients with stages III and IV disease were randomized to receive chemotherapy consisting of the triplet of cisplatin 50 mg/m^2, doxorubicin 45 mg/m^2, and paclitaxel 160 mg/m^2 (TAP) versus the doublet of cisplatin and doxorubicin (AP) at the same dosing for six cycles after volume directed XRT. Eighty percent completed six cycles of chemotherapy. No difference in OS was found. The PFS was 64% for the TAP versus 62% for the AP arm HR 0.9 95% CI: 0.69–1.17 p = .21, one-tail). A subgroup analysis found that TAP was associated with a 50% reduction in recurrence or death if there was gross residual disease.[355]

- GOG 209: This noninferiority trial compared carboplatin AUC 6 and paclitaxel 175 mg/m^2 given every 3 weeks for seven cycles to paclitaxel 160 mg/m^2, doxorubicin 45 mg/m^2, and cisplatin 50 mg/m^2 (TAP) with G-CSF support every 3 weeks for seven cycles in 1,312 patients with metastatic or recurrent endometrial cancer. Patients were allowed to receive volume directed XRT. A 14-month RFS was found in each arm (HR: 1.03), with an OS of 32 months versus 38 months, respectively (HR: 1.01). The neurotoxicity was 26% versus 19% favoring carboplatin and paclitaxel, thus this regimen is not inferior to TAP.[356]

- GOG 238: This is a randomized trial of pelvic XRT with or without concurrent weekly cisplatin in patients with pelvic only recurrence of carcinoma of the uterine corpus. The two arms were (a) WP-XRT dosed at 4500 cGy in 25 fractions with interstitial or intracavitary brachytherapy or an external beam boost versus (b) WP-XRT 4500 cGy in 25 fractions with weekly cisplatin at 40 mg/m^2 with interstitial or intracavitary brachytherapy or an external beam boost. Results pending.

- GOG 258: In this phase III study, 707 patients with FIGO (2009) stage III or IVA cancer were eligible.[357] 346 received chemoradiotherapy (CRT) and 361 received platinum-based chemotherapy (CT) only. The median follow-up was 47 months. At 5Y, the KM estimate of RFS was 59% (95% CI, 53–65) in the CRT group and 58% (95% CI, 53–64) in the CT group (HR, 0.90; 90% CI, 0.74 to 1.10). CRT was associated with a lower 5Y incidence of vaginal recurrence (2% vs. 7%; HR, 0.36; 95% CI, 0.16–0.82) and pelvic and paraaortic LN recurrence (11% vs. 20%; HR, 0.43; 95% CI, 0.28–0.66) than CT group, but distant recurrence was more common in association with CRT (27% vs. 21%; HR, 1.36; 95% CI, 1.00–1.86). G 3, or higher AEs were reported in 202 patients (58%) in the CRT group and 227 patients (63%) in the CT group. CRT was not associated with longer relapse-free survival than CT alone in patients with stage III or IVA endometrial carcinoma. Thus, it appears uterine cancer cannot be sensitized with standard therapies.

- MITOEND-2: This was a randomized phase II trial of 108 patients with Stages III/IV or recurrent endometrial cancer.[358] Carboplatin/paclitaxel for six to eight cycles versus carboplatin/paclitaxel/bevacizumab at 15 mg/kg and maintenance until progression or toxicity was assessed. The primary endpoint of PFS showed 10.5 versus 13.7 months (HR 0.84 p = .43) for the control vs experimental groups. ORR was 53.1% versus 74.4% and the OS was 29.7 versus 40.0 months, respectively (HR 0.71 p = .24). These results showed a nonsignificant improvement in PFS for bevacizumab treated patients with results only became significant when an exploratory analysis was used showing an increase in 6 months disease control rate of 70.4% versus 90.7%. There were more HTN and VTE events in the experimental arm (G ≥2 HTN 21% vs 0% and G ≥2 VTE 11% vs 2%) respectively.

- GARNET Study: This was a phase I/II trial in women with recurrent or advanced endometrial cancer using dostarlimab (a monoclonal anti PD-L1/2 antibody). Cohort assignment was based on MMR IHC results. TMB status as a posthoc exploratory biomarker analysis was determined using Foundation One test. TMB-H status was defined as having 10 or more mutations/megabase, and TMB-L status was defined as having less than 10 mutations/megabase. Part 2B included expansion cohorts of evaluable patients with MMRd/MMRp (n = 105) and MMRp/MSS (n = 156). Dosing was at 500 mg IV q3 weeks for four cycles, then 1000 mg IV q6 weeks. The median age was 64 Y. Patients must have progressed on platinum doublet therapy, have received two or fewer prior lines of treatment, have measurable disease at baseline, and naïve to anti–PD-L1 agents. This study enrolled 161 patients with MMRp/MSS disease with dostarlimab. The median age of patients was 64 Y; 53% of patients with MMRd/MMRp status were FIGO staged I/II disease at primary diagnosis (54.3%); and 62.8% of patients in the MMRp/MSS cohort were FIGO staged III/IV. In this cohort, 67.6% of patients had endometrioid G 1/2 histology for cohort A1 and 37.8% had serous histology for cohort A2. Of those who were MMRd/MMRp: 82.9% (n = 87) were TMB-H, 12.4% (n = 13) were TMB-L, and 4.8% (n = 5) were undetermined. Of those who were MMRp/MSS disease: 90.4% (n = 141) were TMB-L, 7.0% (n = 11) were TMB-H status, and 2.6% (n = 4) were undetermined. The median number of mutations/megabase in patients with MMRd/MMRp endometrial cancer (n = 100) was 20.17 (range, 2.52-428.69). TMB-H status and MMRd/MMRp status were ultimately found to have large overlaps between patient populations, and experienced similar RRs at 44.9% and 44.8% (n = 47/105; 95% CI, 0.35–0.55), respectively. ORR of 44.9% (95% CI, 0.35-0.55) was seen in patients with TMB-H status (n = 44/98) versus 13.0% (95% CI, 0.8.–0.19) in (TMB-L) status (n = 20/154). In those with TMB-H and MMRd/MMRp status (n = 39/87), the ORR was 44.8% (95% CI, 0.34–0.56) versus 23.1% (95% CI, 0.05–0.54) in MMRd/MMRp and TMB-L (n = 3/13). In those with TMB-H and MMRp/MSS disease, the

ORR was 45.5% (95% CI, .17–0.77) versus 12.1% (95% CI, 0.07–0.19) for those with TMB-L/ MMRp/MSS disease (n = 17/141).[359]

- XRT salvage for vaginal recurrent disease: WP and HDR brachytherapy were used: 45 Gy of WP-XRT was delivered in 25 fractions and VB was given to a median dose of 23.75 Gy in five fractions. CCR was seen in 95% of patients. 5Y local control, distant control, RFS, and OS were 95%, 61%, 68%, and 67%, respectively.[360]

- Mundt et al. found evidence to support the continued use of locoregional XRT in combination with chemotherapy for high-risk stage III/IV patients. 43 patients were reviewed retrospectively. Patients treated with doxorubicin and platinum chemotherapy alone were found to have a 67% incidence of recurrence; 31% relapsed in the pelvis, vagina, or both, making the case for adding XRT for multimodality therapy.[361]

- GOG 129F: Single-agent paclitaxel was evaluated in a phase II trial for patients with persistent or recurrent endometrial cancer. Paclitaxel was dosed at 200 mg/m^2, and 175 mg/m^2 for patients with prior WP-XRT, every 3 weeks. A 27.3% overall response rate was seen in 44 patients.[362]

- GOG 139S: This study evaluated histology among different uterine cancer studies totaling 1,203 patients from four randomized trials. The response with different combinations of doxorubicin, cisplatin, and paclitaxel was not associated with histology except for the CC subtype (ORR for type I was 44%; type II serous, 44%; type II CC, 32%). A main predictor of OS was histology with the type II tumors having a HR of 1.2 for serous and 1.5 for CC carcinoma. The breakdown of histology by GOG study is; GOG 122 had 50% endometrioid, 20% serous, 5% CC, and 10% mixed histologies; 80% were G 2, 3; GOG 177 had 15% and 19% serous in each arm; GOG 184 had 13% serous in each arm; GOG 99 had none.[363]

- GOG 229H: Phase II study of cediranib, a multitargeted TKI (VEGF/PDGF/FGF) in endometrial cancer. Forty-eight evaluable patients were administered single-agent cediranib 30 mg PO daily for a 28-day cycle. The median age was 65.5Y, 52% of patients had received prior XRT, and 73% of patients received only one prior chemotherapy regimen. PR was seen in 12.5%, 29% had a 6-month EFS. The median PFS was 3.65 months and median OS was 12.5 months.[325]

- Stage 4B uterine cancer: OS is better with hysterectomy even with distant organ metastasis. In this review, 3,197 patients were identified in a cohort study between 2010-14 evaluating OS for patients with uterine cancer with distant organ involvement treated with chemotherapy alone of in addition to TAH.[307] The mean age was 61.9 Y; most patients had lung metastasis (1,544 patients), liver metastasis (851 patients), LN metastasis (497 patients), bone metastasis (249 patients), and brain metastasis (56 patients). Of patients, 1,809 received chemotherapy alone and 1,388 received chemotherapy plus TAH. At 13.4-month median follow-up 13.4 (1.9-54.9), TAH plus chemotherapy was associated with improved survival (univariate HR, 0.57; 95% CI, 0.53–0.62; multivariate HR, 0.59; 95% CI, 0.54–0.65) compared to chemotherapy alone. Subgroup analyses showed that TAH plus chemotherapy was associated with significantly improved survival versus chemotherapy alone for all except LMS (HR, 0.72; 95% CI, 0.51–1.02) or brain metastasis (HR, 0.47; 95% CI, 0.07–3.16). Among surgical patients, 79% (1,091 of 1,388 patients) underwent TAH followed by chemotherapy and had significantly better survival than patients receiving chemotherapy alone (median [IQR] survival, 18.8 [17.0-20.4] months vs. 10.3 [9.7-11.2] months. Of patients, 228 were identified to have received pelvic XRT and 143 had both TAH and XRT, in addition to chemotherapy. Both groups had improved survival over chemotherapy alone (HR, 0.60; 95% CI, 0.51–0.71 and HR, 0.34; 95% CI, 0.26–0.44)

- KEYNOTE-028: Safety and Antitumor Activity of Pembrolizumab in Advanced Programmed Death Ligand 1-Positive Endometrial Cancer.[364] Seventy-five patients with progressive or refractory endometrial cancer after standard cytotoxic chemotherapy were eligible for this study. Patients received pembrolizumab at 10 mg/kg IV every 2 weeks up to 24 months or until progression or toxicity. The primary endpoint was ORR. Thirty-six (48.0%) patients had PD-L1+ tumors, and 24 (32.0%) were enrolled. Three patients (13.0%) achieved PR (95% CI, 2.8%–33.6%); the median DOR was not reached. Two patients were still receiving treatment and showed continued response at time of data cutoff. Three other patients (13.0%) achieved SD, with a median duration of 24.6 weeks. One patient who achieved PR had a polymerase E mutation. Thirteen patients (54.2%) had treatment-related AEs, with four patients having G 3 treatment-related AEs. The median time to response was 8 weeks, and most patients had SD. Most of those who responded had non-MMRp tumors.

- Keynote-146/Study 111: This was a phase Ib/II study of 108 patients with previously treated recurrent endometrial cancer.[365] Lenvatinib dosed at 20 mg daily PO and pembrolizumab at 200 mg IV every 3 weeks were given every 3 weeks. Follow-up was 18.7 months. The ORR_{Wk24} was 38.0% (95% CI, 28.8%–47.8%). For the subgroup MMRp tumors ($n = 11$), the ORR_{Wk24} (95% CI) was 63.6% (30.8%–89.1%) and 36.2% (26.5%–46.7%) in MMS tumors ($n = 94$). The median DOR was 21.2m (95% CI, 7.6 months to NE), median PFS was 7.4 months (95% CI, 5.3 to 8.7 months), and median OS was 16.7 months (15.0 months to NE) regardless of MSI status. G 3/4 AE occurred 66.9%.

- KEYNOTE-775/Study 309 is the confirmatory trial for KEYNOTE-146/Study 111. It evaluated combination therapy for those with advanced endometrial carcinoma with DP following systemic platinum based chemotherapy and who were not candidates for curative surgery or radiotherapy. The primary endpoint was PFR with secondary endpoint of ORR in the all-comer population (MMRp, MMRd), and the MMRp subgroup. 827 (697 MMRp and 130 with MMRd) women with advanced, metastatic, or recurrent endometrial cancer with progression after receiving one prior platinum-based regimen were enrolled. Patients could have received two regimens if one was given in the neoadjuvant and the other in the adjuvant setting. 1:1 random assignment to either pembrolizumab at 200 mg intravenously every 3 weeks for up to 35 cycles in combination with lenvatinib at 20 mg PO once daily, or the chemotherapy treatment of physician's choice consisting of either doxorubicin at 60 mg/m^2 every 3 weeks up to a maximum cumulative dose of 500 mg/m^2, or paclitaxel at 80 mg/m^2 on a 28-day cycle. At a median follow-up at 11.4 months, the lenvatinib/pembrolizumab combination reduced the risk of DP or death by 44% (p <.0001) and the risk of death by 38% in all patients irrespective of MMR status compared to the standard chemotherapy arm. The median PFS was 7.2 months versus 3.8 months (HR = 0.56, p <.0001) and the median OS was 18.3 months versus 11.4 months (HR = 0.63, p <.0001). The ORR among all comers was 31.9% with the lenvatinib/pembrolizumab combination versus 14.7% with doxorubicin or paclitaxel; CR was seen in 6.6% and 2.6%, respectively (p <.0001), and median DOR was 14.4 months versus 5.7 months. A comparable benefit was seen when the MMRp population was reviewed; it was determined that the combination reduced the risk of DP or death by 40% (p <.0001) and death by 32% (p <.0001).[366] Updates in 2021 showed an ORR of 63.6% in the pembrolizumab/lenvatinib arm in MMRp/MMRd patients and a 36.2% ORR in MMRd/MSS patients. Regardless of tumor MSI status, the median DOR was 21.2 months (95% CI, 7.6 months to NE), median PFS was 7.4 months (95% CI, 5.3 to 8.7 months), and median OS was 16.7 months (15.0 months to NE).[366] The 2022 trial updates found that median PFS and OS for combination biologic/immune checkpoint therapy was longer than with cytotoxic therapy at 7.2 versus 3.8 months and 18.3 versus 11.4 months (HR 0.56; 95% CI, 0.47 to 0.66; p <.001; HR, 0.62; 95% CI, 0.51–0.75; p <.001. For the MMRp population: the PFS was: 6.6 versus 3.8 months; HR 0.60; 95% CI, 0.50–0.72; p <.001; and OS MMRp: 17.4 versus 12.0 months; HR, 0.68; 95% CI, 0.56–0.84; p <.001. AEs G3 or higher happened in 88.9% versuss 72.7%.[367]

- A lower starting dose of lenvatinib at 14 mg daily has also been found to have similar efficacy with less toxicity when used in combination with pembrolizumab for recurrent or refractor endometrial cancer.[368]

- Maintenance therapy: For advanced or recurrent disease after completion of platinum/taxane-based therapy with PR/CR. SIENDO trial was a phase III study of 263 stage IV or recurrent patients who received selinexor (XPOVIO) 80 mg PO weekly as frontline therapy versus placebo. The median PFS was 5.7 months versus 3.8 months, yielding a 50% improvement (HR, 0.70; p = .0486), with a 30% reduction in risk of progression or death. p53WT patients had a 62% reduction in risk of DP or death shown by a median PFS of 13.7 months versus 3.7 months (HR, 0.38; p = .0006). AEs were documented as cause for treatment cessation in 10.5% of patients.[369]

- SIENDO/GOG-3055: Selinexor as maintenance treatment for advanced or recurrent (55%) uterine cancer: This was a phase III 2:1 randomized trial of 171 study patients and 88 controls. PFS was 5.7 versus 3.8 months HR .705 p = .024 CI .499–.996. For endometroid histology (55% represented), a significantly better response was seen and those that were p53WT had a 62% reduction in risk of progression or death.[370]

Serous and Clear Cell Studies

- Serous uterine early stage cancer benefits to CT/VBT: This was a retrospective review from the NCDB categorizing 4,602 patients based on GOG249 risk factors and evaluating them for type of treatment using OS as the primary endpoint.[371] Forty-one percent received CT/VBT and 59% received WPXRT. Of the entire cohort, CT/VBT was associated with improved 3YOS at 89.6 versus 87.8 months (HR 1.24, 95% CI, 1.01–1.52 p = .04. A subset analysis of serous uterine histology, CT/VBT (880 vs. 122 patients) showed improved survival, and those with high-grade endometrial patients without LND had a better survival with WPXRT. Only serous carcinoma patients demonstrated a significantly increased HR for death when treated with EBXRT (HR 1.76 95% CI: 1.18–2.64, p = 0.006) compared to CT/VBT. The 5YOS was 79.3% for endometrioid compared to 69.9% for serous tumors (serous histology HR 1.60; 95% CI 1.25–2.05, p <.001). When serous histologies were removed from analysis, there was no difference associated with cancer type.

- A 2016 SEER analysis reviewed 1,188 patients with stage I to II serous uterine cancer and stratified them by adjuvant treatment with brachytherapy, chemotherapy, and both. The 4Y CSM (cancer specific mortality) was significant for survival p = .03 for brachytherapy as well as for chemotherapy p = .002. The 4Y CSM without brachytherapy or chemotherapy was 25%, was 15% with one modality, and 9% if both modalities were implemented. In 601 stage III patients, chemotherapy was significant at p = .002. LND did not predict CSM for stage I to II patients. Thus, combination therapy is of significant benefit for early stage serous cancers and LND may not be of benefit in this histologic subset of uterine cancers.[372]

- Randomized Phase II Trial of Carboplatin-Paclitaxel Versus Carboplatin-Paclitaxel-Trastuzumab in Uterine Serous Carcinomas That Overexpress EGFR HER2/neu: This was a phase II randomized trial of 61 patients with stage 3/4 or recurrent serous uterine cancer that overexpressed HER2/neu receptor. The trial compared CP for six cycles with and without trastuzumab (CPT) at 8 mg initiation dose and 6 mg for maintenance dose every 3 weeks IV. For all patients the median PFS was 8.0 months in the CP arm versus 12.6 months for the CPT arm (experimental; p = .005; HR, 0.44; 90% CI, 0.26–0.76). The median PFS was 9.3 months in the CP arm versus 17.9 months in the CPT arm in the 41 patients with stage III or IV disease undergoing primary treatment (p = .013; HR, 0.40; 90% CI, 0.20–0.80) and 6.0 months for CP versus 9.2 months for CPT for the 17 patients with recurrent disease (p = .003; HR, 0.14; 90% CI, 0.04–0.53).[373]

MMMT-CS Trials

- GOG 108: 194 patients with stages III/IV and recurrent disease were randomized between ifosfamide versus ifosfamide and cisplatin. The RR was 36% versus 54%. The PFS was 4 months versus 6 months with a OR of response 0.73 (p = .02). PFS and survival data suggest that the combination offers a slight prolongation of PFS (RR, 0.73; 95% upper CI: 0.94; p = .02, one-tailed test), but not significant for OS (RR, 0.80, 95% CI: 1.03; p = .071, one-tailed test).[374]

- GOG 150: This trial evaluated 206 patients with stage I to IV optimally debulked CS, and randomized them to WAR with a pelvic boost versus ifosfamide with mesna and cisplatin. The recurrence rate was 58% in the WAR arm versus 52% in chemotherapy arm (NS). There was a significant survival benefit to chemotherapy (HR 0.67) with a 5YS of 47% versus 37%. Recurrence was vaginal in 3.8% of patients who received WAR compared to 9.9% in the chemotherapy arm. The final recommendation was that chemotherapy and vaginal brachytherapy may be the best combination for CS.[320]

- GOG 161: This trial evaluated 179 patients with stage III/IV, persistent, or recurrent disease. Ifosfamide/mesna dosed at 1.6 g/m^2 IV daily for 3 days plus paclitaxel 135 mg/m^2 every 3 weeks was compared to ifosfamide/mesna 2 g/m^2 IV daily for 3 days every 3 weeks up to eight cycles. A higher response rate of 45% was seen with the doublet compared to 29% with the single agent. The PFS was found to be significant at 5.8 versus 3.6 months (a 31% decrease in the HR of death 0.69; 95% CI: 0.49–0.97, p = .3), as was the OS of 13.5 versus 8.4 months (HR 0.71; 95% CI: 0.51–0.97, p = .3), both favoring the doublet.[375]

- GOG 261: 536 patients with uterine MMMT were enrolled with 40% stage 1, 6% stage II, 31% stage III, and 15% stage IV. Eight percent had recurrent disease. Two-hundred twenty-one were randomized to platinum/ifosfamide and 228 to platinum/paclitaxel. The median OS was 29 months vs. 37 months with a HR of 0.87; 90% CI 0.7-1.075. The PFS was 21 vs 16 months with a HR of 0.73. All patients were chemotherapy-naïve in this noninferiority trial. Dosing was ifosfamide 1.6 g/m^2 days 1,2,3 and paclitaxel 135 mg/m^2 versus carboplatin AUC 6 and paclitaxel 135 mg/m^2. Cycles were every 3 weeks for 6 to 10 cycles.[465]

- SEER study: In this study, 1,891 patients with stages I and II MMMT demonstrated that pelvic XRT was associated with a 21% reduction in cancer specific mortality. For patients who did not have an LND, XRT was associated with a 25% reduction in mortality.[279]

- EORTC 55874: This was a phase III randomized trial for 224 patients of adjuvant pelvic XRT versus observation for all early-stage sarcomas. There were 103 LMS, 91 MMMT, and 28 ESS. All patients underwent TAH BSO and washings (166 patients): Nodal sampling was not required and 25% had an LND. Patients were randomized to either observation or pelvic XRT, 51 Gy in 28 fractions over 5 weeks. 112 patients were in each arm. A reduction in local relapse (14 vs. 24, $p = .004$) was seen but no effect on either OS or PFS was seen. The MMMT patients trended toward better local control versus LMS patients, but they had a higher rate of distant metastasis and there was no change in OS with additional XRT.[376]

Surveillance Trials

- TOTEM: Trial Of Two follow-up regimens in EndoMetrial cancer: FIGO stages I to IV endometrial cancer patients who underwent surgical treatment and had CCR confirmed by imaging, were stratified to low or high risk of recurrence and then randomized to INT or MIN follow-up regimens with the final study outcome being OS. Between 2008 and 2018, 1,847 patients were reviewed (60% low risk).[377] Follow-up compliance for scheduled visits averaged 75.3% and was similar between groups. The mean number of exams (laboratory or imaging) was significantly higher in the INT compared to MIN arms (9.7 vs. 2.9, p <.0001). At a median follow-up of 66 months, the 5YOS was 91.3% (90.6% in the INT am vs. 91.9% in the MIN arm HR = 1.12, 95% CI 0.85–1.48, $p = .429$). Comparing the INT versus MIN arms, the 5-Y OS were 94.1% and 96.8% (HR = 1.48, 0.92-2.37, $p = .104$) in the low-risk and 85.3% and 84.7% (HR = 0.96, 0.68-1.36, $p = .814$) in the high-risk group. No significant differences were seen between groups for RFS, (HR = 1.13, 0.87-1.48, $p = .365$). At the time of the relapse most women were asymptomatic (146/228, 64.0%), with a tendency of higher proportions in the INT than in the MIN arm, both in the low group (78.8% vs. 61.1%, $p = .070$) and in the high-risk group (64% vs. 60%, $p = .754$). HRQL was available only for a subgroup of patients (50% at baseline) and did not differ between arms. Intensive follow-up showed a weak advantage for detection of earlier asymptomatic relapses without an improvement in OS for either group or for QOL. Frequent routine use of imaging and laboratory exams in these patients should be discouraged.

- FIGURE: Follow-up In Gynecological Care Units: This study is addressing whether a routine compared with patient-initiated follow-up strategy is superior in patients with uterine MMMT. Results pending.

- ○ ENDAT: Endometrial cancer TFU trial: This study is assessing whether a nurse-led TFU was non-inferior to standard follow-up care. It includes 259 women post-treatment for stage-I endometrial cancer who were randomly allocated to receive traditional hospital-based follow-up (HFU) or nurse-led TFU. Primary outcomes were psychological morbidity and patient satisfaction. TFU was found to be noninferior to HFU. There was no difference between groups in reported satisfaction with information (OR 0.9; 95% CI 0.4–2.1; p = .83) although women in the HFU group more commonly reported longer waiting times for their appointment (p = .001) and that they did not need any information (p = .003). Thus, TFU provides an effective alternative to HFU for patients with stage I endometrial cancer, with no reported physical or psychological detriment. Patient satisfaction with information was high, with similar levels between groups.[378]

Uterine Sarcomas

Characteristics

- Sarcomas arise from the mesodermal tissues of the body. In gynecology, they most commonly originate in the uterus.
- Sarcomas are estimated to comprise 5% to 6% of the total 65,950 uterine cancers in 2022 in the United States.
- Clinically, patients can present with postcoital bleeding, intermenstrual bleeding, an enlarged uterus, or the cancer can mimic a prolapsed fibroid on examination.
- Risk factors include a history of prior pelvic XRT. There may be a hereditary risk component: Those with retinoblastoma have a cumulative risk of 13.1% for developing any STS. Patients with LiFraumeni syndrome (Tp53 mutation) have a 7% to 8% risk of sarcoma at a median age of 44 Y.
- The route of spread can be lymphatic, peritoneal, or hematogenous. Pretreatment workup includes an EMB or D&C, a CXR, CT of the abdomen, pelvis, and chest with particular attention to the lung and liver as 19% of patients with LMS have lung metastasis. Routine preoperative lab tests are important. MRI nor other imaging modalities have been able to distinguish benign from malignant STS.

Staging

- Staging is surgical. This includes hysterectomy, BSO, exploration of the abdomen and pelvis, possible LND, biopsy of any suspicious extrauterine lesions, and omentectomy. WHO histology was updated in 2014. It differentiates LMS, low-grade and high-grade ESS, and undifferentiated sarcoma from AS.[379]

- ○ Staging for LMS and ESS was last amended by FIGO in 2009 (Table 2.20A–D).
- ○ Stage I: tumor limited to uterus
  - ▪ IA: < 5 cm
  - ▪ IB: > 5 cm

Table 2.20A AJCC Staging 8th Edition for ESS and LMS: T Category

AJCC		FIGO
TX	Unable to assess primary tumor.	
T0	Unable to detect presence of primary tumor.	
T1	Tumor is confined within the uterus.	I
T1	**a** Tumor is no larger than 5 centimeters (5 cm).	IA
	b Tumor is larger than 5 centimeters (5 cm).	IB
T2	Tumor has spread beyond the uterus, confined to the pelvis.	II
T2	**a** Tumor has infiltrated the adnexa.	IIA
	b Tumor has infiltrated other pelvic tissues.	IIB
T3	Tumor has extended into the abdomen:	III
T3	**a** One location	IIIA
	b Tumor has multiple locations	IIIB
T4	Tumor has spread into the rectum or bladder.	IVA

Table 2.20B N Category

N	FIGO	N Criteria
NX		Regional LNs cannot be assessed
N0		No regional LN metastasis
N0(i+)		ITCs in regional LN(s) no greater than 0.2 mm
N1	IIIC	Regional LN metastasis

Table 2.20C M Category

M	FIGO	M Criteria
M0		No distant metastasis
M1	IVB	Distant metastasis

Table 2.20D Stage Grouping

I	
IA	T1aN0M0
IB	T1bN0M0
II	
IIA	T2aN0M0
IIB	T2bN0M0
III	
IIIA	T3aN0M0
IIIB	T3bN0M0
IIIC	(T1-T3)N1M0
IV	
IVA	T4(N0)M0
IVB	(Any T)(Any N)M1

- ○ Stage II: tumor extends to the pelvis
  - IIA: adnexal involvement
  - IIB: extrauterine pelvic tissue
- ○ Stage III: abdominal involvement
  - IIIA: invades the abdomen 1 site
  - IIIB: invades the abdomen >1 site
  - IIIC: involvement of pelvic and/or PA-LN
- ○ Stage IV:
  - IVA: involves bladder or rectum
  - IVB: distant metastasis (Table 2.21A–D)
  FIGO staging for adenosarcoma (AS); see Table 2.21A
- There are four main histologic types of uterine sarcoma: LMS (spindle cell, epithelioid, or myxoid), low-grade and high-grade ESS, and undifferentiated sarcoma. More uncommon uterine sarcoma subtypes are AS, PEComa, rhabdomyosarcoma, IMT, Smarca4 deficient uterine sarcoma (SDU), NTRK rearranged sarcoma, Müllerian AS, and UTROSCT.
- LMS is the most common uterine sarcoma. It originates from the uterine smooth muscle. It represents 40% of uterine sarcomas. It can present at any age but most commonly arises in women in their 50s. Only 15% are diagnosed preoperatively with an EMB or D&C.

Leiomyosarcoma
- Histopathology and molecular analysis:

- ○ Stanford criteria are used for histologic diagnosis and include: necessarily cellular atypia, tumor cell necrosis, and/or high mitotic rate (>10 mitosis/HPF).
- ○ IHC is positive for desmin, alpha-smooth muscle actin, and h-caldesmon. Hormone receptors seen on IHC include estrogen and progesterone, which are positive in 40% to 70% of specimens.

Table 2.21A AJCC Staging 8th Edition for AS: T Category

AJCC		FIGO
TX	Unable to assess primary tumor.	
T0	Unable to detect presence of primary tumor.	
T1	Tumor is confined within the uterus.	I
T1	**a** Tumor is confined to the endometrium/endocervix.	IA
	b Tumor has spread into no more than half of the myometrium.	IB
	c Tumor is confined to the endometrium/endocervix.	IC
T2	Tumor has spread beyond the uterus confined to the pelvis.	II
T2	**a** Tumor has infiltrated the adnexa.	IIA
	b Tumor has infiltrated other pelvic tissues.	IIB
T3	Tumor has extended into the abdomen:	III
T3	**a** One location	IIIA
	b More than one location	IIIB
T4	Tumor has spread into the rectum or bladder.	IVA

Table 2.21B N Category

N	FIGO	N Criteria
NX		Regional LNs cannot be assessed
N0		No regional LN metastasis
N0(i+)		ITCs in regional LN(s) no greater than 0.2 mm
N1	IIIC	Regional LN metastasis

Table 2.21C M Category

M	FIGO	M Criteria
M0		No distant metastasis
M1	IVB	Distant metastasis

Table 2.21D Stage Grouping

I	
IA	T1aN0M0
IB	T1bN0M0
IC	T1cN0M0
II	
IIA	T2aN0M0
IIB	T2bN0M0
III	
IIIA	T3aN0M0
IIIB	T3bN0M0
IIIC	(T1-T3)N1M0
IV	
IVA	T4(Any N)M0
IVB	(Any T)(Any N)M1

- ○ Genetic sequencing shows common losses in tumor suppressor genes RB1(10q) and PTEN(13q) with frequent alterations in TP53, RB, ATRX, and MED12. Somatic copy number alterations have been seen with distinct methylation and mRNA signatures and uLMS was noted to have a higher DNA damage response score.
- ○ Signaling pathways that have been identified and upregulated in uLMS include:
  - PIK3/AKT
  - Insulin-like growth factors -1R and -II
- ○ Gene expression studies have identified 3 uLMS molecular subtypes:
  - Subtype I: The conventional subtype, which expresses most genes associated with smooth muscle differentiation, and has a better OS compared to other subtypes.
  - Subtype II: This a less differentiated form and overlaps with undifferentiated pleomorphic sarcomas.
  - Subtype III: This subtype exhibits a preference for the uterus as the anatomic site.

Treatment

- Primary treatment is complete R0 surgical resection:
  - ○ Hysterectomy
  - ○ BSO for peri and postmenopausal women can be recommended although there is no data to indicate that oophorectomy improves OS. The rate of ovarian metastasis is 3%.[380]

- ○ Additional surgical resection of metastatic extrauterine disease identified: if resectable.
- ○ LND:
  - Complete LND is not recommended but enlarged or suspicious LN should be resected.
  - The rate of LN metastasis is 6.6% to 11%.[381,382] BSO has not been shown to affect outcome. Adjuvant pelvic XRT reduces local recurrence but does not change OS.
  - LND has not shown to be of benefit for staging as up to 70% of women with positive LN already have extrauterine disease.[383]
- ○ Uterine morcellation should always be avoided due to its association with intra-operative tumor dissemination and poor OS.
- If a sarcoma is found incidentally after hysterectomy:
  - ○ A second staging surgery should be considered if there was morcellation of the uterus; a supracervical hysterectomy was performed initially (in these cases, the cervix should be removed on reoperation). A second staging surgery for an LND or BSO has not been found to be beneficial.[384]
  - ○ BSO or removal or residual tube/ovary should be considered for ER positive tumor, LGESS, and AS.
  - ○ Consider BRCA testing for uLMS
- Adjuvant Therapy
  - ○ Stage I: Observe.
  - ○ Stage II, III: Consider systemic therapy +/-EBXRT: observation can be considered if negative margins.
  - ○ IVA: Use systemic therapy +/-EBXRT.
  - ○ Stage IVB: Administer systemic therapy +/-palliative EBXRT.

XRT:

- Usually consists of site-directed EBXRT. No XRT is recommended for stage 1.[376] For recurrent disease, IORT and brachytherapy can be added to treatment regimens.

Chemotherapy:

- Chemotherapy can consist of single-agent doxorubicin with an response rate of 25%, single-agent ifosfamide with an RR of 17%, combination ifosfamide and doxorubicin with an RR of 30%, or combination gemcitabine and docetaxel with an RR of 53%. A phase II trial of adjuvant gemcitabine plus docetaxel for four cycles, followed by doxorubicin for four cycles, in women with stage I/II uLMS showed a 2Y PFS of 78% and a 3Y PFS of 58%; but when compared to historical controls, these PFS rates were not superior.[385]
- Antihormone therapies (for LGESS, AS without SO, and ER/PR + sarcomas):
  Aromatase inhibitors can be used for ER/PR +sarcomas, GnRH analogs, and progestins (megestrol acetate and medroxyprogesterone

acetate) as well as fulvestrant. Letrozole has been used in patients with ER +and/or PR +tumors and showed a 3 month PFS of 50%. Thus, hormonal blockade may also be considered for patients with uLMS with low disease burden and an indolent disease trajectory, if their tumors are ER and PR+.[386]

Despite R0 resection the risk of recurrence for high-grade LMS is 50% to 70%.

Metastatic disease:

- Resectable: When considering surgery for metastatic disease, the DFI and isolated sites of disease amenable to complete resection should be considered balanced with risk of morbidity.
- The standard approach after metastatestecomy is surveillance as there is no second-line/adjuvant systemic treatment recommended.
- Unresectable: Systemic treatment continues to be cytotoxic chemotherapy: There is no most recommended chemotherapy treatment.

Early line therapies include:

- Monotherapy with doxorubicin, DTIC, gemcitabine, trabectedin
- Doublets of doxorubicin/ifosfamide, doxorubicin/olaratumab, gemcitabine/docetaxel, gemcitabine/DTIC, or doxorubicin/trabectedin
- Triplet therapy can include gemcitabine/docetaxel/bevacizumab

For isolated lung recurrences, thoracotomy with resection can yield a survival benefit. The 5YS was 43% in one series.[387]

Low-grade endometrial stromal sarcoma (ESS): This is commonly diagnosed in women aged 42 to 53 Y. This tumor represents about 8% of uterine sarcomas and arises from the stromal cells between the endometrial glandular cells. LGESS are characterized by small cells with low-grade cytology and features resembling stromal cells in proliferative endometrium. Mitotic activity is usually low (<5 MF/10 HPF). It cannot be diagnosed by D&C. Final pathology needs to document LVSI and invasion. If one of these two components is absent, then the diagnosis is an endometrial stromal nodule. There is a 20% risk of pelvic LN metastasis, so consideration of a LND should be entertained. Removal of the ovaries is recommended as these are hormone-dependent cancers and can respond to endogenous estrogen. Reoperation for BSO and LND, if ESS was an incidental finding, should be performed if the ovaries were not initially resected. Stage is the most important prognostic factor. Twenty percent of recurrences have been documented in the pelvis.

- Adjuvant Therapy
  - Stage I: Ensure BSO, consider observation (preferred) versus hormonal therapy.
  - Stage II-IVA: Perform BSO with antihormone therapy +/-EBXRT.

○ Stage IVB: Consider hormonal therapy with or without palliative XRT or systemic therapy.

○ Hormonal therapy can include: Megace (40–160 mg daily), which has shown an 88% RR with a 50% CR (88). Aromatase inhibitors and GnRH agonists may also be considered. ERT may increase the chance of recurrence. For recurrent disease, a 33% RR was seen with ifosfamide and doxorubicin. Aromatase inhibitors can also be considered in these tumors.

Radiation: There are data to show that 33.3% of recurrences are pelvic only, if no adjuvant XRT was given—so pelvic XRT can be considered.

High-grade ESS: This is characterized by small cells with high-grade cytology, frequent necrosis, and brisk mitotic activity (>10 MF/10 HPF). HGESS can contain areas of conventional LGESS. Adjuvant therapy is based on stage:

Stage 1: Observe or consider systemic therapy.
Stage II, III: Consider systemic therapy and/or EBXRT.
Stage IVA: Use systemic therapy +/-EBXRT.
Stage IVB: Use systemic therapy +/-palliative EBXRT.

Undifferentiated uterine sarcoma (UUS): This is characterized by cells with high-grade cytologic features lacking any resemblance to the stromal cells in proliferative endometrium or any other specific type of determination. Adjuvant therapy is based on stage: chemotherapy should be considered with a single agent or combination agents to include doxorubicin, ifosfamide, cisplatin, gemcitabine, and docetaxel. Responses to chemotherapy can occur but at low rates.

• Stage I: Observe.
• Stage II, III: Consider systemic therapy +/-EBXRT. Observation may be considered if negative margins.
• Stage IVA: Use systemic therapy +/-EBXRT
  ○ Stage IVB: Use chemotherapy +/-palliative EBXRT

Adenosarcoma: This represents 1% of uterine sarcomas. The median age of diagnosis is 50 Y old. Abnormal bleeding is common and speculum examination can visualize tumor in 50% of cases. These are mixed tumors with sarcomatous stroma and benign epithelium with a favorable prognosis unless sarcomatous overgrowth (SO) or stromal invasion is present. They stain for CD10 and express ER/PR. Extrauterine disease occurs in 20% of cases, staging is appropriate, and BSO should be considered. These are low-grade malignancies, and if they recur do so locally. Those with SO may have distant metastasis. Twenty percent can recur more than 5 Y after surgery. There is an increased risk of recurrence if deep MI is present. Adjuvant XRT and chemotherapy for the subsets of SO or deep stromal invasion can be considered. Ifosfamide, plus doxorubicin, and/or cisplatin or gemcitabine plus docetaxel have produced a few responses for metastatic or recurrent disease. Consider XRT and chemotherapy for SO, heterologous elements, or deep stromal invasion.

- Stage I: Perform BSO with observation.
- Stage II, III, IV.
  - No SO: Perform BSO, consider antihormone therapy, +/-EBXRT.
  - With SO: Perform BSO, consider systemic therapy (cytotoxic, biomarker, or targeted) and consider EBXRT.

Prognostic factors: R0 resection is the most important prognostic factor. Following that, stage ranks second, but other factors, including grade, tumor size, tumor DOI, morcellation, extrauterine spread, mitotic index, patient age, and hormone receptor status can all affect outcome.
5YS

- Overall by FIGO stage: Stage I is 76%; stage II, 60%; stage III, 45%; and stage IV, 29% (Tables 2.22, 2.23, and 2.24).

Follow-Up
- Every 3 months for the first 2Y
- Every 6 months for the next 3Y
- Annual examinations thereafter

Table 2.22 Uterine LMS 5YS

Stage	LMS 5YS (%)
Localized	63
Regional	36
Distant	14

Table 2.23 Uterine ESS 5YS

Stage	ESS 5YS (%)
Localized	99
Regional	94
Distant	69

Table 2.24 Uterine Undifferentiated Sarcoma 5YS

Stage	Undifferentiated 5YS (%)
Localized	70
Regional	43
Distant	23

- Physical and pelvic examination should occur at each visit. Pap smears have not been found to increase the detection of recurrence. CT imaging of the chest/abdomen/pelvis can occur every 3 to 6 months for 2 to 3 Y, then every 6 months for the next 2 Y, then annually for high-grade sarcomas.

Recurrent disease: Local recurrence in the vagina or pelvis with negative CT of the chest/abdomen/pelvis:

- If prior XRT:
  - Surgical exploration and resection with/without IOXRT with/without systemic therapy *or*
  - Systemic therapy *or*
  - Tumor-directed re-irradiation
- If no prior XRT:
  - Surgical exploration with resection and/or IOXRT
  - Tumor-directed XRT with/without systemic therapy can also be offered.

Isolated distant metastasis:

- If resectable: Consider resection or ablative therapy and consider postoperative systemic therapy with/without EBXRT.
- If unresectable: Consider systemic therapy and/or tumor directed EBXRT or local ablative therapy. If there is response, surgical resection can be considered.

If disseminated disease:

- Systemic therapy with/without palliative XRT:
  - Second-line regimens to consider are:
    - Monotherapy with doxorubicin, trabectedin, DTIC, liposomal doxorubicin, gemcitabine, eribulin, temozolomide, ifosfamide, epirubicin, or eribulin
    - Doublets can include gemcitabine/docetaxel, doxorubicin/ifosfamide, gemcitabine/DTIC, gemcitabine/vinorelbine, and trabectedin/doxorubicin.
    - Or a triplet of gemcitabine/docetaxel/trabectedin can be used.

Targeted, Biologic, and Immunotherapies

- Small molecule agents alone or in combination continue to be evaluated:
- Pazopanib is one that has shown some success. Pazopanid versus placebo showed modest efficacy in a subgroup analysis of uLMS with an RR of 11%, PFS of 3 months, and an OS of 17.5 months. In the larger trial of STS, an overall improvement in PFS of 4.6 months compared to 1.6 months was seen, with no difference in OS, and ORR was observed in only 4% of patients.[388]

- Checkpoint inhibitors/immunotherapy is "not warranted" for general use at this time for uLMS despite case reports of responses to single-agent PD-L1 antibodies.[389] But recent guidelines state pembrolizumab is appropriate for TMB-H tumors, larotrectinib or entrectinib for NTRK gene fusion positive tumors are acceptable.
- Parp-inhibitors can be used for BrCA2 uLMS tumors.

Notable Studies in Sarcoma

- ESS: In a retrospective review, overall there was a 64% recurrence. The 10Y PFS was 43%, with an OS of 85%. Those who received HRT had an ORR of 27% and 53% had SD with a median TTP of 24 months. Of those without BSO, 89% had recurrence, 55% who had a BSO did not recur; 32% had LVSI so LND may be beneficial.[390]
- Another retrospective study evaluated ESS stage I and II. There were no relapses in those who received adjuvant XRT, 13 of 30 relapsed if no XRT was administered. Thus, pelvic EBXRT may improve local control but may not affect OS.[391]
- GOG 277: This was a phase III, double-blind, placebo-controlled trial in patients with chemotherapy-naive, metastatic, unresectable uterine LMS. Of 107 patients enrolled, 54 were randomized to gemcitabine–docetaxel plus placebo and 53 to gemcitabine–docetaxel plus bevacizumab. Accrual was stopped early for futility. The gemcitabine–docetaxel—placebo group compared to the gemcitabine–docetaxel—bevacizumab group had median PFS of 6.2 months and 4.2 months, respectively (HR 1.12; p = .58). Objective responses were seen in 31.5% in the gemcitabine–docetaxel—placebo group and 35.8% in the gemcitabine–docetaxel—bevacizumab group. The mean response duration was 8.6 months versuss 8.8 months. The median OS was 26.9 months versuss 23.3 months (HR 1.07; p = .81).
- PALETTE: In a multicenter, international, double-blind, placebo-controlled phase III trial, patients with metastatic STS (all sites) who were angiogenesis inhibitor-naïve, and had failed at least one anthracycline containing regimen, were eligible. A total of 369 patients were randomized (246 pazopanib, 123 placebo), 2:1 to receive either pazopanib 800 mg once daily or placebo until tumor progression, unacceptable toxicity, death, or patient's request. The median age was 56. Median duration of follow-up at clinical cutoff date was 15 months. The primary endpoint was PFS. PFS was significantly prolonged with pazopanib (median 20 vs. 7 weeks; HR 0.31; 95% CI: 0.24–0.40; p <.0001). The interim analysis for OS showed a NS improvement of pazopanib versus placebo (median: 11.9 vs. 10.4 months; HR 0.83; 95% CI: 0.62–1.09). Main grade 3 to 4 toxicities in the pazopanib versus placebo arm were, respectively, fatigue (13%, 6%), HTN (7%, nil), anorexia (6%, nil), diarrhea (5%, 1%), thromboembolic events (grades 3–5) (3%, 2%), and LVEF decrease of greater than 15% (8% and 3%). Thus, pazopanib is an active drug

in anthracycline-pretreated metastatic STS patients with an increase in median PFS of 13 weeks.[388]

- SAR-3007: This was a subgroup analysis of recurrent uterine LMS patients after prior chemotherapy evaluating trabectedin versus DTIC. This phase III study randomized in a 2:1 fashion 577 LMS and liposarcoma patients; 140 uterine LMS patients were in the trabectedin arm versus 81 uterine LMS in the DTIC group. Dosing was 1.5 mg/m^2 as a 24-hour infusion for every 3 weeks versus DTIC 1 g/m^2 IV every 3 weeks. The PFS was 4.2 months versus 1.5 months with the OS was 13.4 versus 12.9 for trabectedin versus DTIC, respectively.[392]

- Study 309: This trial randomized 452 sarcoma patients to eribulin 1.4 mg/m^2 IV days 1 and 8 q21 days or DTIC 850–1200 mg/m^2 IV day 1 q21 days until progression. 228 patients were randomized to eribulin and 224 patients were given DTIC. OS in the DTIC group was a median of 13.5 months compared to 11.5 months in the eribulin group (95% CI: 10.9–15.6; HR 0.77; 95% CI: 0.62–0.95; p = .0169). Adverse effects were seen in 97% of those in the DTIC group and 99% in the eribulin group.[393]

- From the PALETTE and EORTC 62043 trials: Forty-four uterine sarcoma patients who were treated with pazopanib were reviewed; 61.3% were heavily pretreated with greater than 2 lines of chemotherapy, 11% had a PR. Median PFS was 3 months, median OS was 17.5 months. Response to pazopanib was similar for uterine sarcoma compared to non uterine STS.[394]

- A one-arm study of nivolumab in patients with advanced uLMS, closed after the first stage of accrual (12 patients) for lack of efficacy, as this study demonstrated no objective responses with a median PFS of 1.8 months.[395]

- A single-arm phase II trial that combined pembrolizumab with metronomic cyclophosphamide in STS, showed benefit in patients with LMS and a PFS of 1.4 months.[396]

- This randomized phase II study evaluated nivolumab versus nivolumab/ipilimumab in patients with STS. Patients with LMS comprised one third of 85 total patients. The ORR was 3% in the nivolumab arm and 16% in the nivolumab plus ipilimumab arm. Among the eight patients who achieved a response, three had LMS. The observed PFS was 2.1 months with nivolumab and 4.4 months with nivolumab/ipilimumab.[397]

- TAXOGEM: This was a randomized, phase II trial of gemcitabine versus the doublet gemcitabine/docetaxol in 90 patients with metastatic or relapsed LMS showed ORR of 19% in arm A (gemcitabine) and 24% for arm B (gemcitabine plus docetaxel), which was NS. The median PFS for arm A was 5.5 months and 4.7 months for arm B.[398]

- The phase III trial of gemcitabine and docetaxel versus doxorubicin as first-line treatment in previously untreated advanced unresectable or metastatic soft-tissue sarcoma (GeDDiS) did not observe differences in RR or PFS in 257 patients. Patients were randomized with n = 129 to doxorubicin and n = 128 to combination therapy. The median follow-up was 19 months, 61% were female; and the median age was 55 Y. Of the cohort, 27% had LMS. The median PFS was 23 versus 24 weeks, respectively, but the HR was 1.28 (95% CI 0.98–1.67, p = .07) favoring doxorubicin. The median OS was 71 versus 63 weeks (HR = 1.07; 95% CI 0.77–1.49) again favoring doxorubicin.[399]

- Doxorubicin/olaratumab has demonstrated an OS benefit compared to doxorubicin alone in a large phase II STS study, but the number of LMS patients was low, and a confirmatory phase III trial is pending.[400]

- Trabectedin as second-line therapy was approved via a phase III trial in 518 (345/173)patients with unresectable or metastatic disease who received a prior anthracycline-containing regimen. Trabectedin showed a median PFS compared to DTIC of 4.2 versus 1.5 months; HR, 0.55; p < .001). The OS interim analysis showed a median OS of for trabectedin versus DTIC 12.4 versus 12.9 months; HR, 0.87; p = .37 for trabectedin versus DTIC. Trabectedin superiority over DTIC was shown in PFS, but not in ORR or OS.[392]

- The efficacy and safety of trabectedin in 577 uLMS patients who were randomized 2:1 showed a PFS of 4.0 months compared to 1.5m for DTIC (HR = 0.57; 95% CI 0.41–0.81; p = .0012). The OS was similar (trabectedin 13.4 months compared to DTIC at 12.9 months, HR = 0.89; 95% CI 0.65–1.24; p = .51). The ORR was 11% versus 9% respectively (p = .82). The median DOR was 6.5 months for trabectedin versus. 4.1 months for DTIC (p = .32).[401]

- Another study of 431 patients with LMS of any origin who were treated in a trabectedin expanded access program demonstrated an ORR of 7.5% in patients with LMS compared with 5.9% among patients with all-type STS.[402]

- Patients with L-sarcomas (LMS and liposarcomas) obtained a higher clinical benefit rate (54%) and median OS (16.2 months) than did patients with non–L-sarcomas (38% and 8.4 months, respectively). Trabectedin also demonstrated activity as a first-line treatment in LMS or uLMS, either alone or in combination with doxorubicin in two nonrandomized phase II trials.[403,404]

- A randomized trial of trabectedin plus doxorubicin compared with doxorubicin alone demonstrated no improvement in RRs (17% in both arms) or PFS (5.7 months vs. 5.5 months in 115 patients.[405]

- A phase III trial for L-sarcomas with eribulin (n = 228) demonstrated superior OS benefit compared with DTIC, (n = 224). OS was significantly improved in patients assigned to eribulin versus DTIC (median 13.5 months [95% CI 10.9–15.6] vs. 11.5 months [9.6-13.0]; HR 0.77 [95% CI 0.62–0.95]; p = .0169). The FDA approved eribulin for liposarcoma but not uLMS.[393]

- In this study, 309 patients with LMS were randomized 1:1 to eribulin, n = 157; or DTIC, n = 152. The median age was 57; 42% of patients had uterine disease. The median OS was 12.7 months versus 13 months for eribulin versus DTIC, respectively (HR = 0.93 [95% CI 0.71–1.20]; p = .57). The median PFS was 2.2 versus 2.6 months, HR = 1.07 [95% CI 0.84–1.38]; p = .58) and the ORR (5% vs. 7%) were similar between eribulin and DTIC cohorts. Thus, the efficacy of eribulin in patients with LMS was similar to DTIC.[406]

VULVAR CANCER

Characteristics

- Vulvar cancer represents 3% to 5% of all female genital cancers and 1% of all malignancies in women. In 2022, there are 6,330 new cases and 1,560 deaths predicted. The average age at diagnosis is 65 Y, although it is trending toward a younger age.
- Clinical features include pruritus, ulceration, or a mass. The most common location of lesions is the labia majora (40%), the labia minora (20%), periclitoral region (10%), and perineal area (15%). The route of spread is either by direct extension, lymphatic embolization to the groin nodes, or lymphatic or hematogenous spread to distant sites.
- Risk factors are multifactorial: Age greater than 70 Y, lower SES, HTN, diabetes, prior lower genital tract dysplasia or cancer, immunosuppression, and HPV infection are known to increase the risk of vulvar cancer. Vulvar SIL/dysplasia is the precancerous state and 76% of patients with vulvar HSIL are HPV positive. There is a 22% rate of subclinical invasive disease in vulvar HSIL, usually less than 1 mm DOI.[408]
- Groin LN metastasis: subclinical LN metastasis can occur in 10% to 36% of normally palpated groins.[409] Clinical staging clearly understages patients. On the contrary, 20% of palpably enlarged LNs are pathologically negative; 28% of patients with positive groin LNs will have positive pelvic LNs.
- The risk for nodal metastasis is related to both DOI and tumor size. The risk of positive LNs with 1 mm DOI is minimal at less than 1%. For a DOI of 2 mm, the risk is 7% to 8%. For a DOI of 3 mm, the risk is 12% to 17%. For a DOI of 5 mm, there is a 15% to 17% risk of LN metastasis. The risk of LN metastasis by lesion size is significant: for a size of 0 to 1 cm, there is a 7.7% risk of positive LNs; for a 2-cm lesion, the risk Is 22%; for a 3-cm lesion, the risk is 27%; and for a 5-cm lesion, the risk is 35% to 40%.[410]

Histology

- Squamous cell carcinoma represents 85% of all vulvar cancers. Other histologic types are basal cell carcinoma, AC, sarcoma, verrucous carcinoma and melanoma.

- Malignant melanoma represents 5% of vulvar cancers. There are four histologic subtypes of melanoma: superficial spreading, lentigo, acral, and nodular.
- Vulvar Paget's disease has cutaneous and noncutaneous (bladder/colorectal) subtypes. Underlying invasive AC is present in 4% to 17% of cases; 30% to 42% of patients may have, or will later develop, an AC at another nonvulvar location such as the breast, rectum, colon, or uterus.
- Grading: FIGO grading is the most commonly used grading system and is as follows:
  - G1: Well differentiated
  - G2: Moderately differentiated
  - G3: Poorly differentiated or undifferentiated
- GOG grading in vulvar cancer is slightly different than for other tumors. G1 tumors are well differentiated, G2 tumors are composed of less than one third of G3 cells. G3 tumors are composed of greater than one third yet less than one half of G3 cells. G4 tumors have greater than one half of the tumor composed of G3 cells.
- The DOI is measured from the epithelial–stromal junction of the adjacent most superficial dermal papilla to the deepest point of invasion.

Pretreatment Workup
- Pretreatment workup includes a physical exam with careful evaluation of the vagina and cervix. Five percent of invasive lesions are multifocal. Biopsy for diagnosis should occur at the center of any suspicious area.
- Imaging with CT, MRI, or PET can be obtained if positive groin or pelvic LNs are suspected. If no LN metastases are suspected, CT is not recommended. Preoperative abdominal inguinal CT is of limited value for surgical decision-making and, for tumors <4 cm, may be omitted due to low diagnostic accuracy and unrelated incidental findings.[411] CXR should be obtained, as well as standard laboratory tests. EUA with cystoscopy can assist in determination of the extent of an anterior lesion's involvement of the urethra. Proctoscopy can be helpful in determination of anorectal involvement if there is a large lesion impinging on the posterior perineal triangle.
- SPECT/CT has been shown to improve SLND by preoperative three-dimensional anatomical localization. In preoperative imaging, SPECT/CT was shown to identify more LNs (mean 8.7 LN per patient) versus lymphoscintigraphy (mean 5.9) and led to high spatial resolution and anatomical localization. It also identified aberrant lymphatic drainage in 17.5% of patients. Aberrant LNs were found in the following locations: 31.7% pelvic, 2% paravesical, 7.5% PA, 2% gluteal. Sensitivity

for all who underwent complete groin LND was 100%, NPV 100%, the FN rate was 0%. For dissection, distances were calculated from the ASIS or symphysis based on SPECT/CT.[412]

- If the groin LNs appear positive, FNA can be considered before a groin LND. If cytology from the FNA is positive, then aggressive surgical removal of bulky LNs should be considered because the usual doses of EBXRT are not adequate to control large-volume disease. There is no need to perform a complete LND in light of bulky LNs; instead, remove the bulky disease and mark the area with hemoclips before XRT. If the LNs are fixed and unresectable, consider NACT and XRT.

- The workup for melanoma is CT of the chest/abdomen/pelvis, MRI of the brain, LDH, and baseline PET. *BRAFV600E* gene mutation information should be obtained via IHC on the tumor.

Staging

- Vulvar cancer is staged **surgically** and last updated by FIGO in 2021. FIGO modifies the staging systems and the TNM categories have been defined to correspond to the FIGO stages; however, updated AJCC staging for vulvar cancer has not been updated to correlate with 2021 staging at the time of publication (Table 2.25).

- Melanoma is surgically staged in a similar fashion. There are a few different methods of staging. Stage is the most important prognostic factor. Breslow's staging is used by the AJCC because it is more reproducible and better for ulcerated lesions.
  - Stage (Table 2.26):
    - Chung's staging has replaced Clark's staging because it did not take into account that vulvar skin is non–hair-bearing and contains less SC tissue.
    - **Stage grouping**: See Table 2.27A–D.
    - **Mitotic rate** assessment: A higher mitotic rate is proportional to growth and spread (Table 2.28).

Treatment

- Management of squamous cell and adenocarcinomas has been wide radical excision (radical hemi/vulvectomy) with a 1-cm to 2-cm gross margin with groin (S)LND. For lesions that invade less than a depth of 1 mm, the groin LND can be omitted. If the lesion is lateral (more than 2 cm from the midline), dissection of the contralateral groin can be omitted. If the lesion is midline, or within 2 cm of a midline structure, a bilateral groin (S)LND has standardly been performed.
  - Early-stage T1 and ≤4 cm T2 lesions:
    - Less than 1 mm DOI: wide local resection

Table 2.25 2021 FIGO Staging: Carcinoma of the Vulva

FIGO Stage	Description
Stage I	Tumor confined to the vulva and/or perineum; multifocal lesions should be designated as such
• IA	Lesions 2 cm or less, confined to the vulva and/or perineum, and with stromal invasion of 1.0 mm or less
• IB	Lesions more than 2 cm, or any size with stromal invasion of more than 1.0 mm, confined to the vulva and/or perineum
Stage II	Tumor of any size with extension to adjacent perineal structures (lower/distal third of the urethra, lower/distal third of the vagina, anal involvement) with negative nodes
Stage III	Tumor of any size with extension to upper adjacent perineal structures or with any positive nonulcerated unfixed inguino-femoral lymph nodes
• IIIA • IIIB • IIIC	• Tumor any size with extensin to upper 2/3 of vagina or urethra, bladder or rectal mucosa, or inguino-femoral LN metastases ≤5 mm • Regional LN metastasis > 5mm • Regional LN metastases with extracapsular spread
Stage IV	Tumor of any size with distant metastasis, or fixed to the pelvic bone, or ulcerated, or fixed regional LN metastasis
• IVA	Tumor with disease fixed to the pelvic bone or ulcerated or fixed regional LN metastasis
• IVB	Distant metastasis (including pelvic LN metastasis)

Source: From Olawaiye AB, Cotler J, Cuello MA, et al. FIGO staging for carcinoma of tge vulva. *Int J Gyn Obst*. 2021;155(1),43–47.

Table 2.26 AJCC/FIGO Staging of Vulvar Cancer

Stage	Clark's Level	Chung's Level	Breslow's Level/Depth
I	Intraepithelial	Intraepithelial	<0.76 mm
II	Papillary dermis	<1 mm from granular layer	0.76–1.5 mm
III	Fills dermal papillae	1.1–2 mm from granular layer	1.51–2.25 mm
IV	Reticular layer	>2 mm from granular layer	2.26–3 mm
V	SC fat	SC fat	>3 mm

- Greater than 1 mm DOI: wide radical excision or modified radical vulvectomy with:
  - SLND or complete inguinal–femoral LND
  - SLND should not be offered for tumors >4 cm in size.
- Larger T2 and T3 lesions treat with neoadjuvant chemoradiation stratified by radiology imaging to evaluate LN status.
  - If radiologically negative:
    - Can offer EBXRT to primary tumor/groins/pelvis with concurrent platinum-based chemotherapy.
    - Perform complete groin LND:
      - If positive LN: EBXRT to primary tumor/groins/pelvis with concurrent platinum-based chemotherapy
      - If negative: EBXRT to primary tumor (and selectively omit EBXRT to groin LN) with concurrent platinum-based chemotherapy.

Table 2.27A AJCC 8th Edition Staging: Melanoma T Category

T	Thickness	Ulceration Status
TX: Primary tumor thickness cannot be assessed (diagnosis was by curettage)	NA	NA
T0: No evidence of primary tumor (unknown primary or completely regressed)	NA	NA
Tis: (melanoma in situ)	NA	NA
T1	≤1.0 mm	Unknown or unspecified
T1a	<0.8 mm	Without ulceration
T1b	<0.8 mm 0.8–1.0 mm	With ulceration Without ulceration
T2	>1.0–2.0 mm	Unknown or unspecified
T2a	>1.0–2.0 mm	Without ulceration
T2b	>1.0–2.0 mm	With ulceration
T3	>2.0–4.0 mm	Unknown or unspecified
T3a	>2.0–4.0 mm	Without ulceration
T3b	>2.0–4.0 mm	With ulceration
T4	>4.0 mm	Unknown or unspecified
T4a	>4.0 mm	Without ulceration
T4b	>4.0 mm	With ulceration

Table 2.27B AJCC 8th Edition Staging: Melanoma N Category

N	Number of Tumor-Involved Regional LN (s)	Presence of In-Transit, Satellite, and/or Microsatellite Metastases
NX	Regional nodes not assessed (SLND not performed, regional nodes previously removed for unrelated reason. Exception: pathological N category is not required for T1 melanomas, use clinical N	No
N0	No regional metastases	No
N1	One tumor-involved node or in-transit, satellite, and/or microsatellite metastases with no tumor- involved nodes	No
N1a	One clinically occult LN (i.e., detected by SLND)	No
N1b	One clinically detected LN	No
N1c	No regional LN disease	Yes
N2	Two or three tumor-involved nodes or in-transit, satellite, and/or microsatellite metastases with one tumor-involved node	
N2a	Two or three clinically occult (i.e., detected by SLND)	No
N2b	Two or three, at least one of which was clinically detected	No
N2c	One clinically occult or clinically detected	Yes
N3	Four or more tumor-involved nodes or in-transit, satellite, and/or microsatellite metastases with two or more tumor-involved nodes, or any number of matted nodes without or with in-transit satellite, and/or microsatellite metastases	
N3a	Four or more clinically occult (i.e., detected by SLND)	No
N3b	Four or more, at least one of which was clinically detected, or presence of any number of matted nodes	No
N3c	Two or more clinically occult or clinically detected and/or presence of any number of matted nodes	Yes

Table 2.27C AJCC 8th Edition Staging: Melanoma M Category

M	M Criteria/Anatomic Site	LDH level
M0	No evidence of distant metastasis	NA
M1	Evidence of distant metastasis	See the following
M1a M1a (0) M1a (1)	Distant metastasis to skin and soft tissue, including muscle and/or nonregional LN	Not recorded or unspecified Not elevated Elevated
M1b M1b (0) M1b (1)	Distant metastasis to lung with or without M1a sites of disease	Not recorded or unspecified Not elevated Elevated
M1c M1c (0) M1c (1)	Distant metastasis to non-CNS visceral sites with or without M1a or M1b sites of disease	Not recorded or unspecified Not elevated Elevated
M1d M1d (0) M1d (1)	Distant metastasis to CNS with or without M1a, M1b, or M1c sites of disease	Not recorded or unspecified Normal Elevated

Suffixes for M category: (0) LDH not elevated, (1) LDH elevated. No suffix is used if LDH is not recorded or is unspecified.

Table 2.27D AJCC 8th Edition Staging: Melanoma Clinical Stage Grouping (cTMN)

When T is	And N is	And M is	Then the Clinical Stage Group is
Tis	N0	M0	0
T1a	N0	M0	IA
T1b	N0	M0	IB
T2a	N0	M0	Ib
T2b	N0	M0	IIA
T3a	N0	M0	IIA
T3b	N0	M0	IIB
T4a	N0	M0	IIB
T4b	N0	M0	IIC
Any T, Tis	≥N1	M0	III
Any T	Any N	M1	IV
Tis	N0	M0	0
T1a	N0	M0	IA

Table 2.28 5YS for Melanoma

Stage	5YS for Melanoma %
IA	95
IB	5YS rate of approximately 91
IIA	77–79
IIB	63–67
IIC	45
IIIA	T1-4aN1aM0: 70 T1-4aN2aM0: 63
IIIB	T1-4bN1aM0 or T1-4bN2aM0: 50–53 T1-4aN1bM0 or T1-4aN2bM0 46–59
IIIC	T1-4bN1bM0, (T1-4bN2bM0, or ≥4 metastatic LNs, matted LNs, or in-transit met(s)/satellite(s): 24–29
IV	M1a: 19 M1b: 7 M1c: 10

- □ **After completion of neoadjuvant chemoradiation:** Biopsy of the tumor bed to confirm complete pathologic response is indicated, or resection of residual tumor with wide surgical margins is appropriate. If pathologic margins are still positive, consider re-resection, additional EBXRT, and/or chemotherapy. If unresectable, additional EBXRT can be considered, and/or systemic therapy, or best supportive care.
- □ If bulky inguinofemoral LN are present with an unresectable T3 lesion:
  - Resection of the bulky LN before commencement of chemoradiation can be performed or
  - Chemoradiation alone can be administered, confirm with FNA
- □ For T4a lesions:
  - Neoadjuvant combination chemotherapy and XRT ± LND
  - Radical vulvectomy with bilateral groin LND or
  - Pelvic exenteration
- □ For T4B metastatic disease beyond the pelvis: any T, any N, M1
  - EBXRT for locoregional control and/or chemotherapy and/or immunotherapy for control and symptom palliation, or best supportive care

▫ Management of a positive SLN for primary tumors < 4 cm (preferably < 3 cm):

  – If SLN harbors metastasis ≤2mm in size: completion of IF-LND is recommended. If no other positive LN are identified, management of the contralateral groin can be either: contralateral IF-LND, contralateral (bilateral) groin XRT, or no further treatment (NFT) can be considered

  – If SLN metastasis is >2mm:

    a. Completion IF-LND

    b. EBXRT with concurrent cisplatin chemotherapy to the bilateral groins and WP is preferred if extracapsular involvement is present and variably for 1-2+ positive LN.

  – At completion bilateral inguinofemoral LND:

    a. If LND shows ≥2 + LN or extracapsular disease: EBXRT with platinum-based chemotherapy to the groin and whole pelvis.

    b. If no further + LN: Observation or chemoradiation can be considered.

▫ Management of positive LN from complete IF-LND: adjuvant XRT and cisplatin chemotherapy if:

  – More than two LNs are positive.

  – More than one LN is positive with greater than 2mm-sized metastasis, or

  – Extracapsular LN involvement is present.

▫ Neoadjuvant combination chemotherapy and XRT is considered frontline therapy in larger T2 lesions, as well as T3 and T4 lesions. These patients can be treated with 55–65 Gy groin and WP-XRT with concurrent cisplatin at 40 to 50 mg/m^2 weekly. A groin LND/SLND can be performed before XRT, and if negative, WP XRT can be omitted and XRT fields tailored to the primary tumor, including potential en face therapy. Posttreatment surgical evaluation with resection of residual tumor and/or groin LND (if not done previously) should be performed.

▫ Fixed or ulcerated LN can be surgically resected with XRT to follow; or if unresectable, preoperative chemoradiation with postoperative resection of any macroscopic residual disease.

▫ Margin status: If margins are positive, reexcision is preferred, if they continue to be positive, EBXRT is recommended.

- The femoral triangle is anatomically bordered by the inguinal ligament superiorly, the sartorius muscle laterally, and the adductor longus muscle medially. The incision site for the groin LND starts 2 cm below a line drawn between the ASIS and the pubic tubercle. The skin flap is preserved. The upper flap is dissected toward the inguinal ligament. The LN-bearing tissue, which is attached to the inguinal ligament, is removed, and the superficial epigastric and superficial circumflex vessels should be ligated. The lower flap is then dissected. The saphenous vein, which runs through the medial aspect of the triangle, should be conserved, and its tributaries ligated.

- If an **ipsilateral groin LN** is found to be positive at final pathology for a unilateral tumor, management of the contralateral groin should be considered. Options include dissection of the contralateral groin, adjuvant bilateral groin and pelvic XRT, or a combination of contralateral groin LND and if negative, unilateral groin/pelvic XRT.

- The risk of contralateral positive LN with a negative ipsilateral groin LND is between 0.4% and 2.6%. GOG 74 demonstrated a 2.4% risk of isolated contralateral positive LNs in tumors 2 cm or less in size. If the DOI was less than 5 mm, contralateral LN metastasis occurred in 1.2%.[414] Contralateral positive LNs have been found in 0.9% of patients if the tumor was less than 2-cm wide.[415] In another study, a 1.8% rate of positive contralateral LNs was demonstrated if the ipsilateral groin LNs were found to be negative. In no patients were contralateral positive groin LNs found if the tumor was less than 2-cm wide and invasion was less than 5 mm.[416]

- Sentinel groin LND can potentially decrease the extent and complication rate of the groin LND. The combined sequenced injection of Technetium-99m (^{99m}Tc) radiolabeled albumin and blue dye to the primary tumor, followed by intraoperative scintillation, has proven sensitive and specific enough for sentinel node identification. ICG fluorescence-guided SLN biopsy is safe and has a detection rate similar to current techniques on metaanalysis with a detection rate ranging from 89.7% to100% and was not superior to current standard techniques of 99Technium indigo blue.[417] If frozen section is positive for LN metastasis, a complete bilateral groin LND should be performed. Radiation without completion LND is under investigation. Indications for performing a SLND are:
  - ○ Negative clinical groin examination and imaging
  - ○ Primary unifocal tumor
  - ○ Tumor size less than 4 cm
  - ○ No prior vulvar surgery to have altered lymphatic flow

- Margin status has been revisited. A relationship between margin status and recurrence was reported by Heaps et al[418]: If there was less than 8 mm of paraffin fixed tumor-free tissue at resection, 13 of 23 patients recurred locally, whereas if the margins were greater than 8 mm, only 8 of 112 patients recurred. Thus, for positive or close margins, re-excision, and/or adjuvant XRT to the vulva can decrease the local recurrence rate. Those treated with adjuvant XRT had a 44% recurrence rate versus those observed who had a 75% recurrent rate.[419] Tumor thickness greater than 5 mm, tumor >4 cm in size or LVSI, may also be indications for adjuvant local XRT. Recently, Grootenhuis et al reported that pathologic tumor-free margin distance did not influence the risk on local recurrence (HR 1.03, 95% CI, 0.99–1.06), regardless of a cutoff of 8, 5, or 3 mm. Multivariable analyses showed a higher local recurrence rate in patients with DVIN and LS in the margin.[420]

- Adjuvant groin and WP-XRT is indicated for FIGO stages 3, and 4A. Concurrent radiosensitizing cisplatin chemotherapy should be considered.

- Adjuvant groin and WP-XRT is indicated for micrometastasis identified post-surgically in SLN as an alternative to staged completion of bilateral whole groin LND. Isolated tumor cells are not counted as micrometastasis.[421]

- OTT mirrors the data for cervical cancer in that treatment length has an effect on OS with increased risk of death at 0.4% per day over 104 days, preferably with total treatment under 60 days.

- There are complications of a radical vulvectomy and groin LND. The wound infection rate is 29%. The wound breakdown rate is 38% for triple incision surgery versus 68% for en bloc resection. Lymphedema occurs at a rate of 7% to 19%. Lymphocytes occur at a rate of 7% to 28%. Cellulitis or lymphangitis can occur due to *beta Streptococcus*. Prophylactic antibiotics are warranted in patients with chronic lymphedema and if prone to cellulitis. Nerve injuries or paresthesias can also occur.

- Basal cell carcinomas are rarely metastatic. Treatment is with excisional biopsy to include a minimum margin of 1 cm and no LND.

- Verrucous carcinoma is a low grade tumor that is locally invasive and rarely metastasizes. Treatment is wide radical excision. XRT is commonly avoided due to concerns about aggressive transformation and metastasis.

- Vulvar sarcomas are also treated with wide radical excision. Combination chemotherapy and XRT may assist in disease management.

- Vulvar melanoma patients should undergo a wide radical excision with bilateral groin SLND.
  - There are data to suggest that radical surgery versus wide local excision yields no difference in OS.[422]
  - LND in vulvar melanoma is of prognostic indication only; it is not therapeutic. Removal of enlarged nodes is adequate treatment.
  - Margins: The surgically desired margin for in situ disease is 0.5 mm; for a 1-mm thick tumor, a 1-cm margin; for 1.01- to 2-mm

thick lesions, a 1- to 2-cm margin; for 2.01- to 4-mm thick lesions, a 2-cm margin; and for a lesion greater than 4-mm thick, a 2-cm margin.

- ○ Most failures are distant.
- ○ AJCC stage is the most important prognostic factor.
- ○ Adjuvant therapy for vulvar melanoma can be single-agent chemotherapy, including DTIC, temozolomide, cisplatin, vinblastine, or paclitaxel. Combination chemotherapy can consist of cisplatin and paclitaxel.
- ○ Biological agents can be used with standard cytotoxic drugs or alone. Biologicals include ipilimumab, nivolumab, alpha-interferon, and vemurafenib.
- Paget's disease:
  - ○ For noncutaneous vulvar Paget's disease, there is no benefit to an extensive resection or deep vulvectomy.
  - ○ Treatment: For cutaneous vulvar Paget's, surgical resection is the mainstay. Treatments can include:
    - Surgery: A simple wide resection is recommended, with a 1-cm clinically negative margin. Response rates (RRs) range from 33% to 70%. The risk of recurrence is high at 58% overall. If margins are negative the risk is 18% to 38% and if positive range between 45% and 61%. Frozen section of the margins has not been found to be better than visual inspection (FN rate 35%–38%). Permanent section margin status also did not predict recurrence: with 33% recurrence if negative margins versus 40% recurrence if positive margins.[423]
    - XRT: RR of 62% to 100% with a recurrence rate of 0% to 35%
    - **Topical** chemotherapy with bleomycin or 5FU: RR of 57% to 100%, with a recurrence rate of 25%; AEs can be pain, moist desquamation, allergic reactions
    - Photodynamic therapy: 5-aminolevulinic acid with light wavelengths RR of 14% to 50%, with a recurrence rate of 38% to 56%
    - Laser therapy: RR of 53% to 75% with a recurrence rate of 67%
    - Imiquimod: RR 52% to 80%, recurrence rate 19%

Recurrence
- The risk for local recurrence is close surgical margins. There are data to support that an 8-mm fixed margin (a 1-cm fresh margin) is adequate to diminish local recurrence from 50% if margins were less than 8 mm, to 0% if margins were greater than 8 mm. Surgical margins of 2 cm are still recommended, but if anatomy does not permit (urethral, anal, or vaginal margins that would significantly compromise function), a 1-cm margin can be adequate.[418] Farias-Eisner et al[424] looked at radical local excision and LND for stages I and II vulvar cancers, and found that radical local excision had the

same survival as those treated more radically with vulvectomy, and LN status had the largest impact on survival (98% OS if negative nodes were identified vs. 45% if positive nodes were found).

- For local recurrence, a radical excision should be performed with complete bilateral groin LND if not done previously. If groin LN were previously irradiated and clinically negative at the time of recurrence, resection of vulvar recurrence alone is recommended. If margins are negative, observation or additional XRT can be considered. If margins are positive and LN is negative, re-excision or EBXRT with or without brachytherapy XRT ± chemotherapy can be considered. If margins are negative and LN is positive, then concurrent chemoradiation should be offered, and if margins are positive and LN is positive, EBXRT with/without brachytherapy and concurrent chemotherapy ± re-excision should be considered. If radical re-excision is contraindicated or declined, EBXRT with or without brachytherapy and concurrent chemotherapy is recommended. This can be followed by surgical resection of residual tumor if present.

- Isolated perineal recurrences can be cured 75% of the time with salvage surgery. If the recurrence is central and regional, a pelvic exenteration can be considered.

- If groin nodal recurrence is detected: Resection of the involved LN or a complete LND can be performed, followed by concurrent chemoradiation, if not previously performed. If the groin recurrence is fixed or large, then concurrent chemoradiation should be offered.

- If there is an isolated pelvic nodal recurrence: resection can be considered, and/or concurrent chemoradiation should be offered (to follow).

- If distant metastases are identified on comprehensive workup, systemic therapy and/or EBXRT should be considered to include.
  - Cytotoxic: cisplatin/paclitaxel/bevacizumab, cisplatin gemcitabine, cisplatin/vinorelbine, or substituting carboplatin when cisplatin toxicities are present
  - Targeted: erlotinib
  - Biomarker directed:
    - TMB-H, PD-L1, MMRd tumors can be treated with pembrolizumab or nivolumab.
    - NTRK gene fusion-positive tumors can be treated with larotrectinib or entrectinib.
    - Immunotherapy can be considered. Nivolumab alone for squamous cell cancers (see CheckMate 358 in notable trials) or in combination with ipilimumab for melanoma (see checkmate 067 notable trials) has been shown to be beneficial.

- For LN recurrence in melanoma, pathology should be confirmed via biopsy, and imaging should also be obtained with PET/CT or CT of the chest/abdomen/pelvis. If the LN recurrence is in the groin, the enlarged LN should be resected and consideration of complete groin dissection if not previously performed. If a prior LND was performed, removal of the node itself is adequate. If the disease is completely resected, XRT, alpha interferon, systemic therapy and/or a clinical trial can be offered. If the disease is unresectable, systemic therapy, XRT, or a clinical trial can be offered. If there are clinically positive superficial LNs or there are three or greater positive LNs, iliac and obturator LND should be considered.

Survival

The 2YS for nonmelanoma vulvar cancer patients with positive groin LN is 68%, and for those with positive pelvic LN is 23% (Table 2.29).

Follow-Up

- Every 3 months for the first 2 Y
- Every 6 months for the next 3 Y
- Annual visits thereafter

Notable Trials

- GOG 36: This surgical pathology study evaluated 637 patients with vulvar cancer, all of whom had tumors of less than 5 mm DOI. Risk factors for local recurrence and LN metastasis were studied. Multivariate risk factors that were predictive of groin LN metastasis were tumor size less than 2 cm (18.9% + LN); greater than 2 cm (41.6% + LN). Independent predictors of groin LN metastasis were tumor G, LVSI, DOI, age, and fixed or ulcerated LN. A clinically negative groin examination had a FN rate of 23.9%. Those patients in GOG 36 who were identified with positive groin LNs were randomized to GOG 37.[425,426]
- GOG 37: This study identified 114 patients with positive groin LNs after a radical vulvectomy and bilateral groin LND, and randomized them to an ipsilateral pelvic LND or to groin and pelvic XRT. The XRT was dosed at 45 to 50 Gy. Five percent recurred in the XRT group, and 24% recurred in the pelvic LND group. The 2 YS was 68% for those treated with groin and pelvic XRT versus 54% for those who

Table 2.29 Vulvar Cancer 5YS by Stage	
Stage	5YS (%)
I	95
II	75–85
III	55
IVA	20
IVB	5

received the pelvic LND. The number of positive LNs influenced survival: One positive LN yielded an 80% OS, whereas four or more positive LNs had a 27% OS. The incidence of positive pelvic LNs if groin LNs were positive was 28%. There was a 9% incidence of local vulvar recurrence in both arms. A follow-up analysis was performed[427]: The 6 YS for patients who received XRT was 61% versus 41% for those who received the pelvic LND. The 6 YS for cancer-related deaths was 51% versus 29% for the pelvic XRT versus pelvic LND groups, respectively (HR, 50.49). Poor prognostic factors were clinically suspicious or fixed LNs, or greater than two positive groin LNs. A ratio of 20% positive LNs to total LNs was associated with contralateral metastasis, relapse, and cancer-related death, thus the cutoff for recommending XRT. Of patients in the XRT arm, 44% died secondary to other causes. The actual 3Y disease-specific death rate was 25%.[428]

- GOG 74: This study surgically evaluated the outcomes of 143 patients with early-stage vulvar tumors who underwent a superficial groin LND with a modified radical vulvectomy. Overall, 7% developed isolated groin recurrences, and of those with a groin recurrence, 91.7% died. The median time to recurrence in the vulva was 35.9 months, and 7 months for recurrence in the groin. The median survival time after recurrence was 52.4 months for vulvar recurrence and 9.4 months for groin recurrence. This study is criticized for a high number of G 3 tumors (28%) and that of the nine groin recurrences, three were in an undissected groin (patients who refused groin dissection).[414,429]

- GOG 88: Because patients in GOG 37 with positive groin LNs had favorable outcomes with XRT, the question as to whether a groin LND was necessary if prophylactic XRT was administered was investigated. This study evaluated 50 patients after a radical vulvectomy and randomized them to prophylactic groin XRT or to groin LND. In this study, 0 out of 25 patients recurred if a LND was performed, followed by XRT for positive LN (of which 20% were indeed positive), versus an 18.5% recurrence if prophylactic groin XRT was administered to an undissected groin with, therefore, an unknown LN status. Criticisms of this study were underdosing of the groins as the dose prescription point was to 3 cm, and on review, the average vessel depth was 6.1 cm (range 2–18.6 cm) with an average BMI of 25.6.[430,431]

- GOG 101: This phase II study evaluated 73 patients with T3 or T4 disease treated with NACT and XRT. The XRT total dose was 47.6 Gy administered in 1.7 Gy fractions as a hyper-fractionated split-dose regimen of 23.8 Gy BID for 4 days and daily for 6 days with a 2-week break, with two concurrent cycles of cisplatin 50 mg/m^2 day 1 and 5-FU 1,000 mg/m^2 days 1 to 4 given week 1 of each course of XRT. Sixty-nine of 71 women were converted to a resectable status, with 68 patients keeping urinary and fecal capacity. Forty-seven percent (33 of 71) had a CCR and 70% of these were CPR; 2.8% remained unresectable. There was a 55% OS. A companion study to GOG 101 was done for patients with unresectable positive groin LNs (N2/3 nodes); 38 of 40 patients became resectable, with 15 of 37 patients having a CPR. Overall, 29 of 38 patients had local control of their disease. Nineteen patients recurred: nine locally and eight distant.[432,433]

- GOG 205: This phase II study evaluated 58 patients with T3 or T4 disease treated with NACT and XRT. XRT was dosed at 57.6 Gy with concurrent weekly cisplatin dosed at 40 mg/m^2. Surgical resection followed for residual tumor (or biopsy to confirm CCR). Of patients, 64% had a CCR (37 of 58) and 78% of these had a CPR. In this study, there was no hyper-fractionation, no midtreatment break, and no 5-FU. Management of the groin LNs in these studies was standardized. Clinically negative or resectable groin LNs underwent groin LND before neoadjuvant therapy. If there were unresectable groin LNs, the groin dissection was performed after neoadjuvant therapy.[434]

- GOG 173: In this study, 452 eligible patients with a tumor size ≥2 cm, ≤6 cm, and with at least 1-mm invasion underwent radical vulvectomy with groin lymphatic mapping. 772 groin dissections were performed. An SLN was identified in 418 of 452 patients. LN metastases were found in 132 of 418 patients (31.6%). The SLN was positive in 121 of 418 patients. Eleven (8.3%) patients with a negative SLN were found to have positive LNs identified on final complete dissection pathology (thus 132 total SLN positive patients). Of the TP patients, 23% were detected by IHC analysis of the SLN. The sensitivity of SLN dissection was 91.7% and the FNPV was 3.7% (90% upper confidence bound = 6.1%). In patients with tumors less than 4 cm, the FN rate was 2%.[435]

- GOG 195: In this study, 137 patients were evaluable for analysis of lymphedema after randomization to receive sutured closure versus fibrin sealant applied in the wound followed by sutured closure. The incidence of G 2/3 lymphedema was 67% in the sutured closure arm and 60% in the fibrin sealant arm; thus no benefit to fibrin sealant was found. The incidence of lymphedema was correlated strongly with inguinal infection and not increased in those who received adjuvant XRT.[436]

- DiSaia et al recommended omitting the deep LND to decrease morbidity without compromising survival. Fifty stage I patients with negative superficial nodes were retrospectively reviewed. No deep LND was performed. There were no recurrences after 12 months.[437]

- GROINSS-V-1/GOG 270 (**GRO**ningen **IN**ternational **S**tudy on **S**entinel nodes in **V**ulvar) cancer: This study evaluated 403 patients. In it, 623 groin dissections were performed. All tumors were greater than 1 mm DOI, unifocal, squamous, and less than 4 cm in size with clinically negative groin LN. A radical vulvectomy and sentinel groin LND were performed in all patients. Follow-up was 35 months. A combination of radioactive tracer and blue dye was used.

Of patients, 67% had negative SLN, 32.9% had a positive SLN. Of 259 patients with unifocal vulvar disease and a negative sentinel node (median follow-up time, 35 months), six had groin recurrences diagnosed, for a FN rate of 2.3%. The 3YS rate was 97%. The 3Y DSS rate for patients with SLN metastasis greater than 2 mm was 69.5%, the 3Y DSS of the SLN metastasis less than 2 mm was 94.4%. The short-term morbidity was decreased in the SLN patients compared with those patients with a positive sentinel node who underwent a complete inguinofemoral lymphadenectomy. Wound breakdown in the groin was 11.7% versus 34.0%, and cellulitis occurred at 4.5% versus 21.3%. The long-term morbidity was also less with recurrent erysipelas occurring at a rate of 0.4% versus 16.2%, and lymphedema of the legs seen in 1.9% versus 25.2% of patients. GROINSS-V-I 10-Y follow-up: The median follow-up was 105 months. The overall recurrence rate was 37.2% at 5 Y, at a median time of 27 months. The local recurrence rate was 27.2% at 5Y and 39.5% at 10Y after primary treatment. The primary isolated groin recurrence rate was 4.1% and distant recurrence was 2%. In SLN− patients, the isolated groin recurrence was 2.5%. The local recurrence rate for SLN− patients was 24.6% at 5Y and 36.4% at 10Y. In SLN + patients, the groin recurrence was 8% and distant recurrence 6.8% at 5 and 10Y. Local recurrence was 33.2% at 5Y and 46.4% at 10Y. SLN− patients had 5 and 10Y DSS of 93.5% and 90.8% compared to SLN + patients of 75.5% and 64.5%. For all patients, 10Y DSS decreased from 90.4% to 68.7% for local recurrence. For SLN− patients, 10Y DSS decreased from 96.1% to 80.8%, and SLN + patients, 10Y DSS decreased from 77.7% to 44.6% for local recurrence.[438,439]

- AGO-CaRE-1 (**C**hemo **a**nd **R**adiotherapy in **E**pithelial Vulvar Cancer): This was a retrospective multicenter cohort study in Germany, conducted from 1998 to 2008 that reviewed 1,618 documented patients with primary squamous-cell vulvar cancer stage IB and higher. Of the patients, 1,249 had surgical groin staging and known LN status and were further analyzed. Of the 1,249 patients, 447 (35.8%) had LN metastases (N+). The majority of node (N)+ patients had one (172 [38.5%]) or two (102 [22.8%]) positive nodes. The 3Y PFS of N + patients was 35.2%, and the OS was 56.2% compared with 75.2% and 90.2% in node-negative patients (N−). 244 (54.6%) N + patients had adjuvant therapy, of which 183 (40.9%) had XRT directed at the groins (±other fields). The 3Y PFS and OS rates in these patients were better compared with N + patients without adjuvant treatment (PFS: 39.6% vs. 25.9%, HR 0.67; 95% CI: 0.51–0.88; $p =$ .004; OS: 57.7% vs. 51.4%; HR 0.79; 95% CI: 0.56 to 1.11; $p = .17$). This effect was statistically significant in multivariable analysis adjusted for age, ECOG PS, FIGO stage, G, invasion depth, and number of positive nodes (PFS: HR 0.58; 95% CI: 0.43–0.78; $p < .001$; OS: HR 0.63; 95% CI: 0.43–0.91; $p = .01$). Thus, adjuvant XRT was associated with improved prognosis in N+ patients; however, outcomes after adjuvant XRT remain poor compared with N– patients. Adjuvant chemoradiation should improve therapy beyond XRT alone.[440]

- A subgroup analysis of the AGO-CaRE-1 study was conducted in which 1,162 patients were analyzed. Univariate analyses detected age, ECOG, as well as multiple tumor characteristics such as FIGO stage, grading, DOI, tumor diameter, and LVSI—all of which were related to the prevalence of LN metastases. Only tumor stage, tumor diameter, and depth of infiltration were found to be significantly associated with the number of LN metastases. In multivariate analysis, age (OR 1.03), LVSI (OR 4.97), tumor stage (OR 2.22), and DOI (OR 1.08) showed an association with the prevalence of LN metastases. Regarding the number of metastatic LNs, only tumor stage (OR 2.21) or, if excluded, tumor diameter (OR 1.02), were found to be significant. LVSI, tumor stage, and DOI were factors with the strongest association regarding the prevalence of LN metastasis.[441]

- Impact of adjuvant chemotherapy in addition to XRT for N+ vulvar cancer was studied in an NCDB analysis. A total of 1,792 patients were reviewed: 26.3% received adjuvant chemotherapy in addition to XRT, and 76.6% had one to three involved LN. The median unadjusted survival with and without adjuvant chemotherapy was 29.7 and 44 months, $p = .001$. Delivery of adjuvant chemotherapy resulted in a 38% reduction in the risk of death (HR 0.62; 95% CI: 0.48–0.79; $p < .001$) for N+ vulvar cancer patients in the NCDB. A propensity adjusted analysis was performed and able to show a significant improvement in 3YOS of 53.9% versus 46.9% in patients receiving chemoradiation.[442]

- Margin status revisited in vulvar squamous cell carcinoma.[443] Between 2000 and 2010, 287 patients were reviewed with a median follow-up of 80 months (range 0–204). The actuarial local recurrence rate 10 Y after treatment was 42.5%. Pathologic tumor-free margin distance did not influence the risk on local recurrence (HR 1.03, 95% CI, 0.99–1.06), regardless of a cutoff of 8, 5, or 3 mm. Multivariable analyses showed a higher local recurrence rate in patients with dVIN and LS in the margin (HR 2.76, 95% CI, 1.62–4.71), in patients with dVIN in the margin (HR 2.14 (95% CI 1.11–4.12)), and a FIGO stage II≥ (HR 1.62 (95% CI, 1.05-2.48).

- GROINSS-V-II: This was a prospective phase II single-arm treatment trial from 2005 to 2016. The median follow-up for all patients was 24.3 months. 1,535 patients were eligible: 1,213 had a negative SLND (79.0%) and 322 a metastatic SLN (21.0%). Inclusion criteria were unifocal macroinvasive squamous cell carcinoma of the vulva <4 cm; and negative preoperative imaging of groins. The primary endpoint of the study was the isolated groin recurrence rate at 24 months. SLN biopsy was performed with radioactive tracer using lymphoscintigram localization, and blue dye. If H&E staining was negative, ultrastaging was performed. When the SLN could not be identified, an IF-LND was advised and for midline tumors bilateral SLN were recommended. When the SLN was negative after ultrastaging, NFT followed. If metastasis (including ITC) was identified in the SLN, the groin was regarded as positive for metastatic disease. Total dose XRT was 50 Gy in 25 to 28 fractions at 1.8-2 Gy, five times per week. Chemotherapy with XRT was at provider discretion. A data safety amendment in 2010 allowed only patients with micrometastases to receive XRT, whereas patients with macrometastases extracapsular involvement, or more than one + LN returned to full groin dissection with adjuvant radiotherapy due to a 22% 2Y recurrence rate compared to a 1.6% recurrence rate for LN micrometastasis. Critiques of the study design were that XRT planning was to the whole groin rather than just the vessels and dosing was inadequate for gross residual or extracapsular disease. Of the 322 patients with metastatic SLN: 49.7% had micrometastases ≤2 mm. At 2Y, 3.8% had isolated groin recurrences. Of patients, 78.8% with micrometastasis received XRT as prescribed by protocol (of these 11.1% received chemoradiation), whereas 11 patients with ITC or metastases ≤2 mm underwent no radiotherapy or IF-LND, and one had an ipsilateral groin recurrence. Of patients, 50.3% had macrometastases >2 mm; 51 patients received XRT only to the groin (13.7% had chemoradiation), and of these 12.2% had a groin recurrence at 2 Y (95% CI, 7.1–17.4). Stratifying by treatment, groin recurrence rate at 2 Y was 22.0% (95% CI, 10.5–33.5) in patients who underwent XRT versus 6.9% (95% CI, 2.0–11.8) in patients who underwent IF-LND with or without adjuvant XRT (p = .011). No groin recurrences occurred in a contralateral nonirradiated groin. No groin recurrences were observed in the chemoradiation group. Isolated groin recurrences were diagnosed in 2.7% of SLN-negative patients (95% CI, 1.7–3.6). Side effects included G 1 to 2 toxicities consisting of nausea, vomiting, mucositis, anal and UI, and diarrhea. Lymphedema at 1 Y was 4.1% for SLND, compared with SLND with XRT (10.7%, p <.0001) compared to IFL (with or without XRT) 22.9%, p <.001). The estimated risk at 2Y of DS death was 2.1% (95% CI, 1.3–2.9) for SLN-negative patients, 6.5% (95% CI, 2.6–10.4) for patients with SLN micrometastases, and 25.5% (95% CI, 18.6–32.5) for those with SN macrometastases (p <.0001). The 2YOS for SLN-negative patients was 95.2% (95% CI, 94.0–96.5) compared to 88.3% (95% CI, 83.2–93.4) for those with micrometastasis, and 69.3% (95% CI, 62.0–76.6) for those with macrometastases (p <.0001). For all patients with groin recurrence (n = 56), the 2YOS 39.0%.[421]

- Unilateral IF-LND in early-stage patients with + SLN—Management of contralateral groin: 366 patients were evaluated from the GROINSS V I and II studies. Patients underwent unilateral groin SLND. those where were SLND+ then underwent completion unilateral IF-LND. Patients were then divided into three groups: a) 105 had contralateral IF-LND b) 122 had contralateral XRT c) 139 had NFT. A 4.8% rate of positive contralateral LN was identified in the contralateral groin IF-LND. Recurrence rate was 0.8% in the XRT group and 1.4% in the NFT group. Tumor laterality was studied: for those with a midline tumor, 1.7% had contralateral positive LN, a near midline tumor had 2.7% contralateral positive LN, and for those with a lateral tumor 2.2% had contralateral positive LN. The overall rate of contralateral positive LN was 2.9% if only the unilateral SLN was micrometastatic positive. Tumor size of < 3 cm had 3.6% contralateral positive LN compared to > 3cm with a 1.4% rate. It can be safe to limit groin treatment to unilateral IF-LND or radiation especially when the primary tumor is < 3cm size.[467]

- GROINSS-V III investigates whether treatment efficacy can be increased by adding concurrent chemotherapy to inguinofemoral XRT, also increasing XRT dosing to 56 Gy by applying a (simultaneous integrated) boost dose for SLN macrometastasis. Results pending.

- GOG 279: This is a phase II trial of approximately 52 patients evaluating cisplatin and gemcitabine concurrent with IMRT for the treatment of locally advanced SCC of the vulva. Eligible patients are T2 to T3, N0 to N3 squamous cell cancers not amenable to primary surgical resection. Pretreatment SLND or groin dissection is performed. Patients will be treated with 64 Gy IMRT total dose to the vulva and 50 Gy to the nonmalignant groin or 60 Gy to involved LN (>3 + LN, extracapsular involvement, or close margins), concordant with gemcitabine 50 mg/m^2 and cisplatin 40 mg/m^2 weekly during XRT. Surgical resection of residual disease is scheduled at 6 to 8 weeks post-therapy. Results are pending.

- Debulking of clinically involved LN: followed by XRT (compared to complete groin LND or SLND followed by XRT for node positive disease) had fewer complications. There was no increase in groin recurrences or changes in OS in 68 patients.[444]

- Vemurafenib: In a randomized trial of 675 untreated metastatic melanoma patients stage IIIc or IV who were *BRAF*[V600E] positive, vemurafenib was compared to DTIC. Vemurafenib was dosed at 960 mg PO twice daily and DTIC at 1,000 mg/m^2 IV every 3 weeks. The 6-month OS was 84% in the vemurafenib group and 64% in the DTIC group. RRs were 48% for vemurafenib and 5% for DTIC.[445]

- Optimal treatment time node positive vulvar cancer: OTT of adjuvant XRT is an independent risk factor for death in women with resected, node-positive vulvar cancer.[446] This was a retrospective review between 2004-16 of 1500 women with surgically resected, node-positive vulvar squamous cell carcinomas who were treated with adjuvant XRT. The median was 104 days and shorter OTT was associated with age, facility volume, private insurance, and duration of postoperative hospitalization. Median OS with OTT ≤104 days was 56.1 months versus 45.4 months if ≥105 days (p = .015). On multivariable analysis, OTT was independently associated with an increased risk of death of 0.4% per additional day (95% CI 1.001–1.007, p = .003), age at diagnosis (HR 1.031, 95% CI, 1.024–1.037, p <.001), number of nodes positive (HR 1.031, 95%CI, 1.024–1.037, p = .006), the use of concurrent chemotherapy (HR 0.815, 95% CI, 0.693–0.960, p = .014) and increasing pT/pN stage. Each additional day between surgery and completion of adjuvant radiation contributes to higher risk of death.

- CheckMate 067 Trial: This was a randomized, blinded, phase III trial in which patients with untreated advanced melanoma were randomly assigned to receive one of the following regimens: (a) nivolumab dosed at 1 mg/kg plus ipilimumab at 3 mg/kg every 3 weeks for 4 doses, followed by nivolumab 3 mg/kg every 2 weeks; (b) nivolumab dosed at 3 mg/kg every 2 weeks; or (c) ipilimumab dosed at 3 mg/kg every 3 weeks for 4 doses.[447] The two primary endpoints were PFS and OS. At 60-month follow-up, the median OS was not reached in the nivolumab-plus-ipilimumab group and 36.9 months in the nivolumab group, compared with 19.9 months in the ipilimumab group (HR for death with nivolumab plus ipilimumab vs. ipilimumab, 0.52; HR with nivolumab vs. ipilimumab, 0.63). The 5YOS was 52% in the nivolumab-plus-ipilimumab group and 44% in the nivolumab group, compared to 26% in the ipilimumab group. No significant AEs were identified. Long-term 5YOS was seen in a higher percentage of patients who received combination nivolumab plus ipilimumab or nivolumab alone than in those who received ipilimumab alone.

- Niraparib at 240 mg IV q2 weeks was given to 24 patients in HPV+ tumors for recurrent vaginal, cervical or vulvar carcinomas. The median time to response was 1.7 months.[448]

VAGINAL CANCER

Characteristics

- Vaginal cancer represents 1% to 2% of all female genital tract malignancies. The median age at diagnosis is 60 Y. Most vaginal cancers are metastatic lesions from other sites, including the cervix, uterus, breast, GTD and the GI tract. Primary vaginal cancers are commonly found in the upper one third of the vagina, often in the posterior fornix. There are 8,870 new cases with 1,630 deaths estimated for 2022 to include vaginal/other.

- Symptoms include vaginal discharge, vaginal bleeding, tenesmus, pelvic pain, bladder irritation, and pelvic fullness.

- If the patient has a history of uterine, cervical, or vulvar cancer, the vaginal lesion is considered a recurrent cancer unless proven otherwise by discriminating pathology or greater than 5Y have intervally passed since prior diagnosis.
- Risk factors for vaginal cancer include HPV infection, chronic vaginal irritation, prior treatment for cervical cancer, prior CIN, and a history of in-utero exposure to DES.
- DES was used from 1940 to 1971. Vaginal adenosis and vaginal adenocarcinoma are characteristics of exposure. Other physical representations are a cockscomb cervix. The risk of CCC is 1:1,000 with a history of DES. The peak age at diagnosis was 19Y. Surveillance for women who were exposed to DES in utero includes at least yearly gynecologic exams with cervicovaginal cytology (and colposcopy as indicated) to occur indefinitely.
- The route of spread is direct, lymphatic, or hematogenous. The route of lymphatic spread depends on the location of the lesion. If the lesion is in the upper two thirds of the vagina, metastasis is often directly to the pelvic LNs. If the lesion is in the lower one third of the vagina, metastasis can often be to the inguinal–femoral LNs, and/or to pelvic LNs. Hematogenous spread often occurs late in the disease process.
- The most important prognostic factor is stage of disease. Age is also an important factor. Melanomas and sarcomas have the worst prognosis. Lesions of the distal vagina tend to have a worse prognosis than proximal lesions. Size less than 3 cm has a better prognosis than if larger than 5 cm. LN status also confers prognosis, with a 5YS of 33% for positive LNs compared to 56% for negative LNs.

Pretreatment Workup

The pretreatment workup is colposcopy of the entire lower genital tract and physical examination. Diagnosis is via biopsy often guided with colposcopy. It may be necessary to perform an EUA with cystoscopy and proctoscopy. These procedures may also help with initial staging. CXR, IVP, cystoscopy, proctoscopy, and barium enema are FIGO-approved diagnostic studies. CT, MRI, and PET imaging were approved FIGO imaging modalities starting 2019 and may assist in evaluating extent of disease and aid in treatment planning but are not used to change initial cliinical staging.

Histology

- Eighty percent of vaginal cancers are of squamous cell histology.
- Five to 9% are adenocarcinomas.
- Malignant melanoma represents 2.8% to 5% of vaginal neoplasms. Vaginal melanomas are more often found in the lower one third of the vagina.
- Rhabdomyosarcoma is usually found as the botryoid variant of embryonal rhabdomyosarcoma and is the most common malignant

tumor of the vagina in infants and children; 90% of patients are younger than 5 Y. On clinical examination, grape-like edematous masses may protrude from the vagina. The histologic pearl is the presence of a cambium layer beneath an intact vaginal epithelium.
- LMS can also be found, and this can occur in women with a prior history of XRT.

Staging

Staging continues to be clinical, closely following cervical cancer parameters amended in 2021 (Table 2.30A–D).

If there is clinical involvement of the cervix or the vulva, the tumor should be classified as a primary cervical or vulvar cancer, respectively; tumors limited to the urethra should be classified as urethral cancers.

Treatment

Treatment depends on the location and depth of the lesion, the stage of the cancer, and medical comorbidities.

Table 2.30A AJCC 8th Edition: T Category		
AJCC		**FIGO**
TX	Unable to assess primary tumor	
T0	Unable to detect presence of primary tumor	
T1	Tumor limited to the vagina	I
T1	a Tumor limited to the vagina and measures no larger than 2 cm	I
	b Tumor limited to the vagina and measures more than 2 cm	
T2	Tumor has extended into the paravaginal tissues, but not into the pelvic sidewall	II
T2	a Tumor is no larger than 2 cm and has extended into the paravaginal tissues, but not to the pelvic sidewall	II
	b Tumor measures more than 2 cm and has extended into the paravaginal tissues, but not into the pelvic sidewall	
T3	Tumor has invaded the pelvic sidewall and/or extends to the lower third of the vagina and/or the kidney is blocked/nonfunctional or there is hydronephrosis	III
T4	Tumor extends into the mucosa of the rectum or bladder and/or has invaded past the true pelvis (more than a bullous edema is needed as proof for a T4 tumor classification)	IVA

Table 2.30B AJCC 8th Edition: N Category

AJCC		FIGO
NX	Unable to assess regional lymph nodes	
N0	No presence of metastasis of regional lymph nodes	
N0(i+)	Regional lymph nodes contain ITCs that are 0.2 mm or smaller	
N1	Tumor has metastasized from the pelvic or inguinal LN regions	III

Table 2.30C AJCC 8th Edition: M Category

AJCC		FIGO
M0	Distant metastasis not present	
M1	Presence of distant metastasis	IVB

Table 2.30D AJCC 8th Edition: Stage Grouping

I	
IA	T1aN0M0
IB	T1bN0M0
II	
IIA	T2aN0M0
IIB	T2bN0M0
III	
III	(T1-3)N1M0
III	T3N0M0
IV	
IVA	T4(Any N)M0
IVB	(Any T)(Any N)M1

- Treatment for stage I squamous cell or adenocarcinomas that involve the upper two thirds of the vagina can include a radical hysterectomy with upper vaginectomy and LND, or an upper vaginectomy and parametrectomy with LND if the uterus has previously been removed. XRT without surgery has equivalent outcomes. Concurrent platinum-based chemotherapy has been adopted to follow cervical cancer guidelines. If the lower one third of the vagina is involved, EBXRT fields should include the groins. Dosing is 50.4

Gy EBXRT brought up to a total of 80 to 85 Gy with interstitial or Fletcher-suit brachytherapy.

- Treatment for stages II, III, and IV is definitive XRT with concurrent platinum-based chemotherapy. XRT usually includes EBXRT and intracavitary or interstitial therapy to a total dose of 85 to 90 Gy. If the lower one third of the vagina is involved, the groins should also be irradiated.
- Treatment for melanoma is radical surgical resection if possible. Exenterative surgery has not been found to provide additional survival benefit. Chemotherapy +/– biologic therapy may provide adjuvant benefits.
- The treatment of rhabdomyosarcoma is usually multimodal with therapy consisting of surgical resection, XRT, and systemic chemotherapy. Commonly used agents are VAC. Another regimen is cyclophosphamide, doxorubicin, and DTIC.
- LMS is treated with radical surgical resection and the consideration of adjuvant XRT and/or chemotherapy.

Recurrent Disease

If recurrent disease is identified, a full metastatic workup should be employed. If only local disease is confirmed, a wide local excision or a partial (radical) vaginectomy can be performed. If central disease is identified, a pelvic exenteration can be considered. If there is distant metastasis, chemotherapy with or without XRT can be considered.

Survival

See Table 2.31 for 5YOS for vaginal cancer.

Follow-Up

- Physical and pelvic examinations are recommended: An annual Pap smear may help with detection of recurrence.
  - Every 3 months for the first 2Y
  - Every 6 months for the next 3Y
  - Annual examinations thereafter

Table 2.31 Vaginal Cancer 5YS by Stage	
Stage	**5YS (%)**
I	84
II	75
III	57
IV	10

GESTATIONAL TROPHOBLASTIC DISEASE

Characteristics

- GTD describes a group of tumors that arise from trophoblastic cells. This is usually the result of an abnormal fertilization event and includes molar pregnancy, choriocarcinoma, PSTT, and ETT.

- Hydatidiform molar pregnancy occurs in approximately one out of 1,000 pregnancies in North America. Clinical features of a mole are vaginal bleeding in the first trimester or early second trimester; uterine size large for dates; ovarian theca-lutein cysts (seen in 46% of patients, 2% of which may torse); early preeclampsia at less than 20 weeks (12%–17%); hyperthyroidism due to the similarity between the alpha subunit of both hCG and TSH hormones; hyperemesis gravidarum (20%); passage of vesicles per vagina; and respiratory complaints due to tumor emboli or increased progesterone (27%).

- Risk factors for a molar pregnancy include age (<15 Y or > 45 Y of age), history of a prior mole, and Asian ethnicity.

- The WHO has classified GTD into two states: premalignant and malignant. The premalignant tumors are the complete and the partial moles. The malignant tumors are the invasive mole, gestational choriocarcinoma, ETT, and PSTT. Within the malignant tumors are the categories of nonmetastatic and metastatic. Within the metastatic category are low-risk metastatic and high-risk metastatic disease.

- There is an increased risk for a second mole after a first molar pregnancy. This is usually paternally related. The risk of another molar pregnancy increases from one out of 1,000 (.1%) to one out of 100 (1%), and after a 2nd molar pregnancy increases to 15%–20%. There is a familial recurrent hydatidiform mole (FRHM). This is an autosomal recessive disorder with mutations in NLRP7 (in 70% of cases) or KHDC3L (5% of cases) that results in a diploid complete mole (CM) of biparental origin.

- A mole and fetus have been diagnosed at a rate of one out of 100,000 pregnancies. There are data to suggest a 40% chance of a live birth. Persistent GTD is diagnosed in 55% of these patients, and 22.7% are found to have metastatic disease. There is an increased risk for hemorrhage, preeclampsia, and metastatic disease. The pregnancy should be terminated if these life-threatening complications occur.

- Tumors from other primary sites can produce hCG. Genetic studies should be performed on patients with tumors that are refractory to common first-line and salvage therapies to rule out nongestational choriocarcinoma.

- GTN can occur after any gestational event: 25% after a term pregnancy, 50% after a mole, and 25% after an ectopic or miscarriage.

Histopathology

- Complete and partial moles are usually diagnosed at the time of uterine evacuation. Histopathology is the main diagnostic method.

Other abnormal pregnancies/fetuses can be mistaken for a partial mole. These include Turner's, Beckwith-Wiedemann, and Edward's syndromes.

- A complete mole (CM) has no fetal components. Furthermore, the placental villi are hydropic (or edematous) with no identifiable vasculature. The origin of this mole is considered to arise from fertilization of an anuclear oocyte with either two sperm or one sperm that duplicates itself, thus all nuclear DNA is paternal (most commonly diploid with a 46XX karyotype), whereas the mitochondrial DNA is maternal. FISH can confirm the diagnosis with flow cytometry for ploidy and IHC for CDKp57 (CM is p57 negative). The rate of persistent GTD after a CM is 15% to 20%.

- The partial mole's origin is thought to arise from the dual fertilization of an egg by two sperm, or duplication of a paternal chromosome resulting in triploidy with 2:1 paternal to maternal DNA content. Fetal components can be seen, along with fetal vasculature and hydropic villi. FISH can aid with the diagnosis if necessary, and IHC can add information with positive staining for p57 KIP2. Cytogenetic techniques, to include chromosomal banding and RFLP analysis of DNA, have allowed chromosomal patterns for partial and complete molar pregnancies differentiation. The rate of persistent GTD after partial mole is 0.5% to 5% (Table 2.32).

- Choriocarcinoma is the most aggressive type of GTN, regardless of metastatic status. Incidence is 3/100,000 gestational events in North America, but 23/100,000 in Southeast Asia. Fifty percent of tumors

Table 2.32 Molar Pregnancy Classifications With Characteristics

Characteristic	CM	Partial Mole
Hydatidiform edematous villi	Diffuse	Focal
Trophoblastic hyperplasia	Cyto- and syncytial	Syncytial
Embryo	Absent	Present
Villous capillary	No fetal RBC	Many fetal RBC
Gestational age at diagnosis	8–16 wk	10–22 wk
Beta hCG titer mIU/mL	>50,000 mIU/mL in 75%	<50,000 mIU/mL
Malignant potential	15%–25%	0.5%–5%
Karyotype	Diploid (46XX 95%, 46XY 5%)	Triploid (69XXY) 80%
Size for dates: Small Large	33% 33%	65% 10%

follow a term gestation, 20% occur after molar gestations (both partial and complete), and 25% occur after a spontaneous or elective abortion. These tumors have diverse, nonspecific ploidies and are highly malignant. Both cytotrophoblasts and syncytiotrophoblasts are present, with syncytiotrophoblasts predominating, but there are no chorionic villi. Metastasis occurs frequently to the lung (80% with symptoms such as hemoptysis or dyspnea), vagina (30% with bleeding), brain (10% with focal neurologic deficits, headache, mass effect), and liver (10% pain, hemoperitoneum).

- PSTT may follow a term gestation, a nonmolar abortion, a CM, and, in theory, a partial mole. These tumors are mostly diploid and produce very low amounts of beta hCG as well as serum HPL. This is due to the presence of intermediate cytotrophoblast cells. There is an increased proportion of free β hCG. These tumors stain for HPL, β1-glycoprotein, and Ki-67. PSTTs grow slowly and can be seen years after any type of pregnancy. They can produce a nephrotic syndrome or hematuria. The prognosis depends on the time until diagnosis; if it presents less than 4 Y since a pregnancy, the prognosis is better than if later. WHO scoring is not used to determine treatment of PSTT. These tumors present with lung metastases in 10% to 29% of cases and 10% of patients develop metastases during follow-up. Treatment is recommended with hysterectomy and LND—ovarian conservation does not adversely affect outcomes. Adjuvant chemotherapy is recommended for metastatic disease (also surgically remove primary tumor site) and for adverse prognostic factors such as interval from last known pregnancy greater than 2 Y, deep myometrial invasion, tumor necrosis, mitotic count greater than six/10 HPF. Recommended chemotherapy regimens are EMA-EP or paclitaxel/cisplatin-paclitaxel/etoposide doublet.

- Quiescent GTD is the state of elevated β hCG without documented hyperglycosylated hCG. There has never been a documented case of quiescent GTD with a β hCG level that is higher than 230 mIU/mL. In this disease state, the residual mole lacks a cytotrophoblastic cell population. Therefore, there is no hyperglycosylated hCG production, and as a result, no invasion. Usually the residual mass of tissue dies after 6 months. In 10.4% of cases, however, quiescent GTD can activate and lead to persistent trophoblastic disease. Therefore, when a hyperglycosylated hCG is detected, the patient should be treated with chemotherapy. This is similar to a LMP tumor. There are some data to suggest waiting to treat until a threshold β hCG level of 3,000 mIU/mL is detected.[449,450]

- ETT is an extremely rare subtype derived from chorionic type intermediate trophoblast cells. WHO scoring does not apply. Treatment is best with hysterectomy and LN dissection. Chemotherapy is recommended in addition to surgery for metastatic disease (after removal of the primary tumor site), and for adverse prognostic factors such as interval from last known pregnancy greater than

2 Y, deep myometrial invasion, tumor necrosis, and mitotic count greater than 6/10 HPF. EMA-EP or the paclitaxel/cisplatin-paclitaxel/etoposide doublet are chemotherapy options.

- Distinct microRNA profiles may exist for complete hydatidiform moles at risk of malignant progression.[451] Two significantly altered microRNAs were mir-181b-5p (1.65-fold; adjusted $p = .014$) and mir-181d-5p (1.85-fold; adjusted $p = .014$), both of which regulate expression of BCL2. BCL2 mRNA expression was found to be lower in the CMs progressing to GTN, than in those that regressed (-4.69-fold; $p = .018$). Thus, CMs progressing to GTN are associated with a distinct microRNA profile. miR-181 family members and BCL2 may be prognostic biomarkers for predicting risk of progression.

Diagnosis

- A mole is usually detected by US and serum β hCG level in the first trimester.
- The diagnosis of post molar GTN after evacuation of a complete or partial mole is made if there is:
  ◦ An elevating β hCG (a 10% rise over three values in 2 weeks)
  ◦ A plateauing β hCG (a plateau of 10% over four values in 3 weeks)
  ◦ Evidence of metastatic disease (mainly lung)
  ◦ A histologic diagnosis of choriocarcinoma
  ◦ In addition, some may consider the presence of an hCG value greater than 20,000 mIU/mL 4 weeks after evacuation, diagnostic for an invasive mole.
- It is imperative to perform dual serum and urine hCG testing to rule out phantom hCG/false positive results.
- This is the only malignancy that does not necessarily need histologic confirmation and can be diagnosed via serum assay alone. This can be important as some biopsies can lead to grave hemorrhagic events.

Pretreatment Workup

- The pretreatment workup of GTD is a pelvic US (which can document the primary tumor as a uterine mass and give its dimensions and rule out intrauterine/ectopic pregnancy) and a CXR. If the CXR is negative, a CT of the chest can be obtained, but should not determine upstaging/scoring or chemotherapy administration, as 40% of patients have micrometastasis and this does not affect OS. If CXR or exam show metastatic disease, it is then necessary to obtain a CT of the chest, abdomen, and pelvis and a MRI of the brain. Alternatively, some practitioners routinely obtain a CT of the chest, abdomen, and pelvis for initial evaluation, but only the lesions seen in the liver and brain should be scored. Serum laboratories include a quantitative "total hCG assay" (β, core, C-terminal, nicked-free beta, beta-core, and hyperglycosylated) or at minimum a β and hyperglycosylated hCG. Other laboratories include CBC, renal function tests, LFTs, thyroid function tests, and a physical examination. A lumbar puncture can be considered if central neurologic symptoms are present and the brain MRI is negative. The plasma-to-cerebral spinal fluid ratio of hCG can be less than 60 in cases with cerebral metastasis, but this ratio is not always reliable. A urine hCG should always be done at time of diagnosis as well.

- Repeat D&C is controversial. With a second D&C, the risk of needing chemotherapy is 21%; with a third D&C, the risk of needing chemotherapy more than doubles to 47%, possibly due to hematogenous metastasis induced by curettage.[452] In a 2019 study, there was no difference in number of chemotherapy cycles for the 2nd curettage group vs control group.[453]

- Medically induced pregnancy terminations/evacuations should be avoided.

Serum hCG

- **Serum β hCG** is a very sensitive and specific marker for trophoblastic tissue and thus a good tumor marker for this disease. The half-life of β hCG is 24 to 36 hours. The amount of hCG correlates to the amount of viable tissue: 5 mIU/mL is approximately equal to 10,000 to 100,000 viable cells. However, it is also produced by many other carcinomas, including lung cancer, ovarian cancer, and colon cancer. Genetic testing should be performed on refractory tumors to ensure the primary is GTD and not otherwise.

- Pituitary hCG is produced at small amounts. This becomes significant in menopause for women who are on high-dose multiagent chemotherapy ceasing ovarian function. Distinguishing trophoblastic versus pituitary hCG can be accomplished by administration of a GnRH agonist or high-dose OCPs.

- A urine β hCG and serum β hCG both need to be performed to confirm β hCG presence. False positive results are considered "phantom hCG" when heterophilic antibodies interfere with immunoassays in the serum test, thus dual testing should be performed at the outset.

- The hook effect occurs when significantly high hCG levels > 1,000,000 IU/L saturate the immunoassay antibodies producing a false negative result by preventing sandwich formation between the solid fixed labeled and soluble liquid antibodies. Serial dilution can help distill to correct the results.

Staging

- FIGO 2021 staging is **clinical** incorporating the WHO risk factors to obtain a final modified FIGO/WHO risk score (Table 2.33 A–C). The hCG level at the time of diagnosis not molar evacuation should be used.

Table 2.33A AJCC 8th Edition: T Category

AJCC		FIGO
TX	Unable to assess primary tumor	
T0	Unable to detect presence of primary tumor	
T1	Tumor limited to uterus	I
T2	Invasion of tumor (by metastasis or direct invasion) to other genital areas, such as ovary, tube, vagina, broad ligaments	II

Table 2.33B AJCC 8th Edition: M Category

AJCC		FIGO
M0	Distant metastasis not present	
M1	Presence of distant metastasis	
M1	a Metastasis to the lung	III
	b All types of distant metastasis excluding metastasis to the lung	IV

Table 2.33C AJCC 8th Edition: Stage Grouping

*I: (risk score)	T1M0
*II: (risk score)	T2M0
*III: (risk score)	AnyTM1a
*IV: (risk score)	AnyTM1b

*The stage is noted with risk factor score to follow.

- **Prognostic factors** required for staging: Patients are classified into low risk or high risk categories of metastatic disease based on the WHO score as calculated in Table 2.34. The scores from eight risk factors are summed and incorporated into the FIGO stage, separated by a colon (e.g., stage III:8). If the score is less than seven, the patient considered low risk. If the score is seven or greater, the patient high risk. Ultra-high risk is >13. The modified WHO prognostic scoring system is not applicable to patients with PSTT or ETT (Tables 2.34 and 2.35).

Treatment
- Molar pregnancy GTD:
  - Evacuation via suction D&C is the primary treatment. Some clinicians avoid sharp curettage due to the increased risk of uterine

Table 2.34 WHO Prognostic Scoring System for GTD as Modified by FIGO (2002)

Score	0	1	2	4
Age	≤39	≥40		
Antecedent pregnancy	Mole	Abortion	Term	
Interval months from index pregnancy	<4	4–6	7–12	>12
Pre-treatment serum hCG level (IU/L)	$<10^3$	10^3–10^4	10^4–10^5	$>10^5$
Largest tumor size including uterus	<3 cm	3–5 cm	>5	
Site of metastasis	Lung	Spleen, kidney	GI	Brain, liver
Number of metastases	–	1–4	5–8	>8
Prior failed chemotherapy drugs	–	–	1	≥2

perforation and possible metastasis. If fertility is not desired, a hysterectomy with ovarian preservation can be the primary treatment of a molar pregnancy (but with continued serial hCG surveillance).

○ Weekly surveillance with hCG is recommended after evacuation. Once normalized, surveillance should continue for 1 month for a PM and 3–6 months for a CM.

○ Medications, such as Prostin, have been shown to increase the need for chemotherapy due to hematogenous spread via contraction of the uterine arteries. Pitocin administered after cervical dilation can assist in uterine involution in addition to expression of uterine contents extracorporeally and not into the vascular system. RhoGAM should be given if the patient is Rh negative.

Table 2.35 GTD Metastatic Site Rate

GTD Metastatic Sites	Percentage
Lungs	80
Vagina	30
Pelvis	20
Brain	10
Liver	10
Bowel, kidney, spleen	5

Table 2.36 GTD High-Risk Clinical Features for Metastatic Disease

Clinical Feature	Risk of GTD (%)
Delayed postmolar evacuation hemorrhage	75
Theca lutein cysts >5 cm	60
Acute pulmonary insufficiency following molar evacuation	58
Uterus large for dates (16-wk size)	45
Serum hCG >100,000 mIU/mL	45
Second molar gestation	40
Maternal age >40	25

- o Some patients with molar pregnancies are considered high risk for developing GTN or metastatic disease (Table 2.36). Chemoprophylaxis with a one-time dose of single-agent chemotherapy can be considered. In these patients, data have shown the rates of persistent disease have gone from about 50% to 15%. Chemoprophylaxis in lower-risk patients can also be considered if they are seen as potentially noncompliant.
- Invasive disease/GTN:
  - o Stage I disease can be managed surgically or with chemotherapy.
    - Surgical management:
      - □ A hysterectomy with ovarian preservation can be performed if fertility is not desired, and recommended for women >50 Y, or those 40 to 49 with hCG of 175,000 IU. A single dose of either MTX or Act-D immediately prior to the surgical procedure should be considered for prophylaxis against embolism of tumor cells from surgical manipulation.
      - □ A second uterine curettage can be performed in low risk (score 0–6) patients understanding that there is a high risk of uterine perforation. Of patients treated with a second D&C instead of single-agent chemotherapy, 38% normalized their hCG within 6 months, avoiding any chemotherapy; and 6.3% were recategorized histologically to have PSTT.
    - Single-agent chemotherapy is administered if hysterectomy is not performed. Chemotherapy is either with Act-D or MTX. Act-D was found to be superior to MTX with a risk ratio of 0.65 in a Cochrane review. Biweekly pulsed Act-D showed a CRR of 44% when the WHO score was 5–6.[454] The likelihood of success of weekly MTX is dependent on the WHO score. Weekly IM MXT is successful in 70% of patients with a WHO score of 0–1, but falls to 40% in those with a score of 2 to 4, and 12% in those who score 5 to 6.

- Combination chemotherapy is recommended for those scoring 5 to 6 and the hCG >410,000 IU/L.
  - Stage II disease follows the same chemotherapy principles as those of stage I disease.
    - Combination chemotherapy is recommended for an hCG > 150,000 IU/L with (genital) metastasis.
  - Stage III disease is categorized as either low risk or high risk based on WHO risk scoring.
    - If the patient is considered low risk initial single-agent chemotherapy is administered.
    - If low risk but scoring 5 to 6 and hCG > 410,000 (with metastasis): combination chemotherapy is administered.
    - If the patient is high risk, combination chemotherapy with EMA-CO should be initiated.
  - Stage IV disease is high risk, by definition, and is initially managed with combination chemotherapy. Treatment is usually with EMA-CO, but the MTX dose is increased to 1 g/m^2. If there are cerebral metastases, craniotomy to prevent herniation from mass or hemorrhage may be indicated.
  - Ultra high risk: WHO score > 13: Consider induction chemotherapy.
    - *Induction* chemotherapy consists of EP for one to two cycles, continuing thereafter with EMA-CO. Low-dose induction EP consists of etoposide 100 mg/m^2 and cisplatin 20 mg/m^2 on days 1 and 2 repeating weekly for one to three cycles before starting EMA-CO.
- PSTT optimal therapy is a hysterectomy with pelvic and PA-LN dissection. Ovarian preservation has not been found to be detrimental. This is a relatively chemoresistant tumor, so if the disease is found to be advanced or presents >48 months after any gestational event, surgery with adjuvant chemotherapy is considered the best option. Chemotherapy can consist of EMA-EP or EMA-CO. The only prognostic factor identified regarding survival, is time from the last pregnancy. If this time is less than 4 Y, patients usually do well; if it is greater than 4 Y, this is usually universally fatal.
- ETT is generally more aggressive than PSTT but is treated in a similar fashion.
- Choriocarcinoma is, by definition, high-risk disease and should be treated with combination EMA-CO therapy.
- Atypical placental site nodule: This has been associated with PSTT and ETT, or the development of these tumors within 16 months of diagnosis, in 15% of cases. If identified, whole-body imaging should be obtained and hysterectomy should be considered.

Duration of Chemotherapy

- Single-agent chemotherapy is continued for two to three courses beyond normalization of hCG for low-risk disease. For high-risk disease, choriocarcinoma, stage IV disease or a WHO score greater than 13 (ultra-high-risk), three to four additional courses are recommended after normalization of hCG. This is due to data suggesting that 100,000 viable cancer cells remain when the β hCG becomes undetectable. hCG levels should be checked weekly during chemotherapy or at least D1 of each cycle.

Management of Acute Disease and Induced Complications

- If there is uterine hemorrhage, vaginal packing, blood transfusion, and emergent uterine artery embolization can be performed. Laparotomy may be necessary for hysterectomy.
- Respiratory failure either from tumor embolization, pulmonary embolization, tumor burden, or hemorrhage may occur. Mechanical ventilation is contraindicated due to a high risk of trauma and iatrogenic hemorrhage, but CPAP is a good alternative. Risk factors for respiratory failure are as follows: 50% opacification of lung fields on CXR, dyspnea, anemia, cyanosis, and pulmonary HTN. Consideration for those with a high thorax tumor burden, to decrease the risk of death from pulmonary hemorrhage or respiratory failure within the first 4 weeks of therapy, is to start with induction therapy. High-risk patients receiving induction EP compared to patients not receiving EP had a higher, but NS, relapse rate (9% vs. 6% $p = .44$) and death rate (12% vs. 4%; $p = .88$).[455]
- If cerebral metastases are identified, vigilance for cerebral hemorrhage, edema, and herniation should be maintained. If a solitary lesion is found, site-directed gamma knife or stereotactic radiation can be considered, as well as surgical resection, which can be administered simultaneously with systemic chemotherapy. If multiple lesions are identified, WB-XRT is recommended with dosing to 30 Gy in 200 cGy fractions. Premedication with 24 mg of dexamethasone twice daily during treatment with WB-XRT is important. The MTX dose in the EMA-CO regimen is increased to 1 g/m² and 30 mg of folinic acid every 12 hours for 3 days starting 32 hours after the infusion begins. Induction chemotherapy should be considered for three to four cycles. Intrathecal MTX can be considered and administered at 12.5 mg followed in 24 hours with 15–30 mg of oral folinic acid. This is given once with each course of CO during EMA-CO therapy. Cure rates with brain metastasis approach 50% to 80%.

Resistant Disease

- Diagnosis of resistance to first-line therapy in low-risk GTN is by: a persistent elevation over 3 consecutive samples, or an increase over

2 consecutive samples lasting >2 weeks. Patients with a hCG <100 IU/L can be considered for change to single-agent Act-D after failing MTX or they can be treated with EMA-CO. For patients who fail single-agent treatment with a hCG level >100–300 IU/L, treatment should be with combination EMA-CO chemotherapy.

- In stage I resistant disease a switch to the other single-agent chemotherapy drug is indicated if hCG is ≤3000 IU/L. Change to EMA-CO should be considered if the hCG is >3000 IU/L. A salvage hysterectomy or local uterine resection may be considered in addition to chemotherapy if there is persistent disease.

- Stage II resistant disease is treated in a similar fashion as that for stage I resistant disease.

- Stage III resistant disease:
  - For stage III low-risk resistant disease, treatment with MAC or EMA-CO should follow single-agent chemotherapy.
  - For high-risk stage III resistant disease, treatment with other regimens is indicated. These include EMA-EP, MAC, CHAMOCA, VPB, VIP, or ACE, TE-TP, ICE.
  - For oligometastatic disease, thoracotomy or liver wedge resection can be considered.

- Stage IV resistant disease: Second-line combination chemotherapy with EMA-EP, MAC, CHAMOCA, VPB, VIP, ACE, TE-TP, or ICE is indicated. Hysterectomy with ovarian preservation may be indicated if this appears to be the sole site of resistant disease.

Recurrent Disease

- At diagnosis, reimaging with a CT of the chest, abdomen, and pelvis and MRI of the brain should be obtained. If all are negative, it may be helpful to then perform a lumbar puncture. Rescoring of the WHO risk factors is instrumental in choosing treatment regimens.

- Experimental imaging techniques can be employed to include anti-hCG radioisotope scanning and PET.

- Low-risk patients who relapse can switch to the other single-agent chemotherapy drug if the hCG is ≤3000 IU/L. A change to EMA-CO should occur if the hCG is >3000 IU/L.

- If there are lung metastases and this appears to be the only site of resistant disease on comprehensive workup, a thoracotomy with lobectomy may be considered. If there are isolated liver metastases, a wedge resection may also be considered.

- Avelumab and pembrolizumab may be options for recurrent/resistant disease as well as in PSTT after term pregnancy given that PDL-1 is constitutively expressed in all trophoblast subtypes. It is not recommended for low-risk disease after failed MTX treatment.[456]

- Stem cell transplant can be considered with high-dose chemotherapy for multiagent resistant disease.

Follow-Up

- For stages I to III, weekly quantitative "total hCG assay" levels should be drawn until they normalize for 3 weeks. Monthly quantitative hCG levels should then continue until they are normal for 6 to 12 consecutive months. If a total assay is not available, β-hCG should be followed.
- For stage IV disease it is important to follow β hCG levels monthly for 2 Y after the weekly beta hCG levels have normalized. Two large trials have found that surveillance of hCG levels for more than 10 Y is unnecessary.
- Contraception with OCPs (preferably) or another form of reliable contraception is important. Pregnancy may be attempted after 6 to 12 months of normal β hCGs. IUDs are not recommended due to the risk of uterine perforation.
- An hCG level should be obtained 6 to 8 weeks after completion of any gestation.
- A first-trimester US in any subsequent pregnancy should be obtained between 6 to 8 weeks to localize and assess the pregnancy.

Notable Trials

- GOG 55: In this study, 266 patients were randomly assigned to either OCP versus barrier method contraception after molar evacuation. The median time to spontaneous regression in the OCP group was 9 weeks, compared to the median time to regression in the barrier group of 10 weeks. Twice as many patients in the barrier group became pregnant in the immediate follow-up period; 23% of patients receiving OCPs had postmolar trophoblastic disease versus 33% of patients using barrier methods. OCPs are the preferred method of contraception after evacuation of a hydatidiform mole.[457]
- GOG 79: In this study, Patients with nonmetastatic GTD were initially treated with 30 mg/m^2 of weekly IM MTX. If no major toxicity was encountered, the weekly dose was escalated by 5 mg/m^2 at 3-week intervals until a maximum dose of 50 mg/m^2 each week was achieved. Eighty-one percent had a CR to weekly IM MTX. Duration of therapy ranged from 3 to 19 weeks, with a median of 7 weeks. No major dose limiting toxicity occurred, thus 50 mg/m^2 is acceptable dosing.[458]
- GOG 79 follow-up study: This study evaluated 62 patients with nonmetastatic GTD who were initially treated with 40 mg/m^2 weekly of IM MTX. If no major toxicity was encountered, the weekly dose was escalated by 5 mg/m^2 at 2-week intervals until a maximum dose of 50 mg/m^2 per week was achieved; 74% had a CR. Duration of therapy ranged from 3 weeks to 16 weeks with a median of 7 weeks. No major toxicity occurred. The 40 mg/m^2 dose of weekly IM MTX therapy is no more effective and of similar toxicity to the 30 mg/m^2 regimen.[459]

- GOG 174: This trial evaluated 216 eligible patients with a WHO score of 0 to 6 and metastatic disease limited to lung lesions less than 2 cm, adnexa, or vagina, and/or histologically proven nonmetastatic choriocarcinoma. Patients were randomized to either biweekly IV actinomycin D 1.25 mg/m² versus weekly IM MTX 30 mg/m². Biweekly actinomycin D was superior to weekly MTX (CR 70% vs. 53%; $p = .03$). If the risk score was 5 to 6, or the diagnosis was choriocarcinoma, the CR to MTX was 9% and the CR was 42% with actinomycin D. Primary chemotherapy should then consist of actinomycin D in these intermediate and HiR patients.[460]

- GOG 242: This was a phase II study evaluating efficacy and safety of second uterine curettage in low-risk nonmetastatic GTN. In the study, 64 patients were enrolled and 24 (40%) were cured after second curettage without need for any chemotherapy. One uterine perforation occurred. Surgical failure occurred in 59% of women and was found more commonly in the age extremes. Four uterine hemorrhages occurred, and one new lung metastasis was observed. At the second curettage, histopathologic discrepancy changed the diagnosis (PSTT and placental nodule) for four patients. Higher WHO score trended to lower rate of second curettage cure.[461]

- GOG 275: This was a phase III randomized trial of pulse actinomycin-D versus multi-day MTX for the management of low-risk GTN in 57 patients which showed that multiday MTX had an 88% CR vs. q2 week actinomycin-D with a 79% CR, both arms having a 100% OS. QOL was not different between arms but the MTX arm had more treatment disruptions. There were 2 recurrences in each arm.[466]

- Second Uterine Curettage and the Number of Chemotherapy Courses in Postmolar GTN: A Randomized Controlled Trial.[453] This was a phase III trial in patients with low-risk GTN randomized in a 1:1 fashion either to a second or no curettage before MTX treatment in which 89 patients were included between 2011-16. Eligibility criteria were serum hCG level 5,000< IU/L for treatment with MTX. The primary outcome was the number of chemotherapy courses required for hCG normalization between groups. Secondary outcomes were need for second-line treatment, toxicity, rate of relapse. Forty-three patients were included in the ITT analysis. There were no surgical complications, the mean number of chemotherapy courses required to reach hCG normalization was 4.4 ± 2.2 SD in the control group vs 3.8 ± 2.3 SD in the second curettage group ($p = .14$). Groups were comparable in terms of second-line treatment needed to reach hCG normalization, and relapse within the first Y. Thus, second uterine curettage did not affect the number of chemotherapy courses required or change relapse rate in patients with LoR postmolar GTN.

- Trophimmun (Avelumab in Chemo-resistant GTN) trial: This was a phase II multicenter trial of 15 women with GTT whose disease progressed after monotherapy who received avelumab 10 mg/kg IV q2 weeks until hCG normalization, followed by three consolidation cycles, or progression.[462] The rate of hCG normalization was the primary end-point for the study that ran between 2016-18. The median age was 34 Y; disease stage was I in 53.3% and III in 46.7; FIGO score was 0 to 4 in 33.3%, 5 to 6 in 46.7%, and ≥7 in 20% of patients. Prior single-agent treatment was MTX (100%) and actinomycin D (7%). The median follow-up was 25 months, with eight as the median number of avelumab cycles (range, 2-11). G 1 to 2 AEs happened in 93% of patients, the most common being (≥25%) fatigue (33.3%), nausea and vomiting (33.3%), and infusion-related reaction (26.7%). Eight patients (53.3%) had hCG normalization after a median of nine avelumab cycles; none relapsed. Probability of normalization was not associated with FIGO score, stage of disease, or baseline hCG level. In avelumab-resistant patients (46.7%), hCG was normalized with actinomycin D (42.3%) or combination chemotherapy/surgery (57.1%). Thus, avelumab had a favorable safety profile and cured approximately 50% of patients.

- GTN after hCG normalization following molar pregnancy. A systematic review and meta-analysis.[463] This was a meta-analysis, of 19 studies that found a low incidence of GTN after normalization of hCG levels following both CM (64/18,357, 0.35%, 95% CI 0.27–0.45%), and partial mole (5/14,864, 0.03%, 95% CI 0.01–0.08). There was a higher risk of GTN after CM compared to partial mole (risk ratio 4.72, 95% CI 1.81–12.3, $p = .002$). For GTN cases after hCG normalization following CM 89.6% happened when the time from evacuation to normalization was 56 days or longer, and 60.7% were diagnosed beyond the usual 6-month recommended surveillance interval. There was an overall incidence of GTN of 15.7% for CM (1,354/8,611, 95% CI 15.0–16.5%) and 3.95% for partial mole (221/5,593, 95% CI 3.47–4.50%). Recommendations for frequency and duration of hCG testing can be reduced to decrease the burden on patients guided by the type of molar pregnancy and time interval from uterine evacuation to hCG normalization.

- When to stop hCG surveillance after treatment with chemotherapy for GTN: This was a retrospective review of low-risk and high-risk GTN patients receiving chemotherapy in the UK between 1958-2015.[464] The overall risk of relapse in 4,201 patients was 4.7% (198) with a median time to recurrence of 117.5 days ranging from 9 days to 6.54 Y. The greatest risk time was in the first Y after treatment completion at 72.2% for low-risk GTN and 86.4% in high-risk disease. With no recurrences beyond 7 Y, lifelong hCG surveillance is unnecessary and can be discontinued between 7 and 10 Y.

REFERENCES

1. Massad LS, Calvello C, Gilkey SH, et al. Assessing disease extent in women with bulky or clinically evident metastatic cervical cancer: yield of pretreatment studies. *Gynecol Oncol.* 2000;76(3):383–387. doi:10.1006/gyno.1999.5714

2. Havrilesky LJ, Kulasingam SL, Matchar DB, et al. FDG-pet for management of cervical and ovarian cancer. *Gynecol Oncol.* 2005;97(1):183–191. doi:10.1016/j.ygyno.2004.12.007

3. Amit A, Beck D, Lowenstein L, et al. The role of hybrid PET/CT in the evaluation of patients with cervical cancer. *Gynecol Oncol.* 2006;100(1):65–69. doi:10.1016/j.ygyno.2005.07.013

4. Roma AA, Diaz De Vivar A, Park KJ, et al. Invasive endocervical adenocarcinoma: a new pattern-based classification system with important clinical significance. *Am J Surg Pathol.* 2015;39(5):667–672. doi:10.1097/PAS.0000000000000402

5. Roma AA, Mistretta T-A, Diaz De Vivar A, et al. New pattern-based personalized risk stratification system for endocervical adenocarcinoma with important clinical implications and surgical outcome. *Gynecol Oncol.* 2016;141(1):36–42. doi:10.1016/j.ygyno.2016.02.028

6. Bhatl N, Aoki D, Sharma DN. Cancer of the cervix uteri FIGO cancer report 2018. *Int J Gynecol Obstet.* 2018;143(Suppl. 2):22–36. doi:10.1002/ijgo.12611

7. Olawaiye AB, Baker TP, Washington MK, et al. The new (version 9) American joint committee on cancer tumor, node, metastasis staging for cervical cancer. *CA Cancer J Clin.* 2021;71(4):287–298. doi:10.3322/caac.21663

8. Ramirez PT, Frumovitz M, Pareja R, et al. Minimally invasive versus abdominal radical hysterectomy for cervical cancer. *N Engl J Med.* 2018;379(20):1895–1904. doi:10.1056/NEJMoa1806395

9. Landoni F, Maneo A, Cormio G, et al. Class II versus class III radical hysterectomy in stage IB-IIA cervical cancer: a prospective randomized study. *Gynecol Oncol.* 2001;80(1):3–12. doi:10.1006/gyno.2000.6010

10. Landoni F, Maneo A, Colombo A, et al. Randomised study of radical surgery versus radiotherapy for stage IB-IIA cervical cancer. *Lancet.* 1997;350(9077):535–540. doi:10.1016/S0140-6736(97)02250-2

11. Wolf JK, Levenback C, Malpica A, et al. Adenocarcinoma in situ of the cervix: significance of cone biopsy margins. *Obstet Gynecol.* 1996;88(1):82–86. doi:10.1016/0029-7844(96)00083-X

12. Greer BE, Figge DC, Tamimi HK, et al. Stage IA2 squamous carcinoma of the cervix: difficult diagnosis and therapeutic dilemma. *Am J Obstet Gynecol.* 1990;162(6):1406–1409. doi:10.1016/0002-9378(90)90899-i

13. Sutton GP, Bundy BN, Delgado G, et al. Ovarian metastases in stage ib carcinoma of the cervix: A Gynecologic Oncology Group study. *Am J Obstet Gynecol.* 1992;166(1 Pt 1):50–53. doi:10.1016/0002-9378(92)91828-x

14. Whitney CW, Stehman FB. The abandoned radical hysterectomy: a Gynecologic Oncology Group study. *Gynecol Oncol.* 2000;79(3):350–356. doi:10.1006/gyno.2000.5993

15. Ziebarth AJ, Smith H, Killian ME, et al. Completed versus aborted radical hysterectomy for node-positive stage ib cervical cancer in the modern era of chemoradiation therapy. *Gynecol Oncol.* 2012;126(1):69–72. doi:10.1016/j.ygyno.2012.03.046

16. Potter ME, Alvarez RD, Shingleton HM, et al. Early invasive cervical cancer with pelvic lymph node involvement: to complete or not to complete radical hysterectomy? *Gynecol Oncol.* 1990;37(1):78–81. doi:10.1016/0090-8258(90)90312-9

17. Magrina JF. The prognostic significance of pelvic and aortic lymph node metastasis. *CME J Gynecol Oncol.* 2001;6(3):302–306.

18. Goff BA, Muntz HG, Paley PJ, et al. Impact of surgical staging in women with locally advanced cervical cancer. *Gynecol Oncol.* 1999;74(3):436–442. doi:10.1006/gyno.1999.5472

19. Cosin JA, Fowler JM, Chen MD, et al. Pretreatment surgical staging of patients with cervical carcinoma: The case for lymph node debulking. *Cancer.* 1998;82(11):2241–2248. doi:10.1002/(sici)1097-0142(19980601)82:11<2241::aid-cncr20>3.0.co;2-t

20. Smith KB, Amdur RJ, Yeung AR, et al. Postoperative radiotherapy for cervix cancer incidentally discovered after a simple hysterectomy for either benign conditions or noninvasive pathology. *Am J Clin Oncol.* 2010;33(3):229–232. doi:10.1097/COC.0b013e3181a6500d

21. Rose PG, Ali S, Whitney CW, et al. Impact of hydronephrosis on outcome of stage IIIB cervical cancer patients with disease limited to the pelvis, treated with radiation and concurrent chemotherapy: a gynecologic oncology group study. *Gynecol Oncol.* 2010;117(2):270–275. doi:10.1016/j.ygyno.2010.01.045

22. Piver MS, Rutledge F, Smith JP. Five classes of extended hysterectomy for women with cervical cancer. *Obstet Gynecol.* 1974;44(2):265–272.

23. Boran N, Kayikçioğˇlu F, Tulunay G, et al. Scalene lymph node dissection in locally advanced cervical carcinoma: is it reasonable or unnecessary? *Tumori.* 2003;89(2):173–175. doi:10.1177/030089160308900213

24. Li J, Wu X, Li X, et al. Abdominal radical trachelectomy: is it safe for IB1 cervical cancer with tumors ≥ 2 cm? *Gynecol Oncol.* 2013;131(1):87–92. doi:10.1016/j.ygyno.2013.07.079

25. Chambers SK, Chambers JT, Kier R, et al. Sequelae of lateral ovarian transposition in irradiated cervical cancer patients. *Int J Radiat Oncol Biol Phys.* 1991;20(6):1305–1308. doi:10.1016/0360-3016(91)90242-v

26. Sedlis A, Bundy BN, Rotman MZ, et al. A randomized trial of pelvic radiation therapy versus no further therapy in selected patients with stage ib carcinoma of the cervix after radical hysterectomy and pelvic lymphadenectomy: a gynecologic oncology group study. *Gynecol Oncol.* 1999;73(2):177–183. doi:10.1006/gyno.1999.5387

27. Delgado G, Bundy B, Zaino R, et al. Prospective surgical-pathological study of disease-free interval in patients with stage IB squamous cell carcinoma of the cervix: a gynecologic oncology group study. *Gynecol Oncol.* 1990;38(3):352–357. doi:10.1016/0090-8258(90)90072-s

28. Peters WA, Liu PY, Barrett RJ, et al. Concurrent chemotherapy and pelvic radiation therapy compared with pelvic radiation therapy alone as adjuvant therapy after radical surgery in high-risk early-stage cancer of the cervix. *J Clin Oncol.* 2000;18(8):1606–1613. doi:10.1200/JCO.2000.18.8.1606

29. Obermair A, Cheuk R, Horwood K, et al. Anemia before and during concurrent chemoradiotherapy in patients with cervical carcinoma: effect on progression-free survival. *Int J Gynecol Cancer*. 2003;13(5):633–639. doi:10.1046/j.1525-1438.2003.13395.x

30. Thomas G, Ali S, Hoebers FJP, et al. Phase III trial to evaluate the efficacy of maintaining hemoglobin levels above 12.0 g/dl with erythropoietin vs above 10.0 g/dl without erythropoietin in anemic patients receiving concurrent radiation and cisplatin for cervical cancer. *Gynecol Oncol*. 2008;108(2):317–325. doi:10.1016/j.ygyno.2007.10.011

31. Irie T, Kigawa J, Minagawa Y, et al. Prognosis and clinicopathological characteristics of ib-iib adenocarcinoma of the uterine cervix in patients who have had radical hysterectomy. *Eur J Surg Oncol*. 2000;26(5):464–467. doi:10.1053/ejso.1999.0923

32. Tewari KS, Sill MW, Long HJ, et al. Improved survival with bevacizumab in advanced cervical cancer. *N Engl J Med*. 2014;370(8):734–743. doi:10.1056/NEJMoa1309748

33. Russell AH, Koh WJ, Markette K, et al. Radical reirradiation for recurrent or second primary carcinoma of the female reproductive tract. *Gynecol Oncol*. 1987;27(2):226–232. doi:10.1016/0090-8258(87)90297-6

34. Monk BJ, Walker JL, Tewari K, et al. Open interstitial brachytherapy for the treatment of local-regional recurrences of uterine corpus and cervix cancer after primary surgery. *Gynecol Oncol*. 1994;52(2):222–228. doi:10.1006/gyno.1994.1035

35. Moore DH, Tian C, Monk BJ, et al. Prognostic factors for response to cisplatin-based chemotherapy in advanced cervical carcinoma: a gynecologic oncology group study. *Gynecol Oncol*. 2010;116(1):44–49. doi:10.1016/j.ygyno.2009.09.006

36. Winer I, Kim C, Gehrig P. Neuroendocrine tumors of the gynecologic tract update. *Gynecol Oncol*. 2021;162(1):210–219. doi:10.1016/j.ygyno.2021.04.039

37. Delgado G, Bundy BN, Fowler WC, et al. A prospective surgical pathological study of stage I squamous carcinoma of the cervix: a gynecologic oncology group study. *Gynecol Oncol*. 1989;35(3):314–320. doi:10.1016/0090-8258(89)90070-x

38. Keys HM, Bundy BN, Stehman FB, et al. Radiation therapy with and without extrafascial hysterectomy for bulky stage ib cervical carcinoma: a randomized trial of the gynecologic oncology group. *Gynecol Oncol*. 2003;89(3):343–353. doi:10.1016/s0090-8258(03)00173-2

39. Rotman M, Sedlis A, Piedmonte MR, et al. A phase III randomized trial of postoperative pelvic irradiation in stage ib cervical carcinoma with poor prognostic features: follow-up of a gynecologic oncology group study. *Int J Radiat Oncol Biol Phys*. 2006;65(1):169–176. doi:10.1016/j.ijrobp.2005.10.019

40. Keys HM, Bundy BN, Stehman FB, et al. Cisplatin, radiation, and adjuvant hysterectomy compared with radiation and adjuvant hysterectomy for bulky stage ib cervical carcinoma. *N Engl J Med*. 1999;340(15):1154–1161. doi:10.1056/NEJM199904153401503

41. Whitney CW, Sause W, Bundy BN, et al. Randomized comparison of fluorouracil plus cisplatin versus hydroxyurea as an adjunct to radiation therapy in stage IIB-IVA carcinoma of the cervix with negative para-aortic lymph nodes: a gynecologic oncology group and southwest oncology group study. *J Clin Oncol*. 1999;17(5):1339–1348. doi:10.1200/JCO.1999.17.5.1339

42. Rose PG, Bundy BN, Watkins EB, et al. Concurrent cisplatin-based radiotherapy and chemotherapy for locally advanced cervical cancer. *N Engl J Med*. 1999;340(15):1144–1153. doi:10.1056/NEJM199904153401502

43. Monk BJ, Wang J, Im S, et al. Rethinking the use of radiation and chemotherapy after radical hysterectomy: a clinical-pathologic analysis of A gynecologic oncology group/southwest oncology group/radiation therapy oncology group trial. *Gynecol Oncol*. 2005;96(3):721–728. doi:10.1016/j.ygyno.2004.11.007

44. Varia MA, Bundy BN, Deppe G, et al. Cervical carcinoma metastatic to para-aortic nodes: extended field radiation therapy with concomitant 5-fluorouracil and cisplatin chemotherapy: a gynecologic oncology group study. *Int J Radiat Oncol Biol Phys*. 1998;42(5):1015–1023. doi:10.1016/s0360-3016(98)00267-3

45. Lanciano R, Calkins A, Bundy BN, et al. Randomized comparison of weekly cisplatin or protracted venous infusion of fluorouracil in combination with pelvic radiation in advanced cervix cancer: a gynecologic oncology group study. *J Clin Oncol*. 2005;23(33):8289–8295. doi:10.1200/JCO.2004.00.0497

46. Rotman M, Pajak TF, Choi K, et al. Prophylactic extended-field irradiation of para-aortic lymph nodes in stages iib and bulky ib and IIA cervical carcinomas. ten-year treatment results of RTOG 79-20. *JAMA*. 1995;274(5):387–393.

47. Morris M, Eifel PJ, Lu J, et al. Pelvic radiation with concurrent chemotherapy compared with pelvic and para-aortic radiation for high-risk cervical cancer. *N Engl J Med*. 1999;340(15):1137–1143. doi:10.1056/NEJM199904153401501

48. Eifel PJ, Winter K, Morris M, et al. Pelvic irradiation with concurrent chemotherapy versus pelvic and para-aortic irradiation for high-risk cervical cancer: an update of radiation therapy oncology group trial (RTOG) 90-01. *J Clin Oncol*. 2004;22(5):872–880. doi:10.1200/JCO.2004.07.197

49. Pearcey R, Brundage M, Drouin P, et al. Phase III trial comparing radical radiotherapy with and without cisplatin chemotherapy in patients with advanced squamous cell cancer of the cervix. *J Clin Oncol*. 2002;20(4):966–972. doi:10.1200/JCO.2002.20.4.966

50. Moore DH, Blessing JA, McQuellon RP, et al. Phase III study of cisplatin with or without paclitaxel in stage ivb, recurrent, or persistent squamous cell carcinoma of the cervix: a gynecologic oncology group study. *J Clin Oncol*. 2004;22(15):3113–3119. doi:10.1200/JCO.2004.04.170

51. Long HJ, Bundy BN, Grendys EC, et al. Randomized phase III trial of cisplatin with or without topotecan in carcinoma of the uterine cervix: a gynecologic oncology group study. *J Clin Oncol*. 2005;23(21):4626–4633. doi:10.1200/JCO.2005.10.021

52. Monk BJ, Sill MW, McMeekin DS, et al. Phase III trial of four cisplatin-containing doublet combinations in stage ivb, recurrent, or persistent cervical carcinoma: a gynecologic oncology group study. *J Clin Oncol.* 2009;27(28):4649–4655. doi:10.1200/JCO.2009.21.8909

53. Dueñas-González A, Zarbá JJ, Patel F, et al. Phase III, open-label, randomized study comparing concurrent gemcitabine plus cisplatin and radiation followed by adjuvant gemcitabine and cisplatin versus concurrent cisplatin and radiation in patients with stage iib to IVA carcinoma of the cervix. *J Clin Oncol.* 2011;29(13):1678–1685. doi:10.1200/JCO.2009.25.9663

54. Wang C-C, Chou H-H, Yang L-Y, et al. A randomized trial comparing concurrent chemoradiotherapy with single-agent cisplatin versus cisplatin plus gemcitabine in patients with advanced cervical cancer: an Asian gynecologic oncology group study. *Gynecol Oncol.* 2015;137(3):462–467. doi:10.1016/j.ygyno.2015.03.046

55. Penson RT, Huang HQ, Wenzel LB, et al. Bevacizumab for advanced cervical cancer: patient-reported outcomes of a randomised, phase 3 trial (NRG oncology-gynecologic oncology group protocol 240). *Lancet Oncol.* 2015;16(3):301–311. doi:10.1016/S1470-2045(15)70004-5

56. Gynecologic Oncology Group. Randomized phase III clinical trial of adjuvant radiation versus chemoradiation in intermediate risk, stage I/IIa cervical cancer treated with initial radical hysterectomy and pelvic lymphadenectomy. https://clinicaltrials.gov/ct2/show/NCT01101451

57. Huh WK, Brady WE, Moore KN, et al. A phase ii study of live-attenuated *listeria* monocytogenes immunotherapy (ADXS11-001) in the treatment of persistent or recurrent cancer of the cervix (GOG-0265). *JCO.* 2013;31(15_suppl):TPS3121–TPS3121. doi:10.1200/jco.2013.31.15_suppl.tps3121

58. Kitagawa R, Katsumata N, Shibata T, et al. Paclitaxel plus carboplatin versus paclitaxel plus cisplatin in metastatic or recurrent cervical cancer: the open-label randomized phase III trial JCOG0505. *J Clin Oncol.* 2015;33(19):2129–2135. doi:10.1200/JCO.2014.58.4391

59. Alberts DS, Blessing JA, Landrum LM, et al. Phase II trial of nab-paclitaxel in the treatment of recurrent or persistent advanced cervix cancer: a gynecologic oncology group study. *Gynecol Oncol.* 2012;127(3):S0090-8258(12)00741-X):451–455:. doi:10.1016/j.ygyno.2012.09.008

60. Ryu HS, Sugiyama T. 9Th Korea-Japan gynecologic cancer joint meeting. *J Gynecol Oncol.* 2012;23(1):3–4.

61. Mathevet P. Sentinel lymph node biopsy for early cervical cancer: results of a randomized prospective, multicenter study (Senticol 2) comparing adding pelvic lymph node dissection vs sentinel node biopsy only. Abstract presented at: SGO *Annual Meeting National Harbor Maryland.* 2017.

62. Balaya V, Guani B, Magaud L, et al. Long-term oncological safety of sentinel lymph node biopsy in early-stage cervical cancer. *JCO.* 2020;38(15_suppl):6006–6006. doi:10.1200/JCO.2020.38.15_suppl.6006

63. Sponholtz SE, Mogensen O, Hildebrandt MG, et al. Sentinel lymph node mapping in early-stage cervical cancer—a national prospective

multicenter study (SENTIREC trial). *Gynecol Oncol.* 2021;162(3):546–554. doi:10.1016/j.ygyno.2021.06.018

64. Frumovitz M, Obermair A, Coleman RL. Quality of life in patients with cervical cancer after open versus minimally invasive radical hysterectomy: results from the LACC randomized trial. *Lancet Oncol.* 2022.

65. Melamed A, Margul DJ, Chen L, et al. Survival after minimally invasive radical hysterectomy for early-stage cervical cancer. *N Engl J Med.* 2018;379(20):1905–1914. doi:10.1056/NEJMoa1804923

66. Queensland Centre for Gynaecological Cancer. Laparoscopic approach to cervical cancer (LACC). https://clinicaltrials.gov/ct2/show/NCT00614211

67. Mileshkin LR, Moore KN, Barnes E, et al. Adjuvant chemotherapy following chemoradiation as primary treatment for locally advanced cervical cancer compared to chemoradiation alone: the randomized phase III outback trial (anzgog 0902, rtog 1174, nrg 0274). *JCO.* 2021;39(18_suppl):LBA3–LBA3. doi:10.1200/JCO.2021.39.15_suppl.LBA3

68. Chung HC, Ros W, Delord J-P, et al. Efficacy and safety of pembrolizumab in previously treated advanced cervical cancer: results from the phase II KEYNOTE-158 study. *J Clin Oncol.* 2019;37(17):1470–1478. doi:10.1200/JCO.18.01265

69. Colombo N, Dubot C, Lorusso D, et al. Pembrolizumab for persistent, recurrent, or metastatic cervical cancer. *N Engl J Med.* 2021;385(20):1856–1867. doi: 10.1056/NEJMoa2112435

70. Hyun CC, Willeke R, Jean-Pierre D. EMPOWER-cervical 1/GOG-3016/ENGOT-cx9 trial (NCT03257267). *N Engl J Med.* 2022;386:544–555. doi:10.1056/NEJMoa2112187

71. Coleman RL, Lorusso D, Gennigens C, et al. Efficacy and safety of tisotumab vedotin in previously treated recurrent or metastatic cervical cancer (innovatv 204/GOG-3023/ENGOT-cx6): a multicentre, open-label, single-arm, phase 2 study. *Lancet Oncol.* 2021;22(5):609–619. doi:10.1016/S1470-2045(21)00056-5

72. Doherty K. Balstilimab plus zalifrelimab combo may advance survival in patients with recurrent/metastatic cervical cancer. https://www.cancernetwork.com/view/balstilimab-plus-zalifrelimab-combo-may-advance-survival-in-patients-with-recurrent-metastatic-cervical-cancer. Accessed November 28, 2022.

73. Wu J, Logue T, Kaplan SJ, et al. Less radical surgery for early-stage cervical cancer: a systematic review. *Am J Obstet Gynecol.* 2021;224(4):348–358. doi:10.1016/j.ajog.2020.11.041

74. Sturdza A, Pötter R, Fokdal LU, et al. Image guided brachytherapy in locally advanced cervical cancer: improved pelvic control and survival in retroembrace, a multicenter cohort study. *Radiother Oncol.* 2016;120(3):428–433. doi:10.1016/j.radonc.2016.03.011

75. Tanderup K, Fokdal LU, Sturdza A, et al. Effect of tumor dose, volume and overall treatment time on local control after radiochemotherapy including MRI guided brachytherapy of locally advanced cervical cancer. *Radiother Oncol.* 2016;120(3):441–446. doi:10.1016/j.radonc.2016.05.014

76. Fokdal L, Sturdza A, Mazeron R, et al. Image guided adaptive brachyther-apy with combined intracavitary and interstitial technique improves the therapeutic ratio in locally advanced cervical cancer: analysis from the retroembrace study. *Radiother Oncol.* 2016;120(3):434–440. doi:10.1016/j.radonc.2016.03.020

77. Female Genital Tumours. *WHO Classification of Tumours.* Vol 4. 5th Edition. WHO Classification of Tumours Editorial Board; 978–992.

78. Diaz-Padilla I, Malpica AL, Minig L, et al. Ovarian low-grade serous car-cinoma: a comprehensive update. *Gynecol Oncol.* 2012;126(2):279–285. doi:10.1016/j.ygyno.2012.04.029

79. Previs R, Leath CA, Coleman RL, et al. Evaluation of in vitro chemo-response profiles in women with type I and type II epithelial ovarian cancers: an observational study ancillary analysis. *Gynecol Oncol.* 2015;138(2):267–271. doi:10.1016/j.ygyno.2015.05.038

80. Grabowski JP, Harter P, Heitz F, et al. Operability and chemother-apy responsiveness in advanced low-grade serous ovarian cancer. an analysis of the ago study group metadatabase. *Gynecol Oncol.* 2016;140(3):457–462. doi:10.1016/j.ygyno.2016.01.022

81. Gershenson D. The genomic landscape of low-grade serous ovarian/peritoneal carcinoma (LGSOC) and its impact on clinical outcomes. Abstract presented at: SGO annual meeting; March 18–21, 2022.

82. Duska LR, Garrett L, Henretta M, et al. When "never-events" occur despite adherence to clinical guidelines: the case of venous throm-boembolism in clear cell cancer of the ovary compared with other epithelial histologic subtypes. *Gynecol Oncol.* 2010;116(3):374–377. doi:10.1016/j.ygyno.2009.10.069

83. Diaz ES, Walts AE, Karlan BY, et al. Venous thromboembolism during primary treatment of ovarian clear cell carcinoma is associated with decreased survival. *Gynecol Oncol.* 2013;131(3):541–545. doi:10.1016/j.ygyno.2013.09.005

84. Schmeler KM, Tao X, Frumovitz M, et al. Prevalence of lymph node metastasis in primary mucinous carcinoma of the ovary. *Obstet Gynecol.* 2010;116(2 Pt 1):269–273. doi:10.1097/AOG.0b013e3181e7961d

85. Kleppe M, Wang T, Van Gorp T, et al. Lymph node metastasis in stages I and II ovarian cancer: a review. *Gynecol Oncol.* 2011;123(3):610–614. doi:10.1016/j.ygyno.2011.09.013

86. Powless CA, Aletti GD, Bakkum-Gamez JN, et al. Risk factors for lymph node metastasis in apparent early-stage epithelial ovarian cancer: implications for surgical staging. *Gynecol Oncol.* 2011;122(3):536–540. doi:10.1016/j.ygyno.2011.05.001

87. Bristow RE, Tomacruz RS, Armstrong DK, et al. Survival effect of max-imal cytoreductive surgery for advanced ovarian carcinoma during the platinum era: a meta-analysis. *J Clin Oncol.* 2002;20(5):1248–1259. doi:10.1200/JCO.2002.20.5.1248

88. Kumar A, Janco JM, Mariani A, et al. Risk-prediction model of severe postoperative complications after primary debulking surgery for advanced ovarian cancer. *Gynecol Oncol.* 2016;140(1):15–21. doi:10.1016/j.ygyno.2015.10.025

89. Bristow RE, Montz FJ, Lagasse LD, et al. Survival impact of surgical cytoreduction in stage IV epithelial ovarian cancer. *Gynecol Oncol.* 1999;72(3):278–287. doi:10.1006/gyno.1998.5145

90. Panici PB, Maggioni A, Hacker N, et al. Systematic aortic and pelvic lymphadenectomy versus resection of bulky nodes only in optimally debulked advanced ovarian cancer: a randomized clinical trial. *J Natl Cancer Inst.* 2005;97(8):560–566. doi:10.1093/jnci/dji102

91. Harter P, Sehouli J, Lorusso D, et al. A randomized trial of lymphadenectomy in patients with advanced ovarian neoplasms. *N Engl J Med.* 2019;380(9):822–832. doi:10.1056/NEJMoa1808424

92. Fagotti A, Ferrandina G, Fanfani F, et al. Prospective validation of a laparoscopic predictive model for optimal cytoreduction in advanced ovarian carcinoma. *Am J Obstet Gynecol.* 2008;199(6):642e1–642e6. doi:10.1016/j.ajog.2008.06.052

93. Brun J-L, Rouzier R, Uzan S, et al. External validation of a laparoscopic-based score to evaluate resectability of advanced ovarian cancers: clues for a simplified score. *Gynecol Oncol.* 2008;110(3):354–359. doi:10.1016/j.ygyno.2008.04.042

94. Garcia-Soto AE, Boren T, Wingo SN, et al. Is comprehensive surgical staging needed for thorough evaluation of early-stage ovarian carcinoma? *Am J Obstet Gynecol.* 2012;206(3):242e1–242e5. doi:10.1016/j.ajog.2011.08.022

95. Vergote I, De Brabanter J, Fyles A, et al. Prognostic importance of degree of differentiation and cyst rupture in stage I invasive epithelial ovarian carcinoma. *Lancet.* 2001;357(9251):176–182. doi:10.1016/S0140-6736(00)03590-X

96. Van Le L. Stage IC ovarian cancer: the clinical significance of intraoperative rupture. *Obstet Gynecol.* 2009;113(1):4–5. doi:10.1097/AOG.0b013e318194b5a5

97. Dioun S, Wu J, Chen L, et al. Intraoperative rupture of the ovarian capsule in early-stage ovarian cancer: a meta-analysis. *Obstet Gynecol.* 2021;138(2):261–271. doi:10.1097/AOG.0000000000004455

98. Hamilton CA, Miller A, Miller C, et al. The impact of disease distribution on survival in patients with stage III epithelial ovarian cancer cytoreduced to microscopic residual: a gynecologic oncology group study. *Gynecol Oncol.* 2011;122(3):521–526. doi:10.1016/j.ygyno.2011.04.041

99. Cancer Genome Atlas Research Network. Integrated genomic analyses of ovarian carcinoma. *Nature.* 2011;474(7353):609–615. doi:10.1038/nature10166

100. Konecny GE, Wang C, Hamidi H, et al. Prognostic and therapeutic relevance of molecular subtypes in high-grade serous ovarian cancer. *J Natl Cancer Inst.* 2014;106(10):dju249. doi:10.1093/jnci/dju249

101. Zhao L, Wang W, Xu L, et al. Integrative network biology analysis identifies mir-508-3p as the determinant for the mesenchymal identity and a strong prognostic biomarker of ovarian cancer. *Oncogene.* 2019;38(13):PMC6755993):2305–2319. doi:10.1038/s41388-018-0577-5

102. Lin KK, Harrell MI, Oza AM, et al. *BRCA* reversion mutations in circulating tumor DNA predict primary and acquired resistance to the PARP inhibitor rucaparib in high-grade ovarian carcinoma. *Cancer Discov.* 2019;9(2):210–219. doi:10.1158/2159-8290.CD-18-0715

103. van Driel WJ, Koole SN, Sikorska K, et al. Hyperthermic intraperitoneal chemotherapy in ovarian cancer. *N Engl J Med.* 2018;378(3):230–240. doi:10.1056/NEJMoa1708618

104. Greer BE, Bundy BN, Ozols RF, et al. Implications of second-look laparotomy in the context of optimally resected stage III ovarian cancer: a non-randomized comparison using an explanatory analysis: a gynecologic oncology group study. *Gynecol Oncol.* 2005;99(1):71–79. doi:10.1016/j.ygyno.2005.05.012

105. Chi DS, McCaughty K, Diaz JP, et al. Guidelines and selection criteria for secondary cytoreductive surgery in patients with recurrent, platinum-sensitive epithelial ovarian carcinoma. *Cancer.* 2006;106(9):1933–1939. doi:10.1002/cncr.21845

106. Moore KN. PARP inhibitor associated treatment related myeloid neoplasms: what was a "rare" complication may be less so. *Gynecol Oncol.* 2021;161(3):639–641. doi:10.1016/j.ygyno.2021.05.006

107. Nitecki R, Melamed A, Gockley AA, et al. Incidence of myelodysplastic syndrome and acute myeloid leukemia in patients receiving poly-ADP ribose polymerase inhibitors for the treatment of solid tumors: a meta-analysis of randomized trials. *Gynecol Oncol.* 2021;161(3):653–659. doi:10.1016/j.ygyno.2021.03.011

108. Baldwin LA, Huang B, Miller RW, et al. Ten-year relative survival for epithelial ovarian cancer. *Obstet Gynecol.* 2012;120(3):612–618. doi:10.1097/AOG.0b013e318264f794

109. Cress RD, Chen YS, Morris CR, et al. Characteristics of long-term survivors of epithelial ovarian cancer. *Obstet Gynecol.* 2015;126(3):491–497. doi:10.1097/AOG.0000000000000981

110. Rustin GJS, van der Burg MEL, Griffin CL, et al. Early versus delayed treatment of relapsed ovarian cancer (MRC OV05/EORTC 55955): a randomised trial. *Lancet.* 2010;376(9747):1155–1163. doi:10.1016/S0140-6736(10)61268-8

111. Davidson BA, Broadwater G, Crim A, et al. Surgical complexity score and role of laparoscopy in women with advanced ovarian cancer treated with neoadjuvant chemotherapy. *Gynecol Oncol.* 2019;152(3):554–559. doi:10.1016/j.ygyno.2018.12.011

112. Colombo N, Guthrie D, Chiari S, et al. International collaborative ovarian neoplasm trial 1: a randomized trial of adjuvant chemotherapy in women with early-stage ovarian cancer. *J Natl Cancer Inst.* 2003;95(2):125–132. doi:10.1093/jnci/95.2.125

113. Trimbos JB, Vergote I, Bolis G, et al. Impact of adjuvant chemotherapy and surgical staging in early-stage ovarian carcinoma: European Organisation for Research and Treatment of Cancer-adjuvant chemotherapy in ovarian neoplasm trial. *J Natl Cancer Inst.* 2003;95(2):113–125.

114. Trimbos B, Timmers P, Pecorelli S, et al. Surgical staging and treatment of early ovarian cancer: long-term analysis from a randomized trial. *J Natl Cancer Inst.* 2010;102(13):982–987. doi:10.1093/jnci/djq149

115. ICON2: randomised trial of single-agent carboplatin against three-drug combination of cap (cyclophosphamide, doxorubicin, and cisplatin) in women with ovarian cancer. icon collaborators. international collaborative ovarian neoplasm study. *Lancet.* 1998;352(9140):1571–1576. doi:10.1016/S0140-6736(98)04119-1

116. Parmar MKB, Ledermann JA, Colombo N, et al. Paclitaxel plus platinum-based chemotherapy versus conventional platinum-based chemotherapy in women with relapsed ovarian cancer: the ICON4/AGO-OVAR-2.2 trial. *Lancet.* 2003;361(9375):2099–2106. doi:10.1016/s0140-6736(03)13718-x

117. Bookman MA, Brady MF, McGuire WP, et al. Evaluation of new platinum-based treatment regimens in advanced-stage ovarian cancer: a phase III trial of the gynecologic cancer intergroup. *J Clin Oncol.* 2009;27(9):1419–1425. doi:10.1200/JCO.2008.19.1684

118. Perren TJ, Swart AM, Pfisterer J, et al. A phase 3 trial of bevacizumab in ovarian cancer. *N Engl J Med.* 2011;365(26):2484–2496. doi:10.1056/NEJMoa1103799

119. Oza AM, Cook AD, Pfisterer J, et al. Standard chemotherapy with or without bevacizumab for women with newly diagnosed ovarian cancer (ICON7): overall survival results of a phase 3 randomised trial. *Lancet Oncol.* 2015;16(8):928–936. doi:10.1016/S1470-2045(15)00086-8

120. Hreshchyshyn MM, Park RC, Blessing JA, et al. The role of adjuvant therapy in stage I ovarian cancer. *Am J Obstet Gynecol.* 1980;138(2):139–145. doi:10.1016/0002-9378(80)90024-1

121. McGuire WP, Hoskins WJ, Brady MF, et al. Cyclophosphamide and cisplatin compared with paclitaxel and cisplatin in patients with stage III and stage IV ovarian cancer. *N Engl J Med.* 1996;334(1):1–6. doi:10.1056/NEJM199601043340101

122. Piccart MJ, Bertelsen K, James K, et al. Randomized intergroup trial of cisplatin-paclitaxel versus cisplatin-cyclophosphamide in women with advanced epithelial ovarian cancer: three-year results. *J Natl Cancer Inst.* 2000;92(9):699–708. doi:10.1093/jnci/92.9.699

123. Muggia FM, Braly PS, Brady MF, et al. Phase III randomized study of cisplatin versus paclitaxel versus cisplatin and paclitaxel in patients with suboptimal stage III or IV ovarian cancer: a gynecologic oncology group study. *J Clin Oncol.* 2000;18(1):106–115. doi:10.1200/JCO.2000.18.1.106

124. Bell J, Brady MF, Young RC, et al. Randomized phase III trial of three versus six cycles of adjuvant carboplatin and paclitaxel in early stage epithelial ovarian carcinoma: a gynecologic oncology group study. *Gynecol Oncol.* 2006;102(3):432–439. doi:10.1016/j.ygyno.2006.06.013

125. Chan JK, Tian C, Fleming GF, et al. The potential benefit of 6 vs. 3 cycles of chemotherapy in subsets of women with early-stage high-risk epithelial ovarian cancer: an exploratory analysis of a gynecologic oncology group study. *Gynecol Oncol.* 2010;116(3):301–306. doi:10.1016/j.ygyno.2009.10.073

126. Ozols RF, Bundy BN, Greer BE, et al. Phase III trial of carboplatin and paclitaxel compared with cisplatin and paclitaxel in patients with optimally resected stage III ovarian cancer: a gynecologic oncology group study. *J Clin Oncol.* 2003;21(17):3194–3200. doi:10.1200/JCO.2003.02.153

127. Burger RA, Brady MF, Bookman MA, et al. Incorporation of bevacizumab in the primary treatment of ovarian cancer. *N Engl J Med.* 2011;365(26):2473–2483. doi:10.1056/NEJMoa1104390

128. Vasey PA, Jayson GC, Gordon A, et al. Phase III randomized trial of docetaxel-carboplatin versus paclitaxel-carboplatin as first-line chemotherapy for ovarian carcinoma. *J Natl Cancer Inst.* 2004;96(22):1682–1691. doi:10.1093/jnci/djh323

129. Gonzalez-Martin A, Gladieff L, Tholander B, et al. Efficacy and safety results from OCTAVIA, a single-arm phase II study evaluating front-line bevacizumab, carboplatin and weekly paclitaxel for ovarian cancer. *Eur J Cancer.* 2013;49(18):3831–3838. doi:10.1016/j.ejca.2013.08.002

130. du Bois A, Herrstedt J, Hardy-Bessard A-C, et al. Phase III trial of carboplatin plus paclitaxel with or without gemcitabine in first-line treatment of epithelial ovarian cancer. *J Clin Oncol.* 2010;28(27):4162–4169. doi:10.1200/JCO.2009.27.4696

131. Sabbatini P, Harter P, Scambia G, et al. Abagovomab as maintenance therapy in patients with epithelial ovarian cancer: a phase III trial of the AGO OVAR, COGI, GINECO, and GEICO--the MIMOSA study. *J Clin Oncol.* 2013;31(12):1554–1561. doi:10.1200/JCO.2012.46.4057

132. du Bois A, Kristensen G, Ray-Coquard I, et al. Standard first-line chemotherapy with or without nintedanib for advanced ovarian cancer (AGO-OVAR 12): a randomised, double-blind, placebo-controlled phase 3 trial. *Lancet Oncol.* 2016;17(1):78–89. doi:10.1016/S1470-2045(15)00366-6

133. Meier W, du Bois A, Rau J, et al. Randomized phase II trial of carboplatin and paclitaxel with or without lonafarnib in first-line treatment of epithelial ovarian cancer stage IIB-IV. *Gynecol Oncol.* 2012;126(2):236–240. doi:10.1016/j.ygyno.2012.04.050

134. Pfisterer J, Joly F, Kristensen G. Optimal treatment duration of bevacizumab (BEV) combined with carboplatin and paclitaxel in patients (PTS) with primary epithelial ovarian (EOC), fallopian tube (FTC) or peritoneal cancer (PPC): a multicenter open-label randomized 2-arm phase 3 ENGOT/GCIG trial of the AGO study group, GINECO, and NSGO (AGO-OVAR 17/BOOST, GINECO OV118, ENGOT ov-15, NCT01462890). *JCO.* 2021;39(15_suppl):5501–5501. doi:10.1200/JCO.2021.39.15_suppl.5501

135. Walker JL, Brady MF, Wenzel L, et al. Randomized trial of intravenous versus intraperitoneal chemotherapy plus bevacizumab in advanced ovarian carcinoma: an NRG oncology/gynecologic oncology group

study. *J Clin Oncol.* 2019;37(16):PMC6544459):1380–1390. doi:10.1200/JCO.18.01568

136. Coleman RL, Fleming GF, Brady MF, et al. Veliparib with first-line chemotherapy and as maintenance therapy in ovarian cancer. *N Engl J Med.* 2019;381(25):PMC6941439):2403–2415:. doi:10.1056/NEJMoa1909707

137. Falandry C, Rousseau F, Mouret-Reynier M-A, et al. Efficacy and safety of first-line single-agent carboplatin vs carboplatin plus paclitaxel for vulnerable older adult women with ovarian cancer: a GINECO/GCIG randomized clinical trial. *JAMA Oncol.* 2021;7(6):853–861. doi:10.1001/jamaoncol.2021.0696

138. McGuire WP, Hoskins WJ, Brady MF, et al. Assessment of dose-intensive therapy in suboptimally debulked ovarian cancer: a gynecologic oncology group study. *J Clin Oncol.* 1995;13(7):1589–1599. doi:10.1200/JCO.1995.13.7.1589

139. Fruscio R, Garbi A, Parma G, et al. Randomized phase III clinical trial evaluating weekly cisplatin for advanced epithelial ovarian cancer. *J Natl Cancer Inst.* 2011;103(4):347–351. doi:10.1093/jnci/djq530

140. Kaye SB, Paul J, Cassidy J, et al. Mature results of a randomized trial of two doses of cisplatin for the treatment of ovarian cancer. Scottish gynecology cancer trials group. *J Clin Oncol.* 1996;14(7):2113–2119. doi:10.1200/JCO.1996.14.7.2113

141. Jakobsen A, Bertelsen K, Andersen JE, et al. Dose-effect study of carboplatin in ovarian cancer: a Danish ovarian cancer group study. *J Clin Oncol.* 1997;15(1):193–198. doi:10.1200/JCO.1997.15.1.193

142. Gore M, Mainwaring P, A'Hern R, et al. Randomized trial of dose-intensity with single-agent carboplatin in patients with epithelial ovarian cancer. London gynaecological oncology group. *J Clin Oncol.* 1998;16(7):2426–2434. doi:10.1200/JCO.1998.16.7.2426

143. Omura GA, Brady MF, Look KY, et al. Phase III trial of paclitaxel at two dose levels, the higher dose accompanied by filgrastim at two dose levels in platinum-pretreated epithelial ovarian cancer: an intergroup study. *J Clin Oncol.* 2003;21(15):2843–2848. doi:10.1200/JCO.2003.10.082

144. Eisenhauer EA, ten Bokkel Huinink WW, Swenerton KD, et al. European–Canadian randomized trial of paclitaxel in relapsed ovarian cancer: high-dose versus low-dose and long versus short infusion. *J Clin Oncol.* 1994;12(12):2654–2666. doi:10.1200/JCO.1994.12.12.2654

145. Katsumata N, Yasuda M, Takahashi F, et al. Dose-dense paclitaxel once A week in combination with carboplatin every 3 weeks for advanced ovarian cancer: a phase 3, open-label, randomised controlled trial. *Lancet.* 2009;374(9698):1331–1338. doi:10.1016/S0140-6736(09)61157-0

146. Katsumata N, Yasuda M, Isonishi S, et al. Long-term results of dose-dense paclitaxel and carboplatin versus conventional paclitaxel and carboplatin for treatment of advanced epithelial ovarian, fallopian tube, or primary peritoneal cancer (JGOG 3016): a randomised, controlled, open-label trial. *Lancet Oncol.* 2013;14(10):1020–1026. doi:10.1016/S1470-2045(13)70363-2

147. Chan JK, Brady MF, Penson RT, et al. Weekly vs. every-3-week paclitaxel and carboplatin for ovarian cancer. *N Engl J Med*. 2016;374(8):738–748. doi:10.1056/NEJMoa1505067

148. Pignata S, Scambia G, Katsaros D, et al. Carboplatin plus paclitaxel once a week versus every 3 weeks in patients with advanced ovarian cancer (MITO-7): a randomised, multicentre, open-label, phase 3 trial. *Lancet Oncol*. 2014;15(4):396–405. doi:10.1016/S1470-2045(14)70049-X

149. Clamp AR, James EC, McNeish IA, et al. Weekly dose-dense chemotherapy in first-line epithelial ovarian, fallopian tube, or primary peritoneal carcinoma treatment (ICON8): primary progression free survival analysis results from a GCIG phase 3 randomised controlled trial. *Lancet*. 2019;394(10214):2084–2095. doi:10.1016/S0140-6736(19)32259-7

150. Alberts DS, Liu PY, Hannigan EV, et al. Intraperitoneal cisplatin plus intravenous cyclophosphamide versus intravenous cisplatin plus intravenous cyclophosphamide for stage III ovarian cancer. *N Engl J Med*. 1996;335(26):1950–1955. doi:10.1056/NEJM199612263352603

151. Markman M, Bundy BN, Alberts DS, et al. Phase III trial of standard-dose intravenous cisplatin plus paclitaxel versus moderately high-dose carboplatin followed by intravenous paclitaxel and intraperitoneal cisplatin in small-volume stage III ovarian carcinoma: an intergroup study of the gynecologic oncology group, southwestern oncology group, and eastern cooperative oncology group. *J Clin Oncol*. 2001;19(4):1001–1007. doi:10.1200/JCO.2001.19.4.1001

152. Armstrong DK, Bundy B, Wenzel L, et al. Intraperitoneal cisplatin and paclitaxel in ovarian cancer. *N Engl J Med*. 2006;354(1):34–43. doi:10.1056/NEJMoa052985

153. Armstrong D. Distillation. Abstract presented at: *SGO Annual Meeting*. March 19, 2022.

154. Tewari D, Java JJ, Salani R, et al. Long-term survival advantage and prognostic factors associated with intraperitoneal chemotherapy treatment in advanced ovarian cancer: a gynecologic oncology group study. *J Clin Oncol*. 2015;33(13):1460–1466. doi:10.1200/JCO.2014.55.9898

155. Landrum LM, Java J, Mathews CA, et al. Prognostic factors for stage III epithelial ovarian cancer treated with intraperitoneal chemotherapy: a gynecologic oncology group study. *Gynecol Oncol*. 2013;130(1):12–18. doi:10.1016/j.ygyno.2013.04.001

156. Walker JL, Armstrong D, Huang H. Intraperitoneal catheter outcomes on GOG 172: a gynecologic oncology group study in women with optimally debulked stage III ovarian cancer. *Int J Gynecol Cancer*. 2004;14:19.

157. Dizon DS, Sill MW, Gould N, et al. Phase I feasibility study of intraperitoneal cisplatin and intravenous paclitaxel followed by intraperitoneal paclitaxel in untreated ovarian, fallopian tube, and primary peritoneal carcinoma: a gynecologic oncology group study. *Gynecol Oncol*. 2011;123(2):182–186. doi:10.1016/j.ygyno.2011.07.016

158. Walker JL, Armstrong DK, Huang HQ, et al. Intraperitoneal catheter outcomes in A phase III trial of intravenous versus intraperitoneal chemotherapy in optimal stage III ovarian and primary peritoneal cancer:

a gynecologic oncology group study. *Gynecol Oncol.* 2006;100(1):27–32. doi:10.1016/j.ygyno.2005.11.013

159. Fujiwara K, Aotani E, HamanoT, et al. A randomized phase II/III trial of 3 weekly intraperitoneal versus intravenous carboplatin in combination with intravenous weekly dose-dense paclitaxel for newly diagnosed ovarian, fallopian tube and primary peritoneal cancer. *Jpn J Clin Oncol.* 2011;41(2):278–282. doi:10.1093/jjco/hyq182

160. Fujiwara K, Nagao S, Yamamoto K, et al. A randomized phase 3 trial of intraperitoneal versus intravenous carboplatin with dose-dense weekly paclitaxel in patients with ovarian, fallopian tube, or primary peritoneal carcinoma (a GOTIC-001/JGOG-3019/GCIG, iPocc trial). Abstract presented at: 2022 SGO Annual Meeting on Women's Cancer; March 19, 2022.

161. Provencher DM, Gallagher CJ, Parulekar WR, et al. OV21/PETROC: a randomized gynecologic cancer intergroup phase II study of intraperitoneal versus intravenous chemotherapy following neo-adjuvant chemotherapy and optimal debulking surgery in epithelial ovarian cancer. *Ann Oncol.* 2018;29(2):431–438. doi:10.1093/annonc/mdx754

162. Markman M, Liu PY, Wilczynski S, et al. Phase III randomized trial of 12 versus 3 months of maintenance paclitaxel in patients with advanced ovarian cancer after complete response to platinum and paclitaxel-based chemotherapy: a southwest oncology group and gynecologic oncology group trial. *J Clin Oncol.* 2003;21(13):2460–2465. doi:10.1200/JCO.2003.07.013

163. Markman M, Liu PY, Moon J, et al. Impact on survival of 12 versus 3 monthly cycles of paclitaxel (175 mg/m2) administered to patients with advanced ovarian cancer who attained a complete response to primary platinum-paclitaxel: follow-up of a southwest oncology group and gynecologic oncology group phase 3 trial. *Gynecol Oncol.* 2009;114(2):195–198. doi:10.1016/j.ygyno.2009.04.012

164. McMeekin DS, Tillmanns T, Chaudry T, et al. Timing isn't everything: an analysis of when to start salvage chemotherapy in ovarian cancer. *Gynecol Oncol.* 2004;95(1):157–164. doi:10.1016/j.ygyno.2004.07.008

165. Mannel RS, Brady MF, Kohn EC, et al. A randomized phase III trial of IV carboplatin and paclitaxel × 3 courses followed by observation versus weekly maintenance low-dose paclitaxel in patients with early-stage ovarian carcinoma: a gynecologic oncology group study. *Gynecol Oncol.* 2011;122(1):89–94. doi:10.1016/j.ygyno.2011.03.013

166. du Bois A, Floquet A, Kim J-W, et al. Incorporation of pazopanib in maintenance therapy of ovarian cancer. *J Clin Oncol.* 2014;32(30):3374–3382. doi:10.1200/JCO.2014.55.7348

167. Ledermann J, Harter P, Gourley C, et al. Olaparib maintenance therapy in platinum-sensitive relapsed ovarian cancer. *N Engl J Med.* 2012;366(15):1382–1392. doi:10.1056/NEJMoa1105535

168. Moore K, Colombo N, Scambia G, et al. Maintenance olaparib in patients with newly diagnosed advanced ovarian cancer. *N Engl J Med.* 2018;379(26):2495–2505. doi:10.1056/NEJMoa1810858

169. Helwick C. SOLO-1 trial: After 5 years, maintenance olaparib still keeps ovarian cancer at bay. 2020. https://ascopost.com/issues/november-10-2020/solo-1-trial-after-5-years-maintenance-olaparib-still-keeps-ovarian-cancer-at-bay

170. Despierre E, Vergote I, Anderson R, et al. Epidermal growth factor receptor (EGFR) pathway biomarkers in the randomized phase III trial of erlotinib versus observation in ovarian cancer patients with no evidence of disease progression after first-line platinum-based chemotherapy. *Target Oncol.* 2015;10(4):583–596. doi:10.1007/s11523-015-0369-6

171. Ray-Coquard I, Pautier P, Pignata S, et al. Olaparib plus bevacizumab as first-line maintenance in ovarian cancer. *N Engl J Med.* 2019;381(25):2416–2428. doi:10.1056/NEJMoa1911361

172. González-Martín A, Pothuri B, Vergote I, et al. Niraparib in patients with newly diagnosed advanced ovarian cancer. *N Engl J Med.* 2019;381(25):2391–2402. doi:10.1056/NEJMoa1910962

173. Monk BJ, Colombo N, Oza AM, et al. Chemotherapy with or without avelumab followed by avelumab maintenance versus chemotherapy alone in patients with previously untreated epithelial ovarian cancer (javelin ovarian 100): an open-label, randomised, phase 3 trial. *Lancet Oncol.* 2021;22(9):1275–1289. doi:10.1016/S1470-2045(21)00342-9

174. Ning L, Zhu J, Yin R, et al. SGO annual meeting. 2022.

175. Pfisterer J, Plante M, Vergote I, et al. Gemcitabine plus carboplatin compared with carboplatin in patients with platinum-sensitive recurrent ovarian cancer: an intergroup trial of the AGO-OVAR, the NCIC CTG, and the EORTC GCG. *J Clin Oncol.* 2006;24(29):4699–4707. doi:10.1200/JCO.2006.06.0913

176. Gordon AN, Tonda M, Sun S, et al. Long-term survival advantage for women treated with pegylated liposomal doxorubicin compared with topotecan in a phase 3 randomized study of recurrent and refractory epithelial ovarian cancer. *Gynecol Oncol.* 2004;95(1):1–8. doi:10.1016/j.ygyno.2004.07.011

177. Aghajanian C, Blank SV, Goff BA, et al. OCEANS: a randomized, double-blind, placebo-controlled phase III trial of chemotherapy with or without bevacizumab in patients with platinum-sensitive recurrent epithelial ovarian, primary peritoneal, or fallopian tube cancer. *J Clin Oncol.* 2012;30(17):2039–2045. doi:10.1200/JCO.2012.42.0505

178. Aghajanian C, Goff B, Nycum LR, et al. Final overall survival and safety analysis of OCEANS, a phase 3 trial of chemotherapy with or without bevacizumab in patients with platinum-sensitive recurrent ovarian cancer. *Gynecol Oncol.* 2015;139(1):10–16. doi:10.1016/j.ygyno.2015.08.004

179. Pujade-Lauraine E, Wagner U, Aavall-Lundqvist E, et al. Pegylated liposomal doxorubicin and carboplatin compared with paclitaxel and carboplatin for patients with platinum-sensitive ovarian cancer in late relapse. *J Clin Oncol.* 2010;28(20):3323–3329. doi:10.1200/JCO.2009.25.7519

180. Mahner S, Meier W, du Bois A, et al. Carboplatin and pegylated liposomal doxorubicin versus carboplatin and paclitaxel in very platinum-sensitive ovarian cancer patients: results from a subset analysis of the CALYPSO phase III trial. *Eur J Cancer.* 2015;51(3):352–358. doi:10.1016/j.ejca.2014.11.017

181. Pujade-Lauraine E, Hilpert F, Weber B, et al. Bevacizumab combined with chemotherapy for platinum-resistant recurrent ovarian cancer: the aurelia open-label randomized phase III trial. *J Clin Oncol.* 2014;32(13):1302–1308. doi:10.1200/JCO.2013.51.4489

182. Poveda AM, Selle F, Hilpert F, et al. Bevacizumab combined with weekly paclitaxel, pegylated liposomal doxorubicin, or topotecan in platinum-resistant recurrent ovarian cancer: analysis by chemotherapy cohort of the randomized phase III aurelia trial. *J Clin Oncol.* 2015;33(32):3836–3838. doi:10.1200/JCO.2015.63.1408

183. Pignata S, Scambia G, Bologna A, et al. Randomized controlled trial testing the efficacy of platinum-free interval prolongation in advanced ovarian cancer: the mito-8, mango, BGOG-ov1, AGO-ovar2.16, ENGOT-ov1, GCIG study. *J Clin Oncol.* 2017;35(29):3347–3353. doi:10.1200/JCO.2017.73.4293

184. Pujade-Lauraine E, Fujiwara K, Ledermann JA, et al. Avelumab alone or in combination with chemotherapy versus chemotherapy alone in platinum-resistant or platinum-refractory ovarian cancer (javelin ovarian 200): an open-label, three-arm, randomised, phase 3 study. *Lancet Oncol.* 2021;22(7):1034–1046. doi:10.1016/S1470-2045(21)00216-3

185. Monk BJ, Poveda A, Vergote I, et al. Anti-angiopoietin therapy with trebananib for recurrent ovarian cancer (TRINOVA-1): a randomised, multicentre, double-blind, placebo-controlled phase 3 trial. *Lancet Oncol.* 2014;15(8):799–808. doi:10.1016/S1470-2045(14)70244-X

186. Monk BJ, Poveda A, Vergote I, et al. Final results of a phase 3 study of trebananib plus weekly paclitaxel in recurrent ovarian cancer (TRINOVA-1): long-term survival, impact of ascites, and progression-free survival-2. *Gynecol Oncol.* 2016;143(1):27–34. doi:10.1016/j.ygyno.2016.07.112

187. Westin SN, Randall L. The European Society of Gynecologic Oncology (ESGO) 19th Biannual Meeting: overview and summary of selected topics. *Gynecol Oncol.* 2016;140(3):377–380. doi:10.1016/j.ygyno.2016.01.021

188. Raja F, Perren T, Embleton A. Randomised double-blind phase III trial of cediranib (AZD 2171) in relapsed platinum sensitive ovarian cancer: results of the ICON6 trial. *Int J Gynecol Cancer.* 2013;23:47.

189. Mirza MR, Monk BJ, Herrstedt J, et al. Niraparib maintenance therapy in platinum-sensitive, recurrent ovarian cancer. *N Engl J Med.* 2016;375(22):2154–2164. doi:10.1056/NEJMoa1611310

190. Moore KN, Secord AA, Geller MA, et al. Niraparib monotherapy for late-line treatment of ovarian cancer (QUADRA): a multicentre, open-label, single-arm, phase 2 trial. *Lancet Oncol.* 2019;20(5):636–648. doi:10.1016/S1470-2045(19)30029-4

191. Wu XH, Zhu JQ, Yin RT, et al. Niraparib maintenance therapy in patients with platinum-sensitive recurrent ovarian cancer using an individualized starting dose (NORA): a randomized, double-blind, placebo-controlled phase III trial. *Ann Oncol.* 2021;32(4):512–521. doi:10.1016/j. annonc.2020.12.018

192. Li N. Fuzuloparib PARP-i maintenance therapy improves progression-free survival in patients with recurrent ovarian cancer, society of gynecologic oncology. In: *Annual Meeting on Women's Cancer.* 2021.

193. Poveda A, Vergote I, Tjulandin S, et al. Trabectedin plus pegylated liposomal doxorubicin in relapsed ovarian cancer: outcomes in the partially platinum-sensitive (platinum-free interval 6-12 months) subpopulation of OVA-301 phase III randomized trial. *Ann Oncol.* 2011;22(1):39–48. doi:10.1093/annonc/mdq352

194. Pignata S, Lorusso D, Scambia G, et al. Pazopanib plus weekly paclitaxel versus weekly paclitaxel alone for platinum-resistant or platinum-refractory advanced ovarian cancer (MITO 11): a randomised, open-label, phase 2 trial. *Lancet Oncol.* 2015;16(5):561–568. doi:10.1016/S1470-2045(15)70115-4

195. Thigpen JT, Blessing JA, Ball H, et al. Phase II trial of paclitaxel in patients with progressive ovarian carcinoma after platinum-based chemotherapy: a gynecologic oncology group study. *J Clin Oncol.* 1994;12(9):1748–1753. doi:10.1200/JCO.1994.12.9.1748

196. Monk BJ, Sill MW, Hanjani P, et al. Docetaxel plus trabectedin appears active in recurrent or persistent ovarian and primary peritoneal cancer after up to three prior regimens: a phase II study of the gynecologic oncology group. *Gynecol Oncol.* 2011;120(3):459–463. doi:10.1016/j. ygyno.2010.11.012

197. Monk BJ, Sill M, Walker JL. A randomized phase II evaluation of bevacizumab vs bevacizumab/fosbretabulin in recurrent ovarian, tubal, or peritoneal carcinoma: a Gynecologic Oncology Group study. In: *15th Biennial Meeting of the International Gynecologic Cancer Society*; Melbourne, Australia. ; 2014.

198. Jackson AL, Davenport SM, Herzog TJ. Targeting angiogenesis: vascular endothelial growth factor and related signalling pathways. *Transl Cancer Res.* 2015;491:70–83.

199. Kurzeder C, Bover I, Marmé F, et al. Double-blind, placebo-controlled, randomized phase III trial evaluating pertuzumab combined with chemotherapy for low tumor human epidermal growth factor receptor 3 mrna-expressing platinum-resistant ovarian cancer (PENELOPE). *J Clin Oncol.* 2016;34(21):2516–2525. doi:10.1200/JCO.2015.66.0787

200. Liu JF, Barry WT, Birrer M, et al. Combination cediranib and olaparib versus olaparib alone for women with recurrent platinum-sensitive ovarian cancer: a randomised phase 2 study. *Lancet Oncol.* 2014;15(11):1207–1214. doi:10.1016/S1470-2045(14)70391-2

201. Vergote I, Tropé CG, Amant F, et al. Neoadjuvant chemotherapy or primary surgery in stage IIIC or IV ovarian cancer. *N Engl J Med.* 2010;363(10):943–953. doi:10.1056/NEJMoa0908806

202. Hirte H, Lheureux S, Fleming GF, et al. A phase 2 study of cediranib in recurrent or persistent ovarian, peritoneal or fallopian tube cancer: a trial of the princess margaret, chicago and california phase II consortia. *Gynecol Oncol.* 2015;138(1):55–61. doi:10.1016/j.ygyno.2015.04.009

203. SGO Annual Meeting National Harbor Maryland. 2017.

204. Penson RT, Valencia RV, Cibula D, et al. Olaparib versus nonplatinum chemotherapy in patients with platinum-sensitive relapsed ovarian cancer and A germline BRCA1/2 mutation (SOLO3): a randomized phase III trial. *J Clin Oncol.* 2020;38(11):PMC7145583):1164–1174. doi:10.1200/JCO.19.02745

205. McNeish IA, Oza AM, Coleman RL, et al. Results of ARIEL2: a phase 2 trial to prospectively identify ovarian cancer patients likely to respond to rucaparib using tumor genetic analysis. *JCO.* 2015;33(15_suppl):5508–5508. doi:10.1200/jco.2015.33.15_suppl.5508

206. Ledermann JA, Oza AM, Lorusso D, et al. Rucaparib for patients with platinum-sensitive, recurrent ovarian carcinoma (ARIEL3): post-progression outcomes and updated safety results from a randomised, placebo-controlled, phase 3 trial. *Lancet Oncol.* 2020;21(5):710–722. doi:10.1016/S1470-2045(20)30061-9

207. Kristeleit R. Rucaparib vs chemotherapy in patients with advanced, relapsed ovarian cancer and a deleterious BRCA mutation: efficacy and safety from ARIEL4, a randomized phase 3 study. presented at: ESMO gynaecological cancers virtual congress. *JAMA Oncol.* 2021;4(8):1059–1065. doi:10.1001/jamaoncol.2018.0211

208. Harter P, du Bois A, Hahmann M, et al. Surgery in recurrent ovarian cancer: the arbeitsgemeinschaft gynaekologische onkologie (ago) desktop OVAR trial. *Ann Surg Oncol.* 2006;13(12):1702–1710. doi:10.1245/s10434-006-9058-0

209. Harter P, Sehouli J, Reuss A, et al. Prospective validation study of A predictive score for operability of recurrent ovarian cancer: the multicenter intergroup study desktop II. a project of the AGO kommission OVAR, AGO study group, NOGGO, AGO-austria, and MITO. *Int J Gynecol Cancer.* 2011;21(2):289–295. doi:10.1097/IGC.0b013e31820aaafd

210. Chan J, Brady WE, Brown J, et al. A phase II evaluation of sunitinib (SU11248) in the treatment of persistent or recurrent clear cell ovarian carcinoma: an NRG oncology/gynecologic oncology group (GOG) study. *Gynecol Oncol.* 2015;138(Suppl 1):3. doi:10.1016/j.ygyno.2015.04.021

211. Matulonis UA, Shapira-Frommer R, Santin AD, et al. Antitumor activity and safety of pembrolizumab in patients with advanced recurrent ovarian cancer: results from the phase II KEYNOTE-100 study. *Ann Oncol.* 2019;30(7):1080–1087. doi:10.1093/annonc/mdz135

212. Bonaventura A, O'Connell RL, Mapagu C, et al. Paragon (ANZGOG-0903): phase 2 study of anastrozole in women with estrogen or progesterone receptor-positive platinum-resistant or -refractory recurrent ovarian cancer. *Int J Gynecol Cancer.* 2017;27(5):900–906. doi:10.1097/IGC.0000000000000978

213. Pujade-Lauraine E, Selle F, Weber B, et al. Volasertib versus chemotherapy in platinum-resistant or -refractory ovarian cancer: a randomized phase II groupe des investigateurs nationaux pour l'etude des cancers de l'ovaire study. *J Clin Oncol.* 2016;34(7):706–713. doi:10.1200/JCO.2015.62.1474

214. Senzer N, Barve M, Kuhn J, et al. Phase I trial of "bi-shrnai(furin)/GMCSF DNA/autologous tumor cell" vaccine (FANG) in advanced cancer. *Mol Ther.* 2012;20(3):679–686. doi:10.1038/mt.2011.269

215. van der Burg ME, van Lent M, Buyse M, et al. The effect of debulking surgery after induction chemotherapy on the prognosis in advanced epithelial ovarian cancer. Gynecological Cancer Cooperative Group of the European Organization for Research and Treatment of Cancer. *N Engl J Med.* 1995;332(10):629–634. doi:10.1056/NEJM199503093321002

216. Rose PG, Nerenstone S, Brady MF, et al. Secondary surgical cytoreduction for advanced ovarian carcinoma. *N Engl J Med.* 2004;351(24):2489–2497. doi:10.1056/NEJMoa041125

217. Soo Hoo S, Marriott N, Houlton A, et al. Patient-reported outcomes after extensive (ultraradical) surgery for ovarian cancer: results from a prospective longitudinal feasibility study. *Int J Gynecol Cancer.* 2015;25(9):1599–1607. doi:10.1097/IGC.0000000000000551

218. Nitecki R, Fleming ND, Fellman BM, et al. Timing of surgery in patients with partial response or stable disease after neoadjuvant chemotherapy for advanced ovarian cancer. *Gynecol Oncol.* 2021;161(3):660–667. doi:10.1016/j.ygyno.2021.04.012

219. Vergote I, Harter P, Chiva L. Hyperthermic intraperitoneal chemotherapy does not improve survival in advanced ovarian cancer. *Cancer.* 2019;125 (Suppl 24):4594–4597. doi:10.1002/cncr.32496

220. Lim MC, Chang SJ, Yoo HJ. Randomized trial of hyperthermic intraperitoneal chemotherapy (HIPEC) in women with primary advanced peritoneal, ovarian, and tubal cancer [abstract 5520]. *J Clini Oncol.* 2017;5520(Suppl).

221. Jou J, Zimmer Z, Charo L, et al. HIPEC after neoadjuvant chemotherapy and interval debulking is associated with development of platinum-refractory or -resistant disease. *Gynecol Oncol.* 2021;161(1):25–33. doi:10.1016/j.ygyno.2020.11.035

222. Chi DS, Zhou Q. Hyperthermic intraperitoneal chemotherapy (HIPEC) with carboplatin during secondary cytoreduction. MSI phase 2 trial. *J Clini Oncol.* 2021;39(23):2594–2604.

223. Coleman RL, Brady MF, Herzog TJ, et al. A phase III randomized controlled clinical trial of carboplatin and paclitaxel alone or in combination with bevacizumab followed by bevacizumab and secondary cytoreductive surgery in platinum-sensitive, recurrent ovarian, peritoneal primary and fallopian tube cancer (gynecologic oncology group 0213). *Gynecol Oncol.* 2015;137(Suppl):3–4. doi:10.1016/j.ygyno.2015.01.005

224. Coleman RL, Spirtos NM, Enserro D, et al. Secondary surgical cytoreduction for recurrent ovarian cancer. *N Engl J Med.* 2019;381(20):1929–1939. doi:10.1056/NEJMoa1902626

225. Harter P, Sehouli J, Vergote I, et al. Randomized trial of cytoreductive surgery for relapsed ovarian cancer. *N Engl J Med.* 2021;385(23):2123–2131. doi:10.1056/NEJMoa2103294

226. Du Bois A, Sehouli J, Vergote I, et al. Randomized phase III study to evaluate the impact of secondary cytoreductive surgery in recurrent ovarian cancer: final analysis of ago desktop III/ENGOT-ov20. *JCO.* 2020;38(15_suppl):6000–6000. doi:10.1200/JCO.2020.38.15_suppl.6000

227. Shi T, Zhu J, Feng Y, et al. Secondary cytoreduction followed by chemotherapy versus chemotherapy alone in platinum-sensitive relapsed ovarian cancer (SOC-1): a multicentre, open-label, randomised, phase 3 trial. *Lancet Oncol.* 2021;22(4):439–449. doi:10.1016/S1470-2045(21)00006-1

228. Kehoe S, Hook J, Nankivell M, et al. Primary chemotherapy versus primary surgery for newly diagnosed advanced ovarian cancer (chorus): an open-label, randomised, controlled, non-inferiority trial. *Lancet.* 2015;386(9990):249–257. doi:10.1016/S0140-6736(14)62223-6

229. van Meurs HS, Tajik P, Hof MHP, et al. Which patients benefit most from primary surgery or neoadjuvant chemotherapy in stage IIIC or IV ovarian cancer? an exploratory analysis of the European Organisation for Research and Treatment of Cancer 55971 randomised trial. *Eur J Cancer.* 2013;49(15):S0959-8049(13)00488-7):3191–3201. doi:10.1016/j.ejca.2013.06.013

230. Fagotti A, Vizzielli G, Fanfani F, et al. Phase III scorpion trial (id number: nct01461850) in epithelial ovarian cancer patients with high tumor load receiving PDS versus NACT: an interim analysis on peri-operative outcome. *Gynecol Oncol.* 2015;138(Suppl 1):1–2. doi:10.1016/j.ygyno.2015.04.017

231. Fagotti A, Vizzielli G, De Iaco P, et al. A multicentric trial (olympia-MITO 13) on the accuracy of laparoscopy to assess peritoneal spread in ovarian cancer. *Am J Obstet Gynecol.* 2013;209(5):462e1–462e11. doi:10.1016/j.ajog.2013.07.016

232. Petrillo M, Vizzielli G, Fanfani F, et al. Definition of a dynamic laparoscopic model for the prediction of incomplete cytoreduction in advanced epithelial ovarian cancer: proof of a concept. *Gynecol Oncol.* 2015;139(1):5–9. doi:10.1016/j.ygyno.2015.07.095

233. Tozzi R, Giannice R, Cianci S, et al. Neo-adjuvant chemotherapy does not increase the rate of complete resection and does not significantly reduce the morbidity of visceral-peritoneal debulking (VPD) in patients with stage IIIC-IV ovarian cancer. *Gynecol Oncol.* 2015;138(2):252–258. doi:10.1016/j.ygyno.2015.05.010

234. Rosen B, Laframboise S, Ferguson S, et al. The impacts of neoadjuvant chemotherapy and of debulking surgery on survival from advanced ovarian cancer. *Gynecol Oncol.* 2014;134(3):462–467. doi:10.1016/j.ygyno.2014.07.004

235. Guo C, Chénard-Poirier M, Roda D, et al. Intermittent schedules of the oral RAF-MEK inhibitor CH5126766/VS-6766 in patients with RAS/RAF-mutant solid tumours and multiple myeloma: a single-centre, open-label, phase 1 dose-escalation and basket dose-expansion study. *Lancet Oncol.* 2020;21(11):1478–1488. doi:10.1016/S1470-2045(20)30464-2

236. Rosa K. FDA grants breakthrough therapy designation to VS-6766/ Defactinib for recurrent low-grade serous ovarian cancer. 2021. https:// www.onclive.com/view/fda-grants-breakthrough-therapy-designation -to-vs-6766-defactinib-for-recurrent-low-grade-serous-ovarian-cancer

237. Banerjee SN, Monk BJ, Van Nieuwenhuysen E. ENGOT-ov60/GOG3052/ RAMP 201: a phase 2 study of VS-6766 (dual raf/MEK inhibitor) alone and in combination with defactinib (FAK inhibitor) in recurrent low-grade serous ovarian cancer (LGSOC). *J Clin Oncol. 39*(15_suppl).

238. Monk BJ, Grisham RN, Banerjee S, et al. MILO/ENGOT-ov11: binimetinib versus physician's choice chemotherapy in recurrent or persistent low-grade serous carcinomas of the ovary, fallopian tube, or primary peritoneum. *J Clin Oncol.* 2020;38(32):3753–3762. doi: 10.1200/JCO.20 .01164

239. Gershenson DM, Miller A, Brady WE, et al. Trametinib versus standard of care in patients with recurrent low-grade serous ovarian cancer (GOG 281/ LOGS): An international, randomised, open-label, multicentre, phase 2/3 trial. *Lancet.* 2022;399(10324):S0140-6736(21)02175-9):541–553:. doi:10.1016/S0140-6736(21)02175-9

240. Chekerov R, Braicu I, Castillo-Tong DC, et al. Outcome and clinical management of 275 patients with advanced ovarian cancer International Federation of Obstetrics and Gynecology II to IV inside the European Ovarian Cancer Translational Research Consortium-OVCAD. *Int J Gynecol Cancer.* 2013;23(2):268–275. doi:10.1097/ IGC.0b013e31827de6b9

241. Rocconi RP, Monk BJ, Walter A, et al. Gynecol Oncol. 2021 Jun;161(3):676–680. doi:10.1016/j.ygyno.2021.03.009

242. Rocconi RP, et al. Abstract 5502. Presented at: ASCO Annual Meeting (virtual meeting); June 4–8, 2021.

243. Winter WE, Kucera PR, Rodgers W, et al. Surgical staging in patients with ovarian tumors of low malignant potential. *Obstet Gynecol.* 2002;100(4):671–676. doi:10.1016/s0029-7844(02)02171-3

244. Gershenson DM, Silva EG, Tortolero-Luna G, et al. Serous borderline tumors of the ovary with noninvasive peritoneal implants. *Cancer.* 1998;83(10):2157–2163. doi:10.1002/(sici)1097-0142(19981115)83 :10<2157::aid-cncr14>3.0.co;2-d

245. Crispens MA, Bodurka D, Deavers M, et al. Response and survival in patients with progressive or recurrent serous ovarian tumors of low malignant potential. *Obstet Gynecol.* 2002;99(1):3–10. doi:10.1016/ s0029-7844(01)01649-0

246. Stewart SL, Wike JM, Foster SL, et al. The incidence of primary fallopian tube cancer in the united states. *Gynecol Oncol.* 2007;107(3):392–397. doi:10.1016/j.ygyno.2007.09.018

247. Hu CY, Taymour ML, Hertig AT. Primary carcinoma of the fallopian tube. *Am J Obstet Gynecol.* 1950;59(1):58–67. doi:10.1016/0002 -9378(50)90341-3

248. Sedlis A. Carcinoma of the fallopian tube. *Surg Clin North Am.* 1978;58(1):121–129. doi:10.1016/s0039-6109(16)41439-8

249. Slayton RE, Park RC, Silverberg SG, et al. Vincristine, dactinomycin, and cyclophosphamide in the treatment of malignant germ cell tumors of the ovary. A gynecologic oncology group study (A final report). *Cancer.* 1985;56(2):243–248. doi:10.1002/1097-0142(19850715)56:2<243::aid-cncr2820560206>3.0.co;2-t

250. Williams SD, Blessing JA, Moore DH, et al. Cisplatin, vinblastine, and bleomycin in advanced and recurrent ovarian germ-cell tumors. A trial of the gynecologic oncology group. *Ann Intern Med.* 1989;111(1):22–27. doi:10.7326/0003-4819-111-1-22

251. Li J, Yang W, Wu X. Prognostic factors and role of salvage surgery in che-morefractory ovarian germ cell malignancies: a study in chinese patients. *Gynecol Oncol.* 2007;105(3):769–775. doi:10.1016/j.ygyno.2007.02.032

252. Williams S, Blessing JA, Liao SY, et al. Adjuvant therapy of ovarian germ cell tumors with cisplatin, etoposide, and bleomycin: a trial of the gynecologic oncology group. *J Clin Oncol.* 1994;12(4):701–706. doi:10.1200/JCO.1994.12.4.701

253. Williams SD, Blessing JA, Hatch KD, et al. Chemotherapy of advanced dysgerminoma: trials of the gynecologic oncology group. *J Clin Oncol.* 1991;9(11):1950–1955. doi:10.1200/JCO.1991.9.11.1950

254. Williams SD, Kauderer J, Burnett AF, et al. Adjuvant therapy of com-pletely resected dysgerminoma with carboplatin and etoposide: a trial of the gynecologic oncology group. *Gynecol Oncol.* 2004;95(3):496–499. doi:10.1016/j.ygyno.2004.07.044

255. Williams SD, Blessing JA, DiSaia PJ, et al. Second-look laparotomy in ovarian germ cell tumors: the gynecologic oncology group experi-ence. *Gynecol Oncol.* 1994;52(3):287–291. doi:10.1006/gyno.1994.1050

256. Brown J, Sood AK, Deavers MT, et al. Patterns of metastasis in sex cord-stromal tumors of the ovary: can routine staging lymphadenec-tomy be omitted? *Gynecol Oncol.* 2009;113(1):86–90. doi:10.1016/j.ygyno.2008.12.007

257. Tavassoeli FA, Devilee P. *WHO Classification of Tumours, Pathology and Genetics: Tumours of the Breast and Female Genital Organs.* IARC; 2003.

258. Wolf JK, Mullen J, Eifel PJ, et al. Radiation treatment of advanced or recurrent granulosa cell tumor of the ovary. *Gynecol Oncol.* 1999;73(1):35–41. doi:10.1006/gyno.1998.5287

259. Wilson MK, Fong P, Mesnage S, et al. Stage I granulosa cell tumours: a management conundrum? results of long-term follow up. *Gynecol Oncol.* 2015;138(2):285–291. doi:10.1016/j.ygyno.2015.05.011

260. Homesley HD, Bundy BN, Hurteau JA, et al. Bleomycin, etoposide, and cisplatin combination therapy of ovarian granulosa cell tumors and other stromal malignancies: a gynecologic oncology group study. *Gynecol Oncol.* 1999;72(2):131–137. doi:10.1006/gyno.1998.5304

261. Mangili G, Ottolina J, Cormio G, et al. Adjuvant chemotherapy does not improve disease-free survival in FIGO stage IC ovarian granulosa cell tumors: the MITO-9 study. *Gynecol Oncol.* 2016;143(2):276–280. doi:10.1016/j.ygyno.2016.08.316

262. Billmire DF, Cullen JW, Rescorla FJ, et al. Surveillance after initial surgery for pediatric and adolescent girls with stage I ovarian germ cell tumors: report from the children's oncology group. *J Clin Oncol*. 2014;32(5):465–470. doi:10.1200/JCO.2013.51.1006

263. Lu KH, Broaddus RR. Endometrial cancer. *N Engl J Med*. 2020;383(21):2053–2064. doi:10.1056/NEJMra1514010

264. Kurman RJ, Kaminski PF, Norris HJ. The behavior of endometrial hyperplasia. a long-term study of "untreated" hyperplasia in 170 patients. *Cancer*. 1985;56(2):403–412. doi:10.1002/1097-0142(19850715) 56:2<403::aid-cncr2820560233>3.0.co;2-x

265. Trimble CL, Kauderer J, Zaino R, et al. Concurrent endometrial carcinoma in women with A biopsy diagnosis of atypical endometrial hyperplasia: a gynecologic oncology group study. *Cancer*. 2006;106(4):812–819. doi:10.1002/cncr.21650

266. Talhouk A, McConechy MK, Leung S, et al. A clinically applicable molecular-based classification for endometrial cancers. *Br J Cancer*. 2015;113(2):299–310. doi:10.1038/bjc.2015.190

267. Concin N, Matias-Guiu X, Vergote I, et al. ESGO/ESTRO/ESP guidelines for the management of patients with endometrial carcinoma. *Int J Gynecol Cancer*. 2021;31(1):12–39. doi:10.1136/ijgc-2020-002230

268. Imboden S, Nastic D, Ghaderi M, et al. Implementation of the 2021 molecular ESGO/ESTRO/ESP risk groups in endometrial cancer. *Gynecol Oncol*. 2021;162(2):394–400. doi:10.1016/j.ygyno.2021.05.026

269. Britton H, Huang L, Lum A, et al. Molecular classification defines outcomes and opportunities in young women with endometrial carcinoma. *Gynecol Oncol*. 2019;153(3):487–495. doi:10.1016/j.ygyno.2019 .03.098

270. Stelloo E, Nout RA, Osse EM, et al. Improved risk assessment by integrating molecular and clinicopathological factors in early-stage endometrial cancer-combined analysis of the PORTEC cohorts. *Clin Cancer Res*. 2016;22(16):4215–4224. doi:10.1158/1078-0432.CCR-15-2878

271. Talhouk A, McConechy MK, Leung S, et al. Confirmation of promise: a simple, genomics-based clinical classifier for endometrial cancer. *Cancer*. 2017;123(5):802–813. doi:10.1002/cncr.30496

272. Guntapalli SR, Dreyer G. Meeting report from 2020 annual global IGCS meeting. *Gynecol Oncol*. 2021;161:333–335.

273. Kommoss FK, Karnezis AN, Kommoss F, et al. L1CAM further stratifies endometrial carcinoma patients with no specific molecular risk profile. *Br J Cancer*. 2018;119(4):480–486. doi:10.1038/s41416-018-0187-6

274. Clement PB, Scully RE. Uterine tumors resembling ovarian sex-cord tumors; a clinicopathologic analysis of fourteen cases. *Am J Clin Pathol*. 1976;66(3):512–525. doi:10.1093/ajcp/66.3.512

275. Chan JK, Loizzi V, Youssef M, et al. Significance of comprehensive surgical staging in noninvasive papillary serous carcinoma of the endometrium. *Gynecol Oncol*. 2003;90(1):181–185. doi:10.1016/ s0090-8258(03)00195-1

276. Geisler JP, Geisler HE, Melton ME, et al. What staging surgery should be performed on patients with uterine papillary serous carcinoma? *Gynecol Oncol.* 1999;74(3):465–467. doi:10.1006/gyno.1999.5513

277. Pennington KP, Walsh T, Lee M, et al. BRCA1, TP53, and CHEK2 germline mutations in uterine serous carcinoma. *Cancer.* 2013;119(2):332–338. doi:10.1002/cncr.27720

278. Brinton LA, Felix AS, McMeekin DS, et al. Etiologic heterogeneity in endometrial cancer: evidence from a gynecologic oncology group trial. *Gynecol Oncol.* 2013;129(2):277–284. doi:10.1016/j.ygyno.2013.02.023

279. Cantrell LA, Blank SV, Duska LR. Uterine carcinosarcoma: a review of the literature. *Gynecol Oncol.* 2015;137(3):581–588. doi:10.1016/j.ygyno.2015.03.041

280. Walker JL, Piedmonte MR, Spirtos NM, et al. Laparoscopy compared with laparotomy for comprehensive surgical staging of uterine cancer: gynecologic oncology group study LAP2. *J Clin Oncol.* 2009;27(32):5331–5336. doi:10.1200/JCO.2009.22.3248

281. James JA, Rakowski JA, Jeppson CN, et al. Robotic transperitoneal infra-renal aortic lymphadenectomy in early-stage endometrial cancer. *Gynecol Oncol.* 2015;136(2):285–292. doi:10.1016/j.ygyno.2014.12.028

282. Wright JD, Jorge S, Tergas AI, et al. Utilization and outcomes of ovarian conservation in premenopausal women with endometrial cancer. *Obstet Gynecol.* 2016;127(1):101–108. doi:10.1097/AOG.0000000000001181

283. Burke WM, Orr J, Leitao M, et al. Endometrial cancer: a review and current management strategies: part I. *Gynecol Oncol.* 2014;134(2):385–392. doi:10.1016/j.ygyno.2014.05.018

284. Matsuo K, Mandelbaum RS, Matsuzaki S, et al. Ovarian conservation for young women with early-stage, low-grade endometrial cancer: a 2-step schema. *Am J Obstet Gynecol.* 2021;224(6):S0002-9378(20)32630-2):574–584. doi:10.1016/j.ajog.2020.12.1213

285. Kho KA, Anderson TL, Nezhat CH. Intracorporeal electromechanical tissue morcellation: a critical review and recommendations for clinical practice. *Obstet Gynecol.* 2014;124(4):787–793. doi:10.1097/AOG.0000000000000448

286. Uterine morcellation for presumed leiomyomas. *ACOG Clinical.* 2017.

287. Barlin JN, Khoury-Collado F, Kim CH, et al. The importance of applying a sentinel lymph node mapping algorithm in endometrial cancer staging: beyond removal of blue nodes. *Gynecol Oncol.* 2012;125(3):531–535. doi:10.1016/j.ygyno.2012.02.021

288. Rossi EC, Kowalski LD, Scalici J, et al. A comparison of sentinel lymph node biopsy to lymphadenectomy for endometrial cancer staging (fires trial): a multicentre, prospective, cohort study. *Lancet Oncol.* 2017;18(3):384–392. doi:10.1016/S1470-2045(17)30068-2

289. Mariani A, Webb MJ, Keeney GL, et al. Low-risk corpus cancer: is lymphadenectomy or radiotherapy necessary? *Am J Obstet Gynecol.* 2000;182(6):1506–1519. doi:10.1067/mob.2000.107335

290. Goff BA, Rice LW. Assessment of depth of myometrial invasion in endometrial adenocarcinoma. *Gynecol Oncol.* 1990;38(1):46–48. doi:10.1016/0090-8258(90)90009-a

291. Doering DL, Barnhill DR, Weiser EB, et al. Intraoperative evaluation of depth of myometrial invasion in stage I endometrial adenocarcinoma. *Obstet Gynecol.* 1989;74(6):930–933.

292. Franchi M, Ghezzi F, Melpignano M, et al. Clinical value of intraoperative gross examination in endometrial cancer. *Gynecol Oncol.* 2000;76(3):357–361. doi:10.1006/gyno.1999.5694

293. Cragun JM, Havrilesky LJ, Calingaert B, et al. Retrospective analysis of selective lymphadenectomy in apparent early-stage endometrial cancer. *J Clin Oncol.* 2005;23(16):3668–3675. doi:10.1200/JCO.2005.04.144

294. Chan JK, Cheung MK, Huh WK, et al. Therapeutic role of lymph node resection in endometrioid corpus cancer: a study of 12,333 patients. *Cancer.* 2006;107(8):1823–1830. doi:10.1002/cncr.22185

295. Kilgore LC, Partridge EE, Alvarez RD, et al. Adenocarcinoma of the endometrium: survival comparisons of patients with and without pelvic node sampling. *Gynecol Oncol.* 1995;56(1):29–33. doi:10.1006/gyno.1995.1005

296. Chan JK, Kapp DS, Cheung MK, et al. The impact of the absolute number and ratio of positive lymph nodes on survival of endometrioid uterine cancer patients. *Br J Cancer.* 2007;97(5):605–611. doi:10.1038/sj.bjc.6603898

297. Creutzberg CL, van Putten WLJ, Wárlám-Rodenhuis CC, et al. Outcome of high-risk stage ic, grade 3, compared with stage I endometrial carcinoma patients: the postoperative radiation therapy in endometrial carcinoma trial. *J Clin Oncol.* 2004;22(7):1234–1241. doi:10.1200/JCO.2004.08.159

298. Nelson G, Randall M, Sutton G, et al. FIGO stage IIIC endometrial carcinoma with metastases confined to pelvic lymph nodes: analysis of treatment outcomes, prognostic variables, and failure patterns following adjuvant radiation therapy. *Gynecol Oncol.* 1999;75(2):211–214. doi:10.1006/gyno.1999.5569

299. Ayhan A, Taskiran C, Celik C, et al. Surgical stage III endometrial cancer: analysis of treatment outcomes, prognostic factors and failure patterns. *Eur J Gynaecol Oncol.* 2002;23(6):553–556.

300. Benedetti Panici P, Basile S, Maneschi F, et al. Systematic pelvic lymphadenectomy vs. no lymphadenectomy in early-stage endometrial carcinoma: randomized clinical trial. *J Natl Cancer Inst.* 2008;100(23):1707–1716. doi:10.1093/jnci/djn397

301. Blake P, Swart AM, Orton J, et al. Adjuvant external beam radiotherapy in the treatment of endometrial cancer (MRC ASTEC and NCIC CTG EN.5 randomised trials): pooled trial results, systematic review, and meta-analysis. *Lancet.* 2009;373(9658):137–146. doi:10.1016/S0140-6736(08)61767-5

302. Kitchener H, Swart AMC, Qian Q, et al. Efficacy of systematic pelvic lymphadenectomy in endometrial cancer (MRC ASTEC trial): a randomised study. *Lancet.* 2009;373(9658):125–136. doi:10.1016/S0140-6736(08)61766-3

303. Morrow CP, Bundy BN, Kurman RJ, et al. Relationship between surgical-pathological risk factors and outcome in clinical stage I and II carcinoma of the endometrium: a Gynecologic Oncology Group study. *Gynecol Oncol.* 1991;40(1):55–65. doi:10.1016/0090-8258(91)90086-k

304. Disaia PJ. Predicting parametrial involvement in endometrial cancer: is this the end for radical hysterectomies in stage II endometrial cancers? *Obstet Gynecol.* 2010;116(5):1016–1017. doi:10.1097/AOG.0b013e3181f98202

305. Backes FJ, Felix AS, Plante M, et al. Sentinel lymph node (SLN) isolated tumor cells (itcs) in otherwise stage I/II endometrioid endometrial cancer: to treat or not to treat? *Gynecol Oncol.* 2021;161(2):347–352. doi:10.1016/j.ygyno.2021.02.017

306. Takenaka M, Kamii M, Iida Y, et al. Re-thinking the prognostic significance of positive peritoneal cytology in endometrial cancer. *Gynecol Oncol.* 2021;161(1):135–142. doi:10.1016/j.ygyno.2021.01.007

307. Wang Y, Tillmanns T, VanderWalde N, et al. Comparison of chemotherapy vs chemotherapy plus total hysterectomy for women with uterine cancer with distant organ metastasis. *JAMA Netw Open.* 2021;4(7):e2118603. doi:10.1001/jamanetworkopen.2021.18603

308. Greer BE, Hamberger AD. Treatment of intraperitoneal metastatic adenocarcinoma of the endometrium by the whole-abdomen moving-strip technique and pelvic boost irradiation. *Gynecol Oncol.* 1983;16(3):365–373. doi:10.1016/0090-8258(83)90164-6

309. Goff BA, Kato D, Schmidt RA, et al. Uterine papillary serous carcinoma: patterns of metastatic spread. *Gynecol Oncol.* 1994;54(3):264–268. doi:10.1006/gyno.1994.1208.

310. Bristow RE, Duska LR, Montz FJ. The role of cytoreductive surgery in the management of stage IV uterine papillary serous carcinoma. *Gynecol Oncol.* 2001;81(1):92–99. doi:10.1006/gyno.2000.6110

311. Shih KK, Yun E, Gardner GJ, et al. Surgical cytoreduction in stage IV endometrioid endometrial carcinoma. *Gynecol Oncol.* 2011;122(3):608–611. doi:10.1016/j.ygyno.2011.05.020

312. Chao A, Wu R-C, Jung S-M, et al. Implication of genomic characterization in synchronous endometrial and ovarian cancers of endometrioid histology. *Gynecol Oncol.* 2016;143(1):60–67. doi:10.1016/j.ygyno.2016.07.114

313. Kelly MG, O'malley DM, Hui P, et al. Improved survival in surgical stage I patients with uterine papillary serous carcinoma (UPSC) treated with adjuvant platinum-based chemotherapy. *Gynecol Oncol.* 2005;98(3):353–359. doi:10.1016/j.ygyno.2005.06.012

314. Olawaiye AB, Leath CA. Contemporary management of uterine clear cell carcinoma: A Society of Gynecologic Oncology (SGO) review and recommendation. *Gynecol Oncol.* 2019;155(2):365–373. doi:10.1016/j.ygyno.2019.08.031

315. Bogani G, Ray-Coquard I, Concin N, et al. Uterine serous carcinoma. *Gynecol Oncol.* 2021;162(1):226–234. doi:10.1016/j.ygyno.2021.04.029

316. Nasioudis D, Roy AG, Ko EM, et al. Adjuvant treatment for patients with FIGO stage I uterine serous carcinoma confined to the endometrium. *Int J Gynecol Cancer.* 2020;30(8):1089–1094. doi:10.1136/ijgc-2020-001379

317. Tanner EJ, Leitao MM, Garg K, et al. The role of cytoreductive surgery for newly diagnosed advanced-stage uterine carcinosarcoma. *Gynecol Oncol.* 2011;123(3):548–552. doi:10.1016/j.ygyno.2011.08.020

318. Toboni MD, Crane EK, Brown J, et al. Uterine carcinosarcomas: from pathology to practice. *Gynecol Oncol.* 2021;162(1):235–241. doi:10.1016/j.ygyno.2021.05.003

319. Reed NS, Mangioni C, Malmstrom H, et al. FIRST results of a randomised trial comparing radiotherapy versus- observation post operatively in patients with uterine sarcomas. an EORTC-GCG study. *Int J Gynecol Cancer.* 2003;13(Suppl 1):4. doi:10.1136/ijgc-00009577-200303001-00012

320. Homesley HD, Filiaci V, Markman M, et al. Phase III trial of ifosfamide with or without paclitaxel in advanced uterine carcinosarcoma: a gynecologic oncology group study. *J Clin Oncol.* 2007;25(5):526–531. doi:10.1200/JCO.2006.06.4907

321. Awtrey CS, Cadungog MG, Leitao MM, et al. Surgical resection of recurrent endometrial carcinoma. *Gynecol Oncol.* 2006;102(3):480–488. doi:10.1016/j.ygyno.2006.01.007

322. Scudder SA, Liu PY, Wilczynski SP, et al. Paclitaxel and carboplatin with amifostine in advanced, recurrent, or refractory endometrial adenocarcinoma: a phase II study of the southwest oncology group. *Gynecol Oncol.* 2005;96(3):610–615. doi:10.1016/j.ygyno.2004.11.024

323. Thigpen JT, Brady MF, Alvarez RD, et al. Oral medroxyprogesterone acetate in the treatment of advanced or recurrent endometrial carcinoma: a dose-response study by the gynecologic oncology group. *J Clin Oncol.* 1999;17(6):1736–1744. doi:10.1200/JCO.1999.17.6.1736

324. Fleming GF, Sill MW, Darcy KM, et al. Phase II trial of trastuzumab in women with advanced or recurrent, HER2-positive endometrial carcinoma: a gynecologic oncology group study. *Gynecol Oncol.* 2010;116(1):15–20. doi:10.1016/j.ygyno.2009.09.025

325. Bender D, Sill MW, Lankes HA, et al. A phase II evaluation of cediranib in the treatment of recurrent or persistent endometrial cancer: an NRG oncology/gynecologic oncology group study. *Gynecol Oncol.* 2015;138(3):507–512. doi:10.1016/j.ygyno.2015.07.018

326. Lheureux S, Matei D, Konstantinopoulos PA, et al. A randomized phase II study of cabozantinib and nivolumab versus nivolumab in

recurrent endometrial cancer. *J Clin Oncol.* 2020;38(15_suppl):6010–6010. doi:10.1200/JCO.2020.38.15_suppl.6010

327. Barakat RR, Bundy BN, Spirtos NM, et al. Randomized double-blind trial of estrogen replacement therapy versus placebo in stage I or II endometrial cancer: a gynecologic oncology group study. *J Clin Oncol.* 2006;24(4):587–592. doi:10.1200/JCO.2005.02.8464

328. Curtis RE, Freedman DM, Sherman ME, et al. Risk of malignant mixed mullerian tumors after tamoxifen therapy for breast cancer. *J Natl Cancer Inst.* 2004;96(1):70–74. doi:10.1093/jnci/djh007

329. Aalders J, Abeler V, Kolstad P, et al. Postoperative external irradiation and prognostic parameters in stage I endometrial carcinoma: clinical and histopathologic study of 540 patients. *Obstet Gynecol.* 1980;56(4):419–427.

330. Creutzberg CL, van Putten WL, Koper PC, et al. Surgery and postoperative radiotherapy versus surgery alone for patients with stage-1 endometrial carcinoma: multicentre randomised trial. PORTEC study group. post operative radiation therapy in endometrial carcinoma. *Lancet.* 2000;355(9213):1404–1411. doi:10.1016/s0140-6736(00)02139-5

331. Creutzberg CL, Nout RA, Lybeert MLM, et al. Fifteen-year radiotherapy outcomes of the randomized PORTEC-1 trial for endometrial carcinoma. *Int J Radiat Oncol Biol Phys.* 2011;81(4):e631–8. doi:10.1016/j.ijrobp.2011.04.013

332. Nout RA, van de Poll-Franse LV, Lybeert MLM, et al. Long-term outcome and quality of life of patients with endometrial carcinoma treated with or without pelvic radiotherapy in the post operative radiation therapy in endometrial carcinoma 1 (PORTEC-1) trial. *J Clin Oncol.* 2011;29(13):1692–1700. doi:10.1200/JCO.2010.32.4590

333. Keys HM, Roberts JA, Brunetto VL, et al. A phase III trial of surgery with or without adjunctive external pelvic radiation therapy in intermediate risk endometrial adenocarcinoma: a gynecologic oncology group study. *Gynecol Oncol.* 2004;92(3):744–751. doi:10.1016/j.ygyno.2003.11.048

334. Nout RA, Smit VTHBM, Putter H, et al. Vaginal brachytherapy versus pelvic external beam radiotherapy for patients with endometrial cancer of high-intermediate risk (PORTEC-2): an open-label, non-inferiority, randomised trial. *Lancet.* 2010;375(9717):816–823. doi:10.1016/S0140-6736(09)62163-2

335. de Boer SM, Powell ME, Mileshkin L, et al. Adjuvant chemoradiotherapy versus radiotherapy alone for women with high-risk endometrial cancer (PORTEC-3): final results of an international, open-label, multicentre, randomised, phase 3 trial. *Lancet Oncol.* 2018;19(3):295–309. doi:10.1016/S1470-2045(18)30079-2

336. de Boer SM, Powell ME, Mileshkin L, et al. Toxicity and quality of life after adjuvant chemoradiotherapy versus radiotherapy alone for women with high-risk endometrial cancer (PORTEC-3): an open-label, multicentre, randomised, phase 3 trial. *Lancet Oncol.* 2016;17(8):1114–1126. doi:10.1016/S1470-2045(16)30120-6

337. Anne Sophie VM, Nanda H, Remi AN. PORTEC-4: randomised phase III trial comparing vaginal brachytherapy (two doses schedules: 21 or 15 gy HDR in 3 fractions) and observation after surgery in patients with endometrial carcinoma with high-intermediate risk features. *Int J Gynecol Cancer*. 2020;30(12):2002–2007.

338. Nomura H, Aoki D, Michimae H, et al. Effect of taxane plus platinum regimens vs doxorubicin plus cisplatin as adjuvant chemotherapy for endometrial cancer at a high risk of progression: a randomized clinical trial. *JAMA Oncol*. 2019;5(6):833–840. doi:10.1001/jamaoncol.2019.0001

339. Greven K, Winter K, Underhill K, et al. Final analysis of RTOG 9708: adjuvant postoperative irradiation combined with cisplatin/paclitaxel chemotherapy following surgery for patients with high-risk endometrial cancer. *Gynecol Oncol*. 2006;103(1):155–159. doi:10.1016/j.ygyno.2006.02.007

340. Susumu N, Sagae S, Udagawa Y, et al. Randomized phase III trial of pelvic radiotherapy versus cisplatin-based combined chemotherapy in patients with intermediate- and high-risk endometrial cancer: a japanese gynecologic oncology group study. *Gynecol Oncol*. 2008;108(1):226–233. doi:10.1016/j.ygyno.2007.09.029

341. Todo Y, Kato H, Kaneuchi M, et al. Survival effect of para-aortic lymphadenectomy in endometrial cancer (SEPAL study): a retrospective cohort analysis. *Lancet*. 2010;375(9721):1165–1172. doi:10.1016/S0140-6736(09)62002-X

342. McMeekin DS, Filiaci VL, Aghajanian C, et al. 1A randomized phase III trial of pelvic radiation therapy (PXRT) versus vaginal cuff brachytherapy followed by paclitaxel/carboplatin chemotherapy (VCB/C) in patients with high risk (HR), early stage endometrial cancer (EC): a gynecologic oncology group trial. *Gynecol Oncol*. 2014;134(2):438. doi:10.1016/j.ygyno.2014.07.078

343. Randall ME, Filiaci V, McMeekin DS, et al. Phase III trial: adjuvant pelvic radiation therapy versus vaginal brachytherapy plus paclitaxel/carboplatin in high-intermediate and high-risk early stage endometrial cancer. *J Clin Oncol*. 2019;37(21):1810–1818. doi:10.1200/JCO.18.01575

344. Viswanathan AN, Moughan J, Miller BE, et al. NRG oncology/RTOG 0921: a phase 2 study of postoperative intensity-modulated radiotherapy with concurrent cisplatin and bevacizumab followed by carboplatin and paclitaxel for patients with endometrial cancer. *Cancer*. 2015;121(13):2156–2163. doi:10.1002/cncr.29337

345. Creasman WT, Ali S, Mutch DG, et al. Surgical-pathological findings in type 1 and 2 endometrial cancer: an NRG oncology/gynecologic oncology group study on GOG-210 protocol. *Gynecol Oncol*. 2017;145(3):519–525. doi:10.1016/j.ygyno.2017.03.017

346. Cohen CJ, Bruckner HW, Deppe G, et al. Multidrug treatment of advanced and recurrent endometrial carcinoma: a gynecologic oncology group study. *Obstet Gynecol*. 1984;63(5):719–726.

347. Thigpen JT, Blessing JA, DiSaia PJ, et al. A randomized comparison of doxorubicin alone versus doxorubicin plus cyclophosphamide in

the management of advanced or recurrent endometrial carcinoma: a gynecologic oncology group study. *J Clin Oncol.* 1994;12(7):1408–1414. doi:10.1200/JCO.1994.12.7.1408

348. Sutton G, Axelrod JH, Bundy BN, et al. Adjuvant whole abdominal irradiation in clinical stages I and II papillary serous or clear cell carcinoma of the endometrium: a phase II study of the gynecologic oncology group. *Gynecol Oncol.* 2006;100(2):349–354. doi:10.1016/j.ygyno.2005.08.037

349. Sutton G, Axelrod JH, Bundy BN, et al. Whole abdominal radiotherapy in the adjuvant treatment of patients with stage III and IV endometrial cancer: a gynecologic oncology group study. *Gynecol Oncol.* 2005;97(3):755–763. doi:10.1016/j.ygyno.2005.03.011

350. Thigpen JT, Brady MF, Homesley HD, et al. Phase III trial of doxorubicin with or without cisplatin in advanced endometrial carcinoma: a gynecologic oncology group study. *J Clin Oncol.* 2004;22(19):3902–3908. doi:10.1200/JCO.2004.02.088

351. Randall ME, Filiaci VL, Muss H, et al. Randomized phase III trial of whole-abdominal irradiation versus doxorubicin and cisplatin chemotherapy in advanced endometrial carcinoma: a gynecologic oncology group study. *J Clin Oncol.* 2006;24(1):36–44. doi:10.1200/JCO.2004.00.7617

352. Gallion HH, Brunetto VL, Cibull M, et al. Randomized phase III trial of standard timed doxorubicin plus cisplatin versus circadian timed doxorubicin plus cisplatin in stage III and IV or recurrent endometrial carcinoma: a gynecologic oncology group study. *J Clin Oncol.* 2003;21(20):3808–3813. doi:10.1200/JCO.2003.10.083

353. Fleming GF, Filiaci VL, Bentley RC, et al. Phase III randomized trial of doxorubicin + cisplatin versus doxorubicin + 24-h paclitaxel + filgrastim in endometrial carcinoma: a gynecologic oncology group study. *Ann Oncol.* 2004;15(8):1173–1178. doi:10.1093/annonc/mdh316

354. Fleming GF, Brunetto VL, Cella D, et al. Phase III trial of doxorubicin plus cisplatin with or without paclitaxel plus filgrastim in advanced endometrial carcinoma: a gynecologic oncology group study. *J Clin Oncol.* 2004;22(11):2159–2166. doi:10.1200/JCO.2004.07.184

355. Homesley HD, Filiaci V, Gibbons SK, et al. A randomized phase III trial in advanced endometrial carcinoma of surgery and volume directed radiation followed by cisplatin and doxorubicin with or without paclitaxel: a gynecologic oncology group study. *Gynecol Oncol.* 2009;112(3):543–552. doi:10.1016/j.ygyno.2008.11.014

356. Lorusso D, Ferrandina G, Colombo N, et al. Randomized phase II trial of carboplatin-paclitaxel (CP) compared to carboplatin-paclitaxel-bevacizumab (CP-B) in advanced (stage III-IV) or recurrent endometrial cancer: the MITO END-2 trial. *JCO.* 2015;33(15_suppl):5502–5502. doi:10.1200/jco.2015.33.15_suppl.5502

357. Matei D, Filiaci V, Randall ME, et al. Adjuvant chemotherapy plus radiation for locally advanced endometrial cancer. *N Engl J Med.* 2019;380(24):2317–2326. doi:10.1056/NEJMoa1813181

358. Lorusso D, Ferrandina G, Colombo N, et al. Carboplatin-paclitaxel compared to carboplatin-paclitaxel-bevacizumab in advanced or recurrent endometrial cancer: MITO END-2 - a randomized phase II trial. *Gynecol Oncol.* 2019;155(3):406–412. doi:10.1016/j.ygyno.2019.10.013

359. Oaknin A, Gilbert L, Tinker AV. Analysis of antitumor activity of dostarlimab by tumor mutational burden (TMB) in patients (pts) with endometrial cancer (EC) in the GARNET trial. In: *Presented at: 2021 ESMO Congress.* Virtual. Abstract; 2021.

360. Vargo JA, Kim H, Houser CJ, et al. Definitive salvage for vaginal recurrence of endometrial cancer: the impact of modern intensity-modulated-radiotherapy with image-based HDR brachytherapy and the interplay of the PORTEC 1 risk stratification. *Radiother Oncol.* 2014;113(1):126–131. doi:10.1016/j.radonc.2014.08.038

361. Mundt AJ, McBride R, Rotmensch J, et al. Significant pelvic recurrence in high-risk pathologic stage I--IV endometrial carcinoma patients after adjuvant chemotherapy alone: implications for adjuvant radiation therapy. *Int J Radiat Oncol Biol Phys.* 2001;50(5):1145–1153. doi:10.1016/s0360-3016(01)01566-8

362. Lincoln S, Blessing JA, Lee RB, et al. Activity of paclitaxel as second-line chemotherapy in endometrial carcinoma: a gynecologic oncology group study. *Gynecol Oncol.* 2003;88(3):277–281. doi:10.1016/s0090-8258(02)00068-9

363. McMeekin DS, Filiaci VL, Thigpen JT, et al. The relationship between histology and outcome in advanced and recurrent endometrial cancer patients participating in first-line chemotherapy trials: a gynecologic oncology group study. *Gynecol Oncol.* 2007;106(1):16–22. doi:10.1016/j.ygyno.2007.04.032

364. Ott PA, Bang Y-J, Berton-Rigaud D, et al. Safety and antitumor activity of pembrolizumab in advanced programmed death ligand 1-positive endometrial cancer: results from the KEYNOTE-028 study. *J Clin Oncol.* 2017;35(22):2535–2541. doi:10.1200/JCO.2017.72.5952

365. Makker V, Taylor MH, Oaknin A, et al. Characterization and management of adverse reactions in patients with advanced endometrial carcinoma treated with lenvatinib plus pembrolizumab. *Oncologist.* 2021;26(9):e1599–e1608. doi:10.1002/onco.13883

366. Makker V, Taylor MH, Aghajanian C, et al. Lenvatinib plus pembrolizumab in patients with advanced endometrial cancer. *J Clin Oncol.* 2020;38(26):2981–2992. doi:10.1200/JCO.19.02627

367. Makker V, Colombo N, Casado Herráez A, et al. Lenvatinib plus pembrolizumab for advanced endometrial cancer. *N Engl J Med.* 2022;386(5):437–448. doi:10.1056/NEJMoa2108330

368. How JA, Patel S, Fellman B, et al. Toxicity and efficacy of the combination of pembrolizumab with recommended or reduced starting doses of lenvatinib for treatment of recurrent endometrial cancer. *Gynecol Oncol.* 2021;162(1):24–31. doi:10.1016/j.ygyno.2021.04.034

369. News release. *Karyopharm Therapeutics.* 2022.

370. Vergote I, Fidalgo A, Hamilton E. Prospective double-blink, randomized phase II ENGOT-EN5/GOG-3055/SIENDO study or oral selinexor/placebo as maintenance therapy after first line chemotherapy for advanced or recurrent endometrial cancer. In: *SGO Annual Meeting*. 2022.

371. Tatebe K, Hasan Y, Son CH. Adjuvant vaginal brachytherapy and chemotherapy versus pelvic radiotherapy in early-stage endometrial cancer: outcomes by risk factors. *Gynecol Oncol*. 2019;155(3):429–435. doi:10.1016/j.ygyno.2019.09.028

372. Xiang M, English DP, Kidd EA. National patterns of care and cancer-specific outcomes of adjuvant treatment in patients with serous and clear cell endometrial carcinoma. *Gynecol Oncol*. 2019;152(3):599–604. doi:10.1016/j.ygyno.2018.12.007

373. Fader AN, Roque DM, Siegel E, et al. Randomized phase II trial of carboplatin-paclitaxel versus carboplatin-paclitaxel-trastuzumab in uterine serous carcinomas that overexpress human epidermal growth factor receptor 2/neu. *J Clin Oncol*. 2018;36(20):2044–2051. doi:10.1200/JCO.2017.76.5966

374. Sutton G, Brunetto VL, Kilgore L, et al. A phase III trial of ifosfamide with or without cisplatin in carcinosarcoma of the uterus: a gynecologic oncology group study. *Gynecol Oncol*. 2000;79(2):147–153. doi:10.1006/gyno.2000.6001

375. Wolfson AH, Brady MF, Rocereto T, et al. A gynecologic oncology group randomized phase III trial of whole abdominal irradiation (WAI) vs. cisplatin-ifosfamide and mesna (CIM) as post-surgical therapy in stage I-IV carcinosarcoma (CS) of the uterus. *Gynecol Oncol*. 2007;107(2):177–185. doi:10.1016/j.ygyno.2007.07.070

376. Reed NS, Mangioni C, Malmström H, et al. Phase III randomised study to evaluate the role of adjuvant pelvic radiotherapy in the treatment of uterine sarcomas stages I and II: an European organisation for research and treatment of cancer gynaecological cancer group study (protocol 55874). *Eur J Cancer*. 2008;44(6):808–818. doi:10.1016/j.ejca.2008.01.019

377. Zola P, Ciccone G, Piovano E, et al. Intensive versus minimalist follow-up in patients treated for endometrial cancer: a multicentric randomized controlled trial (the totem study—NCT00916708). *JCO*. 2021;39(15_suppl):5506–5506. doi:10.1200/JCO.2021.39.15_suppl.5506

378. Beaver K, Williamson S, Sutton C, et al. Comparing hospital and telephone follow-up for patients treated for stage-I endometrial cancer (ENDCAT trial): a randomised, multicentre, non-inferiority trial. *BJOG*. 2017;124(1):150–160. doi:10.1111/1471-0528.14000

379. Kurman RJ, Carcangiu ML, Herrington CS. *WHO Classification of Tumours*. Vol 6. IARC WHO Classification of Tumours; 2017. at: cancer.org

380. Leitao MM, Sonoda Y, Brennan MF, et al. Incidence of lymph node and ovarian metastases in leiomyosarcoma of the uterus. *Gynecol Oncol*. 2003;91(1):209–212. doi:10.1016/s0090-8258(03)00478-5

381. Giuntoli RL, Metzinger DS, DiMarco CS, et al. Retrospective review of 208 patients with leiomyosarcoma of the uterus: prognostic indicators, surgical management, and adjuvant therapy. *Gynecol Oncol.* 2003;89(3):460–469. doi:10.1016/s0090-8258(03)00137-9

382. Kapp DS, Shin JY, Chan JK. Prognostic factors and survival in 1396 patients with uterine leiomyosarcomas: emphasis on impact of lymphadenectomy and oophorectomy. *Cancer.* 2008;112(4):820–830. doi:10.1002/cncr.23245

383. Goff BA, Rice LW, Fleischhacker D, et al. Uterine leiomyosarcoma and endometrial stromal sarcoma: lymph node metastases and sites of recurrence. *Gynecol Oncol.* 1993;50(1):105–109. doi:10.1006/gyno.1993.1172

384. O'Cearbhaill R, Hensley ML. Optimal management of uterine leiomyosarcoma. *Expert Rev Anticancer Ther.* 2010;10(2):153–169. doi:10.1586/era.09.187

385. Littell RD, Tucker L-Y, Raine-Bennett T, et al. Adjuvant gemcitabine-docetaxel chemotherapy for stage I uterine leiomyosarcoma: trends and survival outcomes. *Gynecol Oncol.* 2017;147(1):11–17. doi:10.1016/j.ygyno.2017.07.122

386. George S, Feng Y, Manola J, et al. Phase 2 trial of aromatase inhibition with letrozole in patients with uterine leiomyosarcomas expressing estrogen and/or progesterone receptors. *Cancer.* 2014;120(5):738):738–743:. doi:10.1002/cncr.28476

387. Levenback C, Rubin SC, McCormack PM, et al. Resection of pulmonary metastases from uterine sarcomas. *Gynecol Oncol.* 1992;45(2):202–205. doi:10.1016/0090-8258(92)90286-r

388. van der Graaf WTA, Blay J-Y, Chawla SP, et al. Pazopanib for metastatic soft-tissue sarcoma (PALETTE): a randomised, double-blind, placebo-controlled phase 3 trial. *Lancet.* 2012;379(9829):1879–1886. doi:10.1016/S0140-6736(12)60651-5

389. George S, Serrano C, Hensley ML, et al. Soft tissue and uterine leiomyosarcoma. *J Clini Oncol.* 2018;36(2):144–150. doi:10.1200/JCO.2017.75.9845

390. Cheng X, Yang G, Schmeler KM, et al. Recurrence patterns and prognosis of endometrial stromal sarcoma and the potential of tyrosine kinase-inhibiting therapy. *Gynecol Oncol.* 2011;121(2):323–327. doi:10.1016/j.ygyno.2010.12.360

391. Malouf GG, Duclos J, Rey A, et al. Impact of adjuvant treatment modalities on the management of patients with stages I-II endometrial stromal sarcoma. *Ann Oncol.* 2010;21(10):S0923-7534(19)39571-7):2102–2106. doi:10.1093/annonc/mdq064

392. Demetri GD, von Mehren M, Jones RL, et al. Efficacy and safety of trabectedin or dacarbazine for metastatic liposarcoma or leiomyosarcoma after failure of conventional chemotherapy: results of a phase III randomized multicenter clinical trial. *J Clin Oncol.* 2016;34(8):786–793. doi:10.1200/JCO.2015.62.4734

393. Schöffski P, Chawla S, Maki RG, et al. Eribulin versus dacarbazine in previously treated patients with advanced liposarcoma or leiomyosarcoma: a randomised, open-label, multicentre, phase 3 trial. *Lancet.* 2016;387(10028):1629–1637. doi:10.1016/S0140-6736(15)01283-0

394. Benson C, Ray-Coquard I, Sleijfer S, et al. Outcome of uterine sarcoma patients treated with pazopanib: a retrospective analysis based on two european organisation for research and treatment of cancer (EORTC) soft tissue and bone sarcoma group (STBSG) clinical trials 62043 and 62072. *Gynecol Oncol.* 2016;142(1):89–94. doi:10.1016/j.ygyno.2016.03.024

395. Ben-Ami E, Barysauskas CM, Solomon S, et al. Immunotherapy with single agent nivolumab for advanced leiomyosarcoma of the uterus: results of a phase 2 study. *Cancer.* 2017;123(17):3285–3290. doi:10.1002/cncr.30738

396. Toulmonde M, Penel N, Adam J, et al. Use of PD-1 targeting, macrophage infiltration, and IDO pathway activation in sarcomas: a phase 2 clinical trial. *JAMA Oncol.* 2018;4(1):93–97. doi:10.1001/jamaoncol.2017.1617

397. D'Angelo SP, Mahoney MR, Van Tine BA, et al. A multi-center phase II study of nivolumab +/- ipilimumab for patients with metastatic sarcoma (alliance A091401). *JCO.* 2017;35(15_suppl):11007–11007. doi:10.1200/JCO.2017.35.15_suppl.11007

398. Pautier P, Floquet A, Penel N, et al. Randomized multicenter and stratified phase II study of gemcitabine alone versus gemcitabine and docetaxel in patients with metastatic or relapsed leiomyosarcomas: a federation nationale des centres de lutte contre le cancer (FNCLCC) french sarcoma group study (TAXOGEM study). *Oncologist.* 2012;17(9):1213–1220. doi:10.1634/theoncologist.2011-0467

399. Seddon BM, Whelan J, Strauss SJ, et al. GeDDiS: a prospective randomised controlled phase III trial of gemcitabine and docetaxel compared with doxorubicin as first-line treatment in previously untreated advanced unresectable or metastatic soft tissue sarcomas (eudract 2009-014907-29). *JCO.* 2015;33(15_suppl):10500–10500. doi:10.1200/jco.2015.33.15_suppl.10500

400. Tap WD, Jones RL, Van Tine BA, et al. Olaratumab and doxorubicin versus doxorubicin alone for treatment of soft-tissue sarcoma: an open-label phase 1B and randomised phase 2 trial. *Lancet.* 2016;388(10043):488–497. doi:10.1016/S0140-6736(16)30587-6

401. Hensley ML, Patel SR, von Mehren M, et al. Efficacy and safety of trabectedin or dacarbazine in patients with advanced uterine leiomyosarcoma after failure of anthracycline-based chemotherapy: subgroup analysis of a phase 3, randomized clinical trial. *Gynecol Oncol.* 2017;146(3):531–537. doi:10.1016/j.ygyno.2017.06.018

402. Samuels BL, Chawla S, Patel S, et al. Clinical outcomes and safety with trabectedin therapy in patients with advanced soft tissue sarcomas following failure of prior chemotherapy: results of a worldwide expanded access program study. *Ann Oncol.* 2013;24(6):1703–1709. doi:10.1093/annonc/mds659

403. Monk BJ, Blessing JA, Street DG, et al. A phase II evaluation of trabectedin in the treatment of advanced, persistent, or recurrent uterine leiomyosarcoma: a gynecologic oncology group study. *Gynecol Oncol.* 2012;124(1):48–52. doi:10.1016/j.ygyno.2011.09.019

404. Pautier P, Floquet A, Chevreau C, et al. Trabectedin in combination with doxorubicin for first-line treatment of advanced uterine or soft-tissue leiomyosarcoma (LMS-02): a non-randomised, multicentre, phase 2 trial. *Lancet Oncol.* 2015;16(4):457–464. doi:10.1016/S1470-2045(15)70070-7

405. Martin-Broto J, Pousa AL, de Las Peñas R, et al. Randomized phase II study of trabectedin and doxorubicin compared with doxorubicin alone as first-line treatment in patients with advanced soft tissue sarcomas: a spanish group for research on sarcoma study. *J Clin Oncol.* 2016;34(19):2294–2302. doi:10.1200/JCO.2015.65.3329

406. Blay J-Y, Schöffski P, Bauer S, et al. Eribulin versus dacarbazine in patients with leiomyosarcoma: subgroup analysis from a phase 3, open-label, randomised study. *Br J Cancer.* 2019;120(11):1026–1032. doi:10.1038/s41416-019-0462-1

407. Lewin SN, Herzog TJ, Barrena Medel NI, et al. Comparative performance of the 2009 international federation of gynecology and obstetrics' staging system for uterine corpus cancer. *Obstet Gynecol.* 2010;116(5):1141–1149. doi:10.1097/AOG.0b013e3181f39849

408. Modesitt SC, Waters AB, Walton L, et al. Vulvar intraepithelial neoplasia III: occult cancer and the impact of margin status on recurrence. *Obstet Gynecol.* 1998;92(6):962–966. doi:10.1016/s0029-7844(98)00350-0

409. Iversen T, Aalders JG, Christensen A, et al. Squamous cell carcinoma of the vulva: a review of 424 patients, 1956-1974. *Gynecol Oncol.* 1980;9(3):271–279. doi:10.1016/0090-8258(80)90038-4

410. Gonzalez Bosquet J, Kinney WK, Russell AH, et al. Risk of occult inguinofemoral lymph node metastasis from squamous carcinoma of the vulva. *Int J Radiat Oncol Biol Phys.* 2003;57(2):419–424. doi:10.1016/s0360-3016(03)00536-4

411. Bohlin KS, Bruno A-K, von Knorring C, et al. Accuracy of computerized tomography in the preoperative evaluation of metastases in primary vulvar cancer - a population-based study. *Gynecol Oncol.* 2021;161(2):449–453. doi:10.1016/j.ygyno.2021.02.005

412. Klapdor R, Länger F, Gratz KF, et al. SPECT/CT for SLN dissection in vulvar cancer: improved SLN detection and dissection by preoperative three-dimensional anatomical localisation. *Gynecol Oncol.* 2015;138(3):S0090-8258(15)30031-7):590–596. doi:10.1016/j.ygyno.2015.06.011

413. Pecorelli S. Revised FIGO staging for carcinoma of the vulva, cervix, and endometrium. *Int J Gynaecol Obstet.* 2009;105(2):103–104. doi:10.1016/j.ijgo.2009.02.012

414. Stehman FB, Bundy BN, Dvoretsky PM, et al. Early stage I carcinoma of the vulva treated with ipsilateral superficial inguinal lymphadenectomy and modified radical hemivulvectomy: a prospective study of the gynecologic oncology group. *Obstet Gynecol.* 1992;79(4):490–497.

415. de Hullu JA, van der Zee AGJ. Surgery and radiotherapy in vulvar cancer. *Crit Rev Oncol Hematol.* 2006;60(1):38–58. doi:10.1016/j.critrevonc.2006.02.008

416. Gonzalez Bosquet J, Magrina JF, Magtibay PM, et al. Patterns of inguinal groin metastases in squamous cell carcinoma of the vulva. *Gynecol Oncol.* 2007;105(3):742–746. doi:10.1016/j.ygyno.2007.02.014

417. Koual M, Benoit L, Nguyen-Xuan H-T, et al. Diagnostic value of indocyanine green fluorescence guided sentinel lymph node biopsy in vulvar cancer: a systematic review. *Gynecol Oncol.* 2021;161(2):436–441. doi:10.1016/j.ygyno.2021.01.031

418. Heaps JM, Fu YS, Montz FJ, et al. Surgical-pathologic variables predictive of local recurrence in squamous cell carcinoma of the vulva. *Gynecol Oncol.* 1990;38(3):309–314. doi:10.1016/0090-8258(90)90064-r

419. Faul CM, Mirmow D, Huang Q, et al. Adjuvant radiation for vulvar carcinoma: improved local control. *Int J Radiat Oncol Biol Phys.* 1997;38(2):381–389. doi:10.1016/s0360-3016(97)82500-x

420. Te Grootenhuis NC, Pouwer AW, de Bock GH, et al. Margin status revisited in vulvar squamous cell carcinoma. *Gynecol Oncol.* 2019;154(2):266–275. doi:10.1016/j.ygyno.2019.05.010

421. Oonk MHM, Slomovitz B, Baldwin PJW, et al. Radiotherapy versus inguinofemoral lymphadenectomy as treatment for vulvar cancer patients with micrometastases in the sentinel node: results of GROINSS-V II. *J Clin Oncol.* 2021;39(32):JCO2100006):3623–3632. doi:10.1200/JCO.21.00006

422. Trimble EL, Lewis JL, Williams LL, et al. Management of vulvar melanoma. *Gynecol Oncol.* 1992;45(3):254–258. doi:10.1016/0090-8258(92)90300-8

423. Fishman DA, Chambers SK, Schwartz PE, et al. Extramammary paget's disease of the vulva. *Gynecol Oncol.* 1995;56(2):266–270. doi:10.1006/gyno.1995.1044

424. Farias-Eisner R, Cirisano FD, Grouse D, et al. Conservative and individualized surgery for early squamous carcinoma of the vulva: the treatment of choice for stage I and II (T1-2N0-1M0) disease. *Gynecol Oncol.* 1994;53(1):55–58. doi:10.1006/gyno.1994.1087

425. Homesley HD, Bundy BN, Sedlis A, et al. Assessment of current international federation of gynecology and obstetrics staging of vulvar carcinoma relative to prognostic factors for survival (a gynecologic oncology group study). *Am J Obstet Gynecol.* 1991;164(4):997–1003. doi:10.1016/0002-9378(91)90573-a

426. Homesley HD, Bundy BN, Sedlis A, et al. Prognostic factors for groin node metastasis in squamous cell carcinoma of the vulva (a gynecologic oncology group study). *Gynecol Oncol.* 1993;49(3):279–283. doi:10.1006/gyno.1993.1127

427. Kunos C, Simpkins F, Gibbons H, et al. Radiation therapy compared with pelvic node resection for node-positive vulvar cancer: a randomized controlled trial. *Obstet Gynecol.* 2009;114(3):537–546. doi:10.1097/AOG.0b013e3181b12f99

428. Homesley HD, Bundy BN, Sedlis A, et al. Radiation therapy versus pelvic node resection for carcinoma of the vulva with positive groin nodes. *Obstet Gynecol.* 1986;68(6):733–740.

429. Stehman FB, Bundy BN, Ball H, et al. Sites of failure and times to failure in carcinoma of the vulva treated conservatively: a gynecologic oncology group study. *Am J Obstet Gynecol.* 1996;174(4):1128–1132. doi:10.1016/s0002-9378(96)70654-3.

430. Stehman FB, Bundy BN, Thomas G, et al. Groin dissection versus groin radiation in carcinoma of the vulva: a gynecologic oncology group study. *Int J Radiat Oncol Biol Phys.* 1992;24(2):389–396. doi:10.1016/0360-3016(92)90699-i

431. Koh WJ, Chiu M, Stelzer KJ, et al. Femoral vessel depth and the implications for groin node radiation. *Int J Radiat Oncol Biol Phys.* 1993;27(4):969–974. doi:10.1016/0360-3016(93)90476-c

432. Moore DH, Thomas GM, Montana GS, et al. Preoperative chemoradiation for advanced vulvar cancer: a phase II study of the gynecologic oncology group. *Int J Radiat Oncol Biol Phys.* 1998;42(1):79–85. doi:10.1016/s0360-3016(98)00193-x

433. Montana GS, Thomas GM, Moore DH, et al. Preoperative chemoradiation for carcinoma of the vulva with N2/N3 nodes: a gynecologic oncology group study. *Int J Radiat Oncol Biol Phys.* 2000;48(4):1007–1013. doi:10.1016/s0360-3016(00)00762-8

434. Moore DH, Ali S, Koh W-J, et al. A phase II trial of radiation therapy and weekly cisplatin chemotherapy for the treatment of locally-advanced squamous cell carcinoma of the vulva: a gynecologic oncology group study. *Gynecol Oncol.* 2012;124(3):529–533. doi:10.1016/j.ygyno.2011.11.003

435. Levenback CF, Ali S, Coleman RL, et al. Lymphatic mapping and sentinel lymph node biopsy in women with squamous cell carcinoma of the vulva: a gynecologic oncology group study. *J Clin Oncol.* 2012;30(31):3786–3791. doi:10.1200/JCO.2011.41.2528

436. Carlson JW, Kauderer J, Walker JL, et al. A randomized phase III trial of VH fibrin sealant to reduce lymphedema after inguinal lymph node dissection: a gynecologic oncology group study. *Gynecol Oncol.* 2008;110(1):76–82. doi:10.1016/j.ygyno.2008.03.005

437. DiSaia PJ, Creasman WT, Rich WM. An alternate approach to early cancer of the vulva. *Am J Obstet Gynecol.* 1979;133(7):825–832. doi:10.1016/0002-9378(79)90119-4

438. Van der Zee AGJ, Oonk MH, De Hullu JA, et al. Sentinel node dissection is safe in the treatment of early-stage vulvar cancer. *J Clin Oncol.* 2008;26(6):884–889. doi:10.1200/JCO.2007.14.0566

439. Te Grootenhuis NC, van der Zee AGJ, van Doorn HC, et al. Sentinel nodes in vulvar cancer: long-term follow-up of the groningen international study on sentinel nodes in vulvar cancer (GROINSS-V) I. *Gynecol Oncol.* 2016;140(1):8–14. doi:10.1016/j.ygyno.2015.09.077

440. Mahner S, Jueckstock J, Hilpert F, et al. Adjuvant therapy in lymph node-positive vulvar cancer: the AGO-care-1 study. *J Natl Cancer Inst.* 2015;107(3):dju426. doi:10.1093/jnci/dju426

441. Klapdor R, Wölber L, Hanker L, et al. Predictive factors for lymph node metastases in vulvar cancer. an analysis of the AGO-care-1 multicenter study. *Gynecol Oncol.* 2019;154(3):565–570. doi:10.1016/j.ygyno.2019.06.013

442. Gill BS, Bernard ME, Lin JF, et al. Impact of adjuvant chemotherapy with radiation for node-positive vulvar cancer: a national cancer data base (NCDB) analysis. *Gynecol Oncol.* 2015;137(3):365–372. doi:10.1016/j.ygyno.2015.03.056

443. Te Grootenhuis NC, Pouwer AW, de Bock GH. Gynecol oncol. 2019;154(2):266–275

444. Nooij LS, Ongkiehong PJ, van Zwet EW, et al. Groin surgery and risk of recurrence in lymph node positive patients with vulvar squamous cell carcinoma. *Gynecol Oncol.* 2015;139(3):458–464. doi:10.1016/j.ygyno.2015.09.081

445. Chapman PB, Hauschild A, Robert C, et al. Improved survival with vemurafenib in melanoma with BRAF V600E mutation. *N Engl J Med.* 2011;364(26):2507–2516. doi:10.1056/NEJMoa1103782

446. Ashmore S, Crafton SM, Miller EM, et al. Optimal overall treatment time for adjuvant therapy for women with completely resected, node-positive vulvar cancer. *Gynecol Oncol.* 2021;161(1):63–69. doi:10.1016/j.ygyno.2021.01.003

447. Larkin J, Chiarion-Sileni V, Gonzalez R, et al. Five-year survival with combined nivolumab and ipilimumab in advanced melanoma. *N Engl J Med.* 2019;381(16):1535–1546. doi:10.1056/NEJMoa1910836

448. Naumann RW, Hollebecque A, Meyer T, et al. Safety and efficacy of nivolumab monotherapy in recurrent or metastatic cervical, vaginal, or vulvar carcinoma: results from the phase I/II checkmate 358 trial. *J Clin Oncol.* 2019;37(31):2825–2834. doi:10.1200/JCO.19.00739

449. Cole LA, Muller CY. Hyperglycosylated hcg in the management of quiescent and chemorefractory gestational trophoblastic diseases. *Gynecol Oncol.* 2010;116(1):3–9. doi:10.1016/j.ygyno.2009.09.028

450. Cole LA, Laidler LL, Muller CY. USA hcg reference service, 10-year report. *Clin Biochem.* 2010;43(12):1013–1022. doi:10.1016/j.clinbiochem.2010.05.006

451. Lin LH, Maestá I, St Laurent JD, et al. Distinct microrna profiles for complete hydatidiform moles at risk of malignant progression. *Am J Obstet Gynecol.* 2021;224(4):372. doi:10.1016/j.ajog.2020.09.048

452. Pezeshki M, Hancock BW, Silcocks P, et al. The role of repeat uterine evacuation in the management of persistent gestational trophoblastic disease. *Gynecol Oncol.* 2004;95(3):423–429. doi:10.1016/j.ygyno.2004.08.045

453. Hemida R, Vos EL, El-Deek B, et al. Second uterine curettage and the number of chemotherapy courses in postmolar gestational trophoblastic neoplasia: a randomized controlled trial. *Obstet Gynecol.* 2019;133(5):1024–1031. doi:10.1097/AOG.0000000000003232

454. Brown J, Naumann RW, Seckl MJ, et al. 15years of progress in gestational trophoblastic disease: scoring, standardization, and salvage. *Gynecol Oncol.* 2017;144(1):200–207. doi:10.1016/j.ygyno.2016.08.330

455. Alifrangis C, Agarwal R, Short D, et al. EMA/CO for high-risk gestational trophoblastic neoplasia: good outcomes with induction low-dose etoposide-cisplatin and genetic analysis. *J Clin Oncol.* 2013;31(2):280–286. doi:10.1200/JCO.2012.43.1817

456. Polnaszek B, Mullen M, Bligard K, et al. Term pregnancy after complete response of placental site trophoblastic tumor to immunotherapy. *Obstet Gynecol.* 2021;138(1):115–118. doi:10.1097/AOG.0000000000004434

457. Curry SL, Schlaerth JB, Kohorn EI, et al. Hormonal contraception and trophoblastic sequelae after hydatidiform mole (a gynecologic oncology group study). *Am J Obstet Gynecol.* 1989;160(4):805–809. doi:10.1016/0002-9378(89)90295-0

458. Homesley HD, Blessing JA, Rettenmaier M, et al. Weekly intramuscular methotrexate for nonmetastatic gestational trophoblastic disease. *Obstet Gynecol.* 1988;72(3 Pt 1):413–418.

459. Homesley HD, Blessing JA, Schlaerth J, et al. Rapid escalation of weekly intramuscular methotrexate for nonmetastatic gestational trophoblastic disease: a gynecologic oncology group study. *Gynecol Oncol.* 1990;39(3):305–308. doi:10.1016/0090-8258(90)90257-I

460. Osborne RJ, Filiaci V, Schink JC, et al. Phase III trial of weekly methotrexate or pulsed dactinomycin for low-risk gestational trophoblastic neoplasia: a gynecologic oncology group study. *J Clin Oncol.* 2011;29(7):825–831. doi:10.1200/JCO.2010.30.4386

461. Osborne RJ, Filiaci VL, Schink JC, et al. Second curettage for low-risk nonmetastatic gestational trophoblastic neoplasia. *Obstet Gynecol.* 2016;128(3):535–542. doi:10.1097/AOG.0000000000001554

462. You B, Bolze P-A, Lotz J-P, et al. Avelumab in patients with gestational trophoblastic tumors with resistance to single-agent chemotherapy: cohort a of the TROPHIMMUN phase II trial. *J Clin Oncol.* 2020;38(27):3129–3137. doi:10.1200/JCO.20.00803

463. Albright BB, Shorter JM, Mastroyannis SA, et al. Gestational trophoblastic neoplasia after human chorionic gonadotropin normalization following molar pregnancy: a systematic review and meta-analysis. *Obstet Gynecol.* 2020;135(1):12–23. doi:10.1097/AOG.0000000000003566

464. Balachandran K, Salawu A, Ghorani E. A national analysis on over 4,000 patients. *Gynecol Oncol.* 2019;155(1):8–12.

465. Powell MA, Filiaci VL, Hensley ML, et al. Randomized phase III trial of paclitaxel and carboplatin versus paclitaxel and ifosfamide in patients with carcinosarcoma of the uterus or ovary: an NRG oncology trial. *J Clin Oncol.* 2022;40(9):968–977. doi:10.1200/JCO.21.02050

466. Schink JC, Filiaci V, Huang HQ, et al. An international randomized phase III trial of pulse actinomycin-D versus multi-day methotrexate for the treatment of low risk gestational trophoblastic neoplasia; NRG/GOG 275. *Gynecol Oncol.* 2020;158(2):354–360.

467. Van Der Kolk WL, Van der Zee AGJ, Slomovitz BM et al. Unilateral IF lymphadenectomy in patients with early stage vulvar squamous cell carcinoma and a unilateral metastatic sentinal LN is safe. *J Gyn Oncol*. 167, Dec 2022 3-10. doi.org/10.1016/j.ygyno.2022.07.017

468. Vergote I, du Bois A, Floquet A, et al. Overall survival results of AGO-OVAR16: A phase 3 study of maintenance pazopanib versus placebo in women who have not progressed after first-line chemotherapy for advanced ovarian cancer. *Gynecol Oncol*. 2019;155(2):186–191. doi:10.1016/j.ygyno.2019.08.024

469. Monk BJ, Parkinson C, Lim MC, et al. A Randomized, phase III trial to evaluate rucaparib monotherapy as maintenance treatment in patients with newly diagnosed ovarian cancer. *J Clin Oncol*. 2022;JCO2201003. doi:10.1200/JCO.22.01003

470. Coleman RL, Lorusso D, Oaknin A, et al. Clinical benefit of mirvetuximab soravtansine in ovarian cancer patients with high folate receptor alpha expression: results from the SORAYA study. Presented at: 2022 Annual Global Meeting of the International Gynecologic Cancer Society; New York, NY; September 29-October 1, 2022. Abstract O028.

471. Phelippeau J, Koskas M. Impact of Radical Hysterectomy on Survival in Patients with Stage 2 Type1 Endometrial Carcinoma: A Matched Cohort Study. *Ann Surg Oncol*. 2016;23(13):4361–4367. doi:10.1245/s10434-016-5372-3

3 Hereditary Cancer Syndromes

HEREDITARY CANCERS

- HBOC are attributed to genetic mutations, with up to 30% of ovarian cancers having an identified mutation. The most commonly known are *BRCA* mutations 1 and 2, which are found on chromosomes 17q21 and 13q12–13 for *BRCA1* and B*RCA2*, respectively. The *BRCA* gene is known to be a tumor suppressor gene and 80% of patients have a frameshift mutation—this causes a defect in DS DNA repair and E3 ubiquitination. Inheritance is autosomal dominant. Many of these mutations are found in the Fanconi anemia pathway.
- Hereditary cancers include mutations in the genes: *Rad50/51/51C/51D, BRIP1, BARD1, CHEK2, MRE11A, MSH2, MLH1, MSH6, PMS2, PPM1Df, POLE, POL-D1, PALB2, 17SNPs, NBN, PALB2, TP53.*[1]
- The lifetime risk of HGSTOC for *BRCA1* is 25% to 40% and for *BRCA2* is 18% to 27%. Penetrance ranges from 41% to 90%. In the Ashkenazi Jewish population the *BRCA* mutation risk is 1/40 compared to the general population risk: *BRCA1*: 1/300; *BRCA2*: 1/800. For patients who are found to harbor *BRCA1* mutations, BSO is recommended between the ages of 35 and 40 and *BRCA2* between 40 to 45, or when childbearing is completed. PFTC is seen in 2% to 17% of patients at the time of RRSO.
- The risk reduction for HGSTOC with RRSO is over 80% depending on age at time of surgery, but there is still an inherent risk of primary peritoneal cancer, possibly due to unrecognized STIC, which is 2% to 4.3%. OCPs administered for at least 6 Y can provide a 60% risk reduction for HGSTOC for *BRCA*-positive patients.[2]
- The presence of a *BRCA* mutation has been found to alter disease prognosis: The DFI after chemotherapy was 14 months for mutation carriers versus 7 months in sporadic cancer patients. The CR was found to be 3.2 times higher if the patient was *BRCA* positive. The OS was found to be 101 months in *BRCA* carriers versus 51 months in sporadic cancer patients. The age of onset for patients who are *BRCA1* positive was 52 Y.

- Oophorectomy may decrease the incidence of breast cancer for both *BRCA1* and *2* carriers. *BRCA*-positive women are recommended to undergo a BSO by age 40 or after childbearing is completed. *BRCA1* breast cancers are often ER negative and commonly are triple negative (ER, PR, HER2-neu negative). The risk of breast cancer decreased 56% in *BRCA1* patients who underwent a BSO, and decreased 46% in *BRCA2* patients. There was an increase in risk reduction from breast cancer the earlier the BSO was performed.[3]

- Patients who have *BRCA* mutations are categorized as "high risk." If these patients do not opt for surgical management, chemoprophylaxis with OCPs or bilateral salpingectomy, and delayed oophorectomy can be considered. Screening with every 6- to 12-month pelvic examinations, TVUS, and serum CA-125 levels has not proven beneficial.

- Adnexal neoplasia is found on average in 5% to 6% of RRSO (high-risk women). Recurrent/metastatic disease has been seen in up to 9% of women with STIC alone. The lag time from a diagnosis of STIC to invasive disease was 4 Y.[4]

- For those women who undergo RRSO, the SEE-FIM pathological protocol should be applied to the fallopian tubes. The tubes should be examined at 5 micrometer sections per 2-mm thick tissue block; as occult STIC may measure 1 mm or less.

- *Penetrance* refers to the likelihood that a person with a pathologic mutation (genotype) will phenotypically exhibit the disease, or the net risk in the absence of any competing risks.
  - For moderate and high-penetrance genes, refining of risk can be done by accounting for the influence of the gene or gene/environment interactions, and in a lot of cases the information from moderate penetrance genes does not change risk management compared to family history alone.
  - High penetrance is listed as >50% expressivity and moderate penetrance has 20% to 50% expressivity.
  - Pathologic/likely pathogenic LP genes are genetic mutations that have known associations with cancer syndromes.
  - As more genes are tested, there is a higher rate of finding VUS, mosaicism, and CHIP.
  - Tumor testing/somatic testing: Testing cancer cells directly to identify and target actionable genes as part of a tumor treatment protocol.
    - Germline confirmation should be performed when a pathogenic variant is found on tumor genomic testing.
    - Circulating cfDNA/tumor DNA can identify both somatic and germline variants with potentially actionable mutations for treatment.

- Somatic pathogenic/likely pathogenic variants seen in tumor specimens are common in *TP53, SK11,* and *PTEN* genes with germline implications and may not indicate the need for germline testing.
  - Polygenic risk scores should not be used for clinical management at this time.
  - The following genes are considered high penetrance: *BRCA 1/2, CDH1, PALB2, PTEN,* and *TP53.*

Genetic counseling and testing involve discussion, the process of seeking informed consent, testing, and interpretation of testing results; followed by discussion of risk-reducing measures and surgical referral if pathologic mutations are identified.

- Pretest evaluation:
  - Assess the patient's knowledge to include the risks, benefits, and limitations of testing, and to evaluate patient concerns.
  - Obtain a detailed family history up to third-degree relatives (pedigree).
  - Evaluate the pedigree to include the type of cancer, laterality, age at diagnosis, histology, pathology report confirmation, and family ethnicity.
  - Obtain personal medical and surgical history, reproductive history, contraceptive use, hormone use, history of carcinogen exposure (including radiation).
  - A physical exam.
  - Written informed consent should be obtained.
  - A plan for disclosure of results should be held to include a release of information if death or incapacitation happens before disclosure.
  - Discuss different management options if a mutation is identified; the cost of testing; risk of inheritance patterns to relatives; provision of current laws, privacy, and discrimination issues surrounding protection and privacy of genetic information.
  - This part of the intake should generate a differential diagnosis; educate the patient on patterns of inheritance, penetrance, variable expressivity, and genetic heterogeneity.
- Testing: Which test to order:
  - Single-gene testing: If a genetic syndrome is high in likelihood based on the pretest intake and the pedigree, the proband (if alive) should be tested first. This could identify the specific mutation for which to then screen others.
  - Panel testing: If the proband is not available for testing, then multigene testing/panel testing, based on next generation sequencing, should be ordered. Panel testing can evaluate for

pathogenic/LP variants in more than one cancer susceptibility gene, so multigene panels can be run on persons already known to carry a single pathogenic/LP germline variant.

- Cascade testing: when a pathogenic/LP variant is identified through multigene panel testing or full gene testing in the proband. Testing for only the identified pathogenic/LPV is then extended to at-risk relatives. Testing can be repeated as more affected persons or pathogenic variant carriers are identified.
- Commercial tests can differ in the classification of variants, methods of DNA/RNA analysis, and discrimination points for when to reflex from narrow to larger panels, as well as the specific genes they analyze.
- Posttest counseling:
  - Discussion of the test results and associated medical risks
  - Interpretation of these results in the context of individual and family cancer histories
  - Discussion of recommendations for management
  - Highlighting the importance of letting family members know when a mutation has been identified
  - Provide resources for testing those at risk, lead to a discussion of options for prenatal diagnosis and prenatal genetic screening (PGS), assisted reproductive technology (ART) preimplantation genetic testing, and should recommend carrier testing for the partner if the gene is autosomal recessive.
  - It is important not to recommend testing family members when a VUS is identified because VUS's are likely benign.
- Reasons why a negative result occurs:
  - The gene mutation may not yet be recognized by current technology.
  - The mutations that exist were not evaluated by the type of testing or gene sequences used.
  - The family member may carry a mutation that the patient may not have inherited.

  In general, testing is indicated:

- For individuals with any blood relative with a known pathogenic mutation or LPV in a cancer susceptibility gene
- Any individual who previously tested negative with limited testing analysis who is interested in pursuing multigene testing
- When a mutation is identified on somatic tumor testing, the mutation should be confirmed on germline cells
- To assist in systemic treatment and surgical decision-making
- In persons of Ashkenazi Jewish ancestry without additional risk factors
- Or with the following tumor syndromes:

Epithelial Ovarian Cancer

- Genetic testing for ovarian cancer is recommended for those with:
  - A personal history of EOC at any age
  - A family history of EOC: Only needed if a first- or second-degree relative had EOC at any age.
  - A family member with a probability >5% of a *BRCA1/2* pathogenic variant based on probability models

Breast Cancer

- If diagnosed with unilateral breast cancer, the cumulative risk for contralateral breast cancer by age 70 is 83% for *BRCA1* and 62% for *BRCA2*.
- Genetic testing for breast cancer is recommended for those with a:
  - breast cancer susceptibility genes *BRCA1/2, CDH1, PALB2, PTEN,* and *TP53* and can be done for persons with a:
    - Personal history of breast cancer:
      - If diagnosed before age 46
      - If diagnosed between ages 46– to 50 and have:
        - Unknown or limited family history
        - Multiple prior familial breast cancers with either metachronous or synchronous cancers in more than one relative with breast, ovarian, pancreatic, or prostate cancer at any age
      - If diagnosed at age 51 or older and
        - One or more relatives with any breast cancer ≤ 50
        - male breast cancer at any age
      - Diagnosed at any age:
        - To aid in systemic treatment decisions to use PARP inhibitors in the metastatic setting
        - To aid in adjuvant treatment decisions for Olaparib for high-risk HER2/neu breast cancer
        - In triple negative breast cancer
        - In lobular breast cancer with personal or family history of diffuse gastric cancer
        - One or more close blood relatives with male breast cancer
        - Ovarian cancer at any age
        - Pancreatic cancer at any age
        - Three or more total diagnoses of breast cancer in patient and/or close blood relatives
        - Two or more close blood relatives with either breast or prostate cancer at any age
    - Or by ancestry: Ashkenazi Jewish

If none of the preceding criteria are met, the average risk for harboring a high-penetrance gene is around 2.5%.

- Management of those with breast and ovarian cancer mutations:
  - Breast screening and risk reduction:
    - Physician examination
      - Breast awareness at age 18
      - Clinical breast exam every 6 to 12 months starting at age 25
    - Breast screening:
      - Age 25 to 29: annual breast MRI with contrast
      - Age 30 to 75: annual breast MRI with contrast and mammogram with contrast QO6m
      - Age >75: individual management
      - If history of breast cancer with lumpectomy/XRT, continue annual MRI or mammogram
    - Discuss option of risk-reducing mastectomy (RRM).
  - Ovarian/uterine screening:
    - No physical examination, US, or CA-125 testing has been proven useful for screening
    - RRSO between 35 to 40 or after completion of childbearing for *BRCA1*
    - RRSO between 40 to 45 or after completion of childbearing for *BRCA2*
    - Hysterectomy: There is a small risk (2.5%) of serous uterine cancer, so hysterectomy can be discussed. In addition, the need for progestin hormone becomes necessary therapy if estrogen replacement is elected for those with an intact uterus. The increased risk of breast cancer that accompanies progestin hormone therapy is compounded with the pathogenic variant genetic risk[5].
    - If the patient declines RRSO: OCP prophylaxis should be initiated. Salpingectomy alone is not the standard of care. The concern is that women are still at risk for developing ovarian cancer. In premenopausal women, oophorectomy reduces the risk of developing breast cancer by 60%. Interval salpingectomy followed by oophorectomy (a staged procedure) can be considered if patients are highly concerned about early surgical menopause.
    - Management of menopausal symptoms (try to not use hormonal therapies): selective serotonin reuptake inhibitors (SSRIs), clonidine, belladonna, and other therapies
- There was a 25% incidence that germline *BRCA1* and *2* mutations were identified when a histology-based referral specific to

high-grade serous ovarian subtypes was employed. This suggests the genetic assessment of all women diagnosed with HGSC will improve detection rates and capture mutation carriers otherwise missed by referral based on family history alone.[6]

- A 2.5% rate of *BRCA1* mutations was identified in uterine serous cancer patients and up to 16% of serous uterine cancers are HRD. This is compared to the 0.06% rate of *BRCA1* mutations in the general population. Nine percent of women with a history of breast cancer who also have USC, had a *BRCA1/2* mutation. Hysterectomy can be discussed in patients with *BRCA1* mutations although this is less than the accepted PPV.[7] The issue at hand would be HRT and the risk of progestins for breast cancer should the uterus be retained.

- Pregenetic screening, counseling, and testing can be offered to those considering children.

Heredity Nonpolyposis Colon Cancer/Lynch Syndrome

- **Characteristics:** HNPCC can contribute to about 10% of hereditary ovarian cancers. HNPCC is also called *Lynch II syndrome*. There is an increase in colon, endometrial, ovarian, pancreatic, CNS and urothelial cancers. The mutations responsible for these cancers are *MLH1, MSH2, MSH6, PMS1, PMS2,* and *EPCAM* genedeletion. These mutations cause defects in DNA mismatch repair mechanisms. 60% of patients present with colon cancer, and 60% present with endometrial cancer. Twenty percent to 30% of uterine cancers have *MLH1* silenced by non-inherited methylation of the *MLH1* promoter.

- The 2004 *HNPCC Bethesda Guidelines* were modified to include endometrial cancer as a sentinel cancer.

- *Bethesda Guidelines for LS:* This guides tumor testing for MSI in individuals with the following:
  - Diagnosed in a patient who is younger than 50 Y of age
  - Presence of synchronous, or metachronous, CRC or other LS-related tumors, regardless of age
  - CRC with IHC-deficient MSI histology diagnosed in a patient who is younger than 60 Y of age
  - CRC diagnosed in a patient with one or more first-degree relatives with an LS-related cancer with one of the cancers being diagnosed before age 50 Y
  - CRC diagnosed in a patient with two or more first- or second-degree relatives with LS-related cancers regardless of age.

- **Amsterdam Criteria I:** Must have at least three relatives with CRC; all of the following criteria should be present:
  - One should be a first-degree relative of the other two.
  - At least two successive generations must be affected.

- At least one of the relatives with CRC must have received the diagnosis before the age of 50.
- FAP should be excluded.
- Tumors should be verified by pathologic examination.
- **Amsterdam Criteria II**: Must have at least three relatives with a cancer associated with LS (colorectal, endometrial, small bowel, ureter, or renal-pelvis); all of the following criteria should be present:
  - One must be a first-degree relative of the other two.
  - At least two successive generations must be affected.
  - At least one relative with cancer associated with LS should be diagnosed before age 50.
  - FAP should be excluded in the CRC case(s; if any).
  - Tumors should be pathologically verified whenever possible.
- Patients should be screened for LS/HNPCC if:
  - They have an endometrial or ovarian cancer and have a synchronous or metachronous colon or other LS/HNPCC-associated tumors at any age to include stomach, ovarian, pancreas, ureter, renal pelvis, biliary tract, brain glioblastoma as seen in Turcot syndrome, sebaceous gland adenomas and keratoacanthomas in Muir-Torre syndrome, and carcinoma of the small bowel.
  - They have CRC with TIL, peritumoral lymphocytes, Crohn-like lymphocytic reaction, mucinous/signet-ring differentiation, or medullary growth pattern diagnosed before the age of 60.
  - They have endometrial or CRC and a first-degree relative with a LS/HNPCC-associated tumor diagnosed before the age of 50.
  - They have colorectal or endometrial cancer diagnosed at any age with two or more first- or second-degree relatives with LS/HNPCC-associated tumors regardless of age.
- Genetic testing is for the gene mutations of *MLH1, MSH2, MSH6, PMS1, PMS2,* and *EPCAM* gene deletion if a familial defective gene has not been identified. IHC can be a first-line approach on the pathological specimen and provide baseline mutation information on the tumor itself.
- Screening tests and risk reduction usually start around age 25. Screening can be divided by the type of mutation carried if identified.
  - *MLH1, MSH2,* and *EPCAM* mutation carriers:
    - Colonoscopy should start between ages 20 and 25 old, or 2 to 5 Y prior to the earliest diagnosed proband. Screening should occur every 1 to 2 Y.
    - Prophylactic hysterectomy with BSO is a risk-reducing option in women. Annual EMB beginning at age 30 to 35 is recommended for those not having completed childbearing. Any

abnormal uterine bleeding should be investigated. Progestin-based contraception should be used to decrease malignant transformation of reproductive organs.

- Consider prophylactic total colectomy as an alternative to surveillance colonoscopy for individuals with confirmed mutations. Because of incomplete penetrance, 15% to 20% of these procedures may be unnecessary, but this risk reduction option can be discussed.
- There are no data to support annual ovarian US and serum CA-125.
- EGD with extended duodenoscopy should be considered every 2 to 3 Y beginning at age 30 to 35 Y.
- UA with cytology should start at age 25 to 30 and continue annually.
- A CNS annual physical examination should also start at age 25 to 30, but no imaging recommendations have been made.
  - ○ *MSH6* and *PMS2* carriers:
    - Colonoscopy at age 25 to 30 or 2 to 5 Y prior to the earliest proband colon cancer if diagnosed before age 30, and repeat every 1 to 2 Y.
    - Endometrial and ovarian cancer surveillance is the same as for *MLH1*, *MSH2*, and *EPCAM* mutation carriers.
- Pregenetic screening counseling and testing should be offered for those considering children.

Li-Fraumeni Syndrome

- **Characteristics:** Li-Fraumeni syndrome occurs in individuals with a mutation in the gene *TP53*. Tumors in the Li-Fraumeni syndrome spectrum include soft- tissue sarcoma, osteosarcoma, brain tumor, breast cancer, adrenocortical carcinoma, leukemia, and lung bronchoalveolar cancer. There are two sets of criteria for inclusion:
  - ○ Classic criteria: include the combination of an individual diagnosed at age <45 with cancer sarcoma, and a first- or second-degree relative diagnosed at age less than 45 with cancer, and an additional first- or second-degree relative with cancer diagnosed at age <45 or a sarcoma diagnosed at any age.
  - ○ Chompret criteria includes an individual diagnosed with a tumor from the Li-Fraumeni syndrome tumor spectrum before age 46 and:
    - At least one first- or second-degree relative with any of the aforementioned cancers (other than breast cancer if the proband had breast cancer) before the age of 56 or with multiple primaries at any age, or
    - An individual with multiple tumors (except multiple breast tumors), two of which belong to the Li-Fraumeni syndrome tumor spectrum with, the initial cancer occurring before age 46, or

- An individual with adrenocortical carcinoma or choroid plexus carcinoma at any age of onset regardless of the family history
- Early-age (≤31) onset of breast cancer
- Genetic testing should be offered to anyone from a family with a known TP53 pathogenic/likely pathogenic variant (LPV)
- **Screening and risk reduction**: if a *TP53* mutation is identified:
  - Breast cancer screening to follow the same as HBOC patients
    - Breast awareness at age 18
    - Clinical breast exam every 6 to 12 months starting at age 20
  - Breast screening:
    - Age 20 to 29: annual breast MRI with contrast
    - Age 30 to 75: annual breast MRI with contrast and mammogram QO6 months
    - Age >75: individual management
  - Other cancer risks:
    - Alert pediatricians of the risk of childhood cancers in affected families.
    - Annual comprehensive physical exam to include neurologic exam.
    - Avoid therapeutic XRT when possible.
    - Physical exam every 6 to 12 months.
    - Colonoscopy and EGD every 2 to 5 Y starting at age 25.
    - Annual dermatologic exam, beginning at age 18.
    - Annual whole-body MRI.
    - Annual brain MRI.
    - Pregenetic screening counseling and testing suggested for patients considering children.

Cowden Syndrome/PTEN Harmatoma Syndrome

- The genetic mutation for this disease is in the *PTEN* gene. There are familial mutations. If the known familial mutation is not identified, then comprehensive *PTEN* testing of the patient, or, the family member with the highest likelihood of a mutation can be performed. Consideration of multigene testing, if appropriate, can be done.
- **Characteristics:** The lifetime risk for cancer in Cowden Syndrome/PTEN Harmatoma Syndrome (CS/PHTS) varies by site.
  - Breast cancer: The risk is 25% to 50% at age 38 to 50
  - Thyroid cancer: The risk is 30% to 68%.
  - The cumulative lifetime estimate for any cancer is 89%.
- Criteria for testing:
  - From a family with a known *PTEN* pathogenic/LPV
  - A personal history of Bannayan-Riley-Ruvaicaba syndrome (BRRS)

- ○ An individual meeting clinical diagnostic criteria for CS/PHTS
- ○ Individual not meeting clinical diagnostic criteria for CS/PHTS with a personal history of:
  - Adult Lhermitte-Duclos disease (cerebellar tumors) or
  - Autism spectrum disorder and macrocephaly or
  - Two or more biopsy proven trichilemmomas or
  - Two or more major criteria (one must be macrocephaly) or
  - Three major criteria without macrocephaly or
  - One major and ≥ three minor criteria or
  - Four or more minor criteria
- ○ At-risk individuals with a relative with a clinical diagnosis of CS/PHTS or BRRS for whom testing has not been performed. The at-risk individual must have:
  - Any one major criteria or
  - Two minor criteria
- ○ *PTEN* pathogenic/LPV mutation detected by tumor profiling/somatic testing on any tumor type in the absence of germline analysis
- ○ Major criteria: breast cancer, endometrial cancer, follicular thyroid cancer, multiple GI hamartomas or ganglioneuromas, macrocephaly, mucocutaneous lesions (one biopsy proven) trichilemmoma, multiple palmoplantar keratoses, multifocal or extensive oral mucosal papillomatosis, multiple cutaneous facial papules (often verrucous)
- ○ Minor criteria: autism spectrum disorder, colon cancer, more than three esophageal glycogenic acanthoses, lipomas, intellectual disability (IQ <75), papillary or follicular variant of papillary thyroid cancer, thyroid structural lesions (adenoma/nodules/goiter, renal cell carcinoma, single GI hamartoma or ganglioneuromas, vascular anomalies (Table 3.1)
- Screening and risk reduction:
  - ○ Annual physical exam starting at age 18
  - ○ Breast cancer:
    - Breast awareness at age 18
    - Clinical breast exam every 6 to 12 months starting at age 25 or 5 to 10 Y earlier than first known familial breast cancer
    - Breast screening: Annual mammography and breast MRI with contrast QO 6 months
    - Age >75: Individualized screening
    - If patient has had cancer and is status post lumpectomy/XRT: annual mammogram and breast MRI should continue QO 6 months

Table 3.1 Major and Minor Criteria for Cowden's Syndrome

Major Criteria	Minor Criteria
Breast cancer	Autism spectrum disorder
Endometrial cancer	Colon cancer
Follicular thyroid cancer	Esophageal glycogenic acanthoses (≥3)
Multiple GI hamartomas or ganglioneuromas	Lipomas (≥3)
Macrocephaly (i.e., >97% or 58 cm in adult women)	Intellectual disability (i.e., IQ ≤75)
Mucocutaneous lesions	Thyroid structural lesions (adenoma, nodules, goiter)
Multiple trichilemmomas (≥3, with one biopsy proven)	Papillary or follicular variant of papillary thyroid cancer
Multiple (≥3) acral/palmoplantar keratosis, pits, or papules Mucocutaneous neuromas (≥3)	Renal cell carcinoma
Multifocal or extensive oral mucosal papillomatosis (≥3) or biopsy proven or dermatologist diagnosed	Single GI hamartoma or ganglioneuroma
Multiple cutaneous facial papules (often verrucous)	Vascular anomalies

- ▪ Risk-reducing mastectomy
  - ○ Uterine cancer:
    - ▪ EMB should any abnormal bleeding occur.
    - ▪ Risk-reducing hysterectomy after childbearing
    - ▪ US or EMB have no proven benefit.
  - ○ Colon: Colonoscopy starting at age 35 and every 5Y thereafter
  - ○ Kidney: Renal US at age 40 then every 1 to 2Y
  - ○ Neurology: Brain MRI if any symptoms
  - ○ Skin: There is a higher risk of melanoma: annual dermatology exam.
  - ○ Thyroid: Annual thyroid US starting at age 7
- • Pregenetic screening counseling and testing can be offered to for those interested children.

Peutz Jeghers Syndrome

- • Characteristics of Peutz Jeghers Syndrome (PJS) are breast cancer, ovarian cancer (with sex cord tumors the most common), colon cancer, and hamartomatous polyps of the intestine and lips.

- A clinical diagnosis of PJS can be made when an individual has two or more of the following features:
  - Two or more PJ-type hamartomatous polyps of the small intestine
  - Mucocutaneous hyperpigmentation of the mouth, lips, nose, eyes, genitalia, or fingers
  - Family history of PJS
- The *STK11/LKB1* is the main gene mutation.
- Screening and risk reduction:
  - Breast cancer: There is a 45% to 50% lifetime risk. Mammogram and annual breast MRI with contrast with clinical breast exam is recommended QO 6 months starting at age 25.
  - Colon cancer: There is a 39% lifetime risk and colonoscopy every 2 to 3 Y is recommended starting in the late teens.
  - Stomach cancer: There is a 29% lifetime risk. EGD is recommended every 2 to 3 Y beginning in the late teens.
  - Small intestine cancer: There is a 13% lifetime risk. Small bowel visualization with CT or MRI enterography is needed. A baseline test should be obtained at 8 to 10 Y old with follow-up interval based on findings but at least by age 18, then every 2 to 3 Y, or with symptoms.
  - Pancreatic cancer: There is an 11% to 36% lifetime risk. Magnetic resonance cholangiopancreatography or endoscopic US should be obtained every 1 to 2 Y starting at age 30 to 35.
  - Gynecologic cancers: Pelvic examination and HPV/Pap smears can be performed annually starting around age 18 to 20.
    - Ovary: There is an 18% to 21% lifetime risk (sex cord tumors).
    - Cervix: There is a 10% lifetime risk (adenoma malignum).
    - Uterus: There is a 9% lifetime risk.
  - Lung: There is a 15% to 17% lifetime risk. Education about symptoms and smoking cessation should be provided. No other specific recommendations have been made.
  - Pregenetic screening, counseling, and testing can be offered to those considering children.

Effectiveness of Screening and Risk-Reduction Recommendations

- MRI:
  - MRI is recommended if there is greater than 20% risk of breast cancer with any identified gene mutations or genetic syndromes.
  - The sensitivity of MRI is 77% to 94%, compared to the 33% to 65% sensitivity of mammography in the detection of breast cancer.

- Risk-reducing surgery:
  - Risk-reducing mastectomy: Decreases risk by 90%.
  - RRBSO: an 80% reduction in ovarian cancer; reduces breast cancer risk by 50%—the younger the age at which a woman has a BSO, the lower the rates of breast cancer.
- Chemoprevention:
  - Tamoxifen: *BRCA+* women with breast cancer have a 40% chance of contralateral breast cancer at 10 Y. Tamoxifen has been shown to be protective with OR = 0.38 to 0.5 for *BRCA1* mutation carriers and 0.42 to 0.63 for *BRCA2* mutation carriers.
  - OCP use: The EOC risk reduction for *BRCA1* carriers was 45% to 50% and was 60% for *BRCA2* carriers.
- Specific Genes and Risks for Associated Tumor Syndromes
  - ATM gene:
    - Tumor syndrome: EOC
      - Risk: Absolute risk <3%
      - Management: Insufficient evidence for RRSO; manage based on family history.
    - Tumor syndrome: Breast cancer
      - Risk: Absolute risk 15% to 40%
      - Management: Insufficient evidence exists for RRM, instead manage based on family history.
    - Screening requires an annual mammogram and consider MRI with contrast starting at age 40.
  - *BARD1* gene:
    - Tumor syndrome: EOC
      - Risk: There is no established association for increased risk.
    - Tumor syndrome: Breast cancer
      - Risk: Absolute risk is 15% to 40%.
      - Management: Insufficient evidence for RRM, instead manage based on family history.
      - Screening: Annual mammogram needed and consider breast MRI starting at age 40.
  - *BRCA1 (FANCS)* gene:
    - Tumor syndrome: EOC
      - Absolute risk: 39% to 58%
      - Management: RRSO, OCPs
    - Tumor syndrome: Breast cancer
      - Absolute risk: >60%
      - Management: RRM
      - Very strong association with predisposition to triple-negative disease

- *BRCA2 (FANC<u>D</u>) gene:*
  - Tumor syndrome: EOC
    - Absolute risk: 13% to 29%
    - Management: RRSO, OCPs
  - Tumor syndrome: Breast cancer
    - Absolute risk: >60%.
    - Management: RRM
    - Very strong association with predisposition to ER+ disease
- *PALB2 (FANC<u>N</u>) gene:*
  - Tumor syndrome: EOC
    - Absolute risk: 3% to 5%.
    - Management: Insufficient evidence to recommend RRSO
  - Tumor syndrome: Breast cancer
    - Absolute risk: 41% to 60%
    - Management: Begin mammogram and breast MRI screening starting at age 30Y; consider RRM.
- *RAD51C (FANC<u>O</u>) gene:*
  - Tumor syndrome: EOC
    - Absolute risk: >10%
    - Management: Consider RRSO between 45 to 50Y, OCP.
  - Tumor syndrome: Breast cancer
    - Absolute risk: 15% to 40%
    - Management: Insufficient data
    - Predisposition to ER/PR negative breast cancer
- *RAD51D gene:*
  - Tumor syndrome: EOC
    - Absolute risk: >10%
    - Management: Consider RRSO between 45 to 50Y, OCP.
  - Tumor syndrome: Breast cancer
    - Absolute risk: 15% to 40%
    - Management: Insufficient evidence
    - Predisposition for ER/PR negative breast cancer
- *BRIP1 (FANC<u>J</u>) gene:*
  - Tumor syndrome: EOC
    - Absolute risk: >10%
    - Management: Consider RRSO between 45 to 50Y, OCP.
  - Tumor syndrome: Breast cancer
    - Absolute risk: >10%
    - Management:

- □ Breast: Insufficient evidence, instead manage based on family history.
- ○ *TP53* gene:
  - Tumor syndrome: EOC
    - □ Absolute risk: No established association
  - Tumor syndrome: Breast cancer
    - □ Absolute risk: >60%
    - □ Management: Same as LFS
    - □ Predisposition to triple-positive breast cancer
- ○ *PTEN* gene:
  - Tumor syndrome: EOC
    - □ Absolute risk: No established association
  - Tumor Syndrome: Breast cancer
    - □ Absolute risk: 40% to 60%
    - □ Management: See Cowden Syndrome management.
    - □ Predisposition to luminal subtype of breast cancer
- ○ *STK11* gene:
  - Tumor syndrome: EOC
    - □ Absolute risk: No established association
  - Tumor syndrome: Nonepithelial ovarian cancer (sex cord with annual tubules)
    - □ Absolute risk: >10%
    - □ Management: Insufficient evidence for RRSO; screening as per PJS.
  - Tumor syndrome: Breast cancer
    - □ Absolute risk: 40% to 60%.
    - □ Management: As per PJS
- ○ *CDH1* gene:
  - Tumor syndrome: EOC
    - □ Absolute risk: No established association
  - Tumor syndrome: Breast cancer
    - □ Absolute risk: 41% to 60%
    - □ Management: Annual mammogram and consider breast MRI starting at age 30; discuss RRM.
  - Gastric cancer association
- ○ *CDKN2A* gene:
  - Tumor syndrome: EOC
    - □ Absolute risk: No established association

- Tumor syndrome: Breast cancer
  - Absolute risk: No established association
- Tumor syndrome: Melanoma
  - Absolute risk: 28% to 76%
  - Management: annual full-body skin examination and minimize UV exposure.
- *CHEK2* gene:
  - Tumor syndrome: EOC
    - Absolute risk: No established association
  - Tumor syndrome: Breast cancer
    - Absolute risk: 15% to 40%
    - Management: annual mammogram and consider breast MRI starting at age 40.
    - Predisposition to ER+ breast cancer
- *MLH1/MSK2* genes:
  - Tumor syndrome: EOC
    - Absolute risk: >10%
    - Management: Consider RRSO with hysterectomy.
  - Tumor syndrome: Uterine cancer
    - Absolute risk: 60%
    - Management: Consider RR hysterectomy with BSO.
  - Tumor syndrome: Breast cancer
    - Absolute risk: <15%
    - Management: Screen with annual mammogram and consider breast MRI starting at age 40.
  - Tumor syndrome: Colon cancer
    - Absolute risk: 60%
    - Management: Consider RR colectomy and screening colonoscopy starting age 35.
- *MSH6* gene:
  - EOC absolute risk: <13%
  - Breast cancer absolute risk: <15%
- *PMS2* gene:
  - Tumor syndrome: EOC: Absolute risk <3%
  - Tumor syndrome: Breast cancer: Absolute risk <15%
- *EPCAM* gene:
  - Tumor syndrome: EOC: Absolute risk <10%
  - Tumor syndrome: Breast cancer: Absolute risk <15%
- Neurofibromatosis-1:
  - Tumor syndrome: EOC: No established association

○ Tumor syndrome: Breast cancer: Absolute risk 15% to40%
  ▪ Management: Annual mammogram at 30 Y; consider MRI ages 30 to 50; insufficient evidence for RRM.

REFERENCES

1 Walsh T, Casadei S, Lee MK, et al. Mutations in 12 genes for inherited ovarian, fallopian tube, and peritoneal carcinoma identified by massively parallel sequencing. *Proc Natl Acad Sci U S A.* 2011;108(44):18032–18037. doi: 10.1073/pnas.1115052108

2 Narod SA, Risch H, Moslehi R, et al. Oral contraceptives and the risk of hereditary ovarian cancer. *N Engl J Med.* 1998;339(7):424–428. doi: 10.1056/NEJM199808133390702

3 Eisen A, Lubinski J, Klijn J, et al. Breast cancer risk following bilateral oophorectomy in BRCA1 and BRCA2 mutation carriers: an international case-control study. *J Clin Oncol.* 2005;23(30):7491–7496. doi: 10.1200/JCO.2004.00.7138

4 Conner JR, Meserve E, Pizer E, et al. Outcome of unexpected adnexal neoplasia discovered during risk reduction salpingo-oophorectomy in women with germ-line BRCA1 or BRCA2 mutations. *Gynecol Oncol.* 2014;132(2):280–286. doi: 10.1016/j.ygyno.2013.12.009

5 Chlebowski RT, Rohan TE, Manson JE, et al. Breast cancer after use of estrogen plus progestin and estrogen alone: analyses of data from 2 women's health initiative randomized clinical trials. *JAMA Oncol.* 2015;1(3):296–305. doi: 10.1001/jamaoncol.2015.0494

6 Schrader KA, Hurlburt J, Kalloger SE, et al. Germline BRCA1 and BRCA2 mutations in ovarian cancer: utility of a histology-based referral strategy. *Obstet Gynecol.* 2012;120(2 Pt 1):235–240. doi: 10.1097/AOG.0b013e31825f3576

7 Pennington KP, Walsh T, Lee M, et al. BRCA1, TP53, and CHEK2 germline mutations in uterine serous carcinoma. *Cancer.* 2013;119(2):332–338. doi: 10.1002/cncr.27720

4 Surgical Care for Gynecologic Cancers

ANATOMY

Layers of the Abdomen

Layers of the abdomen (from superficial to deep): skin, Camper's fascia, Scarpa's fascia, deep fascia (composed of the aponeuroses of the external oblique, internal oblique, and transversus muscles). The transversalis fascia lies below the transversus muscle. Superior to the arcuate line, the internal oblique aponeurosis splits to envelop the rectus abdominis muscle. Inferior to the arcuate line, the internal oblique and transversus abdominis aponeuroses merge and pass superficially (i.e., anteriorly) to the rectus muscle (Figure 4.1).

Ligaments

- Infundibulopelvic: Contains ovarian vessels and nerves.
- Round: Originates from the uterine cornua, passes through the inguinal ring, the inguinal canal, and inserts into the labia majora. The male counterpart to this ligament is the gubernaculum testis. A small evagination of peritoneum (canal of Nuck) accompanies the round ligament through the inguinal ring.
- Utero-ovarian: These contain the utero-ovarian vessels between the ovary and the uterus. They represent the proximal portion of the gubernaculum testis.
- Cardinal (Mackenrodt's ligaments): Located laterally to the cervix, they originate from thickening of the endopelvic fascia. They are the main support for pelvic organs.
- Uterosacral: Located posterior to the cervix, they originate from thickening of the endopelvic fascia. They insert on the anterior surface of S2 to S4.

Vasculature

- Ovarian vessels: These travel through the infundibulopelvic ligaments. The ovarian arteries arise from the abdominal aorta, below

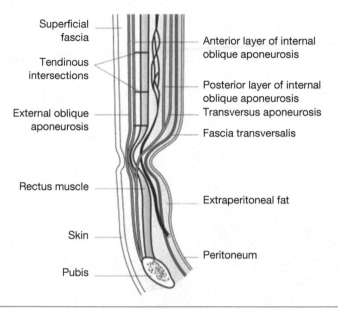

Figure 4.1 The layers of the anterior abdominal wall in transverse section.

Source: From Farthing A. Clinical anatomy of the pelvis and reproductive tract. In: Edmonds DK, ed. *Dewhurst's Textbook of Obstetrics & Gynaecology*, 8th ed. Wiley-Blackwell; 2012.

the renal arteries. The left ovarian vein drains to the left renal vein. The right ovarian vein drains to the IVC (Figure 4.2).

- Artery of Sampson: This travels through the round ligament.
- External iliac artery and vein: These become the femoral vessels after they pass under the inguinal ligament. There are two branches of the external iliac artery and vein: the deep circumflex iliac and the inferior epigastric.
- The internal iliac artery and vein are also known as the *hypogastric* vessels.
  - Branches of the internal iliac artery:
    - Posterior division: Iliolumbar, lateral sacral (superior and inferior), superior gluteal
    - Anterior division: Inferior gluteal, internal pudendal, obturator, middle rectal, uterine, vaginal, inferior vesical, superior vesical, obliterated umbilical
- Branches of the celiac trunk: Left gastric, common hepatic (branches: right gastric, gastroduodenal), splenic
- Omental blood supply: Right and left gastroepiploics, from the gastro-duodenal and splenic vessels, respectively
- Short gastric arteries originate from the splenic artery.

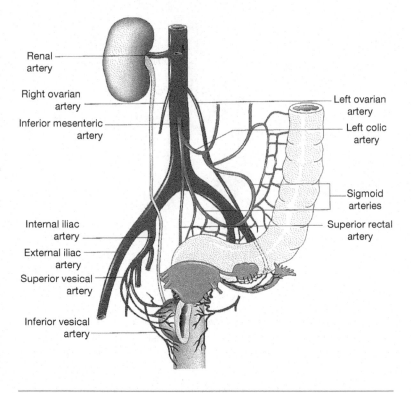

Figure 4.2 Abdomino-pelvic arterial distributions.

Source: From Holschneider CH, et al. Cytoreductive surgery: pelvis and radical oophorectomy. In: Bristow RE, et al., eds. *Surgery for Ovarian Cancer,* 3rd ed. Taylor & Francis Group; 2016.

- Marginal artery of Drummond: Collateral blood supply for the large bowel
- Blood supply the to bowel is from two main arteries, the SMA and IMA.
  - SMA supplies the:
    - Small bowel
    - Right colon: right colic and ileocolic arteries, which are branches of the SMA
    - Appendix: Ileocolic branch of the SMA
    - Transverse colon: Middle colic branch of the SMA
  - IMA supplies the:
    - Descending colon: Left colic branch of the IMA
    - Sigmoid colon and rectum: Sigmoid arteries, superior hemorrhoidal artery branches of the IMA

Nerves

The following nerves are composed of contributing spinal nerve roots:

- Brachial plexus: C5, C6, C7, C8, and T1
  - Injury can cause paresthesias of the radial, ulnar, or median nerves.
  - Etiology of injury is from traction on the extended arm or neck.
- Genitofemoral nerve: L1 and L2
  - This arises on the medial border of the psoas muscle. It is a sensory nerve to the medial thigh, and provides motor innervation to the cremaster muscle.
  - Injury can cause paresthesia or anesthesia of the labia or skin of the superior thigh.
  - Etiology of injury is transection or traction of the nerve along the psoas muscle.
- Ilioinguinal nerve: L1
  - This arises on the anterior abdominal wall between the internal oblique and transversus abdominis muscles. It supplies the skin over the pubic symphysis.
  - Injury can cause paresthesia or anesthesia of the lower abdomen.
  - Etiology of injury is commonly from scar fibrosis.
- Lateral femoral cutaneous nerve: L2 and L3
  - Injury can cause paresthesia or anesthesia to the anterior and lateral thigh.
- Femoral nerve: L2, L3, L4
  - Injury can cause paresthesia or anesthesia to the anterior and medial thigh, groin pain, weakness of knee extension, and thigh flexion.
  - Etiology of injury is often from retractor placement, stirrup positioning, or tumor invasion.
- Obturator nerve: L2, L3, L4
  - This emerges from the medial border of the psoas muscle and traverses the obturator space.
  - Injury can cause sensory loss to the upper and medial thigh, and weakness in hip adductors.
  - Etiology of injury is commonly transection during LND.
- Accessory obturator nerve: L3 and L4
  - This is present in 5% to 30% of patients.
- Internal pudendal nerve: S1, S2, and S3
  - Injury can cause sensory loss to the labia.
- Sciatic nerve: L5 and S1
  - Injury can cause paresthesias of the posterior leg skin and hamstring areas and difficulty with knee flexion.

   ○ Etiology of injury is from stretch injury from poor stirrup positioning.
- Common peroneal nerve: L4, L5, S1, S2
   ○ Foot drop is a symptom.
   ○ Etiology of injury is usually from poor stirrup positioning.
- Autonomic nerves
   ○ Symptoms are large bowel dysfunction and urinary retention.
   ○ Etiology of injury is from radical pelvic surgery or tumor invasion of the autonomic plexus.

Vulvar and Groin Anatomy

- The anatomical boundaries of the groin form the femoral triangle. This is bounded superiorly by the inguinal ligament, the sartorius muscle laterally to medially, and the adductor longus muscle medially to laterally. The base of the triangle consists of the iliacus, iliopsoas, and pectineus muscles, laterally to medially (Figure 4.3).
- Through the triangle run the femoral nerve and three other smaller nerves. The femoral nerve consists of the anterior femoral cutaneous branch and the medial femoral cutaneous branches from the L1, L2, and L3 nerve roots. The lateral femoral cutaneous nerve runs on top of the iliopsoas muscle and originates from L1. The genital–femoral nerve runs medial to the psoas muscle in the abdomen and originates from the L1 and L2 nerve roots. The

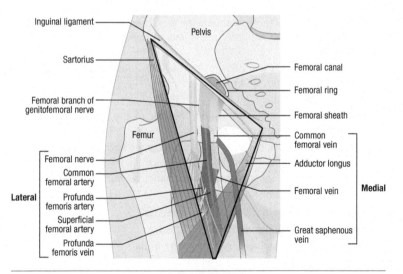

Figure 4.3 Femoral triangle.

ilioinguinal nerve also runs through the triangle and originates in the L1 root.

- Innervation to the vulva is from branches of the genitofemoral nerve and the perineal branch of the posterior femoral cutaneous nerve (a branch of the femoral nerve). The internal pudendal nerve also provides innervation to the vulva.

- The femoral artery gives off branches to form the superficial circumflex, the external pudendal, and the superficial epigastric arteries. The femoral vein receives branches from the superficial circumflex, external pudendal, and superficial epigastric veins. These enter the femoral vein near the saphenous vein, or sometimes drain into the saphenous vein prior to entry into the femoral vein.

- The lymphatics drain first into the superficial inguinal LNs. Around the clitoris and prepuce, the LNs may drain directly into the deep inguinal LNs or the pelvic LN, but this has little clinical relevance. The superficial inguinal LNs lie around the branches of the femoral vein. The deep inguinal LNs lie medial to the femoral vein beneath the cribriform fascia. The most superior deep inguinal node is Cloquet's node, which is medial to the femoral vein. Jackson's node is the most distal of the external iliac nodes; thus, Jackson's node is first exiting the pelvic LNs and last entering from the groin route.

- The blood supply to the vulva is not anomalous. The internal pudendal artery (a branch of the anterior division of the internal iliac) divides to form the perineal, clitoral, and inferior rectal arteries. The SEPA (a branch of the common femoral) supplies the lower abdominal wall, pubis, and labia majora. The deep external pudendal (a branch of the common femoral) supplies the labial fat pad. The veins commonly follow arteries except that the superficial epigastric and superficial and deep external pudendal arteries drain into or near the saphenous and may not drain directly into the femoral vein.

Lymph Nodes

- LN basins should be sentineled/sampled/completely dissected in most gynecologic cancer-staging surgeries.
- The node basins for uterine and cervical cancers:
  - Pelvic to include: External and internal iliac and obturator spaces to the mid-common iliac
  - PA: From the mid-common iliac to the IMA and higher to the renal vessels.
- The node basins for vulvar cancer:
  - Inguinal–femoral groin LNs in the femoral triangle
- The node basins for tubo-ovarian cancers:
  - Pelvic to include: External and internal iliac and obturator spaces up to the mid-common iliac
  - PA: From the mid-common iliac to the renal vessels

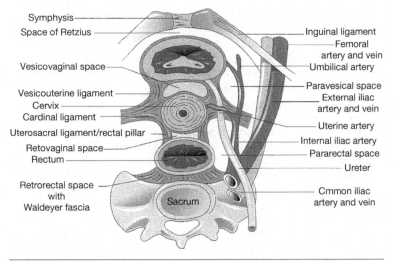

Figure 4.4 Eight potential spaces of the pelvis: retropubic space of Retzius, right and left paravesical spaces, vesicovaginal space, right and left pararectal spaces, rectovaginal space, and presacral space.

Source: From Holschneider CH, et al. Cytoreductive surgery: pelvis and radical oophorectomy. In: Bristow RE, et al., eds. *Surgery for Ovarian Cancer, Third Edition.* Taylor & Francis Group; 2016.

Potential Spaces in the Pelvis

There are eight potential spaces in the pelvis: the space of Retzius, the right and left paravesical spaces, the vesicovaginal space, the right and left pararectal spaces, the rectovaginal space, and the presacral space. These potential spaces are avascular and contain loose areolar or fatty connective tissue and can be developed to aid surgical dissection (Figure 4.4).

PREOPERATIVE RISK ASSESSMENT AND OPTIMIZATION

Recommended Laboratories

Recommended laboratory tests include CBC, PTT, PT, CMP, and LFTs. Other recommended studies include an EKG, a CXR, and pelvic imaging as appropriate. Further workup depends on patient medical history and physical findings.

Bowel Preparation

- The administration of a preoperative bowel preparation is debatable. The pros include easy palpation of the entire colon, improved exposure, a decrease in operative time due to easier handling, and the removal of solid material from the GI tract. The cons include more anastomotic leaks from liquid stool, more sepsis due to trauma from the prep, and nonsignificant differences in operative times or facilitated exposure.

- There are a number of different preparations: PEG can be given in 4 L, magnesium citrate can be given in 300-mL bottles × 2 with or without a Dulcolax suppository, as well as using antibiotic preparations. Antibiotic preparations include erythromycin base 1 g and neomycin 1 g; each given by mouth at 1, 2, and 10 p.m. the day before surgery. The erythromycin is given for both its antibiotic and its stimulant mechanisms of action. Another option is metronidazole 1 g and neomycin 1 g by mouth given at 1, 2, and 10 p.m. the day before surgery.

  o A meta-analysis of bowel preparation and outcomes was reviewed in elective colorectal surgery for effect of type of bowel preparation on anastomotic leak, SSI, and ileus. Three arms were reviewed to include preoperative MBP and antibiotics (MBP+/ABX+), MBP alone (MBP+/ABX−), and no bowel preparation (no-prep). In the study, 8,442 patients were evaluated. Twenty-seven percent were given no bowel preparation, 45.3% were given a MBP without antibiotics (MBP+/ABX−), and 27.5% were given MBP with oral antibiotics (MBP+/ABX+). Patients in the MBP+/ABX+ or MBP+/ABX− had reduced ileus [MBP+/ABX+: OR = 0.57, 95% CI: 0.48–0.68; MBP+/ABX−: OR = 0.78, 95% CI: 0.68–0.91] as well as SSI [MBP+/ABX+: OR = 0.39, 95% CI: 0.32–0.48; MBP+/ABX−: OR = 0.80, 95% CI: .69–0.93] compared to no prep. There was also a lower association with anastomotic leak for the MBP+/ABX− group compared to no prep. On multivariate analysis, the addition of antibiotics to MBP was associated with reduced anastomotic leak rates (OR = 0.57, 95% CI: 0.35–0.94), SSI (OR = 0.40, 95% CI: 0.31–0.53), and postoperative ileus (OR = 0.71, 95% CI: 0.56–0.90). Thus, MBP with oral antibiotics reduced by almost half SSI, anastomotic leak, and ileus after colorectal surgery.[1]

- It is important to rehydrate with electrolytes (Gatorade) after the preparation, and care should be taken in patients with renal, heart, or liver failure.

American Society of Anesthesiologists Score

The ASA score provides risk information regarding surgical patients. There are five score classifications. Gynecologic oncology patients usually fall into classes 2 or 3. Class 1 includes usually healthy and young persons. Class 2 patients have mild to moderate systemic disease. Class 3 patients have severe systemic disease. Class 4 patients have severe life-threatening systemic disease, and class 5 patients are usually moribund.

Table 4.1 Cardiac Risk and Associated Score

Sign/Symptom	Points
S3 gallop or increased JVP	11
Myocardial infarction in last 6 months	10
More than 5 PVCs/min	7
Any rhythm other than sinus or PAC	7
Age greater than 70 Y	5
Emergent noncardiac operative procedure	4
Aortic stenosis	3
Poor general health	3
Abdominal or thoracic surgery	3

Cardiac Risk Score

Cardiac risk evaluation is important because one of 12 patients over the age of 65 will have coronary artery disease. Thirty percent of those undergoing major elective surgery have at least one cardiac risk factor. The Goldman multifactorial index helps to stratify patients based on their history and studies ordered (Table 4.1). The index of cardiac risk factors is listed in Table 4.1.

Functional Status

Functional status is commonly determined by METS. The ability to climb one flight of stairs is equal to 4 METS, and considered a decent functional status.

If a patient has a diagnosis of CHF, a recent echocardiogram can assist in perioperative management. Normal EF is 60% to 70%. Severe CHF is less than 40%. Care with IVF should be taken in these patients so as not to overload them with fluid (Table 4.2).

Frailty Index

- FI = (number of health deficits present) ÷ (number of health deficits measured). Usually 11 factors are included.

Table 4.2 Cardiac Risk Class

Class	Points	Morbidity (%)	Mortality (%)
I	0–5	0.7	0.2
II	6–12	5	1.6
III	13–25	11	2.3
IV	≥26	22	55.6

- Five factors make up the mFI: Functional status, diabetes, history of COPD, history of CHF, and HTN requiring medication
- An mFI score ≥3 predicts severe complications in 29% to 50% of ovarian cancer patients.[2]
- A mFI combined with secondary cytoreduction surgery (SCS) (scored 1–3) can predict morbidity and mortality in ovarian cancer patients.
- Counseling to include discussion of the frailty score can help guide treatment plans for older frail women: as frailty, not chronological age, can be associated with worse clinical outcomes and survival.[3–5]

Subacute Bacterial Endocarditis

Prophylaxis for subacute bacterial endocarditis (SBE) should still be considered. There are three categories of risk that require different levels of antibiotic protection.

- The low-risk category includes isolated secundum ASD; prior surgical repair of an ASD, VSD, or PDA more than 6 months from surgery; a prior CABG, MPV without valve regurgitation; physiologic heart murmurs; prior Kawasaki disease without valve dysfunction; pacemakers and defibrillators; and prior rheumatic fever without valve dysfunction.
- The moderate-risk category includes acquired valve dysfunctions, hypertrophic cardiomyopathy, MVP with valve regurgitation or thickened leaflets, and other congenital cardiac malformations.
- The high-risk category includes patients with prosthetic cardiac valves, prior SBE, complex cyanotic congenital heart disease, tetralogy of Fallot, transposition of the great arteries, patients with a single ventricle, or surgically constructed systemic pulmonary shunts or conduits.
- Treatment is directed at the moderate- and high-risk patients. Those who are at moderate to high risk should get ampicillin 2 g IV within 30 minutes of the procedure. If they are allergic to ampicillin, they should receive vancomycin 1 g IV over 1 hour within 2 hours of starting the procedure. HiR patients should receive ampicillin 2 g and gentamicin 1.5 mg/kg IV 30 minutes prior to surgery and again 8 hours after the surgery. If the patient is allergic to ampicillin, the patient should then receive vancomycin 1 g and gentamicin 1.5 mg/kg IV 2 hours prior to surgery and 8 hours after surgery.

Nutritional Status

- Controlling Nutritional Status (CONUT) score: Preoperative control of nutritional status. This screening tool can assess and help predict surgical outcome and prognosis. Scoring includes serum albumin level, total lymphocyte count, and total cholesterol (Table 4.3).[6]

Table 4.3 Calculation of the CONUT Score

Parameter	None	Light	Moderate	Severe
Serum albumin (g/dL)	≥3.5	3–3.49	2.5–2.99	<2.5
Score	0	2	4	6
Total lymphocyte (count/mm3)	≥1600	1200–1599	800–1199	<800
score	0	1	2	3
Total cholesterol (mg/dL)	>180	140–179	100–139	<100
Score	0	1	2	3
CONUT score (total)	0–1	2–4	5–8	9–12
Grouping (total score)	<3: Low CONUT group ≥3 High CONUT group			

Source: With modifications, from Li, W., Li, M., Wang, T., *et al.* Controlling Nutritional Status (CONUT) score is a prognostic factor in patients with resected breast cancer. *Sci Rep.* 2020;10:6633 (2020). https://doi.org/10.1038/s41598-020-63610-7. Licensed and reprinted under the parameters of the Creative Commons Attribution 4.0 International License.

DVT/VTE Prophylaxis

- Khorana scoring: By definition, most patients with gynecologic malignancies will fall into the high-risk category.
- Hospitalized patients with active cancer and an acute medical illness or reduced mobility should be administered thromboprophylaxis with pharmacologic treatment and mechanical SCDs.
- The estimated rate of PE mortality is 18 % to 20%.
- Dalteparin is the only LMWH approved for prophylaxis in patients with cancer.
- DOACs edoxaban and rivaroxaban are approved for prophylaxis at this time.
- LMWH is more effective than VKAs to reduce the risk of recurrent VTE in cancer patients.
- Vena cava filter placement in addition to LMWH should be a last resort approach due to lack of evidence to a survival benefit. There were increased rates of DVT, with comparable decreased rates of PE with an IVC filter in place.
- For those with renal impairment, measurement of anti-Xa levels is important for dosing adjustments of LMWH. If this test is not available, UFH or VKA are safer options.
- Notable trials:
  - Di Nisio's meta-analysis showed that LMWH reduced the risk of symptomatic VTE by half with a RR of 0.54 (95% CI 0.38–0.75) compared to nonprophylaxis.[7]
  - Cassini trial: In this study, rivaroxaban at 10 mg PO daily (7% had lymphoma) was administered. VTE occurred in 6% on the rivaroxaban arm compared to 8.8% in the placebo arm.[8]
  - The FRAGEM trial of dalteparin 200IU/kg once daily[9]
  - CONKO-004 enoxaparin 1 mg/kg once daily[10]
  - CLOT trial: This study compared dalteparin to VKA. The dalteparin arm had a 2.7 occurrence, which translated to a 17% reduced risk for recurrent VTE (HR, 0.15; 95% CI, 0.03–0.65).[11]
  - Edoxaban was shown to be noninferior to dalteparin with a VTE rate of 12.8% in the edoxaban arm versus 13.5% in the dalteparin arm (HR, 0.97; 95% CI, 0.7–1.36).[12]
  - SELECT-D trial evaluated rivaroxaban versus dalteparin and the 6-month risk for recurrent VTE. A 4% occurrence was seen with rivaroxaban versus 11% with dalteparin (HR, 0.43; 95% CI, 0.19–0.99).[13]
  - A meta-analysis by Young showed DOACs had a lower risk of VTE (RR = 0.65) but had a higher risk of major bleeding events (RR = 1.74) compared to LMWH.[13]

○ The safety and efficacy of apixaban versus enoxaparin for preventing postoperative VTE in women undergoing surgery for malignant gynecologic cancers was reviewed. This was a randomized controlled trial comparing 2.5 mg PO BID of apixaban to enoxaparin at 40-mg SC daily. The primary endpoint was major bleeding. The study was underpowered for VTE. No differences in bleeding events were seen and VTE occurred in two versus three patients (OR, 1.57; 95% CI, 0.26–9.5 p = .68).[14]

○ AVERT trial: Apixaban was use to prevent VTE in patients with cancer.[15] This was a randomized, double-blind placebo-controlled trial of 563 patients (25% had lymphoma) to review the efficacy and safety of apixaban at 2.5 mg BID prophylactic dosing in ambulatory cancer patients at intermediate to high risk for VTE (Khorana score, ≥2) at the time of chemotherapy initiation. The primary outcome was VTE of the first 180 days with the main safety outcome as a major bleeding episode. VTE happened in 12 of 288 patients (4.2%) of those on apixaban and 28 of 275 patients (10.2%) in the placebo group (HR, 0.41; 95% CI, 0.26–0.65; p < .001). Major bleeding occurred in 10 patients (3.5%) on apixaban versus five patients (1.8%) in the placebo group (HR, 2.00; 95% CI, 1.01–3.95; p = .046). Bleeding was mainly from the GI system.

○ Effect of length of surgery on the incidence of VTE after benign hysterectomy.[16] This was a secondary analysis of a prospectively collected database. In this study, 70,606 patients who had hysterectomy for benign conditions were reviewed. The approach was abdominal, vaginal, or laparoscopic. The 30-day VTE incidence was 0.4% (n = 259). Those who had VTE were often obese, inpatient, and had larger uterine weight. For each 60-minute operative time increase, a concomitant 35% chance of VTE occurred (adjusted odds ratio [aOR], 1.35; 95% CI, 1.25–1.45). When surgical route was taken into account, the aOR for VTE with abdominal hysterectomy was 1.49; (95% CI, 1.35–1.65) compared to the laparoscopic approach with an aOR of 1.20 (95% CI, 1.05–1.38) and vaginal approach with an aOR of 1.271 95% CI, 0.97–1.66; p =.01). Larger BMI and older age didn't affect the relationship of operative time and incidence of VTE (p = .66 and p = .58).

Surgical Bundling

This was a retrospective analysis of a prospectively implemented, multidisciplinary team-designed SSI prevention bundle that consisted of chlorhexidine-impregnated preoperative wipes, standardized aseptic surgical preparation, standardized antibiotic dosing, perioperative normothermia, surgical dressing maintenance, removal of sterile dressing between 24 and 48 hours, and direct feedback to clinicians when the protocol was breached. Of 2,099 hysterectomies performed during the 33-month study period, there were 61 SSIs (4.51%) in the pre-full bundle implementation period and 14 (1.87%) in the post-full bundle implementation period; patients were less likely to develop an SSI (OR, 0.46, p = .01). There was no difference in days of postoperative hospital stay (adjusted mean ratio 0.95, p =.09) or rate of readmission (adjusted OR, 2.65, p = .08) between the before and after full-bundle implementation periods. No single component was more effective than another in reducing infection rates. The superficial infections were the most significantly reduced type.[17]

Comorbidity Indices

- **Charleston Comorbidity Index**: This index accounts for the patient age and 16 conditions.
- The Charleston Comorbidity Index predicts the 10-Y mortality for patients presenting with one or more of the conditions in the model. This is an index used in decision-making when short- and long-term benefits of treatment in a patient with comorbid conditions are assessed for long-term risk. Each of the conditions listed is awarded a value-based point of 1, 2, 3, or 6 and combined with an age-based score. The more points given, the more likely the predicted adverse outcome. The total points are then summed. This Charleston Comorbidity Index score is transformed by algorithm into a 10Y survival/mortality percentage taking into account that C is the score result obtained by summing the points.
  - Age—Divided into five age groups of different risk:
    - ≤40 Y (0 points)
    - Between 41 and 50 (1 point)
    - Between 51 and 60 (2 points)
    - Between 61 and 70 (3 points)
    - ≥71 Y (4 points)
- Comorbidity-based score: 1, 2, 3, or 6 points depending on the mortality risk associated with each of the comorbidities.

➤ Myocardial infarction	➤ CHF
➤ PVD	➤ Cerebrovascular disease
➤ Dementia	➤ COPD
➤ Connective tissue disease	➤ Peptic ulcer disease
➤ DM	➤ Moderate to severe chronic kidney disease
➤ Hemiplegia	
➤ Malignant lymphoma	➤ Leukemia
➤ Solid tumor	➤ Liver disease
	➤ AIDS

  - 1-point condition—Myocardial infarction, CHF, PVD, dementia, cerebrovascular disease, connective tissue disease, ulcer, chronic liver disease, DM.

- 2-point condition—hemiplegia, moderate to severe kidney disease, DM with end organ damage, solid tumor, leukemia, lymphoma.
- 3-point condition—Moderate to severe liver disease.
- 6 point condition—Malignant tumor, metastasis, AIDS[18-20]
- **The Cumulative Illness Index Rating Scale** was developed by Linn in 1968. Fourteen systems are evaluated and scored. The scores are then summed and can range from 0 to 56. A higher score predicts a worse outcome.
- Scoring:
  - Less than 6 and CrCl greater than 70 mL/min (GO: suitable for treatment)
  - Greater than 6 and CrCl less than 70 mL/min (SLOW: suitable for reduced treatment)
  - Severe comorbidities and short-life expectancy (NO: suitable for supportive care)
  - Each system is rated as follows:
    - 1 = None: There is no impairment to that organ/system.
    - 2 = Mild: Impairment does not interfere with normal activity; treatment may or may not be required; prognosis is excellent.
    - 3 = Moderate: Impairment interferes with normal activity; treatment is needed; prognosis is good.
    - 4 = Severe: Impairment is disabling; treatment is urgently needed; prognosis is guarded.
    - 5 = Extremely severe: Impairment is life-threatening; treatment is urgent; prognosis is grave

SURGICAL PROCEDURES

Laparotomy Incisions
- The most common vertical incision used for an exploratory laparotomy in oncology is a vertical midline incision. A less commonly used vertical incision is the paramedian incision.
- There are three common transverse skin incisions, with differences in fascial entry:
  - Pfannenstiel: Dissects fascia from rectus muscles.
  - Cherney: Dissects the tendons of the rectus abdominis muscles from the pubic bone. A major complication with this incision is the development of osteomyelitis due to suturing of muscle tendons back to bone.
  - Maylard: Cuts muscle. Involves ligating the inferior epigastrics prior to transection of the muscle bodies. This incision does not separate the transversalis fascia from the rectus muscles.

Incision Closure

- Abdominal wall closure:
  - Mass closure: Made with one continuous length of suture material; includes all body-wall layers, and incorporates fascia, muscles, and peritoneum.
  - Smead-Jones (far-near, near-far): This is a double-loop, interrupted mattress suture technique that incorporates all the body layers in the outside suture ("far") and fascia and peritoneum in the inner suture ("near").
  - Fascial incision strength after surgery: Week 1, 10%; week 2, 25%; week 3, 30%; week 4, 40%; 6 months: 80%.
- SC tissue: If the wound is greater than 2 cm deep, SC suture or placement of a JP drain is indicated.
- Skin closure:
  - Staples
  - SC suture with Monocryl or Vicryl with or without a topical skin adhesive overlay
  - Vertical mattress skin closure: Useful in delayed primary closure of abdominal incisions and in perineal wound closure (places the knot lateral to the line of incision)

Lymph Node Dissection

- Pelvic: The boundaries for the P-LND are the following: superiorly, the distal half of the common iliac vessels; laterally, the anterior and medial aspect of the external and internal iliac vessels; the ureter or the superior vesical artery medially; the circumflex iliac vein inferiorly; and the obturator nerve posteriorly.
- Para-aortic: The boundaries for the PA-LND are the following: the fat pads over and lateral to the IVC and aorta, the IMA (or up to renal vessels) superiorly, the proximal half of the common iliac vessels inferiorly, and the ureters laterally (Figure 4.5).
- For a high PA-LND, the LNs up to the renal vessels are removed medial to the ureters and anterior to the great vessels.
- Sentinel LND (SLND): Radiolabeled albumin with Technetium-99 is injected into the tumoral/peritumoral bed preprocedure (for cervical and vulvar lesions: directly into the tumor; for uterine cancer, injection is into the cervix vaginally at the start of procedure, the fundus via laparoscopic injection, or the corpus via hysteroscopic injection). Alternatively or to-follow, Lymphazurin blue or ICG is injected into the tumoral bed at initiation of surgical procedure and the first LN identified in the drainage basins from that tumor site is dissected. It can be sent for frozen section or considered complete awaiting final pathology adjuvant therapy. If negative on frozen, the procedure is considered complete. If positive, a complete lymphadenectomy is usually recommended. There may be more than one sentinel node. For midline structures/tumors, SLND should be performed bilaterally.

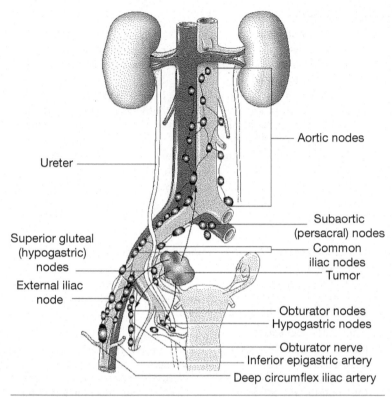

Aortic nodes

Ureter

Superior gluteal (hypogastric) nodes

External iliac node

Subaortic (persacral) nodes

Common iliac nodes

Tumor

Obturator nodes
Hypogastric nodes

Obturator nerve
Inferior epigastric artery
Deep circumflex iliac artery

Figure 4.5 **Lymphatic drainage of the ovary. The three principal routes are to the PA nodal basins accompanying the ovarian vessels, the obturator and iliac nodal basins through the broad ligament, and the external iliac and inguinal nodal basins via the round ligament.**

Source: Reproduced with permission from Holschneider CH, et al. Cytoreductive surgery: pelvis and radical oophorectomy. In: Bristow RE, et al., eds. *Surgery for Ovarian Cancer,* 3rd ed. Taylor & Francis Group; 2016.

Bowel Diversion

- When an ostomy is considered preoperatively, an ostomy consult should be obtained. The consultation should focus on patient education regarding the care and maintenance of an ostomy. In addition, best placement of the ostomy should be identified. This includes evaluation of the patient's waistline, common pant line, and any other individual body factors related to optimal appliance placement.

- A mucous fistula is the distal segment of cut bowel remaining at the time of ostomy creation. It is brought through a separate ostomy site. The mucous fistula is created when the remaining distal bowel is more than 10 cm from the anus. These mucous fistulas have minimal drainage. It is important to ensure that the proximal end ostomy and mucus fistula opening are distant enough from each other so that cross fecal contamination and infection cannot occur.

- Complications:
  - Stricture: There is a 3% stricture rate for all ostomies. Dilation or surgical correction can be performed for strictures.
  - Prolapse: The descending colon has the least risk of prolapse.
  - Hernia
- There are two common types of large bowel ostomy:
  - An end ostomy is performed when a takedown is not planned. A mucous fistula needs to be constructed in most cases. The distal end of resected bowel needs management because it still produces mucus, gas, and sloughed cells, and could become dilated and perforate. Permanent colostomies prolapse in 1% to 3% of cases. If the resection of the colon occurs at the rectosigmoid and 5 to 10 cm remain, this remaining rectum is then called a *Hartmann's pouch* and functions as a mucous fistula with output through the anus.
  - A loop ostomy should be performed when there are plans to take the ostomy down. The bowel is brought through the abdominal wall and opened on its antimesenteric side. Both sides of the opened bowel are sutured to the skin. A Hollister bridge or glass rod is placed under the bowel loop for temporary support until healing occurs. The proximal end functions as the colostomy and the distal opening functions as the mucous fistula. It is easier to take down because it is not mandatory to know which end is proximal and which is distal.
- Ileostomy: Indications include diversion when no distal large bowel is available, when small bowel is too dilated to perform an anastomosis, for protection of a distal anastomosis when an anastomotic leak is likely, or in the presence of a bowel perforation with peritonitis. These are high-output ostomies, so as distal an ostomy as possible is preferred. A Turnbull loop is recommended.
- G-tube: G-tubes are indicated for decompression of the stomach and intestine to avoid long-term use of a NGT. They are also used for intractable SBOs associated with carcinomatosis and fistulas. The body or antrum of the stomach is chosen. A size 18 to 20 Malecot or Foley catheter can be used. The greater curve of the stomach is incised with a scalpel 0.5 cm in length. Two purse-string sutures of 2–0 gauge silk are placed to secure the tube to the stomach. The gastrostomy site is brought to the peritoneal surface and secured with interrupted Vicryl sutures. The catheter is then exteriorized through a skin incision and secured to the skin with 2–0 gauge prolene sutures. The G-tube needs to be changed every 2 months.

Bowel Resection

- Bowel anastomosis can be performed using either the hand-sewn or stapled technique.
  - Types:
    - End to end: The bowel is aligned with cut ends together and hand-sewn together using a two-layer technique (the inner layer using 3–0 gauge Vicryl and the outer imbricating layer using 3–0 gauge Vicryl or silk). Alternatively, using a stapler, the bowel ends are aligned on their antimesenteric borders. An enterotomy is made on the antimesenteric corner of the two bowel sections. One prong of the GIA stapler is then advanced through each enterotomy and fired. The TA stapler is then used to close the connected bowel segments to create a functional end-to-end anastomosis. The mesentery should be closed and silk stay sutures are placed along the antimesenteric borders to reduce tension.
    - Side to side: Five-mm enterotomies are made with the Bovie on each segment of the resected bowel 5 to 10 cm back from the primary transection site. One prong of the GIA stapler is then advanced through each enterotomy and the stapler is then fired. The TA stapler is then applied to close the defect transversely or longitudinally, whichever narrows the lumen least.
    - Low rectal anastomosis is often performed after a rectosigmoid resection. Consider placing a diverting-loop colostomy or loop ileostomy to protect the anastomosis and allow for healing. The anastomosis should preferably be performed out of the irradiated field. The largest staple cartridge available and accommodated by the patient should be used. If a very low anastomosis is performed, consider construction of a J pouch to increase reservoir capacity and to decrease tenesmus.
    - If fistula is present, consider excision of fistulous tract, pelvic rest × 6 weeks, fistulogram after healing and before takedown of diverting ileostomy or secondary reanastomosis.
  - Anastomotic leaks complicate bowel surgery in 0% to 30%. Rectal anastomosis has a higher complication rate of about 6%.
  - Requirements for a good anastomosis include the following: An adequate lumen of at least 2 to 3 cm, the anastomosis must be tension free, there must be adequate vascular supply from the mesentery with evidence of bleeding (viability) of the cut edges, and the presence of peristalsis.
  - Watershed areas of the bowel include the ileocecal junction/terminal ileum, the splenic flexure of colon (Griffith's point), and the rectosigmoid flexure (Sudeck's point).

- Meckel's diverticulum represents persistence of the vitelline yolk sac. It is present in 2% of people. It is twice as common in men as women. It is usually located within 2 feet of the ileocecal valve. It should be removed when found, due to the presence of ectopic gastric tissue in 2% of patients, that is, Zollinger–Ellison syndrome.

Urinary Diversion: Stents, Conduits, and Bladder Reconstructions

- Ureteral stents should be placed in most ureteral injury cases. They can be placed via retrograde cystoscopy, retrograde cystotomy, ureterotomy, or antegrade through a PCN. A 6-French double pigtail stent or a pediatric feeding tube can be placed. These should be changed every 3 to 6 months. They can often be removed 6 weeks after surgery via cystoscopy.

- Urinary conduits/neobladders are often placed in the settings of pelvic exenteration, intractable hemorrhagic cystitis, a neurogenic bladder, or decreased bladder capacitance from surgery or XRT. *Decreased capacity* is defined as an intravesical pressure greater than 30 cm of H_2O with minimum volume.

- Bladder reconstruction can be performed when there has been surgical resection with the urethra safely preserved.

- Principles of urinary conduits are a low-pressure system (<20-cm H_2O), high-volume, antirefluxing system to prevent ascending infection, and low water and solute reabsorption.
  - Universal techniques are needed. There has to be a wide ureterobowel anastomosis, the intestinal segment should be isoperistaltic, the stoma should be protruding, the conduit should be stabilized within the abdominal cavity, and there should be an adequate diameter of the efferent loop with a straight path through the abdominal wall for urine outlet.
  - There are two types of conduits: incontinent and continent.
    - Incontinent types include:
      - PCN tube
      - Cutaneous ureterostomy: The ureters should be brought out 2 cm past the skin, and the skin incision should be an inverted "V" pointing down.
      - Right colon pouch: is made from nonirradiated, detubularized colon. It has an increased risk of ureteral obstruction, angulation of the distal ureters, fibrosis of the submucosal ureteral tunnels, devascularization, and distension of the pouch. The left ureter requires more mobilization to reach the colon.
      - Ileal conduit: uses a longer intestinal segment. The Bricker type incorporates a horizontal internal orientation for the body of the reservoir. The ureters are anastomosed laterally. The Leadbetter modification orients the body of the conduit

vertically. The ureters are brought to the midline for the anastomosis. The ureteroileal anastomoses are end to end. A Turnbull stoma is used to overcome the complications of nipple ischemia. A short ileal segment of 15 to 18 cm is used. The conduit is sutured at its proximal end to the sacral prominence. The Daniels modification is used for obese patients, and the Wallace modification is used for double ureters (where both ureters are split and sewn together).

▫ Jejunal conduit: has a higher incidence of electrolyte imbalances: Hyperchloremic acidosis occurs in 25% to 65% of patients. There is reabsorption of potassium (K) and urea and a concomitant increase in aldosterone. It is more often outside the fields of XRT.

▫ Sigmoid conduit: has the advantages of avoiding small-bowel anastomosis and fewer stomal complications. Disadvantages are that it cannot be used with inflammatory bowel syndromes or diverticulosis. There is an increased risk of secondary cancers inside the conduit. The ureters should be tunneled submucosally if no prior XRT was given.

▫ Transverse colon conduit: has advantages in that it is good for the obese patient, in those with a history of WP-XRT as it is outside the field of XRT, and in those with short ureters.

- Continent diversions are contraindicated in persons with short life expectancies, in those with physical problems accessing/maintaining the conduit (dementia/arthritis), those with right colon diseases (prior bowel cancer, IBD, cecal XRT), those with morbid obesity (making this a short system), and in those with compromised renal function.

▫ Ureterosigmoidostomy maintains continence through the anal sphincter. The ureters are directly tunneled and secured into the sigmoid colon and efflux is through the rectum. There are high rates of pyelonephritis, obstruction, hyperchloremic acidosis, nocturnal incontinence, and frequent bowel evacuation. Secondary carcinomas of the colon can occur.

▫ Ileocolic continent diversion (Indiana pouch): uses 10 to 15 cm of terminal ileum, the cecum, and 30 cm of ascending colon. The right colonic segment is detubularized. The terminal ileum is plicated over a red robin catheter to the level of the ileocolic valve—this provides the continence mechanism. The plicated ileum is brought to the abdominal wall. Intestinal integrity is reestablished after resection. Stents are placed in each ureter, A Malecot catheter is placed into the right colon pouch and exits superior to the ileal stoma.

A red robin/Foley catheter is placed in the plicated ileum maintaining patency from the right colonic pouch through the abdominal wall, and a JP is placed in the abdomen.

▫ Miami pouch: uses the same principles as previously descibed, but extends the intestinal resection to the level of the transverse colon.

▫ Postoperative maintenance includes irrigation of the Malecot every 4 to 6 hours with 40 mL of normal saline, and irrigation of the ureteral stents only if plugged. Both drains are removed at 14 days, after an IVP and pouchogram are normal. If the patient had prior XRT, 21 days of stenting and drainage are recommended. The JP should be removed at the same time as the ureteral stents. Active catheterization is recommended every 2 hours the first week, every 3 hours the second week, every 4 hours the third week, every 5 hours the fourth week, and every 6 hours the fifth week. The pouch should be irrigated daily to weekly with 50 mL of normal saline. An IVP, pouchogram, and CMP should be obtained at 3 months.

▫ Kock ileal pouch: is specifically contraindicated for chronic inflammatory or neoplastic diseases of the colon, as well as in patients with short ureters. A portion of the ileum is isolated and marked into segments measuring 17, 22, 22, and 17 cm; 15 cm of distal ileum remains at the ileocecal junction to protect the watershed area. The 22-cm (central portion) lengths are sutured together, then opened along their antimesenteric borders to make the reservoir. The pouch is then folded over. The 17-cm lengths are then each intussuscepted and secured with a GIA or TA stapler. The ureters are brought in to the proximal end. Mesh is attached to each intussusception to secure the intussuscepted nipples. A Marlex strut is attached from the distal mesh to the rectus muscle. The two ends of the ileal segment become the nipples: The afferent end prevents reflux into the kidneys and the efferent end is the continence mechanism. Complications include stone formation around staples, prolapse, extussusception, and stenosis from ischemia.

• Bladder reconstruction can be performed with:

  ○ Right colon augmentation (enterocystoplasty)

  ○ A hemi-Kock ileal bladder: can also be constructed. With this technique no efferent nipple is constructed.

  ○ Psoas hitch: provides bladder reconstruction by mobilizing the bladder to reach a shortened ureter on the ipsilateral side. The bladder is distended with water, then opened along the dome. A suture is placed through the lateral side of the bladder to the psoas muscle on the affected side, at the level of the proximal external iliac artery. The ureter is anastomosed to the bladder and the cystotomy is closed in two layers.

○ Boari bladder flap: is used in combination with the psoas hitch for a more extensively shortened ureter. The bladder is again distended, and opened in the dome with a U-shaped incision. The base of the created flap is then oriented toward the psoas muscle and the flap is rotated upward. The flap is tubularized around the ureter, and the bladder is then sutured to the psoas muscle. The bladder defect is then closed in two layers. This technique provides 3 to 5 cm of additional length for a shortened ureter.

- There are three methods for ureteral reanastomosis after transection:
  ○ The ureteroureterostomy (UU), which is a primary reanastomosis.
  ○ The transureteroureterostomy, which is an anastomosis to the contralateral ureter.
  ○ The ureteroneocystostomy (UNC), which reimplants the ureter directly into the bladder, with or without psoas hitch or Boari flap.
  ○ All ureteral injuries and diversions should be stented unless minimal crush injury is seen and immediately released.

Reconstructive Surgery

- Reconstructive surgery is useful in gynecologic oncology for coverage of perineal defects and for neovaginal construction. There are different methods of reconstruction.
- Split thickness skin grafts (STSG) are often used to cover epidermal/dermal defects encountered with simple vulvectomy. The Zimmer dermatome can produce an optimal graft thickness of 0.020 inches.
- Tissue expansion can be produced with inflatable balloons and the area harvested after an appropriate time.
- Skin flaps are used to reconstruct deeper resections. There are three types of flaps: rotational, advancement, and transpositional (pass over).
  ○ Common rotational flaps include the rhomboid and perineal thigh flaps. The rotational flap most often used is the rhomboid flap/Limberg flap. This flap can cover anterior, lateral, or posterior vulvar defects in addition to defects of the perianal region. The donor sites are the buttocks and posterior thigh. The blood supply is the inferior gluteal artery. The perineal thigh flap is used to cover a defect to the labial crural fold. The donor site is the medial thigh. This blood supply is unreliable. The length of the flap should be a ratio of 2:1 to the vulvar defect.
  ○ Advancement flaps are used to provide defect coverage when there is enough adjacent skin mobility. This is usually called a *V–Y advancement flap.*

- ○ Transpositional axial flaps move the flap on an axis (its vascular pedicle) to another site.
    - ▪ The Martius/bulbocavernosus flap is used for repair of vaginal fistulas, for vaginal reconstruction, and for repair of fourth-degree lacerations. The donor site is the labial fat pad and the blood supply is the SEPA and the perineal branch of the internal pudendal artery.
    - ▪ The SEPA flap is often used for vulvar reconstruction and repair of urethral defects. The donor site is the area directly above the mons pubis. This type of flap should not be performed if a groin node dissection is planned. The blood supply is related to the flap's name and originates from the common femoral artery. This is a sensate flap.
    - ▪ The SCIA flap is indicated for anterior perineal and vaginal defects. The donor site is the skin around the ASIS to 2.5 cm below the inguinal ligament. The blood supply again relates to its name.
    - ▪ The posterior labial artery flap is also known as the *pudendal thigh flap* and the *Singapore flap*. It too covers perineal defects and is good for vaginal reconstruction. The donor site is the labial crural fold and the inguinal crease. The blood supply is related to its name and originates from the deep external pudendal artery. This flap is sensate and innervation is from branches of the pudendal nerve and the posterior cutaneous nerves.
    - ▪ The inferior gluteal fasciocutaneous flap can cover vulvar, vaginal, and rectal defects. The donor site is the buttocks. The blood supply is the axial artery of the inferior gluteal artery, originating from the internal iliac artery. This flap can be up to 35 cm long. It too is a sensate flap and the nerve supply is from the posterior cutaneous nerve of the thigh.
- • Myocutaneous flaps are distinguished by the number of vascular pedicles that supply the flap. There are five types. Type I flaps consist of a single vascular pedicle. Type II flaps have one dominant vascular pedicle and one or more minor vascular pedicles. Type III flaps obtain their blood supply from two dominant pedicles. Type IV flaps obtain their blood supply from three dominant pedicles. Type V flaps obtain their blood supply from four dominant vascular pedicles. To test flap viability, IV fluorescein (10 mL of 10% solution, or a dose of 15 mg/kg administered over 5 minutes) can be given and a Wood's light can be placed over the flap site. Twice the dose should be used in patients with darker skin tones.
    - ○ The RAM flap is often used for vaginal/pelvic reconstruction. The blood supply is the superior and inferior epigastrics and it is a type III flap.

- ○ The gracilis myocutaneous flap (GMC) flap is used for vaginal, groin, or perineal reconstruction. It can be used as an island flap, or directly rotated into the defect. The blood supply is the medial femoral circumflex artery from the deep femoral artery. It is a type II flap.

- ○ The tensor fasciae latae flap is indicated for vulvar and groin defects, as well as for ischial and deep abdominal wall defects. The donor sites are the gluteus medius and sartorius muscles. The blood supply is the terminal branch of the lateral circumflex femoral artery. It is a type I flap. Side effects can be lateral instability of the knee, a long scar on the medial thigh, thigh pain, and vascular spasm from torsion. It is not a suitable flap for vaginal reconstruction after a supralevator exenteration.

- ○ The latissimus dorsi flap is a good flap for breast reconstruction. It is a type V flap.

- Neovaginal techniques are also varied. These include the following:

- ○ McIndoe STSG: The McIndoe neovagina is constructed using a STSG formed around a mold. It is placed in the perineal defect and the patient should then be immobilized to allow the STSG to anneal. Daily dilation should follow indefinitely.

- ○ The RAM flap is a more reliable neovaginal flap and is less likely to prolapse than other neovaginal flaps.

- ○ Two GMC flaps are needed for neovaginal reconstruction if this procedure is performed. There can be vascular pedicle spasm with this type of flap. It does have a tendency to prolapse.

- ○ The Martius flap is a durable and pliable flap to use for neovaginal reconstruction.

- ○ The posterior labial artery thigh flap is a sensate flap but has a less reliable blood supply.

- ○ The perineal thigh skin flap tends to prolapse and can stenose.

- ○ Intestinal segments, including the cecum, small bowel, sigmoid colon, and rectum, can also be used for neovaginal reconstruction. The sigmoid colon is used the most often. It is important to detubularize it. The benefits of this type of neovagina are its large caliber, and low-volume mucous output. Risks include secondary malignancies, including those that are HPV-related.

Splenectomy

Splenectomy is often indicated with splenic trauma, or when tumor has involved this organ and optimal debulking is feasible if the spleen is removed.

- Anatomy: The splenic artery originates at the celiac trunk. The splenic vein combines with the hepatic veins to join the IVC.

- Technique: When performing a splenectomy, it is necessary to take down the splenogastric, splenocolic, and splenophrenic ligaments. The artery and vein should be clamped and ligated separately to decrease the risk of arteriovenous fistula.
- Complications: There is a risk of thrombocytosis post-splenectomy, as well as an increased risk of DVT.
- Necessary vaccines after splenectomy include immunization against *Meningococcus, Haemophilus influenzae,* and *Pneumococcus.* Ideally, these vaccines should be given 14 days prior to the anticipated splenectomy. If not done prior, they should be done as soon as possible after surgery.

Diaphragmatic Stripping

Diaphragmatic stripping is performed when optimal debulking can be achieved. The peritoneum is removed with varied techniques.

- The liver usually needs to be mobilized inferiorly with release of the falciform and triangular ligaments.
- Complications include pneumothorax when the diaphragm is perforated. To rectify this, a Foley or red rubber catheter is placed through the defect and connected to suction. A purse string suture is placed around the catheter and the patient is placed in Trendelenburg position. The anesthesiologist is asked to perform an expiratory Valsalva for the patient with the ventilator, and the catheter is removed with the suture tied. A chest tube is usually placed and placement checked with a CXR postoperatively.

Minimally Invasive Surgery

Minimally invasive surgery (MIS) has emerged as an area of growth in procedural medicine and is specifically useful in gynecologic surgery.

- Three laparoscopic approaches are typically used: Traditional laparoscopy, robotic-assisted laparoscopy, and laparoendoscopic single-site surgery.
- Advantages of MIS include a shorter hospitalization, a more rapid recovery, smaller incisions, and a trend for fewer analgesics.
  - Limitations of MIS are a longer learning curve and the costs of instrumentation.

Minimally Invasive Radical Hysterectomy

- Data from the LACC trial dissuade a MIS approach to cervical cancer. This trial evaluated mainly stage IB1 patients, but many academic institutions are foregoing MIS approaches altogether. Some trials have evaluated tumors <2 cm for MIS—with mixed results, and these are retrospective in nature. Shared decision-making needs to be done with the patient.[21–23]

Minimally Invasive Ovarian Cancer Surgery

- Staging:
  - ○ Early-stage disease: Feasibility is present for TH-BSO, LND, peritoneal biopsies, and omentectomy for presumed early-stage disease. Pelvic masses/cancers should be reasonably small to fit into an endocatch bag and removed without rupture, or risk of intracorporeal/in-bag rupture must be discussed with the patient preoperatively.
  - ○ Advanced-stage disease: The Fagotti scoring protocol uses an initial laparoscopic assessment.
- Advanced-stage cytoreduction: Laparoscopic approaches to cytoreduction continue to be explored. Primary and secondary cytoreduction has been evaluated in studies with low power and retrospectively. Small reports have shown feasibility in patients after NACT, with 50% to 76.9% achieving ≤R1 disease and with a 3% to 50% conversion rate. Strict selection of patients with low tumor volume on preoperative workup in addition to no contraindications to a laparoscopic approach (BMI, cardiopulmonary status, Fagotti score) should be part of the inclusion criteria. The equivalencies of this approach should be cautioned in line with the LACC data—the ability to perform such procedures does not mean it is in the patient's best interest. Provider surgical skill, competencies, and opinions can also vary greatly.[24,25] There is an ongoing noninferiority clinical trial comparing PDS laparoscopically to laparotomy.

Minimally Invasive Exenteration

- MIS for exenteration is now being explored. Fifty percent of cases were done robotically in one review, but with lower rates of vaginal reconstruction and colostomy when compared to laparotomy patients. Similar complication rates were seen with MIS versus laparotomy, but with fewer postoperative complications.
  - ○ In one study, 49 (3%) of 1,376 women who underwent pelvic exenteration for a multitude of primary gynecologic cancer diagnoses, had the procedure performed laparoscopically and were retrospectively reviewed.[26] The majority of minimally invasive cases were robotic-assisted (51.0%). Women in the minimally invasive group were younger, White, had primary cervical/uterine cancers, and received urinary diversion, but infrequently had vaginal reconstruction or colostomy when compared to those in the open surgery group (*p* <.05). Overall perioperative complication rates were similar between groups (79.6% laparoscopic vs. 77.7% open, *p* = .862). The laparoscopic group had a lower risk of complications (OR, 0.19; 95% CI: 0.07–0.51) to include fewer episodes of sepsis and TE (*p* <.05). The laparoscopic group had a shorter LOS (median, 9 vs. 14 days) and lower total cost (median, $127,875 vs. $208,591) compared to the open group (*p* <.05).

○ This was a prospective evaluation of laparoscopic exenteration and laterally extended endopelvic resection (LEER) in 28 patients with recurrent cervical carcinoma after receiving XRT. Seventeen patients had laparoscopic PE for a central tumor recurrence and 11 had LEERs due to a lateral tumor recurrence.[27] The median operation time and blood loss were 454 minutes and 285 mL in the PE group, and 562 minutess and 325 mL in the LEER group. There were no conversions to laparotomy. R0 resection was achieved in all patients in the PE group and 73% in the LEER group. The morbidity and mortality rates were 41% and 0% in PE group, and 55% and 0% in LEER group, respectively. The 2Y DFS and OS were 68.9% and 76% in the PE group, and 27.3% and 29.6% in the LEER group, respectively.

SURGICAL DEVICES

Drains

- **G-tube:** Indicated for decompression of the stomach to avoid long-term use of a NGT. It can also be used for feeding patients with swallowing difficulties. When placed to gravity, it can be used as an outlet for bowel contents to decrease nausea and vomiting in patients with bowel obstruction.

- **Chest tube:** Indicated for pleural effusions, hemothorax, or pneumothorax (if >15%). When used with pleurovac, negative pressure is set at 20 cm of H_2O. A purse-string stitch is placed SC to secure it to the skin. Petrolatum-impregnated gauze should be placed over the incision to make it airtight. Obtain CXR daily.

  ○ Pneumothorax: Place to suction for 2 days, then to water seal for the third day. A CXR should be obtained daily to evaluate size of pneumothorax. Leave water sealed until the output is less than 100 mL in 24 hours, and check for the presence of an air leak daily. Pull the chest tube when the pneumothorax is <10%, when output is less than 100 mL in 24 hours, and there is no air leak.

  ○ Hemothorax or pleural effusion: Place to suction for 1 day and then to water seal for the second day. Pull when output is less than 100 mL in 24 hours.

  ○ Resolution normally occurs at 10% to 20% per day.

  ○ When it is ready to be pulled, the patient should take a deep breath and then perform the Valsalva maneuver. The tube is then pulled out as the purse-string stitch is secured tightly around the prior incision. A petrolatum gauze should be placed on top.

- **JP:** Indicated for SC or IP wound drainage. Used to decrease the incidence of seroma and infection. It is a closed drain; placed to bulb suction.

  ○ SC: Removal is recommended when output is less than 30 mL per day. SC drainage decreases the incidence of seromas and infections if not used in conjunction with a SC suture.

○ **Peritoneal/intra-abdominal placement:** Removal is recommended when the peritoneal output is less than 50 mL per day. If there was significant preoperative ascites, the drain is removed when the fluid turns mainly serous.

- **Penrose drain and T-tubes:** These are indicated for drainage of pelvic or SC infections; they are passive drains.

- **NGT:** This is indicated for postoperative ileus or for bowel obstruction. It is placed to low intermittent suction or Gomco suction.

Central Venous Catheters

- Used to administer systemic cytotoxic, biologic, and targeted agents, blood products, antibiotics, or in patients with poor peripheral access.

- The Mediport is a SC port and catheter used for central venous access. It is accessed using a Huber needle. It needs a monthly flush with heparin. A CXR is needed after placement unless it is placed under fluoroscopic guidance.

- A peripherally inserted central catheter, or PICC line, is a central venous line placed through a peripheral vein. Indications are for systemic cytotoxic agents, antibiotic therapy, TPN, or in patients with poor peripheral access. A daily flush is needed but it can be left in place for 6 months. A CXR after placement is needed.

- A Hickman catheter is a subclavian catheter used for central venous access. It has no SC pocket reservoir, so the rate of infection is higher. Indications are similar to the PICC line. It necessitates a daily flush. A CXR is needed after placement.

- A Groshong catheter is a semipermanent central venous catheter. It needs a weekly flush. A CXR after placement is needed.

Peritoneal Catheters

- The Tenckhoff catheter is a type of IP port-a-cath. It can be irrigated with 500 units of heparin in a 15-mL normal saline flush QID × 3 days after placement. It needs a weekly maintenance flush.

- The Bardport or Mediport 8–9.6F nonfenestrated port can also be used for IP placement. It does not need a flush.

Catheter Troubleshooting

- If a blood clot obstructs the use of any vascular catheter, attempts at salvage with a thrombolytic agent are indicated. Patency can be checked by injection of Hypaque contrast or visualization under fluoroscopy. An example of a thrombolytic protocol is a urokinase flush with 5,000 units/mL solution. A 1-mL injection into the port is performed followed by a 3-mL normal saline flush. This is allowed to remain for 1 hour, then fluid withdrawal is attempted.

- Fibrin sheath: This occurs and is diagnosed when there is difficulty withdrawing blood but the flush is smooth or has only moderate resistance. Treatment is placement of a new port if difficulty continues.

Instruments

- Robotics platforms: There are a few companies with robotic platforms. The benefits of robotics are 3D laparoscopy, 7° of wrist movement compared to the 3° that conventional laparoscopy is capable of, minimization of tremor, and accentuated nodal dissection techniques. Although the cost of the program is high, the length of patient stay, amortization, and subjectively improved dissection techniques contribute to high-yield outcomes in oncologic surgery practices.
- 3D laparoscopy is now available to enhance depth of vision and facilitate dissection.
- ICG dye: ICG is an indicator substance for medical diagnostics. The patented technology is Firefly. It can be injected into the bloodstream and binds to albumin, or injected into primary tumor and drains to the regional lymphatics. ICG absorbs between 600 and 900 nm and emits fluorescence between 750 and 950 nm in the near-infrared spectrum. When an 803-nm wavelength laser illuminates the surgical field, the dye is excited and fluoresces, documenting lymphatic vessels and nodes. Toxicity is in one out of 42,000 cases to include anaphylactic shock, hypotension, tachycardia, dyspnea, or urticaria. ICG-supported navigation for sentinel LN biopsy is one of the main medical diagnostic uses in gynecologic oncology.
- Potential therapeutic oncologic uses reside in the selectivity of overheating a tumor cell: As ICG absorbs light at 805 nanometers, a laser of that wavelength that can site specifically overheat fluorescing tissue without damaging surrounding tissue could provide an in vivo therapeutic treatment index. Studies have also been performed investigating targeting specific cells by conjugating the ICG to antibodies such as daclizumab, trastuzumab, or panitumumab.

Staplers[28]

Staplers are now mainly disposable instruments that are used to resect and anastamose luminal organs. They create an inverted or everted tissue closure secured by two or more rows of B-shaped titanium, absorbable, or stainless steel staples. The B shape of the staple allows noncompression with a hemostatic and leak-proof seal.

Disposable intestinal devices include the GIA and ILA. The GIA lengths are 50, 60, 80, and 90 mm and the ILA lengths are 52 and 100 mm. The length used is determined by the lumenal width of the organ/bowel. The cartridges that fit into the jaws of the device are filled with titanium staples that fire two double rows of staggered staples. The cartridge can be changed out after each firing and the stapling device reused on the same patient. The GIA staple are 3.5 mm apart and the tissue is cut between the second and third rows of the staples—thus the incision length is 8 mm short of the last staple. The staples are 3.8 or 4.8 mm in length and compress to 1.5 or 2 mm. The smaller size staples are used for small intestine, the larger for large intestine.

Circular stapling devices can be used for intestinal anastamosis, usually for lower colon/rectal/anal sites. The EEA (end-to-end anastomosis) device contains 4-mm wide staples that are 4.8 mm in length and compress to 2.0 mm. Single-use curved EEA devices come with circular cartridge diameters of 21.3, 25, 28.7, 31.6, and 34.1 mm with knife diameters of 11.5, 15, 18, 21.2, and 23.6 mm. Reusable staple devices are straight and come in lengths of 25, 28, and 31 mm. Replaceable circular cartridges are available in 25, 28.6, 31.6 mm and attach to the arm, with knife diameters of 15, 18, and 21.2 mm. To determine cartridge size, the organ lumen is measured by ovoid sizers. The EEA device is passed into the lumen of the intestine (usually through the anus), the two ends of the intestine to be anastomosed, having been secured around the cartridge using a purse-string suture, are then clamped together. When the device is fired, a circumferential double row of B-shaped titanium staples creates an inverted anastomosis between the two ends. The redundant tissue inside the staple line is removed simultaneously by the knife and should be checked to make sure there are two intact doughnuts of tissue sent to pathology. Leaks are tested by filling the pelvis with water and using a bulb syringe filled with air blown into the rectum: If no bubbles are seen, the anastomosis should be leak tight.

The TA staplers can also be reusable or disposable. These staplers usually do not cut on their own after firing staples. There are two rows of B shaped staples with cartridge sizes of 30, 55, or 90mm for the reusable devices and 30, 45, 60, and 90mm for the disposable devices. The cartridges fire 2 rows of staples except for the 90 mm cartridges which can have 3–4 rows of staples. The staples are 4mm in width, with a length of 4.8 and 3.5mm closing down to 2 and 1.5mm. These staples can articulate to accommodate pelvic curves.

Suture

The smallest gauge suture needed to obtain hemostasis is used to decrease the degree of foreign body reaction (Tables 4.4 and 4.5).

INTRAOPERATIVE COMPLICATIONS

Vascular Injury

- Venous lacerations should be repaired using 6–0 gauge Prolene sutures, in an interrupted or running fashion. Irrigation with heparinized saline can be used to visualize the repair. If the vein is large

Table 4.4 Common Suture Material and Properties

	Name	Composition	Indication	Filament	Tensile strength (lb)	Absorption	Number of knots needed	Gauge	Method of degradation
Natural absorbable	Plain catgut	Collagen from animal submucosa	Tubal ligation	Monofilament	4.4–8.4	70% at 7 days; full digestion at 70 days	3	0, 1–0	Enzyme digestion
	Chromic catgut	Collagen and chromic salts from animal submucosa	Serosal, visceral, vaginal tissues	Monofilament	4.4–8.4	50% at 10 days	3	0, 1–0	Enzyme digestion
Synthetic absorbable	Dexon	Glycolic acid	Serosal, visceral, vaginal tissues, fascia in LoR patients	Braided	6.2–11.6	50% at 14 days; 30% at 21 days	4	0, 1–0, 2–0	Hydrolysis
	Vicryl	Polyglactin 910	Serosal, visceral, vaginal tissues, fascia in LoR patients	Braided	6.2–11.6	50% at 14 days; 30% at 21 days	4	0, 1–0, 2–0	Hydrolysis
	Maxon	Polyglyconate	Fascia	Monofilament	6.2–11.6	90% at 7 days; 25% at 6 weeks	8–9	0, 1–0	Hydrolysis
Synthetic absorbable (cont.)	Polydioxanone suture	Polydioxanone	Fascia	Monofilament	6.2–11.6	90% at 7 days; 25% at 6 weeks	8–9	0, 1–0	Hydrolysis
	Monocryl	Poliglecaprone 25	Serosal, visceral, vaginal tissues under no tension	Monofilament	6.2–11.6	50% at 7 days; 30% at 21 days	8–9	0, 1–0	Hydrolysis

(continued)

Table 4.4 Common Suture Material and Properties *(continued)*

	Name	Composition	Indication	Filament	Tensile strength (lb)	Absorption	Number of knots needed	Gauge	Method of degradation
Nonabsorbable natural	Silk	Silk	Serosal, visceral tissues, inappropriate in infected tissue	Braided	3.2–6.0	50% at 1 Y; full degradation at 2 Y	3–4	0, 1–0, 2–0	Hydrolysis
Synthetic nonabsorbable	Neurolon	Nylon	Suture drains and catheters to skin	Braided	2.3–4.0	Degrades 15% per Y	4	0, 1–0, 2–0	Hydrolysis
	Dermalon	Nylon	Suture drains and catheters to skin	Monofilament	2.3–4.0	Degrades 15% per Y	8–9	0, 1–0, 2–0	Hydrolysis
	Mersilene, Dacron	Polyester	Visceral tissues	Uncoated, braided	2.3–4.0	Degrades 15% per Y	4	0, 1–0, 2–0	Hydrolysis
	Ethibond	Polyester	Visceral tissues, hernia repair	Polybutilate coated, braided	2.3–4.0	Degrades 15% per Y	8–9	0, 1–0, 2–0	Hydrolysis
	Polydek	Polyester	Visceral tissues	Teflon coated, braided	2.3–4.0	Degrades 15% per Y	8–9	0, 1–0, 2–0	Hydrolysis
	Prolene	Polypropylene	Fascia, vascular procedures, ureteral anastomosis, sacrospinous fixation	Monofilament	4.0–10.5	Degrades 15% per Y	8–9	0, 1–0	Hydrolysis

Table 4.5 Topical Hemostatic Agents Biologic and Physical Agents (Needs Coagulation Cascade Intact [No DIC])

Agent	Source	Form	Time to absorb	Mechanism of Action	Adverse Effects	Special Factors	Brand Names
Biologic Agent							
Pooled human plasma	Human	Frozen liquid	NA		Blood-borne pathogens (bacterial and viral)	Transfusion reactions, contraindicated if prior reaction	
Thrombin	Multiple	Multiple	Immediate	Converts fibrinogen to fibrin	Varies	Not effective in hypofibrinogenemia	
Recombinant thrombin	Recombinant	Powder (reconstitute with saline)				Avoid if history of snake or hamster protein sensitivity/allergy	Recothrom
Thrombin-gelatin granules	Cow and human	Liquid	4–6 weeks		See thrombin and gelatin	High cost	Surgiflol, Floseal
Bovine thrombin	Cow	Powder (reconstitute with saline)			Can form antibodies and cause coagulopathy	Re-exposure risk of allergy	Thrombin-JMI

(continued)

Table 4.5 Topical Hemostatic Agents Biologic and Physical Agents (Needs Coagulation Cascade Intact [No DIC]) *(continued)*

Agent	Source	Form	Time to absorb	Mechanism of Action	Adverse Effects	Special Factors	Brand Names
Topical tranexamic acid	Synthetic	Liquid	Immediate	Supplants plasminogen from fibrin clots and inhibits the proteolytic activity of plasmin, antifibrinolytic	Possible thromboembolic incidents		
Physical Agent							
Gelatin matrix	Pig	Powder or Sponge	4–6 weeks	Absorbs blood and fluids, forms clot over matrix, is a mechanical barrier	Foreign body formation/ granuloma, nidus for infection/ abscess	Concerns regarding expansion and compression necrosis Can moisten with thrombin	Gelfilm, gelfoam, surgifoam
Microfibrillar collagen	Cow	Powder or sponge	8–12 weeks	Activates the extrinsic coagulation cascade, establishes a framework for clot formation via platelet accumulation	Foreign body formation/ granuloma, nidus for infection/ abscess		Avitene

Oxidized regenerated cellulose	Plant	Mesh or powder	1–2 weeks	Activates the extrinsic coagulation cascade, establishes a framework for clot formation via platelet accumulation	Foreign body formation/granuloma, nidus for infection/abscess	Low pH has antimicrobial impact, do not use with topical thrombin	Surgicel
Fibrin sealant	Human	Frozen liquid	Immediate	Blends thrombin with fibrinogen to allow fibrin clot creation	Blood-borne pathogens (bacterial and viral)		Tisseel, Evicel
Microporous polysaccharide hemispheres	Plant	Powder	48 hours	Absorbs water and concentrates platelets and blood components	NA	Do not use more than 50 grams in diabetic patients as may effect blood glucose levels	Arista

Source: Data from American College of Obstetricians and Gynecologists. (2020). Topical Hemostatic Agents at Time of Obstetric and Gynecologic Surgery. Committee Opinion 812. American College of Obstetricians and Gynecologists; 2020. https://www.acog.org/clinical/clinical-guidance/committee-opinion/articles/2020/10/topical-hemostatic-agents-at-time-of-obstetric-and-gynecologic-surgery

caliber, distal and proximal control should be obtained using pressure or Judd-Allis clamps. If there is a large hole, a lesser vein can be harvested and opened using Potts scissors to create a patch and sewn in place with interrupted sutures. Omentum can be placed on top to help vascularize the site. If sutures start to tear through the vein, pledgets (small pieces of cellulose) can be used to avoid suture tension.

- Arterial damage should be approximated in a similar fashion. If the edges are ragged, consider complete resection and approximation. If there is a large hole, a vein graft can be used to patch the artery; 100 to 150 units/kg of IV heparin can be given before cross clamping the vessel. This dosing can continue every 50 minutes until circulation is re-established.

Nerve Injury
The nerve should be repaired using 7–0 gauge Prolene sutures to align the fascicle bundles. Only the epineurium should be approximated. Nerve growth is estimated at 1 mm per day, or 1 inch per month.

GI Injury
- Small-bowel injuries:
  - Serosal injuries can be observed if they are small, but should be primarily oversewn with 3–0 gauge silk or Vicryl sutures if large. If XRT has been administered, serosal injuries should always be oversewn.
  - A seromuscular injury is evident if bulging of the bowel wall is seen. Repair should be double layered with 3–0 gauge silk or Vicryl.
  - If there is luminal injury, a double-layered closure is indicated. Double-layered repair can be with 3–0 gauge Vicryl for the mucosal layer and either Vicryl or silk for the serosal layer.
- Large bowel injury should be evaluated for a transmural defect. If no transmural defect is identified, a primary single-layered repair can be performed using 3–0 gauge silk or Vicryl. If there is a transmural defect and no evidence of fecal contamination, a primary double-layer closure can be attempted. If there is an extensive defect, consideration should be given to resection with reanastomosis. If no bowel preparation was given, consideration should be given to a diverting loop or end colostomy with mucous fistula.

Urinary Tract Injury
- Urinary tract injury occurs in 1% to 2.5% of gynecologic surgeries. Intraoperative cystoscopy with 1 ampule of IV indigo carmine or 0.25 to 1.0 mg of fluorescein or PO pyridium (given preoperatively) should follow most hysterectomy procedures to detect and provide early repair of these injuries.[29–31]

- Bladder injury should be identified with direct visualization, IV fluorescein, or IV indigo carmine. The bladder should be closed in two layers using absorbable suture. This is usually with an inverting stitch of 2–0 gauge Vicryl or chromic for the first layer, and Vicryl for the second. If there is trigone injury, cystoscopy should be performed to ensure the ureters are intact. The bladder should be drained with a Foley catheter for 5 to 14 days.
- Ureteral injury is recognized at the time of surgery in 20% to 30% of cases. Injury can be via transection, ligation, crush injury, angulation, or ischemia. Injury is commonly at the level of the uterine artery, at the infundibulopelvic ligament, or at the level of the pelvic brim. Ureteral stenting should occur for most ureteral injuries. This is done via cystoscopy, cystotomy, or ureterotomy. A JP drain should be placed in all cases. If there is concern for further ureteral leakage, the JP fluid can be checked for a creatinine level and compared to a serum creatinine. Stenting is maintained for 6 to 12 weeks followed by IVP after stent removal.
  - If a crush injury is identified, the clamp should be released, and the ureter observed and mobilized. An ampule of IV indigo carmine should be given. If no extravasation is seen, consideration should be given to stenting the ureter.
  - A partial transection can be treated with stenting and primary closure using 4–0 gauge to 6–0 gauge delayed absorbable suture (PDS).
  - If there is complete transection, the ends should be dissected out, mobilized, and trimmed. The location of transection dictates repair.
    - A distal transection (below the pelvic brim) can be managed with UNC/reimplantation. There is debate as to the benefit of tunneling the ureter into the bladder. Reimplantation can also be via a Boari flap, a psoas hitch, the Demel technique, or use of intestinal interposition with an ileal segment.
    - If there is middle pelvic transection, UU or ureteroileoneocystostomy can be performed.
    - If the transection is above the pelvic brim, a transureteroureterostomy or ileal intestinal interposition can be performed. Care should be taken with a transureteroureterostomy as this procedure can compromise the opposite kidney.

Intraoperative Hemorrhage

When there is life-threatening, severe intraoperative hemorrhage, the use of a massive transfusion protocol (MTP) may be indicated. This transfusion protocol decreases the use of blood components, as well as turnaround times, costs, and mortality.[30]

- Initiate MTP.
  - Issue four units of PRBC and four units of FFP in cooler.

Table 4.6 MTP

Blood Component Prepared			
First package	4 units PRBC	4 units FFP	
Second package	4 units PRBC	4 units FFP	1 dose platelets
	Prepare cryo after second package issued.		1 dose cryoprecipitate
Third package	4 units PRBC	4 units FFP	1 dose platelets
	Prepare cryo after third package issued.		1 dose cryoprecipitate

- Once the first package is issued, prepare the second package as a "stay ahead" order and add a six-pack (1 dose) of platelets (Table 4.6).
- Once second package is issued (RBC, FFP, and platelets), begin preparing cryoprecipitate dose and set up next "stay ahead" package (RBC, FFP, platelets).
- Repeat as necessary.

POSTOPERATIVE CARE PROTOCOLS

Radical Vulvar Surgery

- Drains:
  - Groin JP drains should be discontinued when output is less than 30 mL per day.
  - Foley catheter: Depending on site of resection and reconstruction, the Foley can be left in for 7 days with prophylactic antibiotics, or removed POD 1.
- Antibiotics: Oral prophylactic antibiotics can be given starting on POD 1 and until groin and vulvar wounds are well healed. Coverage for *Streptococcus* with antibiotics has been shown to decrease the incidence of lymphedema due to beta-hemolytic *Streptococcus*.
- Wound care: This is mainly pericare with soap and water squirt bottle to the perineum TID and after each bowel movement. The area can be blown dry with a hairdryer on cool setting after each cleaning.
- DVT prophylaxis: A combination of injectable anticoagulant and SCDs should be employed until the patient is fully ambulatory. Ambulation should occur as soon as possible with control for pain, physical therapy consultation, and documentation of wound integrity.

- Nutrition: Suggest low-residue diet as tolerated.
- Complications: Lymphocysts—Percutaneous drainage can be performed if symptomatic by palpation or with image guidance; if they are recurrent, they can be sclerosed with talc, tetracyclines, or alcohol.
- Follow-up in 6 weeks

Radical Hysterectomy
- Drains:
    - JP drains: Discontinue when output is less than 30 mL/day.
    - Foley catheter: Should be discontinued POD 3 to 4. A PVR should be checked immediately after the first self-void. The Foley should be replaced if the residual volume is greater than 100 mL, and the Foley is then continued for 1 week. If at recheck, the PVR is still elevated, the patient should be educated on self-catheterization. Bladder dysfunction can occur in up to 10% of patients due to denervation from cardinal and uterosacral ligament resection.
- Antibiotics: Consider daily oral antibiotics for suppression when a Foley catheter is in place.
- Wound care: Keep clean and dry. Remove staples POD 3 for transverse or Maylard incisions. Remove staples POD 10 for midline incisions.
- DVT prophylaxis: A combination of injectable anticoagulant and SCDs should be used until the patient is fully ambulatory. Four weeks of postoperative anticoagulation should be considered. Ambulation should occur as soon as pain is controlled and strength permits.
- Nutrition: Suggest regular diet as tolerated.
- Complications: Lymphocysts can occur in up to 25% of patients, but are symptomatic in about 5% of patients. If infected or symptomatic, broad-spectrum antibiotics should be employed. Percutaneous drainage can be attempted if spontaneous resolution does not occur or if vessel or organ obstruction/compression occurs. They can also be sclerosed with talc, alcohol, or tetracyclines.
- Follow up in 6 weeks.

Urinary Conduits and Pelvic Exenteration
- Drains:
    - If a NGT was inserted during surgery, it should be removed at the end of the operation.
    - Malecot (for continent conduits): These should be placed to dependent drainage for 7 to 10 days. Irrigation every 4 to 6 hours with 40 mL of normal saline should be performed to prevent the accumulation of mucus.

- ○ Red rubber catheter in continent conduits should be left sewn in place until ready to self-catheterize at 7 to 10 days.
- ○ JP drains should be left in place for 7 to 10 days or until output is less than 30 mL/day.
- ○ Gracilis flap JP leg drains should be left in place for 7 days or until output is less than 30 mL/day.
- Antibiotics: If the patient has a conduit, consider discharge home with PO prophylaxis.
- Wound and flap care: Keep clean and dry. Pericare should be performed TID. The area can be blown dry with a hairdryer on cool setting after each cleaning. Staples should be left in place for 10 days, including those on the legs for gracilis flaps.
- DVT prophylaxis: A combination of injectable anticoagulant and SCDs should be employed until the patient is fully ambulatory. Consider 4 weeks of postoperative injectable or PO anticoagulation. Ambulation should occur as soon as pain is controlled, strength permits, and wound integrity is documented.
- Nutrition: TPN should be started postoperatively if the patient is suspected to be on NPO status for greater than 7 days or if the patient was malnourished prior to surgery. Begin PO feedings with bowel sounds.
- Complications: Evaluation of the urinary tract by IVP or US should be part of a postoperative fever workup. Stomas should be checked daily; if they are dusky, endoscopy should be performed.
- Ureteral stents should be sewn in with chromic suture, which will spontaneously dissolve and separate between days 10 and 14.
- On admission to the recovery room, CXR should be obtained if a central line was inserted.
- Follow-up should occur at 2 weeks and 6 weeks.
- Lab tests: BUN and creatinine levels should be obtained at each visit.
- Radiologic studies: an IVP should be obtained at discharge, 6 weeks, 6 months, 18 months, 3 Y, and 5 Y. A CT of abdomen and pelvis can be considered every 6 months to 1 Y.

Bowel Resection
- Drains:
  - ○ NGT can be removed immediately after surgery. If there was obstruction preoperatively, the NGT can remain until bowel function returns.
  - ○ If multiple enterotomies occurred, JP peritoneal drains can be placed to check for bowel leak or fistula. Leave drains in until fluid output is serosanguinous.

- ○ SC JP drains: These can be discontinued when the output is less than 30 mL/day.
- ○ Foley: This can be discontinued on POD 1.
- Antibiotics: These should only be used postoperatively if gross peritoneal contamination occurs with bowel contents. They can be discontinued on POD 2 to 3 if the patient is afebrile.
- Wound care: Vertical midline staples should remain in place for 10 days. Patients with transverse incisions can have their staples removed between days 3 and 5.
- DVT prophylaxis: A combination of injectable anticoagulant and SCDs should be employed until the patient is fully ambulatory. Consider 4 weeks of injectable or PO postoperative anticoagulation. Ambulation should occur as soon as pain is controlled and strength permits.
- Nutrition: Consider TPN if there is prolonged ileus for more than 7 days, postoperative obstruction occurs, or the patient was malnourished preoperatively.

Ovarian Cancer Debulking

- Drains:
  - ○ If a NGT was placed due to obstruction, this can be removed when bowel function returns.
  - ○ JP peritoneal drain: These will always have output, especially if there was a large amount of ascites.
  - ○ SC drains: Discontinue when output is less than 30 mL/day.
  - ○ Foley: Discontinue on POD 1 if adequate urine output. Urine output is commonly low due to third spacing from surgery and ascites removal. Homeostasis tends to return by POD 3, and urine output normalizes around then.
- Antibiotics: These should only be used postoperatively if gross peritoneal contamination occurs with bowel contents. They can be discontinued on POD 2 to 3 if the patient is afebrile.
- Wound care: Vertical midline staples should remain for 10 days. Patients with transverse incisions can have their staples removed between days 3 and 5.
- DVT prophylaxis: A combination of injectable anticoagulant and SCDs should be employed until the patient is fully ambulatory. Consider 4 weeks of postoperative injectable or PO anticoagulation. Ambulation should occur as soon as pain is controlled and strength permits.
- Nutrition: Consider TPN if there is prolonged ileus for more than 7 days, postoperative obstruction occurs, or the patient was malnourished preoperatively.

Enhanced Recovery Pathways

- Enhanced recovery is encouraged for most surgical patients. This includes:
  - Early ambulation
  - Advancement of diet as tolerated
  - Removal of the Foley catheter in uncomplicated patients by 24 hours
  - Use of DVT prophylaxis with SCDs and SC: Q8h heparin 5,000 IU TID, enoxaparin 40 mg/day, or dalteparin 5,000 IU daily. Use of oral VKAs and DOACs has also recently been studied, including apixaban 2.5 mg PO BID
  - Minimal use of NGT decompression
  - Aggressive nausea and emesis prophylaxis
  - Minimization of IV narcotics and early discontinuation of the PCA with transition to oral narcotics as soon as PO nutrition is tolerated

Enhanced Recovery After Surgery

- Goals are to decrease surgical stress and to reduce the consequences of induced stress. This is obtained by implementing and bundling multiple elements, to form a comprehensive perioperative management program.
- The basic principles of ERAS include attention to the following:
  - Preoperative
    - Counseling
    - Nutritional supplementation
    - Avoidance of lengthy perioperative fasting
  - Perioperative attempts for regional anesthetic
    - Nonopioid analgesic approaches
    - Fluid balance
    - Maintenance of normothermia
  - Postoperative recovery strategies
    - Early mobilization
    - Early diet advancement
    - Thromboprophylaxis
- The benefits of ERAS pathways include shorter LOS, decreased postoperative pain and need for analgesia, quicker return of bowel function, decreased complication and readmission rates, and increased patient satisfaction.
- Implementation of ERAS protocols has not been shown to increase readmission, mortality, or reoperation rates.

Notable Studies

- Outcomes of ERAS in gynecologic oncology—A systematic review and meta-analysis[32]: This meta-analysis included 31 studies and 6,703 patients were included. A meta-analysis of 27 studies (6,345 patients) demonstrated a decrease in LOS of 1.6 days (95% CI, 1.2–2.1) with ERAS implementation. Meta-analysis of 21 studies (4,974 patients) demonstrated a 32% reduction in complications (OR, 0.68; 95% CI: 0.55–0.83) and a 20% reduction in readmission (OR, 0.80; 95% CI: 0.64–0.99) for ERAS patients. There was no difference in 30-day postoperative mortality (OR, 0.61; 95% CI: 0.23–1.6) for ERAS patients compared to controls. The mean cost savings for ERAS patients was $2,129 USD (95% CI: $712– $3544). Thus, ERAS protocols decrease LOS, complications, and cost without increasing rates of readmission or mortality in gynecologic oncology surgery[33]

Opiates
- Gynecologic oncologists encounter a broad range of reasons to prescribe opioids: from management of acute postoperative pain to chronic cancer-related pain to end-of-life care.[34]
  - The goals of pain management in cancer care are to optimize the five dimensions of pain management outcomes (The 5 A's)[35]:
    - Analgesia (optimize pain relief)
    - Activities (optimize daily functional activities)
    - Adverse effects (minimize AEs from opiates)
    - Aberrant drug taking (avoid aberrant drug consumption and minimize addiction)
    - Affect: Relationship between pain and mood

POSTOPERATIVE COMPLICATIONS

GI Complications
- Ileus
  - The etiology is often intraoperative manipulation, electrolyte abnormalities, narcotics, peritonitis, abscess, hematoma, or fistula.
  - Signs are nausea and vomiting, hypoactive or absent bowel sounds, and abdominal distension.
  - Workup is with laboratories and physical examination.
  - Treatment: The patient can be put on NPO status, IVF initiated, and consideration given to an NGT. If the ileus does not resolve, imaging can be obtained with a CT scan of the abdomen and pelvis with oral Gastrografin contrast to rule out an obstruction. Abdominal

imaging provides no difference in clinical treatment between obstruction and ileus as they will both be managed with NPO/NGT/electrolyte replacement upfront. If abscess is seen with CT, a percutaneous drain can be placed with antibiotics as indicated.

- Bowel obstructions: Partial obstructions can resolve spontaneously in 50% of cases. Complete obstructions usually need surgical intervention.
  - Small bowel obstruction (SBO)
    - The etiology can be adhesions or herniation from surgery, bowel kinking, tumor, XRT-induced ischemia, and stricture.
    - Signs are nausea and vomiting. Bowel sounds are present and can be high pitched and hyperactive. Abdominal distension is present, and absence of flatus is common.
    - Workup is with lab tests, a physical examination, and CT scan of the abdomen and pelvis with PO Gastrografin contrast.
    - The patient should be made NPO, an NGT placed to LIWS, pain medication administered, and IVF should be initiated. Correction of electrolyte abnormalities is important in addition to antiemetics and pain management. Occasionally, high-dose steroids can reduce periluminal inflammation and have antiemetic properties. Partial obstructions can resolve with conservative management, but fewer than 50% of complete obstructions resolve similarly.
  - Large bowel obstruction (LBO)
    - Etiology can be a mass causing obstruction intrinsically (intraluminal tumor), extrinsically (pelvic tumor compression), or stricture from transmural invasion.
    - Signs: LBO can have a delayed time to presentation with a lower amount of emesis.
    - Workup is indicated with imaging:
      - CT scan of abdomen and pelvis with Gastrografin should be obtained. This can document the site of obstruction and may occasionally be therapeutic.
      - Barium enema: This can occasionally be therapeutic. This study should be performed before a CT scan or SBFT.
    - To manage conservatively: The patient should be made NPO, an NGT should be placed to LIWS, IV fluids and pain control should be instituted, and antiemetics should be given.
    - To manage surgically:
      - IV second-generation cephalosporins should be given prior to surgical correction.
      - Resection with end-to-end anastomosis, loop, or end ostomy with mucous fistula can be performed.

- □ Stenting may occasionally be useful if the patient is a poor surgical candidate.
- Enemas in partial LBO can either be therapeutic or can convert the obstruction to a complete obstruction by inducing colonic spasm.
  - □ If the patient chooses to forego extensive surgery, consider endoscopy with stent placement or diversion via end ostomy.
  - □ When considering whether to perform surgical reduction of an obstruction in a cancer patient, it is important to take into account the patient's social factors, the expected outcome, the patient's life expectancy, and the etiology and the extent of obstruction (e.g., recurrent cancer, XRT stenosis).
- Bowel perforation:
  - ○ Etiology: Perforation can occur from an unrecognized enterotomy, intestinal devascularization, tumor infiltration of the bowel wall, bowel infarction (from thrombus, atrial fibrillation), or even certain chemotherapy agents (bevacizumab up to 1%–11%, paclitaxel 2%).
  - ○ Signs are peritonitis, pain, abdominal distension, and fever.
  - ○ Workup: Imaging is needed with abdominal x-ray or CT demonstrating free air under the diaphragm. Treatment is with emergent surgical exploration and antibiotics. Cecal perforation tends to occur if the cecum is dilated ≥10 cm as seen on imaging.
  - ○ Treatment is with loop or end ostomy with mucous fistula, or ileostomy.
- Pneumoperitoneum after laparotomy should be considered when ruling out a bowel perforation. Table 4.7 demonstrates the time from surgery and the percentage of patients with residual abdominal air present. Table 4.7
- Anastomotic bowel leak after a bowel resection can occur in up to 15% of patients. Prevention is avoidance of the bowel watershed areas. When performing an anastomosis, universal principles should be followed, ensuring adequate vascularization of both ends of the bowel, absence of tumor at the anastomotic site, a tension-free

Table 4.7 Pneumoperitoneum Duration Seen Radiologically After Surgery

Time	Radiograph Positive (%)	CT Scan Positive (%)
POD 3	53	87
POD 6	8	50

anastomosis, and an adequate bowel lumen. Bowel viability can be ascertained with IV fluorescein dye and a Wood's lamp at the time of resection and reanastomosis, or with Doppler US.

- o Signs: Leaks tend to present with nausea, ileus, abdominal pain, fever, and occasionally leakage of feculent material through the wound.

- o Workup: Includes physical exam, lab tests, and a CT of the abdomen and pelvis with PO Gastrografin.

- o Treatment: A drain needs to be placed, the patient made NPO, broad-spectrum antibiotics given, and consideration given to surgical intervention with intestinal diversion. The diversion can usually be taken down in about 2 months, after imaging with PO contrast shows no evidence of continued leakage or after completion of chemotherapy in abdominal cancer patients and no evidence of recurrent disease (6–12 months).

- o Risk factors for anastomotic leak: A retrospective study investigated 695 patients with ovarian cancer who underwent primary anastomosis between 2010 and 2018.[36] Twelve pre-/intraoperative variables were analyzed as potential risk factors for anastomotic leak. The anastomotic leak rate was 6.6% (46 patients; range 1.7%–12.5%). A total of 457 patients were included in the final multivariate analysis. The following variables were found to be independently associated with anastomotic leakage: age at surgery (OR, 1.046; 95% CI: 1.013–1.080, p = .005), serum albumin level (OR, 0.621; 95% CI: 0.407–0.948, p = .027), one or more additional small-bowel resections (OR, 3.544; 95% CI,: 1.228–10.23, p =.019), manual anastomosis (OR, 8.356; 95% CI: 1.777–39.301, p = .007) and distance of the anastomosis from the anal verge (OR, 0.839; 95% CI: 0.726–0.971, p = .018). Thus, a restrictive protective stoma policy based on the presence of risk factors should be the actual recommendation because of the low rate of anastomotic lead and hand-sewn anastomosis should be avoided.

- Bowel fistula (enterocutaneous, enterovaginal, enterovesicle):
  - o Signs: Fistulae can present as feculent discharge from a surgical wound, urine, or the vagina.

  - o Workup: Diagnosis is with a CT of the abdomen and pelvis with PO Gastrografin contrast or a fistulagram. Oral activated charcoal or isosulfan blue can also be given to evaluate for color change that would indicate a fistula.

  - o Treatment: An NGT should be placed, the patient made NPO, and TPN) initiated. Wound care should be performed, and consideration given to administration of somatostatin. If there is no resolution of the fistula with these conservative measures, surgical resection of the fistulous tract with bowel resection and temporary diversion or primary reanastomosis with protective loop ileostomy should be performed. Staged repair with a diverting loop colostomy, primary fistula repair, and ostomy takedown approximately 2 months later is the preferred option as massive inflammation can hamper primary anastomosis and compromise fistula repair.

- Stoma complications usually involve stomal retraction or devitalization.
  - Etiology: This occurs from tension or decreased blood flow to the distal bowel edges.
  - Signs include a dusky appearance, necrosis, or retraction.
  - Workup: Evaluation of viability includes placement of a test tube or blood vial inside the stoma to assess the depth/extent of damage.
  - Treatment is based on location of devitalization. If it is limited to the distal segment above the fascia, observation and wound care are indicated. If there is necrosis beneath the fascia, surgical revision is necessary.
- Ostomy herniation or prolapse usually occurs in patients whose ostomy was placed lateral to the rectus muscles.
  - Prolapse occurs in 1% to 3% of patients with an ostomy.
    - Etiology: Prolapse is often due to a stoma that is too long or wide, increased intra-abdominal pressure, extensive weight loss, or a redundant sigmoid colon.
    - Treatment: Conservative measures are placement of a rigid appliance with a tight belt. Treatment is resection of the protruding segment of colon with nipple reconstruction. Care should be taken to rule out those with a hernia so there is no loop transection risk.
  - Parastomal hernia: One half of patients with a prolapse also have a parastomal hernia.
    - Etiology: Parastomal hernias occur more often with loop ostomies than with end stomas. Two to 3% of all end colostomy patients require hernia repair. Predisposing factors are often too large of an opening in the abdominal wall, placement lateral to the rectus muscle, placement in the laparotomy incision itself, or increased intra-abdominal pressure due to COPD, coughing, heavy lifting, obesity.
    - Repair is indicated if the hernia does not reduce easily, there is evidence of incarceration, or if the hernia interferes with appliance security. If the hernia is small, primary fascial repair without relocation can often be accomplished. If it is large, the ostomy can be placed at a different site (to a higher midrectus

position, to the opposite side, or to the umbilicus) with repair of the primary ventral hernia. Mesh can otherwise be placed over part of the fascial defect to reduce the defect size (Sugarbaker) and the stoma can be brought out in between an aperture between the mesh and the skin. To initiate the repair, the skin should be elliptically excised, and a finger swept circumferentially around the bowel between it and the fascia.

- *Short bowel syndrome* is defined as malnutrition due to the lack of absorptive bowel length.
  - Etiology: This can occur from significant bowel resection or from XRT injury. A length of bowel, approximately 200 cm, is necessary for nutrient absorption.
  - Signs: Symptoms include diarrhea, steatorrhea, fluid depletion, fatigue, and occasionally abdominal pain.
  - Diagnosis is made by malnutrition indices and weight loss.
  - Treatment is with caloric, vitamin, and mineral supplementation. Hyperalimentation with TPN or continuous G-tube nutrition should be considered if there is significant weight loss. In addition, antacids, antidiarrheals, and lactase supplements should be given.
- Blind loop syndrome:
  - Etiology: Occurs after bowel resection and bypass, producing a nonfunctional but retained loop of bowel.
  - Signs: Look for increased flatulence, steatorrhea, weight loss, fatigue, and malabsorption.
  - Diagnosis: A hydrogen breath test using glucose or lactulose can assist in the diagnosis. Bacterial overgrowth causes the majority of symptoms.
  - Treatment: Antibiotics can reduce the bacterial load and decrease symptoms. Vitamin B_{12} supplementation is also often indicated.

Hemorrhage

- Etiology:
  - Blood loss from the GI system can occur from a stomach ulcer, esophageal varices, a Mallory–Weiss tear, a Boerhaave tear, NGT/catheter erosion, tumor erosion, or XRT enteritis.
  - Inadequate hemostasis can arise from a slipped suture, coagulopathy, or overanticoagulation.
  - Tumor can spontaneously bleed from neovascularization.
- Symptoms can include tachycardia, ectopy, pain, abdominal distension, decreased perfusion with mental status changes from hypoxia, low urine output from renal compromise, or extremity cyanosis due to centralization of the blood supply. Diagnosis is geared to identification of the source.

- Workup: laboratoy tests include CBC coagulation profile, and electrolytes. Imaging studies include CT, MRI, US, or angiography.
- Treatment is focused on the "ABCs." Resuscitation is with IVF (in a 3:1 crystalloid replacement ratio to blood loss), blood products, and oxygen. Treatment is surgical (re)-exploration, angiographic embolization, or reversal of coagulopathies.
- If hemorrhage is due to a large cervical tumor, vaginal packing with Monsel's solution is indicated. The packing should be changed every 24 to 48 hours. Embolization can be considered but this can decrease oxygenation needed for XRT to the primary tumor. Emergent hyperfractionated XRT can also be given.
- If hemorrhage is from brachytherapy application, evaluation for perforation versus vascular disruption should be obtained via imaging. If vascular, Monsels applied to vaginal packing is indicated. If perforation is found, proceeding to the operating room is indicated.

Postoperative Fever

Fever is the most common postoperative complication. The definition of *fever* is a temperature elevation taken two times, 6 hours apart. If the fever occurs within the first 24 hours of surgery, the temperature must be above 101.5°F (38.6°C). If the fever occurs more than 24 hours after surgery, the temperature must be greater than or equal to 100.4°F (38.1°C).

- The source of the fever usually follows the "five W's":
  - Wind: This can represent atelectasis or pneumonia. Obtain a CXR.
  - Water: This can represent a UTI or pyelonephritis. Obtain a urine analysis/culture.
  - Wound: This can represent a superficial infection, a seroma, cellulitis, or abscess. Evaluation involves examination, consideration of imaging, and occasionally opening of the incision.
  - Walk: This can represent a DVT, septic pelvic thrombophlebitis, or a PE. Diagnosis is via examination, measurement of calf diameter, Doppler US, and occasionally CT angiogram.
  - Wonder drugs: This can result from drug fevers. This is a diagnosis of exclusion. After ruling out other causes, consideration of discontinuing all drugs and observing the patient may be beneficial. Evaluation of the WBC differential may be helpful by assessing for the degree of eosinophilia.

Wound Infection

- SSIs account for 40% of nosocomial infections. Risk factors for infection include surgery lasting longer than 2 hours, higher blood loss, preoperative anemia, hypothermia, poor nutrition, cancer, prior XRT, diabetes, obesity, PVD, and a history of prior surgical infections.

- ○ Whole-body cleansing with chlorhexidine can reduce bacterial skin counts, but they do not reduce the rate of wound infection. Alternatively, patients may shower normally before surgery.
- ○ Hair clipping, not shaving, reduces the rate of wound infections.
- ○ Antibiotics given 1 hour before the skin incision are recommended, except for vancomycin and the fluoroquines, which should be given 2 hours prior. Cefazolin has a longer half-life and a broad spectrum of coverage. Cefotetan is preferred in longer, radical gynecologic operations and in colorectal surgery. Alternatives are aztreonam and clindamycin, cefazolin plus metronidazole, or ampicillin–sulbactam. If the patient's weight is greater than 70 kg, it is important to weight-base the antibiotics dosage.
- ○ Repeat dosing is recommended if surgery lasts longer than 3 to 4 hours, or if there is greater than 1,000 mL of blood loss. Antibiotics should be stopped within 24 hours of surgery to decrease bacterial resistance and complications.
- ○ Obese patients have a higher risk for postoperative complications due to their body habitus and medical comorbidities. Some providers suggest these patients have baseline PFTs, assisted intubation, and delayed extubation until they are fully awake. Higher weight capacity hospital beds and operating room tables, specialized retractors, and extra-long instruments for surgery are important. A panniculectomy can be performed to improve surgical exposure.
- • Classification of operative wound infections is standardized.
  - ○ **A clean operative wound** has a 1% to 2% risk of a surgical wound infection. This means that the GI, GU, and respiratory tracts were not entered, no drains were placed, and there was no break in aseptic technique. Examples of these surgeries are elective hernia repair.
  - ○ **A clean contaminated wound** has a 4% to 10% risk of a surgical wound infection in uninfected patients. The GI, GU, or respiratory tracts were entered but minimal contamination occurred. This includes hysterectomy, appendectomy, and most elective bowel surgery.
  - ○ **A contaminated operative wound** has a 20% risk of surgical wound infection. This means there may have been a major break in sterile technique, the wound was made through nonpurulent inflammation, there was gross spill from the GI tract, or the wound was in or near contaminated skin. An example of this is a laparotomy in a patient with a colostomy.
  - ○ **An infected/dirty surgical wound** has a 50% risk of wound infection. This occurs in a wound in which purulent infection or a perforated viscus was encountered. An example is a localized bowel perforation.

Urinary Tract Injury

- When injury occurs it is unrecognized in 70% of patients.
  - Signs of injury include flank pain, fever, ileus from urine, hematuria, an elevated creatinine, or serous wound drainage (vaginal or abdominal).
  - Diagnosis is with renal US, IVP, CT with IV contrast, or cystoscopy with an attempt to pass ureteral stents.
  - Treatment is with antibiotics and ureteral stenting or PCN to decompress the kidney and preserve renal function. Delay of definitive repair until 4 to 6 weeks should occur if the patient is unstable from other comorbidities. Recent data support repair at the time of diagnosis if the patient is stable.
- Postoperative fistulae can be either uretero-vaginal or vesico-vaginal. Symptoms are leakage of clear fluid vaginally. Diagnosis is with a tampon test: This is performed with retrograde filling of the bladder using indigo carmine or methylene blue and placement of a vaginal tampon. If the tampon turns blue, the fistula originates in the bladder. If the tampon does not turn blue, phenazopyridine (Pyridium) can be given PO. If the tampon then turns orange, the fistula is most likely of ureteral origin.
  - Uretero-vaginal fistulas tend to become apparent 5 to 14 days postoperatively. Attempts at retrograde stenting should be made first. PCN with antegrade stenting is the next best step. If stenting is not possible, PCN with drainage should be performed.
  - Vesico-vaginal fistulas should first be treated with prolonged bladder drainage in an attempt to allow spontaneous healing. If this does not work, repair is via the vaginal or abdominal approach. Vaginal repairs are with a modified Latzko technique, or a bulbocavernosus flap. If prior XRT was given, a flap is needed to provide vascularized tissue.
  - Fistula that occurs from a neobladder should be managed conservatively. An abdominal drain and PCN should be placed. If surgical intervention is attempted, there is a 9% mortality rate and 53% rate of complications.

Lymphatic Complications

- Lymphedema mainly occurs from surgical LND. Less commonly, it can be due to XRT or tumor infiltration. Woody edema is the main symptom. Treatment is with elevation of the leg, support hose, or pneumatic compression devices.
- Lymphangitis can present as acute erythema of the extremity, fever, and pain. It usually occurs after surgical LND with superimposed infection. Treatment is with elevation of the leg, antibiotics, and NSAIDs.

- Lymphocysts occur after LND. Signs are a palpable cystic mass and pain. Diagnosis is via US, CT, or MRI. Treatment depends on symptoms. If the patient is asymptomatic, observation is enough. If there are symptoms, from pressure or mass effect, the cyst can be aspirated or sclerosed. If there are symptoms from infection, drainage with broad-spectrum antibiotics and NSAIDs is indicated.

Nerve Injury
- Neuropathy can complicate any surgical procedure. Neuropathy stems from positioning, retractors, or direct nerve injury from dissection. Symptoms are sharp or burning pain, paresthesias, and weakness in the affected muscle groups. Treatment is often supportive care with physical therapy. If there is extensive deficit, a neurology consult can be obtained and electromyograms can assist in assessment.
- Nerve transection: See Chapter 7 for more information.

PERIOPERATIVE MANAGEMENT OF MEDICAL COMORBIDITIES

Enhanced Recovery Pathways in Gynecologic Oncology
Accelerated recovery with multimodal postoperative clinical pathways has been shown to improve outcomes. It starts in the preoperative period and continues through hospitalization.

- Bowel prep continues to be controversial: Infection and anastomotic leak were reviewed in patients with a bowel preparation; results were 9.6% and 4.4%, respectively, with a preparation, compared to 8.5% and 4.5%, respectively, for those without a preparation.
- Overnight fasting: Longer fasting causes untoward metabolic changes and depletion of liver glycogen stores. Therefore, a regimen of 6 hours of no solid food and 2 hours of a clear-liquid diet is advised.
- Intraoperative fluid management: Euvolemia is the goal. Seven percent versus 24% of patients had CV complications when zero balance was the goal versus a standard 3-kg to 7-kg increase of fluid. In patients with sepsis, an average 12 L of fluid overload occurred, which took 3 weeks to mobilize. Pulmonary congestion, edema, hyponatremia, and CHF tend to occur with too much IVF.
- Postoperative pain control: Epidural versus PCA have been compared showing earlier discharge with PCA. Those with an epidural had a longer time to first ambulation, higher rate of pressor use during surgery, and pain control was equivalent or lower than those with a PCA (due to a 30% failure rate of epidural analgesia). Toradol has been shown to provide excellent pain control and is equivalent to opioid relief with no increase in postoperative bleeding or anastomotic leaks.

- Prophylactic drains are not indicated except in those with very low anterior resections (an anastomosis within 6 cm of the anal verge). NGT drainage is contraindicated prophylactically.[37]

Vascular Thromboembolism

- DVT/ vascular thromboembolism (VTE) **prophylaxis** should be given to most hospitalized patients. The gynecologic oncology patient population is a high-risk group.
  - Pneumatic SCDs should be used. Use should start preoperatively, continue intraoperatively, and continue postoperatively.
  - A low-dose injectable anticoagulant should be considered prior to surgery. The normal dose of heparin is 5,000 units SC before surgery. Dalteparin dosed at 5,000 units SC can be given before surgery. Enoxaparin can also be used at 40 mg SC before surgery.
  - In-hospital prophylaxis of DVT: The combination of SCDs and injectable anticoagulants is especially helpful for the prevention of VTE complications. The use of SCDs has taken the incidence of VTE from 25% to 8%. The use of combination therapy then took the VTE occurrence from 8% to 2%. Dosing is usually with UFH 5,000 every 8 hours or enoxaparin 30 to 40 mg daily. The risk of DVT with laparoscopic surgery in high-risk cancer patients with appropriate prophylaxis is 1.2%.[38] Care should be taken and SCDs not used if an active SVT or DVT are present because of potential embolization. Graduated compression stockings have not been found to decrease DVTs.[39–41] If there is a contraindication to anticoagulation prophylaxis, mechanical prophylaxis alone should be used.
    - **Contraindications to mechanical prophylaxis:**
      - Absolute: Acute SVT/DVT, severe arterial insufficiency
      - Relative: Large hematoma, skin ulcerations or wounds, thrombocytopenia (platelets <20,000/mcL) or petechiae, mild arterial insufficiency, peripheral neuropathy
    - **Contraindications to prophylactic or therapeutic anticoagulation:**
      - Absolute: Recent CNS bleed, intracranial or spinal lesion at high risk for bleeding, active bleeding (major) with more than two units PRBC transfused in 24 hours.
      - Relative: Chronic clinically significant measurable bleeding is seen for more than 48 hours, thrombocytopenia (platelets <50,000/mcL), severe platelet dysfunction (uremia, medications, dysplastic hematopoiesis), recent major operation at high risk for bleeding, underlying hemorrhagic coagulopathy, and high risk for falls (head trauma).
- Risk factors for VTE include: Known malignancy, surgery, surgical time greater than 2 to 3 hours, postoperative immobility, a past history of VTE, BMI greater than 30, hereditary coagulopathy, age 60 Y

Table 4.8 VTE Risk Factors in Cancer Patients: Khorana Predictive Model for Chemotherapy-Associated VTE

Patient Characteristic	Risk Score
Site of primary cancer	2
Very high risk: stomach, pancreas	1
High-risk lung, lymphoma, gynecologic, bladder, testicular	1
Prechemotherapy platelet count 350,000/mcL or higher	1
Hg level less than 10 g/dL or use of red cell growth factors	1
Prechemotherapy WBC higher than 11,000/mcL	1
BMI 35 kg/m2 or higher	1

Total score	Risk category	Risk of symptomatic VTE
0	Low	0.8%–3%
1.2	Intermediate	1.8%–4%
3 or more	High	1%–41%

Source: Adapted from Kumar A, Langstraat CL, DeJong SR, et al. Functional not chronologic age: Frailty index predicts outcomes in advanced ovarian cancer. *Gynecol Oncol.* 2017;147(1):104–109:S0090-8258(17)31163-0. doi: 10.1016/j.ygyno.2017.07.1265; Zhang G, Zhang Y, He F, et al. Preoperative controlling nutritional status (CONUT) score is a prognostic factor for early-stage cervical cancer patients with high-risk factors. *Gynecol Oncol.* 2021;162(3):763–769:S0090-8258(21)00492-3. doi: 10.1016/j.ygyno.2021.06.012.

or older, HTN, renal disease, pulmonary disease, estrogen use, IBD, and hereditary coagulopathies (MTHFR deficiency, protein C/protein S deficiencies, prothrombin gene mutation, antithrombin III and factor V Leiden gene mutations, antinuclear antibodies, antiphospholipid antibodies; Table 4.8).

- Symptoms of a SVT/DVT are leg edema, erythema, size discrepancy between the legs, pain, heaviness, persistent cramping, cyanosis of extremity, swelling in the neck of supraclavicular area.
- Positive physical signs are: the Pratt's, Homan's, and Moses's tests.
- Diagnosis is with: Doppler US or CT with IV contrast.
- Treatment
  - SVT that is not close to the deep venous system or is a peripheral catheter-related clot: Remove the catheter, treat symptoms with heating pad, anti-inflammatory medications, and elevation of extremity.
  - SVT in close proximity to deep venous system in a surgical or oncologic patient: Strongly consider therapeutic anticoagulation for 6 weeks and up to 12 weeks if close to the femoral system.

○ Pelvic/iliac/IVC/femoral/popliteal DVT:
  ▪ Therapeutic anticoagulation is indicated.
  ▪ If there is contraindication to anticoagulation:
    □ Placement of an IVC filter is indicated.
○ Upper extremity or superior vena cava DVT:
  ▪ Therapeutic anticoagulation is indicated.
  ▪ If there is contraindication to anticoagulation: Follow clinically until contraindication is resolved.
○ Catheter-related DVT:
  ▪ Therapeutic anticoagulation is indicated for as long as the catheter is in place. If the catheter is removed, the total duration of anticoagulation should be at least 3 months. Consider catheter-directed pharmaco-mediated thrombolysis in appropriate patients.
  ▪ If there is a contraindication to anticoagulation, remove the catheter.

- PE can occur following a DVT. If DVT is untreated, 15% to 25% progress to PE. If treated, 1.6% to 4.5% can still progress to PE, with 0.9% being fatal.
  ○ Symptoms include tachypnea (90%), tachycardia (45%), hemoptysis (30%), cyanosis (20%), and a sense of impending doom (50%–65%).
  ○ Workup includes: CT angiogram/spiral CT of the chest, identification of the original thrombus with lower extremity Doppler (if Dopplers are negative a pelvic CT should follow), a CXR, an ELISA D-dimer (which has a NPV of 99.5%), an ABG (the PO_2 is often <80 in 85% of patients) with calculation of the A-a gradient, cardiac enzymes to include troponin, and baseline coagulation studies.
    ▪ A normal A-a gradient is 5 to 10 mmHg but increases with age and FiO_2. A conservative estimate is: (age in Y/4) + 4.
    ▪ A-a gradient = [(FiO_2) × (Atmospheric pressure − H_2O pressure) − ($PaCO_2/0.8$)] − PaO_2
    ▪ A CXR has a sensitivity of 33%, a specificity of 59%. Signs on CXR are an elevated hemidiaphragm (50%), the Hampton's hump due to a pleural-based infiltrate pointed toward the hilum, Westmark's sign (dilated proximal vessels with a distal cutoff), a pleural effusion, and atelectasis.
    ▪ An EKG showing RBBB or a right axis shift can be helpful.
    ▪ If chest spiral CT/CT angiogram is contraindicated, a V/Q scan can be obtained with probabilities of PE represented as low, intermediate, or high. If the probabilities are intermediate or high, it is important to confirm with echocardiogram to evaluate right-heart strain.

- Echocardiogram can contribute to primary workup in the diagnosis of PE documenting increased right heart strain, dilation, and pressures.

- Treatment of PE is with supportive care and therapeutic anticoagulation. Oxygen is titrated to keep saturations greater than 92%. Echocardiogram can evaluate for pulmonary HTN and right-heart failure. Cardiac support can be given with IV or PO medications. Consider thrombolytic therapy for massive PE or submassive PE with moderate to severe right heart enlargement or dysfunction. Embolectomy either via interventional radiology or surgery is another option, with IVC filter placement. Anticoagulants are dosed the same as for DVT. If there is a contraindication to anticoagulation, consider an IVC filter and embolectomy with frequent evaluation for change in clinical status, continually assessing for changed indication to initiate therapeutic anticoagulation. IVC filter removal is recommended if anticoagulation therapy is tolerated. Filters are only permanent for rare patients with contraindications to anticoagulation.
  - Thrombolytic agents:
    - Altplase (tPA) 0.5 to 1 mg/hr IV; or 100 mg IV over 2 hours
    - Reteplase 0.25 to 0.75 units/hr IV
    - Tenecteplase 0.25 to 0.5 mg/hr IV
  - Contraindications to thrombolysis:
    - Absolute: History of hemorrhagic stroke; intracranial tumor; ischemic stroke in prior 3 months; history of major trauma, surgery, or head injury in prior 3 weeks; platelet count below 100,000/mcL; active bleeding; bleeding diathesis
    - Relative: Age greater than 75, pregnancy or first postpartum week, noncompressible puncture sites, traumatic resuscitation, refractory HTN greater than 180/100 mmHg, advanced liver disease, infective endocarditis, GI bleed in last 3 months, short life expectancy less than 12 months
  - An **IVC filter** can be placed to prevent re/embolization: Indications are absolute contradiction to therapeutic anticoagulation, a PE despite adequate anticoagulation, chronic PE with associated pulmonary HTN, the patient is status post a pulmonary embolectomy, baseline cardiopulmonary dysfunction is severe enough to make a new or recurrent PE life-threatening, significant heparin-induced thrombocytopenia, and patient noncompliance with anticoagulation. Another indication is the need for urgent surgery in a patient with a recent history of DVT, on anticoagulation,who needs temporary discontinuation for a procedure.

- **Therapeutic anticoagulation** is achieved with heparin, dalteparin, enoxaparin, or fondaparinux. It is important not to use SCDs when a DVT is diagnosed due to the risk of clot embolization.

- ○ Dosing:
  - Heparin is given IV and dosed at 80 units/kg bolus, then 18 units/hr with a targeted aPTT of 2 to 2.5 × hospital control.
  - Dalteparin is dosed at 200 units/kg SC every 24 hours or 100 units/kg SC every 12 hours.
  - Enoxaparin is dosed at 1 mg/kg SC every 12 hours. It is possible to convert to a daily dosing schedule of 1.5 mg/kg after 3 days of every-12-hour dosing.
  - Fondaparinux is dosed SC daily at 5 mg if less than 50 kg, 7.5 mg if 50 to 100 kg, or 10 mg if greater than 100 kg body weight .
  - Heparin can also be dosed SC 333 units/kg load, then 250 units/kg every 12 hours.
  - DOAC are not recommended.
- Conversion to PO anticoagulation is usually with DOAC's or warfarin. This is to start after 3 days of IV heparin or SC therapeutic anticoagulation with a 5-day overlap for warfarin due to rebound coagulopathy. It is important to follow the INR to keep it 2 to ×3 normal. Duration of treatment is 3 to 6 months for DVT diagnosis, and 6 to 12 months for a diagnosis of PE. Consider lifetime anticoagulation if there is a diagnosis of cancer, hereditary coagulopathy, or arterial thrombosis.
- Drug interactions with Coumadin can affect the INR. These include erythromycin, sulphas, INH, fluconazole, amiodarone, corticosteroids, cimetidine, omeprazole, lovastatin, phenytoin, and propranolol. If the patient is malnourished, is vegetarian, or has liver disease, a lower dose may be needed. If the patient eats large quantities of green leafy vegetables, the patient may have increased levels of vitamin K and be more difficult to anticoagulate.
- There are data to suggest that continued injectable anticoagulation is better in patients with malignancy than warfarin (CANTHANOX and LITE studies).[42,43] There are also data to suggest better PFS and OS in patients receiving injectable anticoagulation (FAMOUS and CLOT studies)[44,45]
- **Postoperative** outpatient primary VTE **prophylaxis** is recommended for 4 weeks, particularly for pelvic and abdominal cancer surgery patients. Dosing is dalteparin 5,000 units SC daily, if BMI is greater than 40 consider 7,500; Enoxaparin 40 mg SC daily, if BMI is greater than 40 consider dosing q12h; fondaparinux 2.5 mg SC, if BMI is greater than 40 consider 5 mg SC daily; UFH 5,000 units SC every 8 hours, if BMI is greater than 40 consider 7,500 units every 8 hours or apixaban 2.5 mg PO BID.
- Duration of treatment for VTE:
  - ○ A minimum of 3 months is recommended for patients with proximal DVT or PE and 3–6 months if there is a cancer diagnosis.

○ In patients with advanced or metastatic cancer, or in patients with risk factors for recurrence (genetic), a minimum of 6 months and preferably lifelong therapy is recommended. LMWH is preferred for the first 6 months as monotherapy. Warfarin can then be substituted with the target INR of 2 to 3. Both therapies should be continued for at least a 5-day overlap and until the INR is greater than 2 for at least 24 hours. DOAC are now considered for patients without luminal GI or GU lesions, gastric ulcer disease, hepatic or renal impairment, or anticancer therapies that affect p-glycoprotein, CYP3A4, or CYP2J2 pathways.

○ Catheter-associated thrombosis: Continue anticoagulation as long as the catheter is in situ or for at least 3 months.

- Reversal of anticoagulation:
  ○ Heparin (unfractionated/UFH): Half-life of 1 hour
    ▪ Reversal with protamine 1 mg/100 units UFH
    ▪ The maximum dose of protamine is 50 mg, and it can cause anaphylaxis if administered too fast.
  ○ LMWH: Half-life of 12 hours
    ▪ Reversal with protamine:
      □ If within 8 hours: 1 mg/mg of enoxaparin or 1 mg/100 units of dalteparin within 8 hours of the dose
      □ If greater than 8 hours from dosing, then 0.5 mg/mg of protamine
      □ If greater than 12 hours, consider the clinical scenario.
  ○ Warfarin: Half-life of 20 to 60 hours
    ▪ INR 4.5 to 10, no bleeding: Hold warfarin dose, when INR approaches therapeutic range less than 4, restart at reduced dose by 10% to 20% and recheck INR within 4 to 7 days.
    ▪ INR greater than 10, no bleeding: Hold warfarin dose, consider small dose of oral vitamin K 1 to 2.5 mg, follow INR every 1 to 2 days, when approaches therapeutic range less than 4, restarted at 20% dose reduction and recheck INR in 4 to 7 days.
    ▪ **Avoid** SC administration of vitamin K because of erratic absorption, IV administration can be used for more rapid absorption than PO.
    ▪ If urgent surgery is needed:
      □ Within 24 hours; hold warfarin and administer vitamin K 1 to 2.5 mg IV over 1 hour and repeat INR presurgery to determine need for prothrombin complex concentrate (PCC). FFP is another option.
      □ Within 48 hours: Hold warfarin and give vitamin K 2.5 mg PO. Repeat INR at 24 and 48 hours to assess need for supplemental vitamin K, PCC, or FFP.
    ▪ Life-threatening bleeding: Hold warfarin and choose from the following options:

- □ Administer vitamin K 10 mg IV, no faster than 1 mg/min.
- □ Administer four-factor PCC IV not exceeding 5 mL/min.
- □ Administer three-factor PCC IV not exceeding 10 mL/min.
- □ Administer recombinant form of human factor VIIa (rhFVIIa) IVP over 2 to 5 minutes.
- □ For patients with a history of heparin-induced thrombocytopenia (HIT), use three-factor PCC without heparin.
- ○ Direct thrombin inhibitors (DTIs):
  - Bivalirudin has a half life of 25 minutes and argatroban has a half-life 45 minutes
    - □ Discontinue drug.
    - □ Consider hemofiltration and hemodialysis.
    - □ May consider aPCC (anti-inhibitor coagulant complex vapor heated 50–100 units/kg IV) or rhFVIIa (90 mcg/kg IV, dDAVP 0.3 mcg/kg).
  - Dabigatran: Half-life of 14 to 17 hours:
    - □ Discontinue drug.
    - □ Consider hemodialysis with or without charcoal filter.
    - □ Use oral charcoal if dose within 2 hours of ingestion at 50 to 100 g followed by doses every 1, 2, 4 hours equivalent to 12.5 g/hr.
    - □ Consider aPCC anti-inhibitor coagulant complex, vapor heated 25 to 50 units/kg IV.
    - □ Consider rhFVIIa 90 mcg/kg IV.
- ○ Fondaparinux: Factor Xa inhibitor half-life of 17 to 21 hours
  - Discontinue drug.
  - Consider rhFVIIa 90 mcg/kg IV.
- ○ Ivaroxaban half-life of 9 to 12 hours: Direct factor Xa inhibitor
  - Discontinue drug.
  - Consider oral charcoal.
  - Consider rhFVIIa 10 to 120 mcg/kg IV, anti-inhibitor coagulant complex vapor heated 25 to 50 units/kg IV.
  - Consider four-factor PCC 25 to 50 units/kg, or if recent history of HIT in last 12 months, three-factor PCC 50 units/kg.
- ○ Apixaban half-life of 12 hours: Direct factor Xa inhibitor
  - Discontinue drug.
  - Consider oral charcoal.
  - Consider rhFVIIa 10 to 120 mcg/kg IV, anti-inhibitor coagulant complex vapor heated 25 to 50 units/kg IV.
  - Consider four-factor PCC 25 to 50 units/kg.
  - If recent history of HIT in last 12 months, consider three-factor PCC 50 units/kg.

- ○ **Four-factor PCC:** Dosing is based on units of factor IX per kilogram of actual body weight.
    - ▪ INR 2 to 4.5: 25 units/kg maximum 2,500 units
    - ▪ INR 4 to 6: 35 units/kg maximum 3,500 units
    - ▪ INR greater than 6: 50 units/kg maximum 5,000 units
- ○ **FFP:** If four-factor PCC unavailable or the patient is allergic to heparin and/or has a history of HIT in the last 12 months:
    - ▪ INR less than 4: 3-factor PCC 25 units/kg + FFP 2 to 3 units
    - ▪ INR greater than 4: 3-factor PCC 50 units/kg + FFP 2 to 3 units
    - ▪ FFP 15 mL/kg if PCC not available
- ○ **rhFVIIa:** Dosed at 25 mcg/kg (use if PCC unavailable or bleeding is not responsive to PCC)
- • Complications from anticoagulation do occur:
    - ○ Hemorrhage from over anticoagulation
    - ○ HIT
        - ▪ Type I: There is a decrease in platelet count to around 100,000/mL. This is not life-threatening but the patient should be removed from heparin treatment.
        - ▪ Type II (immune mediated via PF4 antibodies): There is a significant decrease in the platelet count by 30% to approximately 50–80/mL, and an increased risk of both arterial and venous thrombi. The patient should be removed from heparin treatment.
        - ▪ To diagnose HIT, heparin antibody testing should be ordered. Probability scoring should be calculated according to NCCN guidelines. If the score is four or more, unfractionated and LMWHs as well as warfarin should be discontinued. The INR should be reversed with vitamin K. A DTI or fondaparinux should be administered. If the HIT antibody test is positive, SRA testing should be ordered and DTIs continued for 6 weeks if no VTE is identified, or 6 months if a VTE is found.
- • Mechanisms of action:
    - ○ Heparin binds to antithrombin III. It enhances the inhibition of thrombin, and factors Xa and IXa. It increases the PTT and the level of anticoagulation can be monitored in this fashion. Heparin does not cross the placenta. Reversal is with protamine sulfate dosed at 1 mg/100 units of heparin. FFP can also be used if there is acute bleeding.
    - ○ Enoxaparin binds to and accelerates the action of antithrombin III. It preferentially potentiates the inhibition of factors Xa and IIa. Enoxaparin also has bleeding complications, but there is a lower incidence of induced thrombocytopenia. Monitoring is through antifactor Xa.

- ○ Warfarin inhibits the synthesis of vitamin K-dependent clotting factors II, VII, IX, and X. It also inhibits proteins C and S. It is usually effective in 48 hours. It does cross the placenta. It increases the PT and INR, and the level of anticoagulation can be monitored in this way. Reversal is with PO or IV vitamin K given at 1 to 10 mg depending on the INR.
- Preoperative anticoagulation:
  - ○ Preoperative discontinuation: anticoagulants such as warfarin should be stopped 5 to 7 days prior to surgery if the desired PT is 1 to 1.5 and the patients were maintained at an INR of 2 to 3. Aspirin should be stopped 7 days prior to surgery due to the irreversible binding to platelets. Clopidogrel should be stopped 10 days prior to surgery.
  - ○ **Perioperative management of anticoagulation** should be determined by the patient's medical comorbidities and urgency of surgery.
    - If emergent, PCC is the treatment of choice to reverse warfarin anticoagulation. It is a combination of blood clotting factors II, VII, IX, X, protein C and S. It is prepared from fresh frozen human plasma. For patients on oral factor Xa inhibitors who require immediate surgery, it is currently recommended to proceed with surgery as specific antidotes for reversal of the anticoagulant are not available and the half-life of these agents is between 5 and 13 hours, except for neurosurgical procedures. Idarucizumab (Praxbind) is used for treatment of patients with dabigatran-induced anticoagulation when emergent surgical procedures, life-threatening, or uncontrolled bleeding is present. The recommended dose for idarucizumab is 5 g (2.5 g/vial) administered IV as two consecutive 2.5 g infusions or a bolus of both vials.
    - For non-emergent surgery:
      - □ An IVC filter should be considered if VTE occurred within 4 weeks of the surgery.
      - □ If there is a very low risk of bleeding with surgery, continue anticoagulation.
      - □ If risk is low: No bridging is recommended.
      - □ If moderate risk (major abdominal/pelvic and thoracic surgeries fall into this category): Bridging should occur and consider therapeutic dosing to restart at 24 to 48 hours after surgery.
      - □ If the risk is high: Bridging is recommended and therapeutic dosing to restart at 24 to 48 hours after surgery.
      - □ Medical indications for bridging should occur in the moderate- and high-risk categories (Table 4.9):

Table 4.9 Risk Stratification of VTE in Surgical Patients With CV Comorbidity

VTE Risk	Events/Y	Mechanical Heart Valves	Atrial Fibrillation	Recent VTE	Thrombophilia
High risk	>10%	Mitral valve prosthesis Caged ball, tilting disc, aortic valve prosthesis Stroke or TIA within 6 months	CHADS >5 Stroke or TIA within 3 months Rheumatic valvular heart disease	VTE within 3 months	Protein C deficiency Protein 2 deficiency Antithrombin deficiency Homozygous factor V Leiden gene mutation Homozygous prothrombin gene mutation Antiphospholipid syndrome
Moderate risk	5%–10%	Bileaflet aortic valve plus: Atrial fib Prior stroke or TIA, HTN, DM, CHF Age >75	CHADS score 3 or 4	VTE within 3–12 months, recurrent DVT or PE, active cancer or cancer treatment within 6 months	Heterozygous factor V Leiden gene mutation, prothrombin gene homozygous mutation
Low risk	<5%	Bileaflet aortic valve prosthesis and no other risk factors for stroke	CHADS 0–2 and no prior stroke or TIA	Single VTE even >12 months prior and no other risk factors	Hyperhomocysteinemia elevated factors VIII, IX, XI

- Bridging:
  a. Stop chronic anticoagulation agent.
     i. Stop warfarin 5 to 7 days before procedure: If INR is greater than 1.5, 1 to 2 days prior to procedure, give 1 mg vitamin K PO.
     ii. Stop fondaparinux 5 days before surgery.
     iii. Stop dabigatran 2 days before surgery if CrCl is greater than 80 mL/min, 3 days if 50 to 79 mL/min, and 4 to 5 days if 31 to 49 mL/min.
     iv. Stop rivaroxaban 3 days prior if CrCl is greater than 30 mL/min.
     v. Stop apixaban 3 days before surgery if CrCl is greater than 50 mL/min or 4 days if CrCl 30 to 49 mL/min.
     vi. If using therapeutic adjusted IV UFH: Discontinue 4 to 6 hours before surgery.
  b. Start LMWH therapeutic dosing every 12 hours, 2 days after stopping warfarin.
  c. Stop LMWH 24 hours before surgery and, if using the 1.5 mg/kg once-daily dosing, the last dose should be half the total daily dose.
  d. May give VTE prophylaxis with UFH or LMWH at 12 to 24 hours after surgery.
  e. Restart:
     i. Administer warfarin with normal diet no sooner than 24 to 48 hours after surgery.
     ii. Administer dabigatran, rivaroxaban, apixaban, or fondaparinux no sooner than 7 days' postoperation.
  f. Naturopathic supplements are commonly used and it is important to discontinue the following prior to surgery as they can alter clotting time: vitamin E, garlic, gingko, and ginseng.

- **Arterial embolic** events:
  ○ Arterial occlusion usually occurs from direct injury or trauma to a vessel or extremity. It may also represent a thrombotic insult from the left heart or a patent foramen ovale.
  ○ Symptoms are related to the arterial occlusion and the extremity usually has pallor, pulselessness, paresthesia, pain, and is cold. The diagnostic workup includes a Doppler US and an angiogram.
  ○ Treatment is via vascular surgery with a thrombectomy, followed by anticoagulation as soon as the diagnosis is made.

○ Acute mesenteric ischemia is a medical emergency. Characteristics are abdominal pain out of proportion to the examination, and a history of atrial fibrillation. Diagnosis is via EKG and CT. Treatment is emergency laparotomy with bowel resection if indicated and surgical revascularization followed by anticoagulation.

- Neuraxial anesthesia/lumbar puncture and anticoagulation parameters: UFH 5,000 every 12 hours and enoxaparin 40 mg daily is fine. Enoxaparin 30 to 40 mg q12 hours, fondaparinux 2.5 mg daily, and therapeutic dosing should be used with extreme caution. Placement of neuraxial catheter should be delayed for at least 12 hours after administration of prophylactic doses of enoxaparin. A postneuraxial placement dose of enoxaparin should be given no sooner than 4 hours after last dosing of enoxaparin.

Nutrition

- Fifty percent of gynecologic oncology patients are malnourished at the time of their diagnosis and ensuing surgery. A weight loss of over 10% from the patient's normal weight usually means the patient is malnourished. There are a few ways to measure the level of malnutrition.

  ○ The prognostic nutritional index includes measurement of the triceps skin fold, the serum albumin level, the serum transferrin level, and assessment of the delayed hypersensitivity response to mumps, TB, and Candida antigen.

  ○ Laboratory measurements of malnutrition can include the total lymphocyte count, or the serum albumin level (which has a half-life of 20 days). The serum albumin test is the single test with the most predictive value: Levels less than 2.1 mg/dL are associated with morbidity from 10% to 65%.

- **Perioperative nutrition:** Immunonutrition has been investigated to improve outcomes. Immunonutrition includes supplementation with arginine, dietary nucleotides, omega-e fatty acids.

  ○ "Impact" nutritional support: When initiated 5 days before the scheduled surgery, given TID and continued for 5 days after surgery if PO was tolerated found that patients receiving Impact had fewer wound complications (19.6% vs. 33%; $p = .049$). There was a 78% reduction in incidence of class 2 and 3 SSIs (OR, 0.22; 95% CI: 0.05 to 0.95; $p = .044$). ASA classification, BMI, DM, history of XRT, length of surgery, and blood loss did affect outcomes. Insurance companies may resist coverage for this as it may be seen as a "food."[46]

  ○ A rapid postoperative feeding schedule has proven benefits and is usually encouraged in gynecologic surgeries. Clear liquids given PO are started as soon as the patient is alert and without nausea, vomiting, or significant abdominal distension. Advancement to a regular diet after proven tolerance to liquids follows. Rapid postoperative feeding has been shown to decrease hospital LOS with no additional AEs.

- The Harris–Benedict equation calculates the daily basal caloric need: BEE = 655 + (9.6 × kg) + (1.8 × cm height) − (4.7 × age in Y). Stress factors should be added to this caloric need as indicated: 1.2× for a minor insult, 1.3× for an elective surgical patient or with moderate stress (SIRS, sepsis), and 1.5× for severe stress (burn patients).

- TPN composition includes glucose at 3.4 kcal/g to yield 70% of the calculated calories. The remaining 30% is from lipids (at 9 kcal/kg). Protein is added at 1 to 1.5 g nitrogen/kg. TPN should be considered if the patient has a nonfunctioning GI tract due to ileus or obstruction, is unable to tolerate PO status for 7 days or more after surgery, has short bowel syndrome, or is severely malnourished.

Endocrine Management

- Diabetes: Diabetes researchers estimate that in 50 Y the incidence of diabetes in women will increase 178% to 351%.
  - ○ DM can increase perioperative complications. It is important to get a preoperative echocardiogram for baseline cardiac function, renal labs, an HgA1c, and a urine analysis to check for protein.
  - ○ Postoperative infections cause 20% of deaths in diabetics. To optimize glycemic control, the serum glucose should be maintained between 80 and 110 mg/dL using a weight-based sliding scale insulin (SSI) regimen. This yields a 46% reduction in septicemia and 34% reduction in hospital mortality. It is recommended to stop metformin and sulfonylurea medications 24 to 48 hours before surgery and restart when the patient tolerates a regular American Diabetes Association diet.
  - ○ Hyperglycemia doubles the risk of SSI and this also affects those who are prediabetic. Optimal perioperative glycemic control should reduce infectious complications 40% to 50%.

- Adrenal support: Steroid therapy is indicated for patients who have medical comorbidities that need additional adrenal support.
  - ○ Indications for stress dosing of steroids would be more than 3 weeks of, or an equivalent to, 20 mg of prednisone daily within 1 Y of surgery.
  - ○ Stress dosing is administered preoperatively with IV hydrocortisone or methylprednisolone 100 mg. Postoperative treatment is 100 mg IV every 8 hours for three doses. When the patient can tolerate PO status, it is okay to resume scheduled dosing or to start a steroid taper. If the patient is clinically Cushingoid, the patient also then requires stress dosing (Table 4.10).

Table 4.10 Postoperative Steroid Taper Protocol

Steroid Taper	Hydrocortisone (IV)	Prednisone (PO)
POD 0	100 mg IV q8h	—
POD 1	100 mg IV q8h	37.5 mg PO q12h
POD 2	80 mg IV q8h	30 mg PO q12h
POD 3	60 mg IV q8h	22.5 mg PO q12h
POD 4	40 mg IV q 8h	15 mg PO q12h
POD 5	20 mg IV q8h	7.5 mg PO q12h
POD 6	May discontinue	

- ○ It is important to perform Accu-Check measures and place the patient on a SSI due to the risk of diabetic insult and systemic hyperglycemia.

- **Thyroid disease:** It is important to check TSH and a T4 levels prior to surgery in patients with a known thyroid disorder, in diabetic patients, or in undiagnosed patients who are symptomatic.
  - ○ Patients who are hypothyroid have more ileus, delirium, and infection without fever.
  - ○ If the patient is severely hypothyroid, it is important to give IV thyroxine, and stress-dose steroids. The half-life of thyroxine is 5 to 9 days.
  - ○ Patients who are hyperthyroid can have major complications as well. These can be cardiac related to both inotropic and chronotropic factors. Atrial fibrillation can occur in 10% to 20% of patients.
  - ○ Thyroid storm should be suspected if there is fever, tachycardia, confusion, CV collapse, or death. Preoperative treatment is with a beta blocker, initiation of or continuation of PTU or methimazole, and administration of stress-dose steroids.

Hepatic Disease

Hepatitis is divided into acute and chronic diseases. It is important to check for coagulopathies in liver disease. It is also important to reduce narcotic dosing by 50% in these patients.

- Surgery should be delayed if there is acute hepatitis. The mortality ranges up to 58% if surgery is pursued in the acute phases.
- If the hepatitis is chronic, there is no change in mortality and surgery does not need to be delayed.
- The Child–Turcotte–Pugh classification system predicts mortality in patients with liver disease.
  - ○ Encephalopathy—None: 1, mild to moderate: 2, severe: 3.

○ Ascites—None, 1; mild to moderate (responsive to diuretics), 2; severe (refractory to diuretics), 3.

○ Bilirubin level—Less than 2 mg/dL, 1; 2 to 3 mg/dL, 2; greater than 3 mg/dL, 3.

○ Albumin level—Less than 3.5 g/dL, 1; 2.8 to 3.5 g/dL, 2; less than 2.8 g/dL, 3.

○ INR—Less than 1.7, 1; 1.7 to 2.3, 2; greater than 2.3, 3.

○ Total points are added and the score then falls into a class. Class A, 5 to 6 points; class B, 7 to 9 points; class C, 10 to 15 points. Class A has a 10% postoperative mortality, class B has 30% mortality, and class C has 80% mortality.

Neurologic Disease

- There are a number of different etiologies that may explain altered mental status. Common causes include metabolic abnormalities, sepsis, meningitis, brain metastasis, or stroke. The initial treatment for a patient with acute-onset altered mental status is to maintain an airway, establish IV access, and provide oxygen, if necessary; laboratories and imaging follow.

  ○ Workup for metabolic causes includes CBC, CMP, UA, urine drug screen, cardiac enzymes, pulse oximetry, and blood cultures.

  ○ Workup for sepsis or meningitis includes CBC, CMP, blood, and urine cultures. Lumbar puncture is appropriate for cell count, culture, and cytology, but should only be performed after a CT of the head demonstrates no brain lesions causing mass effect.

  ○ Workup for metastatic disease or stroke: CT of the head is usually ordered without contrast to evaluate for evidence of an acute hemorrhagic stroke. If negative, a study with contrast is better for evaluation of metastatic lesions. MRI is the most sensitive and specific study to evaluate for evidence of brain metastasis or stroke.

- Treatment for specific clinical situations:

  ○ Narcotic drug overdose: Naloxone: 1 ampule (0.01 mg/kg IV)

  ○ Seizure: Dilantin 1,000 mg load then 200 to 300 mg QD, Valium 5 mg IV.

  ○ Brainstem herniation: Hyperventilate PCO_2 to 25 to 30 mmHg, dexamethasone 10 mg IV then 4 mg IV every 6 hours, mannitol 12 g/kg IV then 50 to 300 mg/kg IV every 6 hours. Surgical intervention may be necessary.

Alcohol Withdrawal

Alcohol withdrawal can cause significant morbidity. Patients with a history of alcohol abuse should be assessed for withdrawal. A well-lit room, social support, and reassurance are first steps. Seizures can occur 12 to 48 hours after alcohol cessation. Delirium tremens complicates 5% to 10% of alcohol withdrawal cases, and mortality can approach 15%. Beer can be ordered while a patient is hospitalized (Table 4.11).

Table 4.11 CIWA Scoring

Nausea and vomiting score:
0 No nausea and no vomiting
1 Mild nausea with no vomiting
4 Intermittent nausea with dry heaves
7 Constant nausea, frequent dry heaves, and vomiting

Tremor score:
0 No tremor
1 Not visible, but can be felt fingertip to fingertip
4 Moderate, with patient's arms extended
7 Severe, even with arms not extended

Paroxysmal sweats score:
0 No sweat visible
1 Barely perceptible sweating, palms moist
4 Beads of sweat obvious on forehead
7 Drenching sweats

Anxiety score:
0 No anxiety, at ease
1 Mildly anxious
4 Moderately anxious, or guarded, so anxiety is inferred
7 Equivalent to acute panic states as seen in severe delirium or acute schizophrenic reactions

Agitation score:
0 Normal activity
1 Somewhat more than normal activity
4 Moderately fidgety and restless
7 Paces during most of the interview, or constantly thrashes about

Tactile disturbances score:
0 None
1 Very mild itching, pins and needles, burning or numbness
2 Mild itching, pins and needles, burning or numbness
3 Moderate itching, pins and needles, burning or numbness
4 Moderately severe hallucinations
5 Severe hallucinations
6 Extremely severe hallucinations
7 Continuous hallucinations

Auditory disturbances score:
0 Not present
1 Very mild harshness or ability to frighten
2 Mild harshness or ability to frighten
3 Moderate harshness or ability to frighten
4 Moderately severe hallucinations
5 Severe hallucinations
6 Extremely severe hallucinations
7 Continuous hallucinations

Visual disturbances score:
0 Not present
1 Very mild sensitivity
2 Mild sensitivity
3 Moderate sensitivity
4 Moderately severe hallucinations
5 Severe hallucinations
6 Extremely severe hallucinations
7 Continuous hallucinations

(continued)

Table 4.11 CIWA Scoring *(continued)*

Headache, fullness in head score:	Orientation and clouding of sensorium score:
0 Not present	0 Oriented and can do serial additions
1 Very mild	
2 Mild	1 Cannot do serial additions or is uncertain about date
3 Moderate	
4 Moderately severe	2 Disoriented for date by no more than 2 calendar days
5 Severe	
6 Very severe	3 Disoriented for date by more than 2 calendar days
7 Extremely severe	
	4 Disoriented for place and/or person

Cumulative score:

0–8 No medication is necessary.

9–14 Medication is optional for patients with a score of 8–14.

15–20 A score of 15 or over requires treatment with medication.

>20 A score of over 20 poses a strong risk of delirium tremens.

Maximum possible cumulative score is 67.

- CIWA scoring is a cumulative score that provides the basis of a treatment plan for patients undergoing alcohol withdrawal.
- Basic orders include seizure precautions, aspiration precautions, and restraints if the patient has safety risks. Admission lab tests include: CBC, CMP, LFTs, PTT, INR, and a urine analysis. Blood alcohol levels should also be drawn. A urine toxicology screen is usually indicated. A CXR to evaluate for pneumonia should be considered. A daily CMP is important.
- IV fluids should be initiated with normal saline. D5 should be added if the patient is NPO but thiamine should be given first. When the patient becomes euvolemic, the IVF should be switched to 1/2 normal saline (or D5 1/2 normal saline) at 125 mL/hr.
- Medications should include vitamins, benzodiazepines, and antipsychotics as indicated.
  - Vitamins include thiamine dosed at 100 mg IV for 3 days, then daily by mouth; folate 1 mg daily by mouth; and a multivitamin daily.
  - Benzodiazepines include chlordiazepoxide and lorazepam. Chlordiazepoxide (Librium) is dosed at 25 to 100 mg PO q4 to 6

hours. Lorazepam (Ativan) is dosed at 1 to 4 mg PO/SL/IM/IV. It may be given every 4 to 6 hours or every 15 to 30 min in cases of severe withdrawal. Lorazepam should be first choice in patients with liver compromise (AST >200, INR >1.5), in patients who need IV dosing and cannot take PO well, and in patients who exceed the maximum chlordiazepoxide dose of 600 mg in 24 hours.

- Treatment per CIWA score:
  - For a CIWA score of less than 8, scheduled doses of benzodiazepine should be considered. Patients should be assessed and assigned a CIWA score every 6 hours. Total benzodiazepine dose should be tapered by 25% per day after an initial 72-hour period. Initially, this can be achieved by decreasing the q6h dose. Once the dose is at the smallest unit (0.5–1 mg lorazepam, or 25 mg chlordiazepoxide), the dosing interval should be lengthened.
  - For patients in active withdrawal with a CIWA score of 8 to 25, symptom-triggered treatment should be initiated. These patients are categorized according to the severity of their current symptoms: mild = CIWA 8 to 13; moderate = CIWA 14 to 20; marked = CIWA 21 to 25. Patients should be assessed every 4 hours, in addition to 1 hour after medication administration.
  - For patients with severe withdrawal who are assigned a CIWA score greater than 25, ICU admission is required. Nursing staff assessment is every 2 hours. Treatment is with lorazepam and these patients may require a continuous infusion of lorazepam. The initial rate may be estimated by averaging the hourly dose of benzodiazepine delivered over the first 6 hours. The infusion rate should then be titrated with the goal of sedation scale of 3 to 4.
  - Treatment of disorientation or hallucinations without autonomic signs of alcohol withdrawal (such as tremor and diaphoresis): Patients may benefit from the addition of haloperidol instead of additional benzodiazepine use.

Blood Transfusion
- Transfusion is recommended in an asymptomatic patient if the Hg level falls below 6 g/dL. If a perioperative patient has an Hg of 7 g/dL and surgery is expected to have significant blood loss, or if the risks associated with anesthesia are high, the patient may be transfused before the procedure. For a postoperative Hg of 6 to 7 g/dL, transfusion is likely/indicated. For an Hg 7 to 8 g/dL—transfusion can be considered, including those with stable CV disease. For an Hg of 8 to 10 g/dL, transfusion should be considered for some populations such as those with symptomatic anemia, ongoing bleeding, and acute coronary syndrome with ischemia. If the patient is expected to receive adjuvant therapies, an optimal Hg is 10 g/dL. If the patient is symptomatic with orthostatic hypotension, dizziness, or has new physical symptoms such as cardiac murmur, transfusion should be

entertained. In general, the AABB guidelines have recommended that transfusion is not indicated solely for an Hg level <10 g/dL.

- The current risk of infection from transfusion:
  - Viral:
    - HIV, one in 1,467,000
    - Hepatitis B, one in 282,000
    - Hepatitis C, one in 1,149,000
    - West Nile virus, uncommon
    - Cytomegalovirus, 50% to 85% of donors are carriers: leukocyte reduction is protective.
  - Bacterial: One in 2,000–3,000 (mostly platelets)
  - Parasitic diseases: Babesiosis, Chagas, and malaria are uncommon.
- Allogeneic blood transfusions are an alternative to standard transfusions, but need to be obtained 6 weeks prior to surgery and are screened in the same fashion as all other blood donations.
- Normovolemic hemodilution is an alternative to blood transfusion.

Potential Adverse Effects of Blood Transfusion
- Immunomodulation from blood transfusion may lead to higher postoperative infections as well as increased morbidity and mortality from:
  - Acute hemolytic transfusion reaction (HTR): Preformed antibodies react to incompatible product (1:76,000).
  - ABO incompatibility occurs in 1:40,000 and is fatal in $1:1.8 \times 10^6$. Symptoms are chills, fever, hypotension, hemoglobinuria, renal failure, back pain, DIC. Treatment: IVF to keep urine output greater than 1 mL/kg/hr, pressors as needed, and treatment of DIC.
  - Delayed HTR: The cause is an anamnestic immune response to incompatible red cell antigens. Symptoms are fever, jaundice, falling Hg newly positive antibody screen 1 to 2 weeks after transfusion. Treatment is transfusion as needed with compatible RBCs. The offending antibody should be identified in the blood bank.
  - Febrile non-HTR: Occurs in 0.1% to 1.0%. The cause is preformed anti-WBC antibodies in the recipient. The risk is minimized with leukocyte-reduced products. Symptoms are a ≥1°C (2°F) rise in body temperature within 2 hours of transfusion initiation with no other explanation for fever. Treatment is with acetaminophen premedication if reactions are recurrent.
  - Allergic (urticarial) reactions: Occur in 1% to 3% of patients. The cause is an antibody to donor plasma proteins. Symptoms are urticaria, pruritus, flushing, and mild wheezing. Treatment is suspension of the transfusion and antihistamines. The transfusion may resume if the reaction resolves.

- o Anaphylaxis: Occurs in 1:20,000 to 50,000. The cause is an antibody to donor plasma proteins (imunoglobulin A [IgA], haptoglobin, C4). Symptoms are hypotension, urticaria, bronchospasm, angioedema, anxiety. Treatment is with epinephrine 1:1,000, 1 ampule SC, antihistamines, and corticosteroids.
- o TRALI: Occurs in 1:10,000; 10% to 20% are fatal. The cause is preformed HLA or neutrophil antibodies in the donor product. Symptoms are hypoxemia, hypotension, bilateral pulmonary edema, transient leukopenia, and fever within 6 hours of transfusion. Treatment is supportive care.
- o Transfusion-associated graft-versus-host disease: This is rare but almost always fatal. The cause is an immunosuppressed recipient who receives a transfusion from an HLA-similar donor (usually a family member). Symptoms are pancytopenia, maculopapular rash, diarrhea, hepatitis presenting 1 to 4 weeks after transfusion. Treatment is supportive care. It can be prevented by irradiating blood products[47]

- For most patients, a restrictive transfusion strategy (i.e., giving less blood, transfusing at a lower Hg level, and aiming for a lower target Hg level) is preferred rather than a liberal transfusion strategy. Restrictive transfusion strategies have resulted in the following: a 39% decrease in the probability of receiving a transfusion (46% vs. 84%; RR = 0.61; 95% CI: 0.52–0.72); fewer units (1.19) transfused per patient; a trend toward a lower 30-day mortality (RR = 0.85; 95% CI: 0.70–1.03); a trend toward a lower overall infection rate (RR = 0.81; 95% CI: 0.66–1.00); although no difference was seen with pneumonia. No difference was seen in functional recovery, hospital, or ICU LOS. There was no increased risk of MI when all trials were included (RR = 0.88; 95% CI: 0.38–2.04).
- A post-transfusion Hg level can be performed as early as 15 minutes following transfusion, as long as the patient is not actively bleeding.
- Acute coronary syndrome: The optimal transfusion threshold in the setting of acute coronary syndrome (ACS; i.e., acute MI, unstable angina) remains unanswered. A standard practice in patients with ACS is to transfuse when the Hg is less than 8 g/dL and to consider a transfusion when the Hg is between 8 and 10 g/dL. If the patient has ongoing ischemia or other symptoms, an Hg can be maintained ≥10 g/dL. The threshold of 8 g/dL is considered safe for asymptomatic medical patients with stable coronary artery disease.

CRITICAL CARE

Pulmonary Complications

- Complications related to pulmonary factors occur in 20% to 30% of postoperative patients. The FRC is reduced 20% when patients are supine, or have had a laparotomy and the vital capacity is decreased 45%.

- Risk factors are obesity, surgery longer than 2 hours, COPD, CHF, renal failure, poor mental status, immunosuppression, NGT use, narcotics, smoking, sleep apnea, and asthma. COPD patients can benefit from a preoperative ABG and PFT.

- Atelectasis usually occurs postintubation and is due to surgical pain with its associated decreased inspiratory effort. Dyspnea, tachypnea, and fever can be present. Examination reveals crackles at the lung bases. Diagnosis is with CXR. Treatment is incentive spirometry.

- Pneumonia can present with dyspnea, tachypnea, fever, and decreased O_2 saturation. Examination reveals decreased breath sounds segmentally. Diagnosis is via CXR and documentation of infiltrate or consolidation. Aspiration pneumonia may take 24 hours to show on CXR. Treatment is with antibiotics, incentive spirometry, chest physiotherapy, and pulmonary hygiene.

- *Respiratory failure* is defined as altered pulmonary function that yields hypercarbia, acidemia, or hypoxemia.
  - The etiology can be a decreased respiratory drive, airway obstruction, decreased pulmonary function, COPD, asthma, anaphylaxis, pulmonary edema from CHF, ARDS, pneumonia, abscess, TB, pneumothorax, pleural effusion, hemothorax, cancer, anemia, or PE.
  - Diagnosis is via physical examination, imaging, and laboratories. It is important to obtain a CXR, oxygen saturation, an ABG, a CBC, electrolytes, a CT angiogram if a PE is suspected, and potentially an echocardiogram to rule out cardiogenic etiology.

- Oxygen is not as good as we think. Administration of 100% O_2 for more than 6 hours has been shown to decrease macrophage activity, mucus velocity, CO, and can cause irreversible pulmonary damage if given for greater than 60 hours. Oxygen can be delivered via nasal prongs, a rebreathing face mask, a nonrebreathing face mask, CPAP, BiPAP, and intubation with mechanical ventilation. Delivery via nasal prongs has been shown to be as good as a rebreathing face mask.

- Parameters
  - PaO_2: Arterial oxygen tension
    - Normal: 70 to 100 mmHg
  - PAO_2: Alveolar oxygen tension ($FiO_2 \times 713$) – ($PaCO_2/0.8$)
    - Normal: 100 mmHg
  - $PaCO_2$: Arterial CO_2 tension
    - Normal: 35 to 44 mmHg
  - A-a gradient: Alveolar – arterial O_2 tension where $PAO_2 = [(FiO_2) \times$ (Atmospheric pressure – H_2O Pressure) – ($PaCO_2/0.8$)]
    - Normal: 3 to 16 mmHg or (Age/4) + 4

- ○ Vital capacity: Volume of expired air after maximal inspiration
  - ▪ Normal: 3 to 5 L
- ○ Tidal volume: Volume of inspired air for each peak breath
  - ▪ Normal: 6 to 7 mL/kg
- ○ FEV1: Maximum volume of air forcefully expired in 1 second
  - ▪ Normal: Greater than 83% of vital capacity
- ○ PEF:
  - ▪ Normal: Greater than 400 L/minute
- ○ NIF:
  - ▪ Normal: 60 to 100 cm H_2O

- Indications for mechanical ventilation include: hypoxemia, hypercarbia, respiratory acidosis, the inability to maintain or protect the airway, including changes in mental status and respiratory fatigue. The largest endotracheal tube possible should be chosen: This is usually a 7.5 to 8 for women. This is to decrease airway resistance. Vitals and laboratory benchmarks are listed in Table 4.12.
- The A-a gradient is calculated to determine shunt and help rule out a PE. The A-a gradient = $PAO_2–PaO_2$ where PAO_2 = [(FiO$_2$) × (Atmospheric pressure – H_2O pressure) – (PaCO$_2$/0.8)]. A normal gradient estimate = (Age/4) + 4.
- Ventilation by machine can be run by volume or by pressure. The volume-cycled setting has a preset tidal volume. The pressure-cycled setting stops the cycle at a preset pressure; this setting is useful in hypoxic patients and those with reduced lung compliance like ARDS.
  - ○ CMV delivers a preset minute ventilation determined by a set respiratory rate and tidal volume. It is useful in heavily sedated patients, those given paralytic agents, and those who do not tolerate assisted ventilation.

Table 4.12 Parameters for Intubation in Respiratory Failure

Mechanics	Results
PaO$_2$	<60 mmHg
PaCO$_2$	>55–60 mmHg
Respiratory rate	>30–35 bpm
Arterial pH	<7.25
NIF	<20 cm H_2O
Vital capacity	<10 mL/kg
FiO$_2$	>60
PaO$_2$/FiO$_2$	<200
FEV1	<10 mL/kg

- ○ Assist control (A/C) or volume controlled ventilation presets the tidal volume, and this tidal volume is delivered when a breath is initiated by the patient. This is the most common mode of mechanical ventilation used in the ICU. A control backup rate is set to prevent hypoventilation.
- ○ IMV has a set rate and tidal volume, but allows unassisted spontaneous breaths and provides a full breath in relation to the amount of patient effort.
- ○ SIMV delivers breaths at regular intervals that are based on a preset tidal volume and rate, which are synchronized with the patient's respiratory efforts.
- ○ PS ventilation provides constant airway pressure, which is delivered during inspiration. It is the most frequently used mode during "weaning." In this mode, each time the patient inhales, the ventilator delivers a pressure-limited breath. The patient controls the rate, volume, and duration of the breaths.
- To initially set the ventilator, either IMV or A/C cycles are chosen. The FiO_2 is started at 60% (maximum), and weaned down to a patient O_2 saturation of 90% to 95% and an FiO_2 of 21% (RA). The rate is usually initiated at eight to 12 breaths per minute. The tidal volume is chosen at 8 to 12 mL/kg, but should be lower at 6 mL/kg if the patient is suspected or diagnosed with ARDS. A PEEP of 5 cm H_2O is also chosen. It is important to check an ABG and adjust the settings further after initial stabilization.
- Extubation should be a rapid goal. A spontaneous breathing trial or t-tube trial should be performed daily to assess patient status. Weaning settings on the ventilator are with SIMV or PS ventilation. To be extubated, the patient must be conscious and can protect the airway, the FiO_2 must be less than 50% (optimally at 21% RA), the PEEP should be less than 5 cm H_2O, the NIF should be greater than 20 cm H_2O (Table 4.13).

Table 4.13 Extubation Parameters

Weaning Parameters	Acceptable for Extubation
Respiratory rate	<30–35 (>8) bpm with FiO_2 <0.5
PaO_2	>60 mmHg with FiO_2 <0.5
$PaCO_2$	<50 with respiratory rate <25 bpm
NIF	More negative than 20–25 cm H_2O
Vital capacity	>10–15 mL/kg
Tidal volume	>3 mL/kg
The patient is awake and can protect the airway	

- VAP occurs in 30% of patients after 72 hours of intubation. The mortality of VAP is 25% to 50%.
- Monitoring of pulmonary and cardiac status can be with a central line. The CVP is an assessment of volume status and crude cardiac function. It consists of multiple measurements, and is not a single number. A normal CVP is 8 to 10 cm H_2O, or 2 to 6 mmHg.
- A PA or Swan catheter can be helpful when it is important to know critical CO or fluid status. Complications of a Swan include pneumothorax, arrhythmia, line sepsis (2%), or PA rupture. CO is calculated thermodynamically. An estimation of preload is obtained by wedging the end of the catheter into an afferent pulmonary capillary. This is called the *PAOP* or *PCWP*. A normal PCWP is 6 to 12 mmHg. The PCWP is a crude reflection of the left arterial pressure. If the PCWP is elevated, then the preload is adequate or excessive; if it is low, then the patient is likely volume depleted. The mixed venous blood sample is blood obtained from the tip of the PA catheter and reflects the most desaturated blood in the body.
- ARDS occurs after a defined insult to the lungs. This can include hemorrhage, sepsis, shock, or pneumonia. An ABG should be drawn.
  - Symptoms are tachypnea, dyspnea, and respiratory failure.
  - There are several criteria for the diagnosis of ARDS:
    - Bilateral diffuse infiltrates are seen on CXR.
    - CHF and iatrogenic volume overload are ruled out by echocardiogram (showing an EF >35%).
    - There is impaired oxygenation with documented oxygen saturation less than 92%.
    - The calculated PaO_2/FiO_2 of less than 300 torr, if greater, the diagnosis is acute lung injury ALI.
  - The mortality of ARDS is 30% to 40%.
  - Management is with intubation, mechanical ventilation, antibiotics, and treatment of the underlying cause. Steroids have not been proven beneficial. Better survival has been seen with ventilatory support maintaining low tidal volumes to prevent barotrauma (6 mL/kg), and elevated PCO_2-permissive hypercapnia.

Cardiac Complications
- Myocardial infarction (MI) can occur at any time during hospitalization. Any chest pain, arrhythmia, SOB, persistent dyspepsia, or arm pain should be worked up with cardiac enzymes and an EKG (serially) as well as a CXR to start.
- Reinfarction can occur after a recent MI. Rates have decreased from 37% to now 5% to 10% due to better medications used for reperfusion. The rate further decreases the length of time from the

initial insult. The rate is 2% to 3% after 4 to 6 months, and 1% to 2% if greater than 6 months have elapsed after a recent MI.

- Perioperative prophylactic beta blockers have been studied. Laughton, in 2005, showed there were fewer infarctions and lower mortality when beta blockers were used after surgery. The rates of infarction with use were 24% versus 39% without. The 2-Y mortality was 16% with use versus 32% without. A more recent study, the POISE study in 2008, refutes the benefit of beta blocker use postoperatively. There were fewer MIs in the beta blocker group (4.2% vs. 5.7%; $p < .05$), but there were more deaths (3.1% vs. 2.3%; $p < .05$) and more CVAs (1% vs. 0.5%; $p < .05$) with beta blocker use.[48]

- The role of a PA catheter (Swan-Ganz) for surgery remains controversial and its use has decreased in modern clinical practice. There are no definitive studies that provide evidence of benefit in the surgical setting. The current indications are active CHF, severely depressed LV function, and critical aortic stenosis.

- Parameters
  - CO: heart rate × stroke volume
    - Normal: 4 to 8 L/min
  - Cardiac index: CO/BSA m^2
    - Normal: 2.5 to 4 L/min
  - MAP = 1/3 × (SBP − DBP) + DBP
    - Normal: 70 to 105 mmHg
  - PAP systolic
    - Normal: 15 to 30 mmHg
  - PAP diastolic
    - Normal: 5 to 12 mmHg
  - PAP mean
    - Normal: 5 to 10 mmHg
  - PAWP = LA and LV filling pressure
    - Normal: 5 to 12 mmHg
  - SVR: (MAP − MRAP) (80)/CO
    - Normal: 900 to 1,400 dynes/sec/cm^{-5}
  - PVR: (mean PAP − PAWP)/CO.
    - Normal: 100 to 240 dynes/sec/cm^{-5}
  - VO_2: O_2 consumption
    - Normal: 115 to 1,165 mL/min/m^2
  - DO_2: O_2 delivery
    - Normal: 640 to 1,000 mL O_2/min

- Ischemic heart disease (IHD)
  - IHD (myocardial infarction) can oftentimes be identified by its symptoms. Angina, nausea, vomiting, dyspnea, sweating, diaphoresis, SOB, weakness, anxiety, elevated BP, tachycardia, bradycardia, JVD, or tachyarrhythmias are often present.
  - Workup includes an EKG, cardiac enzymes × 3 every 6 to 8 hours (CK, CKMB, troponin I), BNP, CXR, and consideration of coronary angiography, especially if an STEMI is diagnosed.
  - Medical treatment is with transfer to the critical care unit for telemetry. Myocardial infarctions are classified as STEMI, non-STEMI, and unstable angina. Pulse oximetry should be obtained, aspirin administered, and oxygen placed to keep saturations greater than 90%. A CXR should be obtained in addition to an EKG and laboratories. Initial stabilization should include administration of SL NTG at 5-minute intervals for three doses if there is chest pain. IV morphine dosed at 4 to 8 mg repeated every 5 to 15 minutes is recommended for chest pain and to decrease the myocardial workload. Atropine can be given to increase BP if hypotension is present due to bradycardia. Beta blockers should be administered in the absence of contraindications. Contraindications include SBP less than 90, bradycardia, findings suggesting right ventricle infarction.
    - Treatment of patients with **STEMI** include: IV thrombolysis within 30 minutes or cardiac catheterization with per cutaneous transluminal coronary angioplasty within 90 minutes of arrival or occurrence.
    - Treatment of patients with **NSTEMI** includes observation and monitoring in a CCU with administration of stool softeners, stress ulcer prophylaxis, aspirin as and bedrest. Oxygen is recommended for saturations less than 90%. Beta blockers should be administered in the absence of contraindications. ACE inhibitors may be additionally beneficial in limiting infarct size and high dose statins should be started. If chest pain continues, angiography and revascularization via PTCA, stenting, or surgery is indicated. Unfractionated heparin infusion or other strategies and with antiplatelet therapies can be initiated. IV NTG titrated to 10 to 200 mg/min to prevent hypotension can be given to alleviate coronary artery spasm and decrease infarct size. Fibrinolytic therapy is not indicated in NSTEMI myocardial infarction.
    - Treatment of patients with **unstable angina** is angiography with PTCA, stenting, or surgery. An EKG should be obtained with each set of enzymes. An echocardiogram is usually ordered as well for EF and ventricular assessment. Angiography should be considered in the timing of PTCA based on refractory or recurrent angina, new or evolving signs of CHF, hemodynamic

instability, new arrhythmias, a temporal change in troponins, or a history of PTCA in the last 6 months. For severe LV dysfunction and cardiogenic shock, angioplasty, thrombolysis, and revascularization with multivessel stenting may be indicated.

○ Interventional treatment:

- Angioplasty is used to dilate a stenosed artery mechanically with a balloon catheter.

- A stent can also be placed simultaneously. The stent can be mechanical alone or medicated (impregnated with paclitaxel). The medicated stents keep occluded arteries open and decrease local plaque. Noncardiac surgery can be performed 6 weeks after a medicated stent as antithrombotics are needed for this duration. A nonmedicated/bare metal stent is indicated if surgery is urgent. Surgery can be performed 2 weeks after bare metal stent placement.

- Thrombolysis is another option for removing coronary artery occlusion. This occurs after localization with angiography and if the diagnosis occurs within 6 hours of the onset of pain. The clot is lysed with antithrombotics.

- *Heart failure* is defined as an EF less than 35% to 40%. The etiology is most commonly a myocardial infarction, but can be viral, hereditary, or drug induced (chemotherapies, targeted therapies, or biologics).

  ○ Symptoms are SOB, lower extremity edema, or JVD. There can be ascites if there is significant right-heart failure, progressing to anasarca if not managed.

  ○ Workup includes a CXR, which will show bilateral infiltrates, an EKG, an echocardiogram, cardiac enzymes × 3 every 6 to 8 hours, BNP, electrolytes, and a CBC. A spiral CT can help rule out a PE.

  ○ Treatment is with O_2 supplementation, water restriction to 2 L/day, morphine, and diuretics (furosemide to start at 20 mg IV, doubling of the dose is indicated if minimal response is seen). If there is a need to increase the CO, inotropes, such as dopamine or dobutamine, can be considered. Digoxin can be administered to improve contractility (0.5 mg IV, then 0.25 mg every 6 hours × 2, maintenance 0.125 mg/day, checking the level the first day, then every 5 days). A daily weight and strict sodium management (<2 g/day) are important.

- Pulmonary edema

  ○ Characterized by SOB

  ○ Diagnosis is with a physical examination demonstrating bilateral rales and low oxygen saturation. Confirmation is with CXR showing bilateral infiltrates. An EKG, an echocardiogram, cardiac enzymes × 3 every 6 to 8 hours, BNP, an ABG, and CT angiogram to rule out PE should be obtained.

Table 4.14 HTN Categories and When to Treat

Category	Systolic (mmHg)	Diastolic (mmHg)	Follow-up	Status
Mild	140–159	90–99	2 month	
Moderate	160–179	100–109	1 month	
Severe	180–209	110–119	1 week	Urgent
Crisis	210	120	Immediate	Crisis

- ○ Treatment is diuresis, O_2 supplementation, and correction of the underlying cause.
- HTN is often not symptomatic (Table 4.14).
  - ○ When symptomatic, symptoms can be headache or change in vision.
  - ○ Diagnosis is via BP assessment. If symptomatic, an EKG, cardiac enzymes × 3 every 6 to 8 hours, and CT head without contrast or MRI are indicated to rule out stroke.
  - ○ Parameters: Grading of HTN is per Table 4.14.
  - ○ Treatment for crisis-range HTN can include: nitroprusside (Nipride) 1 to 10 mcg/kg/min IV; ACE inhibitor (enalapril) 12.5 mg PO or 1.25 to 2.5 mg IV every 6 hours; a beta blocker (labetalol) 20 mg IV, repeated at 40 to 80 mg q10 minutes with a maximum dose of 300 mg and a maintenance dose of 0.5 to 2 mg/min; an alpha blocker (hydralazine) dosed at 5 to 20 mg IV.
  - ○ Management of HTN, other than crisis range, is with single-agent or combination agents. First-line drugs are often diuretics (hydrochlorothiazide). Beta-blockers can be first or second line, as can be calcium channel blockers (a better response is seen with these drugs in African Americans). ACE inhibitors and ARBs can be used if there are contraindications to other medications, or they can be used in combination.
- Arrhythmias are abnormal rhythms of the heart rate. It is important to always rule out a myocardial infarction. If the patient is unstable, cardioversion should always be performed. Secondary investigation is directed at abnormal electrolytes, endocrine issues (TSH), and drug toxicity. Most arrhythmias are transient.
  - ○ Atrial fibrillation is a tachyarrhythmia. Diagnosis is via EKG, which shows an irregularly irregular rhythm with no P wave. Acute Treatment is with IV diltiazem. A beta blocker can be helpful if there is a rapid ventricular response. Amiodarone has a lower incidence of recurrent atrial fibrillation. Digoxin can also be used if low BP accompanies the arrhythmia. If there is persistent atrial fibrillation, chronic anticoagulation should be considered based on the CHADS2 score. The CHADS2 score is based on patient

Table 4.15 Annual Risk of CVAs Based on CHADS2 Score

Score	CVA Risk
0	1.9
1	2.8
2	4
3	5.9
4	8.5
5	12.5
6	18.2

risk factors. These include HTN greater than 140/90 mmHg; age greater than 75; DM; history of CVA or TIA; or history of VTE. All risk factors are given a score of 1 except for the CVA and VTE components, which are scored at 2 each. If the score is a 2 or higher, anticoagulation is recommended (Table 4.15, Table 4.16).

○ Atrial flutter is a tachyarrhythmia. Diagnosis is via EKG, which shows a saw-tooth pattern. Aspirin (ASA) prophylaxis is indicated.

○ Supraventricular tachycardia is a tachyarrhythmia. Diagnosis is via EKG, which shows tachycardia with no P waves. Treatment is initiated with vagal maneuvers. If this is unsuccessful, adenosine can be administered up to three times (given IV at 6 mg, then at 12 mg if no initial response, and 12 mg again if refractory).

○ *Bradycardia* is defined as a pulse less than 60 bpm. Diagnosis is via EKG. If the patient is symptomatic and not stable, the patient should be paced transcutaneously until a permanent pacemaker can be placed or the etiology diagnosed. If the patient is stable, treatment is with atropine dosed at 1 mg IV.

○ Postoperative atrial fibrillation after noncardiac surgery: The differential diagnosis includes hypovolemia, intraoperative hypotension, trauma, pain, acute anemia, hypoxia, hypokalemia, low magnesium, hypervolemia or myocardial infarction. A goal is HR

Table 4.16 CHADS2 Scoring

Age: 65–74	1 pt
>75	2 pt
CHF 1 pt	1 pt
HTN 1 pt	1 pt
DM	1 pt
CVA	2 pts

of 80 to 100 bpm, not rhythm control. The AFFIRM trial was the largest trial to compare rate with rhythm control; 80.1% (NS) of AEs were observed in the rhythm management versus 73% in the rate control arms with more mortality in the rhythm treated arm. Management pathways are determined by symptoms.[49]

- Symptomatic (unstable BP, pulmonary edema, chest pain, change in level of consciousness): Direct cardioversion. If the patient declines electrical cardioversion, then IV medication should be administered: metoprolol, diltiazem, amiodarone, or digoxin.
- Asymptomatic: Determine the EF (order echocardiogram). Consider direct cardioversion. If the EF is:
  □ Greater than 45%: Then administer oral metoprolol, diltiazem, amiodarone, digoxin.
  □ Less than 45%: Consider IV medications to start and convert to oral after rhythm is controlled: IV medications include diltiazem, amiodarone, or digoxin. IV flecainide and propafenone can be used if the duration is less than 7 days. Amiodarone, dofetilide, or ibutilide should be used if there are cardiac comorbidities.
- It is important to restart beta blockers or calcium channel blockers that were used as maintenance preoperatively.
- If atrial fibrillation persists greater than 48 hours, the need for chronic anticoagulation should be assessed.
- Postoperative patients have a high risk of hemorrhage with anticoagulation: The **HAS-BLED** surgical risk scoring system assesses for hemorrhage. A score ≥3 indicates high risk of bleeding: some versions include alcohol use and antiplatelet medications, which are assigned one point each[50] (Table 4.17).

Shock and Sepsis

- *Shock* is defined as a decrease in tissue perfusion.[51] There are five types of shock: septic, cardiogenic, hemorrhagic, neurogenic, and iatrogenic. Diagnosis is via physical examination, vitals, EKG, and lab tests. Treatment generally consists of IVF and type-directed support.

Table 4.17 HAS-BLED Scoring System	
HTN	1 pt
Abnormal renal/liver function	1 pt
CVA	1 pt
Bleeding history	1 pt
Labine INR	1 pt
Age >65	1 pt

- ○ Cardiogenic shock can be due to myocardial infarction, HTN yielding a heavy afterload and severe cardiac strain, or pump failure from too much volume. Cardiogenic shock is managed by diuretics to reduce the preload, dopamine or dobutamine to increase cardiac function, norepinephrine if dopamine fails, and nitroprusside or a NTG drip for venous capacitance. Angiography with angioplasty, stent placement, LVAD, or CABG surgery can be employed for acute management.
- ○ Hemorrhagic shock is managed by IVF replacement (3:1 ratio of IVF to blood loss) and blood products, surgery for hemostasis, or embolization.
- ○ Neurogenic shock often occurs from embolic or hemorrhagic stroke, head trauma, or metastatic disease. It is managed by IVF, pressor support, hyperventilation with intubation if necessary, XRT with steroids to reduce local inflammation, and potential surgery if a mass effect is present.
- ○ Iatrogenic shock is usually related to anaphylaxis. Treatment is to stop the offending medication/infusion, administration of steroids, epinephrine, antihistamines, O_2, and pressor support as indicated.
- ○ Septic shock, see the text that follows.
- SIRS occurs when two or more of the following are documented in the setting of a known cause of inflammation: a body temperature greater than 38°C or less than 36°C; a pulse greater than 90 bpm; a respiratory rate greater than 20 bpm or a $PaCO_2$ ≤32; a WBC greater than 12×10^3/mcL, or less than 4×10^3/mcL, or greater than 10% band forms. In 2001, additional criteria were added for an inclusive approach to SIRS. These include an altered mental status, oliguria, skin mottling, coagulopathy, hypoxemia, and hyperglycemia without a diagnosis of diabetes, thrombocytopenia, and altered LFTs.
- A high level of suspicion should be maintained for SIRS with suspicion of organ dysfunction determined by:
  - ○ Decreased perfusion: Capillary refill greater than 3 seconds, skin mottling, cold extremities
  - ○ Circulatory: SBP less than 90 mmHg, MAP less than 65 mmHg, decrease in SBP greater than 40 mmHg
  - ○ Respiratory: PaO_2/FiO_2 less than 300; PaO_2; SaO_2 less than 90%
  - ○ Hepatic: Jaundice; total bilirubin greater than 4 mg/dL; increased LFTs; increased PT
  - ○ Renal: Creatinine greater than 0.3 mg/dL; urine output less than 0.5 mL/kg/hr for at least 2 hours
  - ○ CNS: Altered consciousness, confusion, psychosis
  - ○ Coagulopathy: INR greater than 1.5 or a PTT greater than 60 seconds, thrombocytopenia (platelets less than 100,000/mm3)
  - ○ Splanchnic circulation: Absent bowel sounds
  - ○ Consider Lactate > 2 mmol/L

- **Sepsis** is the clinical syndrome of organ dysfunction caused by response to infection.
- **Septic shock**: is sepsis with hypotension and reduction in organ perfusion despite adequate fluid resuscitation. There are two stages: early hyperdynamic and late hypodynamic. The crude mortality is 28% to 50%. Three- and 6-hour time marks are used to mark and respond to interventions.
- Screening tools: Recommended tools include SIRS, NEWS, or MEWS to determine extent of organ dysfunction. SOFA scoring is not recommended. Lactate levels are listed as a weak recommendation for sepsis screening (Table 4.18).
- Management: Intervention is needed with transfer or admission to the ICU.
- Lines: An arterial line is needed to measure the MAP; consider use of a PA catheter for measurement of the CO and a Foley catheter to measure urine output. Capillary refill should guide resuscitation as an adjunct measure.
- Laboratories: An ABG to measure the $PaCO_2$ and PaO_2; CBC, coagulation profile, D-dimer, fibrinogen, LFTs, total bilirubin, albumin, CMP, magnesium, phosphorus, calcium, 1,3 beta-D-glucan assay, and mannan and antimannan antibody assays if candidiasis is in the differential diagnosis. The serum lactate (≥2 mmol/L) or POC lactate can be followed to see whether resuscitation is trending appropriately. Lactate as a screening test alone is not sensitive nor specific enough to rule in/out the diagnosis and should only be used as an adjunct if chosen. Procalcitonin levels are not recommended.
- Cultures are needed for bacteria, fungus, and virus. These should be obtained from blood, urine, sputum, and wound before antimicrobial therapy is initiated. At least two sets of blood cultures (aerobic and anaerobic) with at least one drawn percutaneously and one drawn through each vascular access devices, unless it was inserted less than 48 hours prior, are necessary. Prompt removal of source lines should occur after other vascular access has been obtained. Antibiotic initiation should be within 45 minutes to 1 hour of recognition if shock is determined to be septic.
- Imaging should be performed to rule out the site of infection.
- Goals are a CVP of 8 to 12, an MAP ≥65, CVP of 8 to 12 mmHg (12–15 if intubated), a urine output ≥0.5 mL/kg/hr, an $ScvO_2$ (central venous O_2 saturation) ≥70% or a mixed venous oxygen saturation ≥65%, and a normalized lactate level if initially elevated. Goal attainment is desired within 6 hours. If oxygen saturation goals are not met in 6 hours, it may be beneficial to transfuse PRBC to achieve a Hg greater than 10 g/dL.
- Management: Hemodynamic management is achieved through invasive monitoring with an arterial line or a central line.

Table 4.18 MEWS Scoring Table

Score	3	2	1	0	1	2	3
Systolic BP (mmHg)	≤70	71–80	81–100	101–199		≥200	
Heart rate (bpm)		<40	41–50	51–100	101–110	111–129	≥130
Respiratory rate (bpm)		<9		9–14	15–20	21–29	≥30
Temperature (°C / °F)		<35 / 95°	35.1–36	36.1–38	38.1–38.5	≥38.6 / 101.3	
AVPU score				Alert	Reacts to voice	Reacts to pain	Unresponsive
Hourly urine for 2 hours (mL/h)	<10	<30	<45				

0 points: .9%, 2 points: 7.9%, 3 and 4 points 12.7%, 5, 6, 7, 8 points 30% chance of ICU admission or death within 60 days.
AVPU: awake/verbal/pain/unresponsive.

○ Initial treatment is 30mL/kg of IV fluid given within the first 3 hours of resuscitation using balanced crystalloids. Fluid administration is continued as long as there is hemodynamic improvement either based on preferred dynamic (e.g., change in pulse pressure, passive leg raise, stroke volume variation) or static (e.g., arterial pressure, heart rate) variables. Albumin can be used for those receiving large volumes of crystalloids. Normal saline, gelatin, or starches should not be used.

○ For an MAP <65: Vasopressors are recommended with a MAP goal of 65 to 70 mmHg. Initiation through a peripheral line is recommended rather than waiting on a central line. Norepinephrine is recommended as first-line use in the range of 0.25 to 0.5 μg/kg/min, followed by vasopressin at 0.03 U/min (not usually titrated) if the MAP continues to be inadequate (rather than increase NE). Epinephrine and dopamine are recommended as second-line agents.

○ For those with cardiac dysfunction despite adequate volume and normal MAP: Inotropic therapy with dobutamine infusion up to 20 mcg/kg/min can be given or added to a vasopressor in the presence of:

  ▪ Myocardial dysfunction as suggested by elevated cardiac filling pressures and low CO, or

  ▪ Ongoing signs of hypoperfusion, despite achieving adequate intravascular volume and adequate MAP.

○ The cardiac index should not be "improved" by pharmacologic or fluid infusion strategies to predetermined super-normal levels. Thus, dobutamine with NE is recommended, or use epinephrine alone. Terlipressin and levosimendan are not recommended.

● Antimicrobial therapy: Administration of broad-spectrum IV antimicrobials within the first hour of recognition of septic shock or severe sepsis without septic shock is indicated. This should include one or more drugs that have activity against all likely pathogens to include bacterial and/or fungal and/or viral. Antimicrobials with methicillin-resistant *Staphylococcus aureus* (MRSA) coverage should be prioritized if the patient is at risk. Use of only one Gram-negative agent, using prolonged infusion regimens of beta-lactams (over boluses) should be followed. Low procalcitonin levels can assist the clinician in the discontinuation of empiric antibiotics in patients who initially appeared septic, but have no laboratory evidence of infection. Combination empirical antimicrobial therapy should be started for neutropenic patients with severe sepsis. Empiric combination therapy should not be administered for more than 3 to 5 days. Antimicrobial regimens should be reassessed daily for potential de-escalation to the most appropriate single therapy as soon as the susceptibility profile is known. Duration of therapy is the shortest amount of time possible and can be 5 to 8 days. Longer courses may be appropriate in patients who have a slow clinical response, undrainable foci of infection, bacteremia with *Staphylococcus aureus*, some fungal and viral infections, or immunologic deficiencies, including neutropenia. Empiric antifungal coverage should be evaluated by risk factors, including immunosuppression, prior colonization and infection, a vascular access device, neutropenia, prior exposure to prophylactic therapy, and (cancer) comorbidities. Antiviral therapy should be initiated as early as possible in patients with severe sepsis or septic shock of viral origin and considered in immunocompromised patients. For patients with difficult-to-treat, multidrug-resistant bacterial pathogens:

- *Pseudomonas aeruginosa* bacteremia infections associated with respiratory failure and septic shock require combination therapy with an extended spectrum beta-lactam and either an aminoglycoside or a fluoroquinolone.
- *Streptococcus pneumoniae* bacteremia infections: A combination of a beta-lactam and macrolide is recommended.

- Source control: A specific anatomical diagnosis of infection requiring consideration for emergent source control should be identified or excluded as rapidly as possible, and intervention be undertaken for source control within the first 12 hours after the diagnosis is made. All catheters should be changed and cultured. Any site of infection should be explored and drained if possible (there is up to an 80% percutaneous success rate). Surgical exploration can potentially access those sites not amenable to needle drainage. Fever and leukocytosis, respectively, are absent in 35% and 5% of peritoneal infections. An eye examination should also be part of the workup.

- Corticosteroids: If adequate fluid resuscitation and vasopressor therapy are able to restore hemodynamic stability, corticosteroids should not be used. If this is not achievable, IV hydrocortisone alone can be dosed at 200 mg/day, continuous infusion. Hydrocortisone should be tapered when vasopressors are no longer required. An ACTH stimulation test should not be used to determine which patients to treat with steroids. Corticosteroids should not be administered for the treatment of sepsis in the absence of shock.

- Blood product and management: A target Hg concentration is 7.0 to 9.0 g/dL in adults. An RBC transfusion can be considered when the Hg is less than 7.0 g/dL (restrictive transfusion policy). A higher transfusion threshold for patients with myocardial ischemia, severe hypoxemia, acute hemorrhage, or IHD can be considered. Platelet transfusion should only be given prophylactically when counts are less than 10,000/mm^3 to reduce the risk of spontaneous bleeding in therapy-induced hypoproliferative thrombocytopenia. Prophylactic platelet transfusion can be considered when counts are less than 20,000/mm^3, if the patient has a significant risk of bleeding, if there is active bleeding, or there is a planned invasive procedure. The goal is 50,000/mm^3. For elective surgical patients with thrombocytopenia and platelets <50,000/mm^3, it is recommended to transfuse platelets preoperatively. Erythropoietin should not be used as a specific treatment of anemia associated with severe sepsis. FFP should not be used to correct laboratory clotting abnormalities in the absence of bleeding or planned invasive procedures. Antithrombin should not be used for the treatment of severe sepsis and septic shock.

- Mechanical ventilation of sepsis-induced ARDS: The SpO$_2$ should be maintained ≥92% with oxygen. The tidal volume for mechanically ventilated patients with ALI/ARDS is 6 mL/kg. Plateau pressures should be measured and the initial upper limit goal for plateau pressures in a passively inflated lung should be ≤30 cm H$_2$O. PEEP should be applied at 5 cm H$_2$O to avoid alveolar collapse at end expiration (atelecto-trauma), with higher levels of PEEP for patients with moderate to severe ARDS. Prone positioning can be used in sepsis-induced ARDS patients with a PaO$_2$/FiO$_2$ ratio ≤100 mmHg for more than 12 hr/day. Intermittent NMBA boluses should be used instead of continuous infusion. ECMO can be used when conventional ventilation fails. The head of the bed should be elevated 30° to 45° to limit aspiration risk and to prevent the development of VAP. A weaning protocol should be in place daily with daily spontaneous breathing trials. A conservative fluid strategy should be maintained for patients with established sepsis-induced ARDS who do not have evidence of tissue hypoperfusion. Beta 2-agonists are not recommended unless bronchospasm is present.

- Sedation, analgesia, and neuromuscular blockade in sepsis: Continuous or intermittent sedation should be minimized in mechanically ventilated patients. NMBAs should be avoided if possible in the septic patient without ARDS due to the risk of prolonged neuromuscular blockade following discontinuation. If NMBAs must be maintained, either intermittent bolus as required or continuous infusion with peripheral nerve stimulator/train-of-four monitoring of the depth of blockade should be used. A course of NMBA, not greater than 48 hours, can be used for patients with early sepsis-induced ARDS and a PaO$_2$/FiO$_2$ less than 150 mmHg.

- Glucose control: Glucose levels should be checked every 1 to 2 hours upon diagnosis. Insulin dosing should be initiated when two consecutive blood glucose levels are greater than 180 mg/dL. A target upper blood glucose is ≤180 mg/dL. Glucose values should be monitored every 1 to 2 hours until values and insulin infusion rates are stable, then every 4 hours.

- Renal replacement therapy: Continuous renal replacement therapies (CCRT) and intermittent hemodialysis have been shown to be equivalent in patients with severe sepsis and acute renal failure. The use of continuous therapies has been shown to facilitate management of fluid balance in hemodynamically unstable septic patients.

CCRT is intended to be applied for 24 hr/day in an ICU and describes a variety of blood purification techniques, which differ according to the mechanism of solute transport, the type of membrane, the presence or absence of dialysate solution, and the type of vascular access. CRRT provides slower solute clearance per unit time as compared with intermittent therapies but over 24 hours may even exceed clearances with hemodialysis. Solute removal with CRRT is achieved either by convection (hemofiltration), diffusion (hemodialysis), or a combination of both these methods (hemodiafiltration). Hemodialysis most efficiently removes small molecular weight substances such as urea, creatinine, and potassium. Middle and larger molecular weight substances are more efficiently removed using hemofiltration as compared with dialysis.

- Feeding: For those who can be fed enterally, feeding within 72 hours is recommended.
- Bicarbonate therapy: Sodium bicarbonate therapy has not been shown to improve hemodynamics or reduce vasopressor requirements in patients with hypoperfusion-induced lactic acidemia with pH ≥7.2. It can be used with severe metabolic acidemia (pH <7.2) and an AKIN (Acute Kidney Injury Network) score 2 or 3.
- DVT prophylaxis: A combination of pharmacologic therapy and SCD's should be used whenever possible. Daily pharmacoprophylaxis is recommended with SC LMWH versus administering three-times- daily UFH. If the CrCl is less than 30 mL/min, dalteparin is recommended. Patients who have a contraindication to heparin use (e.g., thrombocytopenia, severe coagulopathy, active bleeding, recent intracerebral hemorrhage) should receive SCDs alone. When the risk decreases, pharmacoprophylaxis should start.
- Stress ulcer prophylaxis: Stress ulcer prophylaxis using an H_2 blocker or proton pump inhibitor should be given to patients with severe sepsis/septic shock with preference given to proton pump inhibitors.
- Immunoglobulins, vitamin C, polymyxin B hemoperfusion, and selenium are not recommended for use.

- **Antibiotic by site (overview)**[55]: Note: Please consult current institutional guidelines and sensitivity charts.
  - Fever of unknown origin (Unidentified site of infection/sepsis):
    - Community-acquired: Vancomycin plus ceftriaxone or ertapenem or piperacillin/tazobactam
    - Healthcare-acquired: Vancomycin and either meropenem, piperacillin/tazobactam, or cefepime; an add tobramycin if poor response to antibiotic doublet.
  - Abdominal:
    - *C.difficile colitis*: Administer vancomycin 125 mg PO q6h x 10 days. If severely immunocompromised: fidaxomicin 200 mg PO BID x 10 days, vancomycin 500 mg PO/NGT q6h and

metronidazole 500mg IV q8h +/- rectal vancomycin 500 mg in 100 mL 0f 0.9% NaCl instilled q6h as an enema retained for 1 hour.

- Spontaneous bacterial peritonitis: Ceftriaxone
- Diverticulitis: Ceftriaxone and metronidazole
- Moderate abdominal abscess: Ceftriaxone with metronidazole or ertapenem
- Healthcare-acquired moderate abdominal abscess: Ertapenem or piperacillin/tazobactam
- Severe abdominal abscess: Vancomycin and piperacillin/tazobactam or meropenem, consider antifungal if bowel perforation.

○ Pneumonia:
  - Healthcare-acquired: Administer vancomycin plus ertapenem or cefepime or piperacillin/tazobactam, add azithromycin if ICU admission. If a history of *Pseudomonas*: Administer cefepime 2gIV q8h or piperacillin/tazobactam 4.5g IV q6h; duration is to 7 days.
  - VAP:
    □ Early vancomycin and levofloxacin or ertapenem
    □ Late vancomycin and piperacillin/tazobactam or cefepime or vancomycin and meropenem.
  - Community-acquired: Administer ceftriaxone and doxycycline for 5 days.
○ Necrotizing fasciitis: Administer vancomycin and clindamycin and either piperacillin/tazobactam or ertapenem.
○ Soft tissue or skin abscess: Incise and drain and IV vancomycin
○ Neurology:
  - Meningitis: Administer ceftriaxone 2g IV q12h and vancomycin with or without ampicillin 2g IV q4h.
  - Brain abscess: Administer ceftriaxone 2gIV q12h and metronidazole with or without vancomycin.
○ Renal/Urinary: Pyelonephritis
  - Community acquired: Administer ceftriaxone or ertapenem.
  - Healthcare-acquired: Use ertapenem or piperacillin/tazobactam.
○ Endometritis: Administer cefoxitin, second-line therapy would be an ertapenem.

- **Algorithms:**
  ○ Completed within **3** hours:
    - Invasive monitoring established.
    - Obtain blood cultures prior to antibiotic administration.

- Administer broad-spectrum antibiotics.
- Obtain labs and consider lactate level
- Administer IVF 30 mL/kg for hypotension or a lactate ≥4 mmol/L.
  - To be completed within **6** hours:
    - Remeasure lactate level if initially elevated (≥2 mmol/L).
    - Administer vasopressors if still hypotensive to obtain an MAP ≥65 mmHg and assess CV status with one of the following:
      - Measure CVP, measure ScvO₂, use bedside echocardiogram, or assess fluid responsiveness with passive leg raise or fluid challenge.
  - CV management:
    - MAP: <65 mmHg
      - Fluid challenge: NS or LR 30 mL/kg over 30 to 60 minutes
        - If EF <40%, reduce the volume of the fluid challenge. Consider colloid if pulmonary edema or liver failure. Repeat every 30 minutes until CVP ≥8 mmHg.
      - If MAP still will not respond, then vasopressors should be initiated.
        - Norepinephrine 2.5–5 mcg/kg/min, titrate 2.5 mcg/min every 5 minutes. If MAP is suboptimal at 5 mcg/kg/min, add vasopressin at a fixed dose of 0.03 to 0.06 U/min. If norepinephrine is not available, epinephrine 1 mcg/kg/min titrated by 0.5 mcg/kg/min every 5 minutes or dopamine can be used.
      - If MAP still will not respond: consider hydrocortisone 50 mg IV every 6 hours.
    - CVP:
      - Administer NS or LR bolus over 30 minutes at 30 mL/kg.
      - Consider albumin if pulmonary edema or liver failure.
      - Repeat every 30 minutes until CVP ≥8 mmHg.
  - Pulmonary management:
    - If ScvO₂ is less than 70%, check Hg: If Hg is < 10g/dL, consider transfusion, if Hg ≥10 g/dL administer dobutamine as a continuous infusion until ScvO₂ ≥70%.[52]
    - Multiple organ dysfunction syndrome (MODS) is the development of the progressive physiologic dysfunction of two or more organ systems. This usually occurs after an acute threat to systemic homeostasis. Treatment is support of individual organ function and aggressive therapies aimed at correcting the underlying process.

Neutropenia

- ANC < 1,500 cells/uL; severe neutropenia, ANC is < 500 cells/mL or ANC is expected to fall below 500 cells/uL in the next 2 days; profound neutropenia, ANC is < 100 cells/uL. If the ANC <500/uL, or <1000/uL and likely to fall to <500/uL within 48 hours (and is expected to be low for >7 days), bacterial prophylaxis can be initiated with levofloxacin 500 mg PO daily. Consider antifungal prophylaxis with an oral triazole if profound neutropenia. Consider a nucleoside reverse transcription inhibitor if at high risk of HepB virus reactivation. Consider TMP-SMX if >3.5% risk for pneumocystis pneumonia.

Febrile Neutropenia

- Neutropenic fever: a single oral temperature ≥38.3, or a temperature ≥ to 38.0 degrees C sustained for over an hour, with an ANC of < 500 cells/uL. Calculate ANC: multiple total WBC count by the % of polymorphonuclear cells and band neutrophils.
- **Risk scoring:** It is important to risk stratify all patients into low- or high-risk categories by calculating the **MASCC risk score** (Table 4.19): a score of ≥21 is considered low and a score <21 as high risk (with a PPV of 91%, specificity of 68%, and sensitivity of 71%).[53]
  - **Low risk:** Has outpatient status at time of fever; no acute comorbid illness; anticipated short duration of severe neutropenia (<100 cells/mcL for <7 days); good performance status (ECOG 0–1); no hepatic or renal insufficiency.
  - **High risk:** Includes any of the following risk factors: inpatient at time of fever development; clinically unstable; anticipated prolonged severe neutropenia of less than 100 cells/mcL for greater than 7 days; and significant medical comorbidity to include hepatic insufficiency 5x the upper limit of normal for LFT's; renal insufficiency with CrCl of less than 30 mL/min; uncontrolled or

Table 4.19 The MASCC Risk Index
5 points:
No to few symptoms Normal BP
4 points:
No COPD Solid tumor or blood malignancy without prior fungal infection
3 points:
Moderate symptoms Normovolemic outpatient management
2 points:
Age <60

progressive cancer; pneumonia or other complex infection at presentation; alemtuzumab use; mucositis G 3 to 4.

- Management: All patients should receive **broad-spectrum** antibiotics; **then the source** should be identified. If high risk, the patient needs to be hospitalized and IV therapy instituted. If the patient scores as low risk: PO or IV/sequential PO therapy can be administered. Discharge can be to home if patients are compliant and have established care. If intermediate to high risk, consider adding PCP and candida prophylaxis with fluconazole.

- If unstable: Transfer to the ICU and initiate meropenem 1 g IV q8h and vancomycin dosed to a trough of 15 to 20 uL/mL. Discontinue levofloxacin.

- **Source/Site Management**
  - Abdominal pain: Workup: abdominal CT, LFTs, bilirubin, amylase, lipase, *C. difficile* PCR
  - Perirectal pain: Workup: visual examination, consider CT abdomen/pelvis. Treatment: Ensure adequate anaerobic therapy, consider enterococcal coverage, local care with sitz baths, stool softeners, mesalamine enema.
  - Diarrhea: Workup: *C. difficile* PCR, consider testing for rotavirus, norovirus, consider stool bacterial and parasite cultures, consider adenovirus. Treatment: Administer oral vancomycin, fidaxomicin, or metronidazole if highly suspected or confirmed *C. difficile*.
  - Renal/urinary tract symptoms: Workup: urine analysis and culture. Treatment based on specific pathogen identified.
  - Mouth/mucosal membrane:
    - White coating: Workup: thrush likely, needs fungal culture. Treatment: Fluconazole is first line, voriconazole, posaconazole, or echinocandin if refractory.
    - Vesicular lesions: Workup: viral diagnostics. Treatment is anti-HSV therapy.
    - Necrotizing ulceration: Workup: viral diagnostics, culture and Gram stain, biopsy suspicious lesions, consider leukemic infiltrate. Treatment: Ensure adequate anaerobic activity, consider anti-HSV therapy, and consider systemic antifungal activity.
  - Esophagus: Workup: viral diagnostics, culture suspicious oral lesions for both fungal and bacterial etiology, consider endoscopy if no response to therapy, consider CMV esophagitis. Treatment is guided by clinical findings, fungal versus viral, with ongoing broad-spectrum antibiotics.
  - Sinus/nasal: Workup: CT or MRI of the sinus or orbit, ears, nose, throat, ophthalmology consultation, culture and stain, biopsy if indicated. Treatment: Add vancomycin if periorbital cellulitis, add amphotericin B to cover aspergillosis and mucormycosis in high-risk patients with suspicious CT/MRI findings.

○ Cellulitis/skin and soft-tissue infections: Workup: aspirate or biopsy for culture. Treatment is Gram-positive active agent.

○ Vascular access device: Workup: if there is entry-site inflammation, swab entry-site drainage for culture, blood culture from each port of access device. Treatment: Administer vancomycin initially or add if not responding within 48 hours of empiric therapy. If tunnel infection/port pocket infection, or septic phlebitis: Workup: blood culture from each port. Treatment: cover for the positive culture, remove catheter, add vancomycin if not responding.

○ Vascular lesions: Workup: aspirate or scrape for varicella or HSV PCR or direct fluorescent antibody, herpes virus culture if PCR unavailable. Treatment: Consider acyclovir.

○ Disseminated papules or other lesions: Workup: aspirate or biopsy for bacterial, fungal, mycobacterial cultures, and histopathology, consider VZV evaluation. Treatment: Consider vancomycin, add active antifungal therapy in HiR patients.

○ Central nervous system symptoms: Workup: CT and/or MRI, LP if possible, neurology consult. Treatment: Initial empiric therapy pending ID consult. If suspected meningitis, include antipseudomonal beta-lactam agent that enters CSF plus vancomycin, plus ampicillin unless using meropenem. For encephalitis, add high-dose acyclovir.

○ Lung infiltrates: Workup: blood and sputum cultures, consider nasal wash for viruses, *Legionella* urine Ag test, and serum galactomannan or beta-glucan test if at risk for mold. CT of the chest should be obtained. Consider bronchial–alveolar lavage if poor response or diffuse infiltrates. Consider diagnostic lung biopsy. Treatment: azithromycin or fluoroquinolone. Consider adding antifungal in moderate- to high-risk patients. Add antiviral therapy during influenza outbreaks. TMP/SMX coverage should be added if PCP is possible. Add vancomycin or linezolid if MRSA is suspected.

- **General antimicrobial recommendations:**
  ○ Uncomplicated patient with febrile neutropenia:
    ▪ IV antibiotic monotherapy to include either cefepime, imipenem/cilastatin, meropenem, piperacillin/tazobactam, ceftazidime.
    ▪ Oral antibiotic therapy for low-risk patients to include either ciprofloxacin and amoxicillin/clavulanate, or moxifloxacin, but none if quinolone prophylaxis was used.
  ○ Complicated febrile neutropenic patient: IV antibiotic monotherapy is preferred, but combination therapy should be used if resistance is identified.
- **Duration of treatment** for documented infections in cancer patients is usually 7 to 14 days, and when the patient is clinically stable, and afebrile for at least 48 hours. The antibiotic regimen should be continued until ANC ≥500 cells/mcL and increasing.

○ Skin/soft tissue: 7 to 14 days
○ Bloodstream uncomplicated: Gram negative: 10 to 14 days; Gram positive: 7 to 14 days; *Staphylococcus aureus*: at least 2 weeks after first negative blood culture; yeast 2+ weeks after first negative blood culture. Consider catheter removal for *S. aureus, Pseudomonas aeruginosa, Corynebacterium jeikeium, Acinetobacter, Bacillus* organisms, atypical mycobacteria, yeasts, molds, *vancomycin-resistant enterococci, and Stenotrophomonas maltophilia*.
○ Bacterial sinusitis: 7 to 14 days
○ Catheter removal needed for septic phlebitis, tunnel infection, or port pocket infection.
○ Pneumonia:
  ▪ Bacterial 7 to 14 days
  ▪ Fungal (mold and yeast):
    ▫ *Candida* should be treated for a minimum of 2 weeks after first negative blood culture.
    ▫ Mold (*Aspergillus ex*): Minimum of 12 weeks
  ▪ Viral HSV/VZV: Uncomplicated, skin disease: Administer for 7 to 10 days; influenza: oseltamivir for 5 days if immunocompetent and healthy, 10 days if unhealthy.

Renal Complications

The definition of acute renal failure is not standardized.

• A patient is usually diagnosed with a rising creatinine, or with a urine output of less than 400 mL/24 hr.
• There are three types of acute renal failure: prerenal, renal (intrinsic), and postrenal. Lab tests should be ordered to include a CMP, urine analysis for microscopy, urine electrolytes to include Na and creatinine, SG, and urine osmolality. The next step is to calculate the fractional excretion of sodium (FENa): The equation is UNa × SCr/SNa × UCr × 100%. The renal failure index is another calculation: (Urinary Na concentration × Plasma Cr concentration)/Urinary Cr concentration.
  ○ If the FENa is less than 1% and the urine SG is greater than 1.025, the diagnosis is prerenal failure and often due to hypoperfusion. If the FENa is greater than 4% and the urine SG is less than 1.01, the diagnosis is often due to renal ischemia. It is important to remember that a FENa cannot be calculated if diuretics, mannitol, or IV contrast material have been given.
  ○ Prerenal failure: The etiology is often volume depletion from surgical blood loss, third spacing from removal of ascites, extensive bowel preparation and NPO status, CHF, severe liver disease, or other edematous states. Laboratory findings include a urinary sodium concentration less than 20 mEq/L, a urine:plasma creatinine ratio greater than 30, urine osmolality greater than 500 mOsm/kg. The renal failure index is less than 1.

- ○ Intrinsic renal failure: The etiology can be aminoglycoside anti-biotics, IV contrast material, cytolytic drug exposure, statin medication, rhabdomyolysis, hyperuricemia, multiple myeloma, and streptococcal infection. Findings include a urinary sodium concentration > 40 mEq/L, a urine:plasma creatinine ratio < 20, and urine osmolality < 400 mOsm/kg. The UA can show eosino-phils (acute interstitial nephritis), RBC casts (glomerulonephritis or vasculitis), or renal tubular epithelial cells and muddy brown casts (acute tubular necrosis). The cause is sloughing of renal tubular cells into the lumen, demonstrating casts called *Tamm–Horsfall bodies*. Management is with support, including volume repletion until euvolemia is reached, with monitoring and restriction of potassium agents. A diuretic challenge can be offered if volume overload becomes evident. Dialysis should be consid-ered if volume overload, acidosis, uremia, or EKG changes occur. Treatment is to stop the offending drug. A desired urinary output is ≥0.5 mL/kg/hr.

- ○ Postrenal failure is usually obstructive. This can occur with bilat-eral hydronephrosis from cervical cancer, nephrolithiasis, ure-thral obstruction, bladder compression from tumor, or ureteral obstruction from tumor/stone/surgery. Lab tests include serum BUN:Cr > 20:1, a urine osmolality < 400 mOsm/kg, and a urinary sodium concentration > 40 mEq/L. The Foley catheter should be checked and flushed. A renal US can be obtained to document hydronephrosis. A CT urogram can be obtained to evaluate for ureteral obstruction from surgical injury or tumor. Nephrolithiasis and retroperitoneal fibrosis can also cause this complication. Reduction of the obstruction with surgical correction or place-ment of a PCN tube is indicated. It is important to follow for postobstructive diuresis: *postobstructive diuresis* is defined as diuresis of > 200 mL/hr for at least 2 hours. Electrolytes should be checked every 8 hours and the urine output replaced with IVFs in the form of 1/2 saline at 80% of the hourly urine volume for the first 24 hours, then 50%. Postobstructive diuresis usually lasts 24 to 72 hours. Cardiac status should be observed for potential tachycardic failure.

- *Chronic kidney disease* is defined as a GFR of < 60 mL/min/1.73 m². ESRD is often caused by DM and HTN (68%). These patients are con-sidered immunocompromised. The morbidity from surgery can be up to 54%, with a mortality of 4%. For renal patients, it is important to obtain a cardiac workup, manage fluids and electrolytes vigilantly, exercise caution for anemia and bleeding diatheses, and maintain both glycemic and BP control.

- Cardiac disease causes the most deaths in patients with ESRD, and 23% to 40% have no cardiac symptoms. Patients need to be euvole-mic prior to surgery. They need dialysis without heparin 24 hours prior to surgery, and they need postoperative dialysis the day of surgery if a large fluid load was given.

- It is important to check electrolytes immediately after surgery and every 6 to 8 hours until they are normalized.

- If the patient is uremic, platelets do not work well. Cryoprecipitate or dDAVP should be considered to prevent bleeding during surgery. IV estrogen can also be administered (0.6 mg/kg) 4 to 5 days prior to surgery.

- Indications for dialysis include (AEIOU): acidemia, electrolyte abnormalities (hyperkalemia resistant to prior interventions), EKG changes, intoxication with dialyzable substances (aspirin, lithium), volume overload, uremia, and mental status changes. A large central venous catheter may need to be placed if there is an acute need for dialysis.

- Daily management of renal complications include: Strict intake/output (I/O), daily weight, and a low-sodium and low-nitrogen diet.

ACID–BASE DISORDERS

- Metabolic acidosis: The anion gap is calculated by subtracting the serum concentrations of chloride and bicarbonate (anions) from the concentrations of sodium and potassium (cations): = ([Na+] + [K+]) – ([Cl–] + [HCO3–]).

  - Anion gap: The etiology is based on the mnemonic "PLUMSEEDS." These stand for paraldehyde, lactate, urremia, methanol, salicylates, ethylene glycol, ethanol, DKA, starvation. Another mnemonic is "MUDPILES": methanol, uremia (chronic renal failure), diabetic ketoacidosis, propylene glycol, (infection, iron, INH, inborn errors in metabolism), lactic acidosis, ethylene glycol, salicylates.

  - Nonanion gap: The two main causes are diarrhea or renal tubular acidosis. Other causes include acetazolamide, saline administration, hyperalimentation, and ureteral conduit.

- Metabolic alkalosis: Usually occurs from renal dysfunction due to the loss of hydrochloric acid from nausea/vomiting, volume contraction, exogenous bicarbonate administration, hypokalemia, or hyponatremia.

- Respiratory acidosis occurs when there is a failure of ventilation often due to mental status changes. These changes can occur because of a mass effect in the brain, medications, stroke, infection, or inappropriate mechanical ventilation settings.

- Respiratory alkalosis occurs as a result of hyperventilation, including iatrogenic causes from excessive mechanical ventilation (Table 4.20).

Table 4.20 Acid–Base Disorders

Disorder	Primary Change	pH	Compensatory Change
Metabolic acidosis	Decreased HCO_3	Decreased	Decreased pCO_2
Metabolic alkalosis	Increased HCO_3	Increased	Increased pCO_2
Respiratory acidosis	Increased PCO_2	Decreased	Increased HCO_3
Respiratory alkalosis	Decreased PCO_2	Increased	Decreased HCO_3

Electrolyte Abnormalities

- Sodium abnormalities
  - Hyponatremia (serum sodium <135 mEq/L):
    - Pseudohyponatremia is an erroneously low measurement of sodium caused by elevations of plasma lipids, sugars, or proteins.
    - Hypotonic hyponatremia is an increase in free water relative to sodium in extracellular fluids.
    - Hypovolemic hyponatremia is characterized by loss of sodium and water, with a net loss of sodium relative to water; caused by diuretics, adrenal insufficiency, diarrhea, or vomiting.
    - Isovolemic hyponatremia is characterized by increase in water with the same sodium content; caused by inappropriate ADH secretion or psychogenic polydipsia.
    - Hypervolemic hyponatremia is characterized by excess of sodium and water, with a net gain of water relative to sodium; it is caused by heart, renal, or hepatic failure.
    - Signs/symptoms: Hyponatremic encephalopathy is associated with cerebral edema, increased intracranial pressure, and seizures.
    - Treatment is based on low, normal, or high extracellular volume. Avoid rapid correction to prevent central pontine myelinolysis.
  - Hypernatremia (serum sodium >145 mEq/L):
    - Hypovolemic hypernatremia is caused by inadequate intake of water, excessive loss from urinary tract, sweating or diarrhea. Treatment: volume replacement.
    - Hypertonic syndromes are characterized by impaired renal water conservation. This can be caused by diabetes insipidus, either central or nephrogenic. Treatment is to replace free water deficits.

- Hypervolemic hypernatremia is characterized by an increase in hypertonic fluid. This is caused by excessive hypertonic saline resuscitation, sodium bicarbonate infusions, ingestion of seawater, or excessive amounts of table salt. Treat with sodium restriction or diuretic with fluid replacement.
- It is important to avoid rapidly lowering the sodium concentration with free water to avoid cerebral edema.
- Potassium abnormalities
  - Hypokalemia (serum potassium <3.5 mEq/L):
    - Causes:
      - Transcellular shift of potassium into cells from insulin, beta agonists, furosemide, or alkalosis
      - Diminished intake
      - Increased potassium losses from GI or urinary tracts
    - Signs/symptoms: Fatigue, myalgia, muscular weakness, hypoventilation, paralysis, and arrhythmias
    - EKG changes include: T wave inversion, U waves, ST depression, prolonged QT interval, prolonged PR interval, widening of the QRS complex
    - Treatment: Address the underlying cause:
      - Each 0.1 mEq/L of deficiency on laboratory value needs replacement with 10 mEq of potassium chloride (KCl).
      - The maximum rate of KCl in a peripheral IV is 10 mEq/hr; for a central line the rate is 20 mEq/hr.
      - Magnesium: Magnesium depletion can promote urinary loss of potassium, so it is recommended to also correct for magnesium deficit.
  - Hyperkalemia (serum potassium >5.5 mEq/L):
    - Causes:
      - Pseudohyperkalemia is caused by hemolysis from a traumatic blood draw.
      - Transcellular shift from acidosis; rhabdomyolysis; cytotoxic cell death or drugs such as digitalis or beta receptor antagonists
      - Impaired renal excretion from adrenal insufficiency or drugs such as ACE inhibitors, ARBs, NSAIDs, or potassium-sparing diuretics
      - Massive blood transfusions
    - Signs/symptoms: Cardiac toxicity, paralysis, and hypoventilation
    - EKG changes, including increased T waves, peaked T waves, prolonged PR and QRS intervals, loss of P waves
    - Active treatment is recommended if the serum K is greater than 6.5 mEq/L, the patient is acidotic, fluid overloaded, mental status changes are present, or EKG changes are present.

- Kayexalate PO 15 g daily to QID or PR 30 to 50 g q4 hours
- Sodium bicarbonate: 44 to 132 mEq IV
- Calcium chloride or calcium gluconate 10 to 30 mL of a 10% solution IV
- Glucose: 50 g IV
- Regular insulin: 10 units IV
- Dialysis is needed if the patient does not respond to the these measures.

- Magnesium abnormalities
  - Hypomagnesemia:
    - Causes: Diuretic therapy, antibiotics, alcohol-related illness, diarrhea, DM, acute MI, drugs such as digitalis or cisplatin
    - Signs/symptoms: Patient exhibits generalized weakness and altered mentation. It is commonly associated with other electrolyte abnormalities, including hypokalemia, hypophosphatemia, hypocalcemia. It is also associated with hypokalemia that is refractory to treatment.
    - EKG changes: Torsades de pointes, increased PR and QT intervals, atrial and ventricular arrhythmias
    - Treatment: Magnesium sulfate IV or magnesium oxide PO
  - Hypermagnesemia:
    - Causes: Iimpaired renal function or excessive administration
    - Signs/symptoms: Hyporeflexia and EKG changes to include first-degree AV block, complete heart block
    - Treatment: IV or PO calcium gluconate, IV fluids with Lasix, and hemodialysis if refractory
- Calcium abnormalities
  - Hypocalcemia:
    - Causes: Hypoalbuminemia, tumor lysis syndrome, renal failure, hypoparathyroidism, hypomagnesemia, hypermagnesemia, acute pancreatitis, rhabdomyolysis, or blood transfusion (due to citrate chelating calcium).
    - Signs/symptoms: Tetany, Trousseau's sign, Chvostek's sign
    - EKG changes: increased QT interval, ventricular tachycardia
    - Treatment: IV calcium gluconate or calcium chloride 10 mL of a 10% solution; PO calcium carbonate; or calcium gluconate 1 to 2 g PO 3 times a day with meals
  - Hypercalcemia:
    - Causes: Bone metastasis, hyperparathyroidism, CC cancer of ovary or cervix, small cell cancers
    - Signs/symptoms: GI disturbances, hypotension, polyuria, confusion, depressed consciousness, coma.

- EKG changes: shortened QT interval
- Treatment: Rehydration with NS or 1/2 NS IV; diuresis with Lasix 40 mg IV every 2 hours after IV hydration; pamidronate (Aredia) 60 to 90 mg IV over 2 to 24 hours for 7 days; gluco-corticoids such as hydrocortisone 250 to 500 mg IV every 8 hours; calcitonin which lowers calcium by 1 to 3 mg/dL for 6 to 8 hours (perform skin test first to check for hypersensitivity, start at 4 IU/kg SC or IM q12–24 hours); or mithramycin dosed at 25 mcg/kg via slow IV push daily.

- Phosphorus abnormalities
  - Hypophosphatemia:
    - Causes: Impaired intestinal absorption, increased renal excretion, redistribution of phosphate into cells, DKA, glucose loading, oncogenic osteomalacia, hyperparathyroidism, and the diuretic phase of acute tubular necrosis
    - Signs/symptoms: Muscular weakness, heart and respiratory failure, anemia
    - Treatment: Sodium or potassium phosphate IV or PO
  - Hyperphosphatemia:
    - Causes: Renal failure, tumor lysis syndrome, metabolic and respiratory acidosis, hypoparathyroidism
    - Signs/symptoms: Deposition of calcium-phosphate complexes into soft tissue and tetany
    - Treatment: Promote phosphorus binding with sucralfate or aluminum-containing antacids; dialysis if needed for patients with renal failure.

Fluids and Blood Products

- TBW = 0.5 × kg body weight
- Intracellular fluid = 0.4 × kg body weight
- Extracellular fluid = 0.2 × kg body weight
- Interstitial fluid = 0.15 × kg body weight
- Plasma volume = 0.5 × kg body weight
- Blood volume = 75 mL/kg

Electrolytes

- Daily fluid management (Tables 4.21 and 4.22):
  - Daily physiologic fluid intake is composed of the following: Endogenous water production from oxidation (approximately 250 mL/day) and healthy PO intake (approximately 2,000 to 2,500 mL/day).
  - Daily physiologic fluid losses: 2,000 to 2,500 mL. This is composed of water from the urine 800 to 1,500 mL; stool 200 mL; insensible losses to include respiratory 200 mL and skin 800 mL.

Table 4.21 Common Electrolyte Distribution Within the Body

Electrolyte	Plasma	Interstitial	Intracellular
Na	142	145	10 mEq/L
K	4	–	156 mEq/L
Cl	104	114	2 mEq/L
HCO3	27	31	8 mEq/L
Ca2+	5	0	3.3 mEq/L
Mg2+	2	0	26 mEq/L
Phos	2	–	0.97 mmol/L

- ○ Daily fluid requirement: 1,500 mL/m^2 BSA
- ○ Daily body weight loss if maintenance is with IVF only is 0.5 kg/day.
- ○ Increased fluid is needed when the patient is febrile. There should be a 15% increase in IVF for each degree above normal body temperature.
- IV Fluids (Table 4.23):
  - ○ D5W: 50 g dextrose in 1,000 mL of fluid; provides 170 calories per liter.
  - ○ LR: Multiple electrolyte concentration, similar to that of plasma. Used to expand the plasma volume in hypovolemic states in the first 24 hours.
  - ○ NS (0.9% NaCl): This is an isotonic solution is used to expand volume and correct mild hyponatremia.
  - ○ ½ NS (0.45% NaCl): This is a hypotonic solution used for postoperative IVF replacement after the first 24 hours. It is used when volume expansion is not required.
  - ○ NaCl 3%: This is a hypertonic solution and is used to treat severe hyponatremia.

Table 4.22 Body Fluid Composition

Fluid	Na	Cl	K	HCO$_3$	Daily Production
Gastric juices	60–100	100	10	0	1,500–2,000 mL
Duodenum	130	90	5	0–10	300–2,000 mL
Bile	145	100	5	15–35	100–800 mL
Pancreatic	140	75	5	70–115	100–800 mL
Ileum	140	100	5	15–30	2,000–3,000 mL

Table 4.23 Fluid Composition

	Na	Cl	K	HCO$_3$	Ca	Glu	AA	Mg	PO$_4$	Ac	Osm
Plasma	140	102	4.0	28	5			2			290
NS	154	154									308
½ NS	77	77									154
¼ NS	34	34									78
LR	130	109	4.0	28	3						272
D5W						50 g					252
D10W						100 g					505
PPN	47	40	13			100 g	35 g	3	3.5	52	500
TMP	25	30	44			250 g	50 g	5	15	99	1,900
D50						500 g					2,520

Fluid Deficits
- Presurgical deficit: From being NPO there is a 2 mL/kg/hr loss.
- Intraoperative fluids: The rule of 1:3 blood loss to crystalloid fluid replacement should be followed. Blood transfusion should occur based on NIH transfusion guidelines, medical comorbidities, and anticipated adjuvant therapies. Third spacing fluid loss: removal of significant ascites and water retained as tissue edema is difficult to quantify.
- It is usually assumed:
  ○ 4 mL/kg/hr for minimal surgical procedures (e.g., wide local excision)
  ○ 6 mL/kg/hr for moderate surgical procedures (e.g., appendectomy, hernia repair)
  ○ 8 mL/kg/hr for major surgical procedures (e.g., radical hysterectomy, bowel resection)
  ○ Insensible losses intraoperatively are 2 mL/kg/hr.
- Postoperative fluid replacement: The calculation should include output from surgical drains, urine, and insensible losses. Diuresis from extensive third spacing takes 1 to 3 days. Management can be with D5LR for the first 24 hours. No potassium is added to the IVF because of the possibility of tumor cell lyses and extracellular release from operative cell destruction. Then D5½ NS is started POD 2 for continued volume replacement. Serum potassium should be checked daily. 10 mEq of potassium is added for each 1,000 mL of NGT drainage obtained.

Blood Component Therapy
- Whole blood has a volume of 517 mL. It is only indicated for acute blood loss that is severe enough to cause hypovolemic shock.
- PRBC has a volume of 300 mL. One unit can survive 21 days if refrigerated. The Hct increases 3% to 5% per unit. It contains plasma (78 mL), citrate (22 mL), plasma protein (42 g), Na (15 mEq), potassium (5 mEq), and acid (25 nanoEq). It is important to check a Ca^{2+} level after significant transfusion due to citrate chelation of divalent ions.
- Platelets: One unit has a volume of 20 to 50 mL. One unit has 5.5 × 1,010 platelets. They can be stored for only 72 hours. One unit increases the platelet count 7,000/mcL in 1 hour. The guideline for transfusion is 0.1 unit/kg; so a normal transfusion is 6 to 8 units. Equivalences: one unit is equal to one pack. A six pack of platelets is equal to one dose.
- FFP contains all clotting factors except platelets. FFP should be given after 10 to 12 units of blood. Components are 250 mL of plasma, 200 units of factor VIII, and 200 units of factor IX.

- Cryoprecipitate is obtained from the thawing of FFP at 4°C. Factors VIII, XIII, and fibrinogen are the main factors in cryoprecipitate. Cryoprecipitate is mainly used for factor replacement in the treatment of hemophilia and von Willebrand's disease. It is transfused in a pack of 4 to 6 units each having a volume of 15 mL.

- Albumin is used for volume resuscitation and hypoproteinemia. It is infused as a 5% or 25% solution and 25 g are commonly infused. The volume effects last for 12 hours. It increases the intravascular volume by 500 mL.

- Artificial colloids are not recommended to include Hetastarch and Dextran (Tables 4.24 and 4.25).

Neurologic Care

- Neuromuscular blockage is often used to paralyze the patient. Pancuronium is chosen for its long-acting properties. It lasts for up to 90 minutes after an IV dose of 0.06 to 0.1 mg/kg. Continuous infusion is vagolytic and can cause a heart rate increase of 10 bpm or more. It is important to use vecuronium if the patient cannot tolerate an increased heart rate. An electronic twitch monitor is used to assess the degree of paralyzation. Acute quadriplegic myopathy is a potential adverse event causing post paralytic quadriparesis, which consists of the triad of acute paresis, myonecrosis with increased CPK, and abnormal electromyography.

- Delirium is often seen in ICU patients. Haldol can be used to counteract delirium because of its minimal anticholinergic and hypotensive effects. It is given at a loading dose of 2 to 10 mg IV every 20 minutes, followed by scheduled dosing every 4 to 6 hours at 25% of the necessary loading dose.

- Sedation is used to medically control the ICU patient for rest, recovery, and safety in the ICU environment. Daily interruption of sedation is necessary. This is associated with a shortened duration of ICU stay, less PTSD, and shorter mechanical ventilation. Propofol is used often as a sedative. It has no analgesic properties. It does count as lipid calories at 1.1 kcal/mL. Care should be taken in patients with hypertriglyceridemia, and so it is necessary to monitor TG after 2 days of use (Table 4.26).

- Abdominal compartment syndrome can occur due to ascites, bowel obstruction, ileus, peritonitis, or pancreatitis. It can also occur after massive fluid resuscitation in the setting of septic or hypovolemic shock. Diagnosis is by measurement of the intra-abdominal pressure via a Foley catheter with documentation of a pressure of greater than 12 mmHg on three or more occasions 4 to 6 hours apart, or a single pressure of 20 mmHg or greater. It can manifest as systemic hypotension, reduced urinary output, or decreased pulmonary compliance. On occasion, surgery to decompress the abdomen and temporary closure with a vacuum pack may be necessary.

Table 4.24 Blood Products: Composition and Indication

Blood Products	Contents	Volume	Indication
PRBC	Red cells	1 unit = 250 mL, raises Hct 3%	Acute or chronic blood loss
Platelets	Platelets	One unit = 50 mL, raises platelets by 6×10^3	Platelets <20 nonbleeding patient, <50 in bleeding patient
FFP	Fibrinogen, factors II, VII, IX, X, XI, XII, XIII, and heat labile V and VII	1 unit = 150 – 250 mL, 11 g albumin, 500 mg fibrinogen, 0.7–1.0 units clotting factors	DIC, treatment >10 units of blood, liver disease, IgG deficiency, 1 unit raises fibrinogen by 10 mg/dL
Cryoprecipitate	Factors VIII, XIII, von Willebrand's disease, fibrinogen	1 unit = 10 mL, 250 mg fibrinogen, 80 units Factor VIII	Hemophilia A, von Willebrand's disease, fibrinogen deficiency
PCC 3 or 4 factors	A combination of factors II, VII, IX, and X	9–25–50 IU/kg can be given	Acute or chronic blood loss or reversal of warfarin

Table 4.25 Risk of Infection per Unit of Blood Transfused

Hepatitis C	1:2 million
Hepatitis B	1:350,000
HIV	1:2.3 million
Bacterial	1:5,000 per unit of platelets 1:1 million PRBC

Table 4.26 Glasgow Coma Scale

Response	Score
Eye opening	
Spontaneous	4
To verbal	3
To pain	2
None	1
Verbal response	
Oriented and talking	5
Disoriented and talking	4
Inappropriate talking	3
Incomprehensible	2
None	1
Motor response	
Obeys commands	6
Localizes pain	5
Normal flexion withdrawal	4
Decortical signs (flexion)	3
Decerebrate signs (extension)	2
None	1
Score	
15 = Normal	
11 = Normal if intubated	
8 or less = coma	

Risk Stratification of Morbidity and Mortality

Risk stratification of morbidity and mortality in the ICU as determined by different quantitative scales has been documented as reliable and reproducible in gynecologic oncology patients. Two scales are used the most often: the APACHE IV and the SOFA. An increase of the SOFA score during the first 48 hours of ICU admission predicts a mortality of 50% or more.

Correlation of operative time to complications has been reviewed and increased rates of UTI, organ space SSI, sepsis/septic shock, prolonged intubation, pneumonia, rate of DVT, deep incisional infection, and wound disruption were found. Per 1,000 cases, there were 116 occurrences per additional operating room hour.[54]

REFERENCES

1. Kiran RP, Murray ACA, Chiuzan C, et al. Combined preoperative mechanical bowel preparation with oral antibiotics significantly reduces surgical site infection, anastomotic leak, and ileus after colorectal surgery. *Ann Surg.* 2015;262(3):416–425. doi: 10.1097/SLA.0000000000001416

2. Di Donato V, Caruso G, Bogani G, et al. Preoperative frailty assessment in patients undergoing gynecologic oncology surgery: A systematic review. *Gynecol Oncol.* 2021;161(1):11-19. doi:10.1016/j.ygyno.2020.12.030

3. Di Donato V, Di Pinto A, Giannini A, et al. Modified fragility index and surgical complexity score are able to predict postoperative morbidity and mortality after cytoreductive surgery for advanced ovarian cancer. *Gynecol Oncol.* 2021;161(1):4–10. doi: 10.1016/j.ygyno.2020.08.022

4. Di Donato V, Caruso G, Bogani G, et al. Preoperative frailty assessment in patients undergoing gynecologic oncology surgery: a systematic review. *Gynecol Oncol.* 2021;161(1):11–19. doi: 10.1016/j.ygyno.2020.12.030

5. Kumar A, Langstraat CL, DeJong SR, et al. Functional not chronologic age: frailty index predicts outcomes in advanced ovarian cancer. *Gynecol Oncol.* 2017;147(1):104–109. doi: 10.1016/j.ygyno.2017.07.126

6. Zhang G, Zhang Y, He F, et al. Preoperative controlling nutritional status (CONUT) score is a prognostic factor for early-stage cervical cancer patients with high-risk factors. *Gynecol Oncol.* 2021;162(3):763–769. doi: 10.1016/j.ygyno.2021.06.012

7. Di Nisio M, Porreca E, Candeloro M, De Tursi M, Russi I, Rutjes AW. Primary prophylaxis for venous thromboembolism in ambulatory cancer patients receiving chemotherapy. *Cochrane Database Syst Rev.* 2016;12(12):CD008500. Published 2016 Dec 1. doi:10.1002/14651858.CD008500.pub4

8. Khorana AA, Soff GA, Kakkar AK, et al. Rivaroxaban for Thromboprophylaxis in High-Risk Ambulatory Patients with Cancer. *N Engl J Med.* 2019;380(8):720–728. doi:10.1056/NEJMoa1814630

9. Maraveyas A, Waters J, Roy R, et al. Gemcitabine versus gemcitabine plus dalteparin thromboprophylaxis in pancreatic cancer. *Eur J Cancer*. 2012;48(9):1283–1292. doi:10.1016/j.ejca.2011.10.017

10. Pelzer U, Opitz B, Deutschinoff G, et al: Efficacy of prophylactic low-molecular weight heparin for ambulatory patients with advanced pancreatic cancer: outcomes from the CONKO-004 trial. *J Clin Oncol*. 33:2028–2034, 2015

11. Woodruff S, Feugère G, Abreu P, et al: A post hoc analysis of dalteparin versus oral anticoagulant (VKA) therapy for the prevention of recurrent venous thromboembolism (rVTE) in patients with cancer and renal impairment. *J Thromb Thrombolysis*. 42:494–504, 2016

12. Raskob GE, van Es N, Verhamme P, et al: Edoxaban for the treatment of cancer-associated venous thromboembolism. *N Engl J Med*. 378:615–624, 2018

13. Young AM, Marshall A, Thirlwall J, et al: Comparison of an oral factor Xa inhibitor with low molecular weight heparin in patients with cancer with venous thromboembolism: results of a randomized trial (SELECT-D). *J Clin Oncol*. 36:2017–2023, 2018.

14. Guntupalli SR, Brennecke A, Behbakht K, et al. Safety and efficacy of apixaban vs enoxaparin for preventing postoperative venous thromboembolism in women undergoing surgery for gynecologic malignant neoplasm: a randomized clinical trial. *JAMA Netw Open*. 2020;3(6):e207410. doi: 10.1001/jamanetworkopen.2020.7410

15. Carrier M, Abou-Nassar K, Mallick R, et al. Apixaban to prevent venous thromboembolism in patients with cancer. *N Engl J Med*. 2019;380(8):711–719. doi: 10.1056/NEJMoa1814468

16. Moulder JK, Moore KJ, Strassle PD, et al. Effect of length of surgery on the incidence of venous thromboembolism after benign hysterectomy. *Am J Obstet Gynecol*. 2021;224(4):364. doi: 10.1016/j.ajog.2020.10.007

17. Andiman SE, Xu X, Boyce JM, et al. Decreased surgical site infection rate in hysterectomy: effect of a gynecology-specific bundle. *Obstet Gynecol*. 2018;131(6):991–999. doi: 10.1097/AOG.0000000000002594

18. Li W, Li M, Wang T, et al. Controlling nutritional status (CONUT) score is a prognostic factor in patients with resected breast cancer. *Sci Rep*. 2020;10(1):6633. doi: 10.1038/s41598-020-63610-7

19. Charlson ME, Pompei P, Ales KL, et al. A new method of classifying prognostic comorbidity in longitudinal studies: development and validation. *J Chronic Dis*. 1987;40(5):373–383. doi: 10.1016/0021-9681(87)90171-8

20. Miller MD, Paradis CF, Houck PR, et al. Rating chronic medical illness burden in geropsychiatric practice and research: application of the cumulative illness rating scale. *Psychiatry Res*. 1992;41(3):237–248. doi: 10.1016/0165-1781(92)90005-n

21. Chen X, Zhao N, Ye P, et al. Comparison of laparoscopic and open radical hysterectomy in cervical cancer patients with tumor size ≤2 cm. *Int J Gynecol Cancer*. 2020;30(5):564–571. doi: 10.1136/ijgc-2019-000994

22. Chen C, Liu P, Ni Y, et al. Laparoscopic versus abdominal radical hysterectomy for stage IB1 cervical cancer patients with tumor size ≤ 2 cm: a case-matched control study. *Int J Clin Oncol*. 2020;25(5):937–947. doi: 10.1007/s10147-020-01630-z

23. Kim SI, Lee M, Lee S, et al. Impact of laparoscopic radical hysterectomy on survival outcome in patients with FIGO stage IB cervical cancer: a matching study of two institutional hospitals in korea. *Gynecol Oncol.* 2019;155(1):75–82. doi: 10.1016/j.ygyno.2019.07.019

24. Nezhat FR, Cho JE, Liu C, et al. Laparoscopic cytoreduction for advanced primary and recurrent ovarian, fallopian tube, or primary peritoneal cancer. *J Minim Invasive Gynecol.* 2009;16(6):S39–S40. doi: 10.1016/j.jmig.2009.08.146

25. Nezhat FR, DeNoble SM, Liu CS, et al. The safety and efficacy of laparoscopic surgical staging and debulking of apparent advanced stage ovarian, fallopian tube, and primary peritoneal cancers. *JSLS.* 2010;14(2):155–168. doi: 10.4293/108680810X12785289143990

26. Matsuo K, Matsuzaki S, Mandelbaum RS, et al. Utilization and perioperative outcome of minimally invasive pelvic exenteration in gynecologic malignancies: a national study in the united states. *Gynecol Oncol.* 2021;161(1):39–45. doi: 10.1016/j.ygyno.2020.12.036

27. Kanao H, Aoki Y, Omi M, et al. Laparoscopic pelvic exenteration and laterally extended endopelvic resection for postradiation recurrent cervical carcinoma: technical feasibility and short-term oncologic outcome. *Gynecol Oncol.* 2021;161(1):34–38. doi: 10.1016/j.ygyno.2020.12.034

28. Dart AJ, Dart CM. Comprehensive biomaterials II. 2017.

29. Ibeanu OA, Chesson RR, Echols KT, et al. Urinary tract injury during hysterectomy based on universal cystoscopy. *Obstet Gynecol.* 2009;113(1):6–10. doi: 10.1097/AOG.0b013e31818f6219

30. O'Keeffe T, Refaai M, Tchorz K, et al. A massive transfusion protocol to decrease blood component use and costs. *Arch Surg.* 2008;143(7):686–690. doi: 10.1001/archsurg.143.7.686

31. Doyle PJ, Lipetskaia L, Duecy E, et al. Sodium fluorescein use during intraoperative cystoscopy. *Obstet Gynecol.* 2015;125(3):548–550. doi: 10.1097/AOG.0000000000000675

32. Bisch SP, Jago CA, Kalogera E, et al. Outcomes of enhanced recovery after surgery (ERAS) in gynecologic oncology - A systematic review and meta-analysis. *Gynecol Oncol.* 2021;161(1):46–55. doi: 10.1016/j.ygyno.2020.12.035

33. ACOG committee opinion no. 750: perioperative pathways: enhanced recovery after surgery. *Obstet Gynecol.* 2018;132(3):e120–e130.

34. Lefkowits C, Buss MK, Ramzan AA, et al. Opioid use in gynecologic oncology in the age of the opioid epidemic: part I - effective opioid use across clinical settings, a society of gynecologic oncology evidence-based review. *Gynecol Oncol.* 2018;149(2):394–400. doi: 10.1016/j.ygyno.2018.01.027

35. Swarm RA, Paice JA, Anghelescu DL, et al. Adult cancer pain, version 3.2019, NCCN clinical practice guidelines in oncology. *J Natl Compr Canc Netw.* 2019;17(8):977–1007. doi: 10.6004/jnccn.2019.0038

36. Lago V, Fotopoulou C, Chiantera V, et al. Risk factors for anastomotic leakage after colorectal resection in ovarian cancer surgery: a multicentre study. *Gynecol Oncol.* 2019;153(3):549–554. doi: 10.1016/j.ygyno.2019.03.241

37. Nelson G, Kalogera E, Dowdy SC. Enhanced recovery pathways in gynecologic oncology. *Gynecol Oncol*. 2014;135(3):586–594. doi: 10.1016/j.ygyno.2014.10.006

38. Nick AM, Schmeler KM, Frumovitz MM, et al. Risk of thromboembolic disease in patients undergoing laparoscopic gynecologic surgery. *Obstet Gynecol*. 2010;116(4):956–961. doi: 10.1097/AOG.0b013e3181f240f7

39. Kahn SR, Shapiro S, Wells PS, et al. Compression stockings to prevent post-thrombotic syndrome: a randomised placebo-controlled trial. *Lancet*. 2014;383(9920):880–888. doi: 10.1016/S0140-6736(13)61902-9

40. Khorana AA, Kuderer NM, Culakova E, et al. Development and validation of a predictive model for chemotherapy-associated thrombosis. *Blood*. 2008;111(10):4902–4907. doi: 10.1182/blood-2007-10-116327

41. Tafur AJ, Kalsi H, Wysokinski WE, et al. The association of active cancer with venous thromboembolism location: a population-based study. *Mayo Clin Proc*. 2011;86(1):25–30. doi: 10.4065/mcp.2010.0339

42. Meyer G, Marjanovic Z, Valcke J, et al. Comparison of low-molecular-weight heparin and warfarin for the secondary prevention of venous thromboembolism in patients with cancer: a randomized controlled study. *Arch Intern Med*. 2002;162(15):1729–1735. doi: 10.1001/archinte.162.15.1729

43. Hull RD, Pineo GF, Brant RF, et al. Long-term low-molecular-weight heparin versus usual care in proximal-vein thrombosis patients with cancer. *Am J Med*. 2006;119(12):1062–1072. doi: 10.1016/j.amjmed.2006.02.022

44. Kakkar AK, Levine MN, Kadziola Z, et al. Low molecular weight heparin, therapy with dalteparin, and survival in advanced cancer: the fragmin advanced malignancy outcome study (FAMOUS). *J Clin Oncol*. 2004;22(10):1944–1948. doi: 10.1200/JCO.2004.10.002

45. Dennis M, Cranswick G, Deary A, et al. Thigh-length versus below-knee stockings for deep venous thrombosis prophylaxis after stroke: a randomized trial. CLOTS (CLOTS in legs or stockings after stroke) trial collaboration. *Ann Intern Med*. 2010;153(9):553–562. doi: 10.7326/0003-4819-153-9-201011020-00280

46. Chapman JS, Roddy E, Westhoff G, et al. Post-operative enteral immunonutrition for gynecologic oncology patients undergoing laparotomy decreases wound complications. *Gynecol Oncol*. 2015;137(3):523–528. doi: 10.1016/j.ygyno.2015.04.003

47. Carson JL, Grossman BJ, Kleinman S, et al. Red blood cell transfusion: a clinical practice guideline from the AABB*. *Ann Intern Med*. 2012;157(1):49–58. doi: 10.7326/0003-4819-157-1-201206190-00429

48. Devereaux PJ, Yang H, Yusuf S, et al. Effects of extended-release metoprolol succinate in patients undergoing non-cardiac surgery (POISE trial): a randomised controlled trial. *Lancet*. 2008;371(9627):1839–1847. doi: 10.1016/S0140-6736(08)60601-7

49. Saksena S, Slee A, Waldo AL, et al. Cardiovascular outcomes in the AFFIRM trial (atrial fibrillation follow-up investigation of rhythm management). an assessment of individual antiarrhythmic drug therapies compared with rate control with propensity score-matched analyses. *J Am Coll Cardiol*. 2011;58(19):1975–1985. doi: 10.1016/j.jacc.2011.07.036

50. Danelich IM, Lose JM, Wright SS, et al. Practical management of post-operative atrial fibrillation after noncardiac surgery. *J Am Coll Surg.* 2014;219(4):831–841. doi: 10.1016/j.jamcollsurg.2014.02.038

51. Evans L, Rhodes A, Alhazzani W, et al. Surviving sepsis campaign: international guidelines for management of sepsis and septic shock 2021. *Crit Care Med.* 2021;49(11):e1063–e1143. doi: 10.1097/CCM.0000000000005337

52. Dellinger RP, Levy MM, Rhodes A, et al. Surviving sepsis campaign: international guidelines for management of severe sepsis and septic shock, 2012. *Intensive Care Med.* 2013;39(2):165–228. doi: 10.1007/s00134-012-2769-8

53. Klastersky J, Paesmans M. The multinational association for supportive care in cancer (MASCC) risk index score: 10 years of use for identifying low-risk febrile neutropenic cancer patients. *Support Care Cancer.* 2013;21(5):1487–1495. doi: 10.1007/s00520-013-1758-y

54. Daley BJ, Cecil W, Clarke PC, et al. How slow is too slow? correlation of operative time to complications: an analysis from the tennessee surgical quality collaborative. *J Am Coll Surg.* 2015;220(4):550–558. doi: 10.1016/j.jamcollsurg.2014.12.040

55. University of California San Francisco. Infection diseases management program at UCSF. https://idmp.ucsf.edu/

5 Gynecologic Cancer Systemic Treatment Modalities

CHEMOTHERAPY

One Letter and Combination Chemotherapy Abbreviations
A: Act-D actinomycin D
ABVD: Adriamycin/doxorubicin, bleomycin, vinblastine, DTIC
AcFucy: Act-D, 5-FU, cyclophosphamide
AI: Aromatase inhibitor
B: Bleomycin
BEP: Bleomycin, etoposide, cisplatin
C: Cyclophosphamide
CDDP: Cisplatin; cis-diamminedichloroplatinum
CHOPP-R: Cyclophosphamide, hydroxyurea, vincristine, procarbazine, prednisone, rituximab
CMFV: Cyclophosphamide, MTX, 5-FU, vinblastine
D: Doxorubicin
E: Etoposide, VP-16
Epi: Epirubicin
F: 5-FU
H: Hydroxyurea
L: Chlorambucil
Lev: Levamisole
L-PAM: L-phenylalanine mustard
M: MTX
MAC: MTX, Act-D, cyclophosphamide or chlorambucil
MMC: Mitomycin
MOPP: Nitrogen mustard, vincristine, procarbazine, prednisone
MVPP: Nitrogen mustard, vinblastine, procarbazine, prednisone
O: Oncovin/vincristine
P: Cisplatin
Pr: Prednisolone
T: Tamoxifen
TVPP: Thiotepa, vinblastine, procarbazine, prednisone
V: Vinblastine
VAC: Vincristine, doxorubicin cyclophosphamide

VBM: Vinblastine, bleomycin, MTX
VBP: Vinblastine, bleomycin, cisplatin
VDC: Vincristine, doxorubicin, cyclophosphamide

Chemotherapy Definitions

- Dose: Amount of chemotherapy administered
- Intensity: The amount of drug administered over time
- Schedule: Time interval for delivery of chemotherapy
- Chemotherapy cycle: One treatment of single or combination agents in the full course of therapy
- Planning of treatment: Must take into consideration tumor type, extent of disease, patient's comorbidities, age, social and emotional function, or whether therapy is primary or salvage.

Delivery

Routes are IV, IM, PO, IP, or regional. Most cytotoxic chemotherapy is administered systemically, by IV. IP chemotherapy is administration of chemotherapy directly into the abdominopelvic cavity. Regional chemotherapy can be used to treat solitary organ lesions, like liver metastasis. This occurs by obstruction of the outflow tract for a limited amount of time so that the chemotherapy can penetrate the tumor mass directly. It can also be directly administered to a cavity such as for pleural or pericardial lesions.

Metabolism

- Pro-drugs can be bio-transformed into active metabolites. This includes cyclophosphamide. It is important to know those drugs that are activated by the liver because IP administration may have no effect.
- Excretion: Hepatobiliary or renal excretion are the main routes of excretion. Drugs can be metabolized to pro-drugs, to inactive states, remain unchanged, or accumulate in body tissues.

Principles of Chemotherapy Tumor Kill

The patient needs two cycles after resolution of tumor markers and/or no evidence of disease with CCR to eliminate microscopic systemic disease.

Chemotherapy Regimens

- Primary: Chemotherapy is the initial treatment (also referred to as Front Line).
- Adjuvant: Chemotherapy is used following primary treatment with surgery or XRT.

- Neoadjuvant chemotherapy (NACT): used for initial treatment to be followed by surgery, XRT, or a combination of therapies.
- Secondary: Any chemotherapy regimen that is given after primary chemotherapy.
- Salvage: Chemotherapy is used in the treatment of recurrent or persistent disease after previous chemotherapy.
- Consolidation: Chemotherapy that is continued/used for a defined interval after primary or adjuvant chemotherapy to decrease the chance of cancer recurrence in patients with CCR. This is usually a short duration of treatment (4–6 more cycles).
- Maintenance: Chemotherapy that is continued/used after primary or adjuvant chemotherapy for an indefinite interval to decrease the chance of cancer recurrence in patients with CCR. This is usually of a longer duration than consolidation therapy and used until progression or toxicity. Some protocols specify 18 cycles or 22 months of treatment after primary adjuvant therapy.

Platinum Sensitivity/Resistance in HGSTOC or Ovarian GCTs
Tumors are classified as platinum sensitive, resistant, or refractory.

- Platinum sensitive: If the tumor recurs 6 or more months after the completion of primary platinum-based chemotherapy, it is said to be platinum sensitive.
- Platinum resistant (Pl-R): If the tumor recurs within 6 months of primary platinum-based chemotherapy, it is considered Pl-R.
- Platinum refractory: If the tumor does not respond to initial platinum chemotherapy and growth continues during the primary treatment, it is considered platinum refractory.
- For GCTs, the time interval is different and resistance is specified at 6 weeks. GCTs are designated as refractory if no response is seen at 4 weeks of ongoing chemotherapy.

Toxicity
- Side effects from chemotherapy are graded according to severity. The most commonly affected organ systems are the GI system, the hematopoietic system, and the integumentary system. Please refer to the CTC website (https://ctep.cancer.gov/protocoldevelopment/electronic_applications/ctc.htm) for the full classification of toxicity grades. Management of toxicity due to chemotherapy is with a reduction in the total dose of drug per cycle, called a dose reduction. This is usually a 20% to 25% dose reduction, or a decrease in the AUC by one level.
  - Cardiac toxicity mainly occurs with doxorubicin and trastuzumab. A history and exam can diagnose CHF symptoms. Confirmation is with an echocardiogram or with a MUGA scan.

○ Pulmonary toxicity has been seen mainly with bleomycin. A pretreatment DLCO is recommended. A 15% change in the FEV indicates toxicity. Pulmonary toxicity can also be determined clinically with an examination. Clinical symptoms, such as rales, hypoinflation, or a lag in the inspiratory phase on exam, as well as dyspnea, occur before a documented drop in FEV.

○ Secondary malignancies can occur after the administration of chemotherapeutic agents and PARP-inhibitors. The rate is about 1% to 2%. Leukemias and myelodysplastic syndromes can occur from alkylating agents, which include melphalan, the podophyllotoxins, etoposide, cyclophosphamide, and the platinum compounds. The development of leukemias is dose dependent (2 g for etoposide). The median latency is 4 Y after chemotherapy for EOC, with an overall incidence of 0.17%.[1]

The Cell Cycle

- The cell cycle is broken into interphase and mitosis. Interphase consists of the G1, S, and G2 phases. G1 is a variable period, during which protein, RNA, and DNA repair occur. The cell can terminally differentiate or continue in the cell cycle from this phase. S phase is when new DNA is synthesized. The G2 phase occurs after the S phase and thus the cell contains two times the amount of DNA. This is a short phase. It is the variation in the length of the G1 phase that affects the proliferative behavior of cell populations.

- Mitosis consists of five phases. Prophase, the first phase, is when chromosomes condense. Metaphase is when chromosomal division occurs. This is the most radiosensitive phase. Anaphase is when sister chromosomes move to opposite cell poles. Telophase demonstrates polarization of chromosomes and disassembly of the cytoskeleton occurs. Cytokinesis follows with division of the cell into separate daughter cells. Cell cycle times vary from 10 to 31 hours.

- Masses are usually palpated at 10^9 cells or 1 cm in size. The 1-cm size usually occurs after 30 doublings of one tumor cell.

Growth Fraction

This consists of the fraction of cells in a tumor that is actively proliferating. This fraction ranges from 25% to 95%.

Cell Death

Cell death has been seen with some tumors. This has been documented in some breast cancers associated with febrile episodes[2] or when tumors outgrow their vascular supply.

Log Kill

A constant fraction of cells are killed with each dose of therapy—not a constant number of cells. To achieve substantial tumor reduction, a repetitive insult has to be delivered to the tumor. Single-agent chemotherapy can be curative in this fashion, but is not as effective as multiagent chemotherapy. Multiagent chemotherapy uses different drugs that target separate cellular pathways. The effect can be additive or synergic.

Cell-Cycle Nonspecific Chemotherapeutic Agents

These agents kill cells in all phases of the cell cycle.

Cell-Cycle Specific Agents

These agents depend on the proliferative fraction of the tumor and a specific cell-cycle phase. These agents are usually more effective against tumors with a high proliferative rate and a high growth fraction.

Cell Growth

Growth is usually demonstrated via a Gompertzian log tumor growth curve.

- There are four phases to cell growth:
  - ○ Lag growth phase
  - ○ The log growth phase
  - ○ Stable growth phase
  - ○ Death phase

Mechanisms of Cytotoxicity

Chemotherapeutic agents can target cellular DNA, proteins (such as enzymes, receptors, or the metabolic respiratory chain), and RNA.

Mechanisms of Resistance

- The Goldie–Coldman hypothesis is a mathematical model that predicts the probability of a tumor harboring drug-resistant clones. The number of drug-resistant clones depends on the mutation rate and the size of the tumor.
- Documented mechanisms of drug resistance include:
  - ○ The MDR-1 and MDR-2 P-glycoproteins, which are components of the ATP-ABC transporters. These proteins transport drugs out of cells.
  - ○ Cells can decrease the entry of the drug into the cell via downregulation of cellular receptors.
  - ○ Metabolic inactivation of the drug can occur via upregulation of the GSH sulfate and DHFR enzymes.
  - ○ There can be altered binding affinity of the drug to albumin or intracellular targets.
  - ○ Genomic change can occur via:

- Altered DNA repair mechanisms
- Gene point mutation
- Gene frameshift mutation
- Gene deletion
- Gene amplification
  - Gatekeeping mutation: The initial genetic change that gives a single cell a selective growth advantage, allowing the subsequent acquisition of driver mutations, which alter the proliferation rate, invasion capability, cellular signaling, and DNA repair of a tumor.
  - Passenger mutations: These have no effect on the neoplastic process and accumulate with age.
  - *BRCA* reversion mutations

Prior to Chemotherapy Administration

The patient should have adequate assessment of laboratory values; these are considered to be:

- WBC greater than 3×10^3/mcL with an ANC greater than 1.5×10^3/mcL
- Platelets greater than 100×10^3/mcL
- Normal LFTs
- Creatinine less than 2 mg/dL or CrCl greater than 50 mL/min
- GOG performance status of either 0, 1, or 2 with an estimated survival of more than 2 months

Classes of Chemotherapeutic Agents and Independent Mechanisms of Action of Alkylating Agents

These work by intercalating or cross-linking DNA to make DNA adducts. They are cell-cycle nonspecific.

- **Carboplatin (Paraplatin):** This is a platinum compound. It is dosed with the following equation: carboplatin total dose (mg) = AUC $\times$ (GFR + 25). It can be given at an AUC of 7 as single agent or at an AUC of 5 to 6 in combination therapy. Its mechanism of action is intercalation with DNA and is administered via the IV or IP route. It is eliminated via the renal system. Its toxicities are primarily thrombocytopenia, hypersensitivity reactions, leukopenia, nausea, and vomiting. The platelet nadir is usually around 21 days. Secondary toxicities can include nephrotoxicity 7%, peripheral neuropathy 6%, and ototoxicity 1%. Vitamin B_6 can prevent some neurotoxicity. Hypersensitivity can occur in 25% of patients if more than six cycles are received. There is an increased risk of leukemia with a RR of 6.5. Amifostine can reduce the amount of thrombocytopenia at a dose of 910 mg/m^2.

- **Cisplatin (Platinol):** This is a platinum compound that works by intercalating with DNA and creating G–G adducts. It is administered either IV or IP. It can be given as a single agent to radiosensitize certain tumors at 40 to 50 mg/m² weekly. It can be given as single-agent therapy at 50 to 100 mg/m², or at 75 mg/m² in combination with other drugs every 3 weeks. Ninety percent is eliminated by the renal system and 10% by the hepatic/biliary system. Primary toxicities are leukopenia and anemia. Nephrotoxicity occurs in 21%, ototoxicity in 10%, and some patients have peripheral or autonomic neuropathy. Secondary toxicities are allergic reactions, low sodium (Na), potassium (K), calcium (Ca), and magnesium (Mg). The pancytopenia nadir occurs between 18 and 23 days. To reduce some nephrotoxicity, prehydrate with normal saline IVF and consider mannitol diuresis with an additional 3 g of $MgSO_4$.

- **Cyclophosphamide (Cytoxan):** This is a pro-drug that is activated by liver metabolism and then the active drug intercalates with DNA. It is administered either IV or PO. It can be given as a single agent or in combination with other agents. The dosing is usually 10 to 50 mg/kg IV every 1 to 4 weeks or 600 to 1,000 mg/m² every 4 weeks. Eighty-five percent is eliminated by the liver and 15% by the renal system. Primary toxicities include pancytopenia (this is the most marrow-suppressive drug), nausea, vomiting, and alopecia. Secondary toxicities are hemorrhagic cystitis from the acrolein metabolite, SIADH if the dose is greater than 50 mg/kg, interstitial pneumonia, cardiomyopathy, and leukemia with a RR of 5.4 after 10 Y. The nadir occurs at days 8 to 14. To diagnose hemorrhagic cystitis, obtain a urine analysis: confirmation is with gross hematuria or 20 RBC/HPF. Mesna should be coadministered to decrease the incidence of hemorrhagic cystitis. Methylene blue bladder irrigation can also decrease the complications of hemorrhagic cystitis.

- **Dacarbazine (DTIC):** This is administered IV, usually at a dose of 2 to 4.5 mg/kg/day for 5 to 10 days every 4 weeks. Elimination is via the renal system. Primary toxicities include pancytopenia, nausea, vomiting, and alopecia. Secondary toxicities include mucositis, stomatitis, myalgias, and hepatotoxicity. The nadir occurs 2 to 4 weeks after administration.

- **Ifosfamide (Ifex):** This is a pro-drug; it is activated by hepatic metabolism and is administered IV at a dose: of 1.2 to 1.6 g/m²/day for 5 days every 3 to 4 weeks; 700 to 900 mg/m²/day for 5 days every 3 weeks; or 1,000 mg/m² on days 1 and 2 every 28 days as part of the ICE protocol. Elimination is via the renal system for 73% of the drug. Primary toxicities are hemorrhagic cystitis, pancytopenia, nausea, vomiting, and alopecia. Secondary toxicities are nephrotoxicity, SIADH, and CNS toxicity. CNS toxicity is increased with baseline dementia or a low serum albumin. The neurotoxin chloroacetaldehyde is a byproduct of this drug. The nadir is days 5 to 10 after administration and this drug also needs coadministration of mesna to decrease the incidence of hemorrhagic cystitis.

- **Melphalan (Alkeran):** This drug cross-links DNA and can be administered IV, PO, or IP. Dosing occurs at 16 mg/m^2 IV every 2 weeks for four doses then at 4-week intervals, or 1 mg/kg IV every 4 weeks. The PO dose is 6 mg/day for 2 to 3 weeks followed by a 4-week holiday. There is 63 x greater exposure via the IP route. Elimination is 99% renal. Primary toxicity is pancytopenia with secondary toxicities to include nausea, vomiting, and leukemia (11.2% cumulative 10-Y risk). The nadir occurs at days 28 to 35 and there is increased drug bioavailability if taken after fasting for 8 hours. Drug resistance is via increased intracellular GST, and buthionine sulfoximine can reverse this resistance.

- **Temozolomide (Temodar):** This is a triazene analog of DTIC with antineoplastic activity. As a cytotoxic alkylating agent, temozolomide is converted at physiologic pH to the short-lived active compound, MTIC. The cytotoxicity of MTIC is due primarily to methylation of DNA at the O6 and N7 positions of guanine, resulting in inhibition of DNA replication. Unlike DTIC, which is metabolized to MTIC only in the liver, temozolomide is metabolized to MITC at all sites. Temozolomide is administered PO and penetrates well into the CNS. Dosing varies by tumor protocol but commonly is calculated: BSA x 75 then rounded to the nearest 5 mg. It is administered PO BID days 1 to 14 every 28 days. Another regimen is 150 mg/m^2 IV daily for 5 days of a 28-day cycle.

- **Altretamine (Hexalen, Hexamethylmelamine):** This is a pro-drug that is metabolically activated by the liver. It is important not to take B$_{12}$ supplements because this inactivates the drug. It is administered PO at a dose of 260 mg/m^2/day in four daily divided doses for 14 to 21 days every 4 weeks. Eighty-five percent is eliminated via the renal system. Primary toxicities are pancytopenia, neuropathy, nausea, vomiting, and nephrotoxicity. Secondary toxicities include rash, neurotoxicity, and seizures. The nadir occurs at days 21 to 28.

Antitumor Antibiotics

These agents intercalate with DNA, inhibit RNA synthesis, and interfere with DNA repair. They are cell-cycle nonspecific except for bleomycin.

- **Bleomycin (Blenoxane):** Complexes with iron to form an oxidase that produces free radicals. These free radicals produce DNA strand breaks in the G2 and M phases. It can be administered either IV, IM, or intracavitary for effusions. Dosing is calculated at 1 unit = 1 mg. The IV dose is bolused at 30 mg/week for 12 weeks, or 10 mg/m^2/day for 4 days every 4 weeks. Do not exceed 400 mg total lifetime dose. For pleural effusions, 60 to 120 mg can be instilled into the cavity. Seventy percent is eliminated by the kidneys. Primary toxicities are interstitial pneumonitis (10%), pulmonary fibrosis (1%), alopecia, mucositis, and non-neutropenic fever. Secondary toxicities are nausea, vomiting, pancytopenia, hyperpigmentation, and allergic reactions. The nadir occurs at day 12. Pulmonary toxicity occurs due to the iron free radicals targeting the type I alveoli first, followed by the type II alveoli. DLCO is the test used to determine pulmonary toxicity. A 15% change from pretreatment value signifies toxicity and thus the need to discontinue treatment. A CXR should be obtained prior to each course, along with a DLCO, but it is important to rely on physical examination and patient symptoms. Risk factors for pulmonary toxicity are prior mediastinal irradiation, age greater than 70, and hyperoxia during surgical anesthesia. Steroid therapy may help with acute pneumonitis.

- **Doxorubicin (Adriamycin):** This inhibits the strand-passing activity of topoisomerase-II and also intercalates with DNA. It is administered via IV and chelates with iron and copper. These heavy metal chelations contribute to the cardiotoxicity of the drug. It is dosed at 60 to 75 mg/m^2 as a single agent or 40 to 60 mg/m^2 in combination every 3 to 4 weeks. Elimination is hepatobiliary for 40% of the drug. It is a vesicant. Primary toxicity is pancytopenia and secondary toxicities are XRT recall, cardiomyopathy, and PPE. To avoid PPE, consider treatment with vitamin B$_6$, avoid hot tubs and high-friction activities. The nadir is at days 10 to 14. With a total dose greater than 500 mg/m^2, the patient has an 11% risk of cardiomyopathy. If the total dose is greater than 600 mg/m^2, there is a 30% risk. Dexrazoxane (Zinecard) is a cardioprotective agent. It is administered at a 10:1 ratio, but if there is renal compromise, the dose should be reduced (to a 5:1 ratio). Risk factors for development of cardiomyopathy are age greater than 70 Y, prior cardiac disease, and prior mediastinal XRT. Pretreatment tests include a baseline MUGA scan or echocardiogram, EKG, and a CXR. If symptoms present during treatment, obtain a MUGA scan or an echocardiogram.
- **Liposomal Doxorubicin (Doxil):** The mechanism of action is similar to the nonliposomal form. It is given IV every 4 weeks at 40 to 50 mg/m^2. It is not a vesicant. The drug is found highly concentrated in tumor tissue (4 x the serum amount). Toxicity is primarily pancytopenia. Secondary toxicity is PPE.
- **Act-D (Actinomycin D):** The mechanism of action is DNA intercalation and it is administered IV. Dosing can be 9 to 13 mcg/kg IV per day for 5 days every 2 weeks or 1.25 mg/m^2 every 2 weeks for nonmetastatic GTD; 90% is eliminated via the hepatobiliary system. Primary toxicities are pancytopenia, nausea, vomiting, and mucositis. Secondary toxicity is alopecia. The nadir is days 7 to 10. The mode of resistance is via MDR P-glycoprotein.
- **Mitomycin C (Mutamycin):** This is a pro-drug that cross-links DNA. It is selectively activated by hypoxic cells. It is administered IV and dosed as a single agent at 10 to 20 mg/m^2 or in combination at 10 mg/m^2 every 6 to 8 weeks. Elimination is by the hepatobiliary system

for 90% of the drug. Primary toxicity is pancytopenia and secondary toxicities are nausea, vomiting, nephrotoxicity, microangiopathic hemolytic anemia, HUS, and multiorgan failure. The nadir is 4 to 6 weeks. There is cumulative myelosuppression so the total lifetime dose should be less than 60 mg/m^2.

- **Mitoxantrone (Novantrone):** This drug inhibits topoisomerase-II and is administered IV or IP at a dose of 12 to 14 mg/m^2 IV, or 10 mg/m^2 in 2 L of NS IP every 3 weeks. Elimination is hepatobiliary and primary toxicities are nausea, vomiting, diarrhea, and myelosuppression. The nadir is day 10. This drug may cause the "Smurf" syndrome and can turn the bowel and sclera blue.

- **Levamisole (Ergamisol):** This synthetic imidazothiazole derivative was initially used for helminthic infections. It is administered PO at a dose of 50 mg PO TID × 3 days per week, weekly in combination with chemotherapy (5-FU). It is eliminated via the renal system. Primary toxicities are stomatitis, diarrhea, nausea, vomiting, and a metallic taste. Secondary toxicities are fever, chills, fatigue, myalgias, agranulocytosis, telangiectasia, seizures, edema, and chorea. The nadir is days 7 to 10. The tablets contain lactose: Lactaid may be necessary in those with lactose intolerance.

Antimetabolites

These drugs antagonize folate, purines, pyrimidines, or ribonucleotide reductase. They therefore interfere with DNA synthesis. These agents are cell cycle specific for the S phase.

- **5-FU (Efudex):** This is a pro-drug that is metabolized to FUDR. FUDR is a pyrimidine antimetabolite that inhibits thymidylate synthase and is incorporated into DNA and RNA. Administration is IV or topical. Dosing as a single agent is with a loading dose of 12 mg/kg (maximum of 800 mg) IV daily for 4 to 5 days, then after 28 days, a weekly maintenance dose of 200 to 250 mg/m^2 every other day for 4 days, every 4 weeks. It can also be dosed at 800 to 1,000 mg/m^2 IV daily for 4 days, repeated every 3 to 4 weeks. Oral dosing as **capecitabine**, of 15 to 20 mg/kg/day for 5 to 8 days can be used. Topical/vaginal application is given as a 5% cream; apply ½ vaginal applicator of 5% 5-FU (2.5 g) deep in the vagina at bedtime every 2 to 3 weeks. Elimination is 80% by the liver and 15% by the kidneys. Primary toxicities are granulocytopenia, thrombocytopenia, mucositis, nausea, vomiting, alopecia, and hyperpigmentation. Secondary toxicities are photosensitivity, cerebellar syndrome from the metabolite fluorocitrate, PPE (occurs in 42%–82% and can be reversed with vitamin B$_6$ dosed at 50 to 150 mg), and cardiotoxicity. The nadir is days 9 to 14. Patients with a genetic deficiency of DHFR should not receive this drug.

- **Capecitabine (Xeloda):** This is a pro-drug that is metabolized to 5-FU. It is administered PO with a starting dose of 1,250 mg/m^2 given as a divided BID dose. A reduced starting dose (950 mg/m^2 BID) is required for patients with a CrCl equal to 30 to 50 mL/min. It is given for 14 days of a 21-day cycle. Elimination is renal and primary toxicities are diarrhea, nausea, and vomiting. Secondary toxicities are hand-and-foot syndrome, rash, dry skin, and fatigue. If the patient is taking warfarin concomitantly, frequent monitoring of the INR is recommended.

- **Methotrexate: MTX (Trexall):** This drug blocks DHFR and can be administered IV, PO, IM, or intrathecally. The dose can be weekly at 30 to 50 mg/m^2 IM or IV; 0.4 mg/kg IV or IM daily × 5 days every 14 days; 1 mg/kg IM or IV, days 1, 3, 5, and 7 with leucovorin given 15 mg PO on days 2, 4, 6, and 8 every 14 days; or 100 mg/m^2 IV bolus followed by 200 mg/m^2 12-hour continuous IV infusion with leucovorin given 15 mg PO every 12 hours × four doses (beginning 24 hours after start of MTX infusion) every 14 days; or 12 to 15 mg/m^2/week intrathecally. Elimination is mainly renal. Primary toxicities are nausea, vomiting, pancytopenia, mucositis, and hepatotoxicity. Secondary toxicities are nephrotoxicity, alopecia, and interstitial pneumonitis. The nadir is days 4 to 7. Resistance is via elevated DHFR or mutated transport mechanisms into the tumor cells. MTX accumulates in pleural effusions, so it is necessary to drain effusions before administration. It is also helpful to alkalinize the urine with 3 g PO or 40 to 50 mEq per L of IVF of sodium bicarbonate 12 hours before therapy.

- **Hydroxyurea (Hydrea):** This is S-phase specific and inhibits ribonucleotide reductase. It is administered IV or PO. Dosing is 1 to 3 mg/m^2/day every 2 to 6 weeks; 80 mg/kg twice weekly; or 2 to 3 g/m^2 twice weekly. Elimination is mainly renal and toxicity is myelosuppression. The nadir occurs at 10 days.

- **Gemcitabine (Gemzar):** This is a synthetic nucleoside analog. It is a pro-drug and is metabolized to its active diphosphate and triphosphate states by the liver. These metabolites are then incorporated into DNA and cause masked chain termination. In addition, it is a radio-sensitizing agent and can cause radiation recall. Dosing is IV. It can be given as a single agent at 800 to 1,000 mg/m^2 IV weekly for 7 weeks of an 8-week cycle; 1,000 mg/m^2 weekly for 3 weeks of a 4-week cycle; or at 1,000 to 1,250 mg/m^2 days 1 and 8 with cisplatin at 75 to 100 mg/m^2 on day 1 of a 3-week cycle. Elimination is 90% renal. Primary toxicities are neutropenia, elevated LFTs, alopecia, and mucositis. Secondary toxicities are SC edema, HUS, and ARDS.

- **Pemetrexed (Alimta):** This a folate analog metabolic inhibitor. It is packaged with mannitol and comes in 500-mg vials. It can be used as a single agent or in combination with platinum or pembrolizumab. Dosing is 500 mg/m^2 IV over 10 minutes every 21 days. Elimination is renal and should not be administered for those whose CrCl is less than 45mL/min. Folate supplementation of 400 to 1,000 mcg

PO daily starting 7 days prior to the first dose and continuing 21 days after the last is recommended. B_{12} 1 mg IM is recommended 1 week prior to the first dose. Dexamethasone 4 mg PO BID for 3 days before each infusion is also recommended. Dose reductions are by 25%.

Plant Alkaloids

These agents are cell-cycle specific.

- **Etoposide (VP-16, VePesid):** The mechanism of action is inhibition and stabilization of topoisomerase-II. It arrests cells in the G2 phase. There are multiple regimens but it can be given at a dose of 100 mg/m^2 days 1 to 5 the first week of a 3-week cycle or 50 mg/m^2/day × 21 days PO. Elimination is primarily renal with 98% being cleared by the kidneys. Primary toxicities are pancytopenia, nausea, and vomiting. Secondary toxicities are alopecia, neurotoxicity, and hypotension; therefore, give over 30 minutes. It can also cause secondary leukemia above a total dose of 2 g/m^2. The nadir is day 16.

- **Paclitaxel (Taxol):** This drug stabilizes microtubules and promotes their formation. It can be given IV or IP and should be administered before platinum agents. Single-agent dosing is usually 175 to 250 mg/m^2 but in combination it is usually dosed at 175 mg/m^2 every 3 weeks or 80 mg/m^2 weekly every 3 weeks. Dose reduction is usually to 135 mg/m^2. Elimination is 90% hepatic/biliary and 10% renal. Primary toxicities are neurotoxicity (distal extremities), pancytopenia, hypersensitivity reactions to the vehicle cremophor, arrhythmias, and alopecia. Secondary toxicities are nausea, vomiting, mucositis, arthralgias, and an abnormal EKG. The nadir is days 8 to 11. Always premedicate before chemotherapy with dexamethasone 12-20 mg PO 12 and 6 hours prior to administration, Benadryl 50 mg IV/PO, and cimetidine 300 mg IV both 30 minutes before initiation.

- **Albumin-Bound Paclitaxel (Abraxane, ABI-007):** This stabilizes microtubules and promotes their formation. The albumin-bound drug has a superior toxicity profile because it lacks the castor oil/cremophor base that paclitaxel is mixed with. Dosing is 260 mg/m^2 IV every 3 weeks without needed premedications. Cardiotoxicity occurs in 3% of patients, neutropenia occurs in 9% of patients, and neuropathy is dose dependent.

- **Topotecan (Hycamtin):** This inhibits topoisomerase-I and is usually given IV. Dosing as a single agent is 1.25 to 1.5 mg/m^2/day for 3 to 5 days/week every 3 weeks. Elimination is both renal and hepatic. Primary toxicities are myelosuppression and alopecia with secondary toxicity being asthenia. The nadir is days 9 to 15.

- **Irinotecan (Camptosar):** This is a pro-drug and inhibits topoisomerase-I. It is given IV at doses of 125 mg/m^2 every week, 240 mg/m^2 every 3 weeks, or 350 mg/m^2 every 3 weeks. Elimination is hepatobiliary. Primary toxicities are anemia, nausea, vomiting, elevated liver enzymes, and alopecia. Secondary toxicity is diarrhea. Use antimotility agents (e.g., loperamide at 16 mg/day) as soon as diarrhea appears. The nadir is days 15 to 27.

- **Docetaxel (Taxotere):** This inhibits the depolymerization of tubulin and stabilizes microtubules. It is given IV as a single agent at 60 to 100 mg/m² every 3 weeks; or in combination at 75 to 100 mg/m² every 3 weeks. Its elimination is primarily hepatobiliary at 99.4%. Primary toxicities are neutropenia, edema, and hypersensitivity reactions. Secondary toxicity is a maculopapular rash. The nadir occurs at 5 to 9 days. To decrease the rate of hypersensitivity reactions and third spacing edema, premedicate with corticosteroids 8 mg PO BID starting 1 day prior to, and continuing up to 4 days after, administration.

- **Vinblastine (Velban):** This inhibits microtubule assembly by binding to tubulin and is given IV at a dose of 0.1 to 0.5 mg/kg/week (4 to 20 mg/m²); 6 mg/m² days 1 and 15 every 3 weeks; or 0.15 mg/kg days 1 and 2 every 3 weeks. It is eliminated via both the renal (30%) and the hepatobiliary (80%) systems. Primary toxicities are pancytopenia, constipation, abdominal pain, and adynamic ileus. Secondary toxicities are nausea, vomiting, mucositis, alopecia, neurotoxicity, Raynaud's syndrome, and transient hepatitis. The nadir is days 4 to 10.

- **Vincristine (Oncovin):** This inhibits microtubule assembly. It is administered IV at a dose of: 1 mg/m² or 0.01 to 0.03 mg/m² given every 1 to 2 weeks. Elimination is primarily renal (90%), with hepatobiliary elimination at 10%. Primary toxicities are neurotoxicity, and alopecia. Secondary toxicities are pancytopenia, constipation, and SIADH. The nadir is day 7.

- **Vinorelbine (Navelbine):** This inhibits microtubule assembly and is given IV as a single agent at a dose of 30 mg/m² every week, or in combination at 25 mg/m² weekly. Elimination is hepatobiliary. Primary toxicities are granulocytopenia, neurotoxicity, nausea, vomiting, alopecia, and chest pain. Secondary toxicities are arthralgias, SOB, and constipation. The nadir is days 7 to 14. It is incompatible with 5-FU, mitomycin C, thiotepa, antibiotics, antivirals, and can exacerbate pulmonary toxicity.

Hormonal Agents

These agents bind hormone receptors and either stimulate or inhibit DNA transcription depending on the agonist/antagonist properties of the drug. They are cell-cycle nonspecific.

- **Leuprolide Acetate (Lupron):** This a GnRH superagonist administered as a depot IM injection. Dosing can be 3.5 to 7.5 mg monthly or 11.25 to 22.5 mg every 3 months. Elimination is renal. Primary toxicity is hot flashes with secondary toxicities of headache, edema, and bone pain.

- **Megestrol (Megace):** This is a progestin given PO at doses of 160 to 380 mg daily. Elimination is renal. Primary toxicity is edema and weight gain. Secondary toxicities are DVT/VTE and a Cushing-like syndrome.

- **Tamoxifen (Nolvadex):** This is an ER agonist/antagonist administered PO at a dose of 20 mg/day. Elimination is hepatobiliary and primary toxicity is hot flashes. Secondary toxicities are vaginal bleeding, DVT/VTE, rash, and endometrial cancer.

- **Anastrozole (Arimidex):** This is a nonsteroidal aromatase inhibitor given PO. The dose is 1 mg/day. Elimination is renal. Primary toxicities are anorexia, vaginal dryness, and hot flashes. Secondary toxicities are DVT/VTE, osteopenia, and osteoporosis.

- **Letrozole (Femara):** This is a nonsteroidal aromatase inhibitor. It is given PO at a dose of 2.5 mg/day. Primary toxicities are bone pain and hot flashes, arthralgias, and dyspnea in 20% of patients. It does not increase serum FSH and does not impact adrenal steroid synthesis.

- **Exemestane (Aromasin):** This is a steroidal aromatase inhibitor. It is an irreversible inhibitor that is dosed at 25 mg/day. Primary toxicities are hot flashes, fatigue, and arthralgias.

- **Giredestrant (CDC-9545):** This is a selective ER degrader. Dosing is PO 30mg daily. Used in HR-positive HER2-negative cancers For the phase-2 coopERA Breast Cancer trial, giredestrant showed an average Ki67 reduction of 80% versus 67% compared to anastrozole (95% CI; 95% CI: –75%, –56% p = .0222). Greater than 20% Ki67 suppression was seen in 83% versus 71% for anastrozole; baseline Ki67 <20% was 65% versus 24% respectively; and 25% of tumors showed complete cell cycle arrest at 2 weeks versus 5% with anastrozole (Δ 20%; 95% CI: –37%, –3%). Side effects were 28% versus 38% comparatively for anastrozole.[3]

Novel Drugs

- **Eribulin (Halaven):** This is a microtubule dynamics inhibitor. It is the mesylate salt of a synthetic analogue of halichondrin B, a substance derived from a marine sponge (*Lissodendoryx sp.*). It binds to the vinca domain of tubulin and inhibits the polymerization of tubulin and the assembly of microtubules, resulting in inhibition of mitotic spindle assembly, of vascular remodeling, reversal of epithelial–mesenchymal transition, suppression of migration and invasion, induction of cell cycle arrest at the G2/M phase, and, potentially, tumor regression. Dosing is 1.4 mg/m^2 IV days 1 and 8 of a 21-day cycle.

- **Trabectedin (Yondelis):** This is a tetrahydroisoquinoline alkaloid isolated from the marine tunicate *Ecteinascidia turbinata* that binds to the minor groove of DNA and interferes with the transcription-coupled nucleotide excision repair machinery to induce lethal DNA strand breaks and block the cell cycle in the G2 phase. It also inhibits the differentiation of monocytes into macrophages. Dosing is 1.5 mg/m^2 IV over 24 hours once every 21 days.

- **Lurbinectedin (Zepzelca):** This is an alkylating agent that is an analog of trabectedin. It was approved for platinum-refractory small cell lung cancer. Dosing is 4m IV every 21 days.

- **Ixabepilone (Ixempra):** This is a microtubule-stabilizing agent that evades paclitaxel resistance via retention of tumor-binding affinity despite upregulation of class III beta-tubulin and maintenance of intracellular concentrations as a nonsubstrate for the p-glycoprotein drug efflux pump. It is a PO bioavailable semisynthetic analogue of epothilone B with antineoplastic activity. Ixabepilone binds to tubulin and promotes tubulin polymerization and microtubule stabilization, thereby arresting cells in the G2-M phase of the cell cycle and inducing tumor cell apoptosis. It demonstrates antineoplastic activity against taxane-resistant cell lines. Dosing is 40 mg/m^2 IV every 3 weeks, usually in combination therapy.

Protective Agents

These agents protect against the cytotoxic effects of chemotherapeutic drugs.

- **Leucovorin:** This drug has two mechanisms of action. It is protective against MTX and it modulates and prolongs the effects of 5-FU. Dosing is 370 mg/m^2/day for 5 days during 5-FU infusion plus an additional infusion of 500 mg/m^2/day beginning 24 hours before the first dose of 5-FU and continuing 12 hours after completion of 5-FU therapy; or 5 to 15 mg PO or 10 to 20 mg/m^2 given IV 10 minutes before 5-FU infusion. It is eliminated by the renal system. Primary toxicities are pancytopenia, nausea, and vomiting. The nadir is days 7 to 14.

- **Dexrazoxane (Zinecard):** This is chemoprotective against doxorubicin-induced cardiomyopathy. It chelates divalent heavy metals and is administered IV, 30 minutes prior to chemotherapy at a dose of 10:1 (500 mg/m^2 dexrazoxane to 50 mg/m^2 of doxorubicin). Consider administration when the cumulative dose of doxorubicin rises to 300 mg/m^2. Elimination is primarily renal with toxicities of granulocytopenia, nausea, vomiting, and alopecia.

- **Amifostine:** This is a radioprotective and cytoprotective compound. It has a highly selective transport mechanism into normal cells and there it scavenges free radicals. It can reduce the renal toxicity of cisplatin as well as the neurotoxicity of other agents. It is administered IV 30 minutes prior to chemotherapy at a dose of 740 to 910 mg/m^2. Toxicity is mucositis, nausea, vomiting, arterial hypotension, and hypocalcemia. The dosing interval is with chemotherapy and elimination is renal.

- **Sodium thiosulfate:** This protects against cisplatin-induced nephro-toxicity. It is administered IV at a dose of 16 to 20 mg/m² given 2 hours after cisplatin. The dose interval is with chemotherapy and elimination is renal.

- **Mesna:** This drug is chemoprotective against hemorrhagic cystitis and it inactivates the metabolite acrolein. It can be administered IV or SC at a dose that is 20% of the total cytotoxic alkylator dose. Dosing is prior to chemotherapy with two additional doses 4 and 8 hours after chemotherapy treatment. Elimination is renal.

- **Buthionine sulfoximine:** This enhances the cytotoxicity of alkylator agents by modifying GSH and GST, thus depleting intracellular lev-els of GSH. It is administered IV. Dosing is with a loading dose of 3 g/m² over 30 minutes, followed by three consecutive 24-hour infu-sions at 18 mg/m². Chemotherapy should be given 48 hours after buthionine sulfoximine. Elimination is via the renal system.

Antiangiogenesis, Targeted Therapies, and Immunotherapy

Antiangiogenesis

Antiangiogenesis therapy: All members of the VEGF family of ligands stimulate cellular responses by binding to tyrosine kinase receptors on the cell surface and causing dimerization and activation through transphosphorylation. VEGFR-1,2,3 are membrane-bound receptors and have an extracellular portion consisting of seven immunoglobu-lin (Ig)-like domains, a single transmembrane-spanning region, and an intracellular portion containing the split tyrosine kinase domain. Inhibition can be direct or indirect (Figure 5.1).

- Direct VEGF inhibitor:
  - Bevacizumab (Avastin): This is a recombinant humanized mAb directed against the VEGFR-1,2,3. Bevacizumab binds to VEGF and inhibits VEGF receptor binding, preventing the activation of the VEGFR-1,2,3 by sequestering it. Dosing is 5 to 7.5 mg/kg IV every 2 weeks or 7.5 to 15 mg/kg every 3 weeks. Elimination is renal. Primary toxicities are HTN (28%), nephrotic syndrome, GI perforation (1% to 11%), wound dehiscence, and CHF.
  - Cediranib (Recentin): is an anti-angiogenic multi-TKI targeting VEGFR-1,2,3. It competes with ATP, and binds to and inhibits VEGFR-1,2,3 thus blocking the VEGF signaling, angiogenesis, and tumor cell growth. Dosing: 30 mg PO daily for a 28 day cycle.

- Indirect VEGF inhibitor :
  - Aflibercept (Zaltrap): This works as a VEGF trap. It is a fusion protein that prevents VEGF receptor binding. This protein is composed of segments of the extracellular domains of human VEGFR-1 and -2 fused to the constant region (Fc) of human IgG1 Aflibercept functions as a soluble decoy receptor, binding to pro-angiogenic VEGFs, preventing VEGFs from binding to their cell

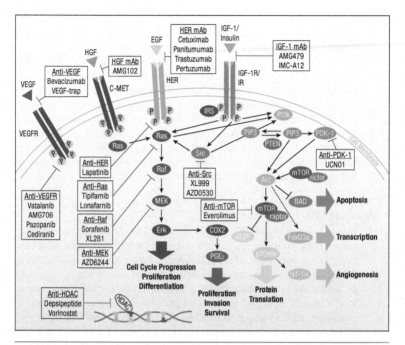

Figure 5.1 Overview of interlinked cellular signaling pathways involved in the proliferation and progression of CRC.

Source: From Siena S, et al. Biomarkers predicting clinical outcome of epidermal growth factor receptor—targeted therapy in metastatic colorectal cancer. *J Nat Can Inst.* 2009;101(19):1308–1324.[4]

receptors. Disruption of the binding of VEGFs to their cell receptors results in the inhibition of tumor angiogenesis, metastasis, and ultimately tumor regression. Dosing is 4 mg/kg IV every 2 weeks.

○ Trebananib (AMG 386): This is a peptide-Fc fusion protein neutralizing peptibody that inhibits binding of angiopoietin 1 and 2 to the Tie2 receptor. Trebananib targets and binds to Ang1 and Ang2, preventing the interaction of the angiopoietins with their target Tie2 receptors. This inhibits angiogenesis and may lead to inhibition of tumor cell proliferation. Dosing is 15 mg/kg IV weekly.[5]

● Vascular disrupting agents:

○ CA4P (Fosbretabulin): This a pro-drug that comes either in a disodium salt or a tromethamine salt form derived from the African willow bush (*Combretum caffrum*). After administration, the pro-drug fosbretabulin is dephosphorylated to its active metabolite, the microtubule-depolymerizing agent combretastatin A4, which binds to the colchicine binding site of beta-tubulin dimers and prevents microtubule polymerization, resulting in mitotic arrest and apoptosis in endothelial cells. This agent also disrupts the engagement of the endothelial cell-specific junctional molecule VE-cadherin and the ensuing activity of the VE-cadherin/β-catenin/AKT signaling pathway, which may result in the inhibition of endothelial cell migration and capillary tube formation. As a result of fosbretabulin's dual mechanism of action, the tumor vasculature collapses, resulting in ischemic necrosis of tumor tissue. Dosing is 45 to 60 mg/m^2 IV weekly for 3 weeks of a 4-week cycle for a total of 6 maximum cycles.

Targeted Therapies
- Multiple target therapies:
  - Nintedanib (Vargatef/OVEF): This is an PO bioavailable multitargeted RTK inhibitor (TKI) with potential antiangiogenic and antineoplastic activities. It selectively binds to and inhibits VEGFR, FGFR, and PDGFR tyrosine kinases, which results in the induction of endothelial cell apoptosis, a reduction in tumor vasculature, and the inhibition of tumor cell proliferation and migration. In addition, this agent also inhibits members of the Src family of tyrosine kinases, including Src, Lck, Lyn, and FLT-3. Dosing is 200 mg PO BID.
  - Pazopanib (Voltrient): This is the hydrochloride salt of a small molecule inhibitor of multiple protein tyrosine kinases and selectively inhibits VEGFR-1,2,3, c-kit, and PDGF-R, which results in inhibition of angiogenesis in tumors in which these receptors are upregulated. Dosing is 800 mg PO BID.
  - Sorafenib (Nexavar): This blocks the enzyme RAF kinase, a critical component of the RAF/MEK/ERK signaling pathway that controls cell division and proliferation; it also inhibits the VEGFR-2/PDGFR-beta signaling cascade, thereby blocking tumor angiogenesis. Dosing is 400 mg PO q12 hours.[6]
  - Rebastinib: This peptibody is an PO bioavailable small-molecule inhibitor of multiple tyrosine kinases. It inhibits angiopoietin-1/ang 1 binding to the Tie2 receptor. It binds to and inhibits the Bcr–Abl fusion oncoprotein by changing the conformation of the folded protein to disallow ligand-dependent and ligand-independent activation. It also binds to and inhibits Src family kinases LYN, HCK, and FGR and the RTKs TIE-2 and VEGFR-2. Rebastinib may exhibit more potent activity against T315I Bcr-Abl gatekeeper mutant kinases than other Bcr-Abl kinase inhibitors. The TIE-2 and VEGFR-2 RTKs regulate angiogenesis, respectively, whereas the Src family kinases Abl, LYN, and HCK Src regulate a

variety of cellular responses, including differentiation, division, adhesion, and the stress response. Dosing is 150 mg PO BID.

○ Vandetanib (Caprelsa): This is an PO bioavailable 4-anilinoquinazoline that selectively inhibits the tyrosine kinase activity of VEGFR-2. It blocks VEGF-stimulated endothelial cell proliferation and migration and reduces tumor vessel permeability. This agent also blocks the tyrosine kinase activity of EGFR. Dosing is 300 mg PO daily.[7]

○ Volasertib: This is a dihydropteridinone derivative and cell-cycle kinase inhibitor with selectivity for Polo-like kinase 1 (Plk1) and half maximal inhibitory activity for Plk2/3. It can induce G2-M arrest and subsequent apoptosis in tumors. Dosing is 300 mg IV every 21 days in heavily pretreated patients. Dose reductions are in 50-mg steps. Side effects are mainly hematologic.

○ Cabozantinib (Cabometyx): This is a small-molecule inhibitor of VEGFR-2 and c-Met among other tyrosine kinases. Dosing is 60 mg PO daily.

○ Defactinib (VS-6063): This is an PO active ATP competitive, reversible inhibitor of FAK. Defactinib has shown synergistic activity with BRAF and MEK inhibitors. Dosing is 200 to 400 mg PO BID every 21 days of a 28-day cycle.

○ Avutometinib VS-6766: This is a small molecule inhibitor that blocks MEK kinase activity and RAF phosphorylation of MEK. This limits compensatory MEK activation, potentially enhancing efficacy of MEK inhibition. A third of patients with recurrent LGSOC harbor somatic KRAS mutations. FAK inhibition has been shown to induce tumor regression when combined with RAF, MEK or RAF/MEK inhibitors in in vivo models of KRAS mutant ovarian cancer. Dosing is 3.2 mg twice weekly 21 days of a 28-day cycle.

○ Trametinib: This is a selective, reversible, allosteric inhibitor of MEK1 and MEK2, effective for use in LGSTOC. It has also been approved for use in combination with dabrafenib for unresectable or metastatic $BRAF^{V600E}$ (i.e., Val600Glu) or $BRAF^{V600K}$ mutation melanoma, metastatic $BRAF^{V600E}$ mutation NSC lung cancers, and metastatic $BRAF^{V600E}$ mutation anaplastic thyroid cancer. Dosing is 2 mg PO daily.

○ Repotrectinib: This is a multiple kinase inhibitor that includes the RTK, ALK; ROS1; the NTRK types 1, 2, and 3; the proto-oncogene SRC; and FAK. Dosing is 160 mg PO daily.

• mTOR inhibitors:

○ Temsirolimus (Torisel): This is an ester analog of rapamycin. Temsirolimus binds to and inhibits the mTOR, resulting in decreased expression of mRNAs necessary for cell-cycle progression and arresting cells in the G1 phase of the cell cycle.

mTOR is a serine/threonine kinase that plays a role in the PI3K/AKT pathway that is upregulated in some tumors. Dosing is 25 mg IV weekly.

○ Everolimus (Afinitor): This is an mTOR serine–threonine kinase inhibitor, and binds to intracellular FKBP-12 resulting in inhibition of formation with mTOR complex 1, thus inhibiting translation of 4EBP-1 and S6K1, which regulate proteins in the cell cycle, angiogenesis, and glycolysis. Dosing is 10 mg PO daily.

○ Ridaforolimus (AP23573): This is an mTOR kinase inhibitor. Dosing is 40 mg PO daily for 5 days/week or 12.5 mg IV daily for 5 days every 2 weeks.

○ Sirolimus (Rapamune): This is an mTOR kinase inhibitor. Dosing is 5 mg PO daily if patient weight is greater than 40 kg, or 1 mg/m²/day if patient weight is less than 40 kg after a loading dose of 3 mg/m² if weight is less than 40 kg or 15 mg if weight is greater than 40 kg.

- Notch inhibitors: The Notch signaling pathway plays an important role in cell-fate determination, cell survival, and cell proliferation.

○ MK0752: This is a synthetic small gamma secretase inhibitor that inhibits the Notch signaling pathway, which results in growth arrest and apoptosis of tumor cells in which the Notch signaling pathway is overactivated. Dosing is 1,200 mg PO weekly.

○ Demcizumab: This is a humanized mAb directed against the N-terminal epitope of Notch ligand DLL4 with potential antineoplastic activity. Demcizumab binds to the membrane-binding portion of DLL4 and prevents its interaction with Notch-1 and Notch-4 receptors, inhibiting Notch-mediated signaling and gene transcription, which impedes tumor angiogenesis. Activation of Notch receptors by DLL4 stimulates proteolytic cleavage of the NICD; after cleavage, NICD is translocated into the nucleus and mediates the transcriptional regulation of a variety of genes involved in vascular development. The expression of DLL4 is highly restricted to the vascular endothelium. Dosing is 3.5 to 5 mg/kg IV weekly days 1, 8, 15 of a 28-day cycle.

○ REGN421 (Enoticumab): This an anti-DLL4 mAb, a human mAb directed against DLL4 preventing its binding to Notch receptors and inhibiting Notch signaling, which may result in defective tumor vascularization and the inhibition of tumor cell growth. DLL4 is the only Notch ligand selectively expressed on endothelial cells. Dosing is 3 mg/kg IV every 2 weeks.

- EGFR inhibitors: EGFR is overexpressed on the cell surfaces of various solid tumors.

○ Cetuximab (Erbitux): This is a recombinant, chimeric mAb directed against EGFR. Cetuximab binds to the extracellular domain of EGFR, preventing the activation and subsequent dimerization of the receptor; the decrease in receptor activation and dimerization results in an inhibition in signal transduction and antiproliferative effects. This agent may inhibit EGFR-dependent primary tumor growth and metastasis. Dosing is 400 mg/m^2 1 week before starting cytotoxic chemotherapy, then 250 mg/m^2 weekly.

- ○ Trastuzumab (Herceptin): This is a recombinant humanized mAb directed against HER2. After binding to HER2 on the tumor cell surface, trastuzumab induces an ADCC against tumor cells that overexpress HER2. Elimination is renal and toxicities are a rash or CHF (1% to 29%). Dosing begins with a 4 mg/kg IV loading dose with maintenance dosing at 2 mg/kg IV once weekly for 12 to 18 weeks. Maintenance dosing continues at 6 mg/kg IV every 3 weeks starting 1 week after completion of combination cytotoxic therapy.

- ○ Pertuzumab: This is a humanized mAb inhibiting HER-2 binding with HER family members HER1, HER3, and HER4 preventing downstream signal transduction to PI3K. Elimination is renal and toxicities are rash or CHF. Dosing is an 840-mg loading dose IV day 1, then 420 mg IV every 21 days subsequently, in combination with other chemotherapies. Low HER3 mRNA expression has been shown to be a positive predictive factor for response.

- ○ Erlotinib (Tarceva): This targets EGFR. It is dosed at 150 mg PO daily. It is not recommended in combination with platinum therapy.

- TKIs:
  - ○ Sunitinib (Sutent): This is a selective TKI that blocks the tyrosine kinase activities of VEGFR-2, PDGFRb, and c-kit, thereby inhibiting angiogenesis and cell proliferation. This agent also inhibits the phosphorylation of FLT3, another RTK expressed by some leukemic cells. Dosing is 50 mg PO daily for 4 weeks, then 2 weeks off.

  - ○ Crizotinib (Xalkori): This is an PO available aminopyridine-based inhibitor of the RTK, ALK. Crizotinib also binds to c-MET/HGFR, disrupting c-MET signaling. It binds in an ATP-competitive manner, and inhibits ALK kinase and ALK fusion proteins. It has activity in ALK-positive patients and vaginal sarcoma ALK mutation-positive patients. Dosing is 250 mg BID.

  - ○ Lenvatinib: This is an oral multitargeted TKI of VEGFR 1 to 3, FGFR 1 to 4, PDGFR beta, RET, and KIT, and antagonizes neovascularization via downregulating angiopoietin signaling by binding to ligands ANG 1-2. Dosing is 24 mg PO daily.

  - ○ Cediranib: This is a TKI and single-agent response is 17% in recurrent EOC administered at 20 to 30 mg PO daily.

  - ○ Larotrectinib (Vitrakvi): This agent targets NTRK gene fusion tumors. It is a tropomyosin receptor kinase inhibitor. Dosing is 100 mg PO BID and comes in a capsule or oral solution.

○ Entrectinib (Rozlytrek): This is a TKI (tropomyosin), which acts as an ATP competitor to inhibit TRH A/B/C as well as proto-oncogene tyrosine protein kinase ROS1 and ALK. Dosing is 600 mg PO daily.

- Serine/threonine kinase inhibitors:

○ XL418: This is a selective, PO active small molecule, targeting protein kinase B (PKB or AKT) and ribosomal protein S6 Kinase (p70S6K), with antineoplastic activity. XL418 inhibits the activities of PKB and p70S6K, both acting downstream of PI3K. Inhibition of PKB induces apoptosis, wereas inhibition of p70S6K results in the inhibition of translation within tumor cells. Dosing is 6.4 mg/kg PO daily.

- Multikinase inhibitors: PI3K/mTOR inhibitors:

○ SF1126: Administer 1,110 mg/m² twice weekly for 4 weeks of a 28-week cycle.

○ BEZ235: Administer 300 mg PO BID for 8 days every 4 weeks.

○ Gedatolisib (PF-05212384): This is an inhibitor of PI3K and mTOR (TORC1/2) kinase activity. It is given once weekly IV with a MTD of 154 mg. Side effects are mucosal inflammation, nausea, and hyperglycemia. It has shown to be effective in recurrent uterine cancer.

- Dual mTOR/AKT:

○ MKC1: This is an oral cell-cycle inhibitor that binds to and inhibits the importin-beta proteins and tubulin-preventing mitotic spindle formation. Dosing is 150 mg PO daily for a 28-day cycle.

- CHK1 inhibitor: KRAS mutation:

○ Prexasertib: used as monotherapy dosed IV at 105 mg/m2 as a 1 hour infusion on day 1 of a 14 day cycles or at 70 mg/m2 IV in combination therapy with a PARP inhibitor. Toxicities are pancytopenias.

- WEE1 inhibitors: Inhibition of WEE1 activity prevents the phosphorylation of CDC2 and impairs the G2 DNA damage checkpoint. Unlike normal cells, most p53-deficient or mutated human cancers lack the G1 checkpoint, as p53 is the key regulator of the G1 checkpoint and these cells rely on the G2 checkpoint for DNA repair to damaged cells. Termination of the G2 checkpoint may therefore sensitize p53-deficient tumor cells to genotoxic/antineoplastic agents through deregulation of the G2/M checkpoint and enhancement of their cytotoxic effects.

○ Adavosertib AZD1775: This selectively targets and inhibits WEE1, a tyrosine kinase that phosphorylates cyclin-dependent kinase 1 (CDK1, CDC2) at the G2 checkpoint to inactivate the CDC2/cyclin B complex. Dosing is 225 mg daily to BID 5 days/week for 14 days of a 21-day cycle. Activity may be enhanced in *BRCA*-mutated patients.

- TolR agonists:
  - Entolimod (TLR5 agonist CBLB502): This is a polypeptide derived from the *Salmonella* filament protein flagellin with potential radioprotective and anticancer activities. As a TLR5 agonist, entolimod binds to and activates TLR5, stimulating TNF production and activating NF-kB. This induces NF-kB-mediated signaling pathways and inhibits the induction of apoptosis. This may prevent apoptosis in normal, healthy cells during XRT and may allow for increased doses of ionizing XRT. In addition, entolimod may inhibit XRT-independent proliferation in TLR5-expressing tumor cells. Dosing is 30 mcg/day days 1, 4, 8, and 11 via IV every 2 weeks.
  - Motolimod (VTX2337): This is a small-molecule agonist of toll-like receptor 8. This molecule mobilizes the immune system by directly activating myeloid DCs, monocytes, and NK cells, resulting in production of mediators that integrate both the innate and adaptive antitumor responses to cancer. Dosing in phase II studies is 2.5 mg/m² SC weekly days 1, 8, and 15 of a 28-day regimen with cetuximab.
  - ANA773 tosylate (TLR7). The tosylate salt form of ANA773, this is a TLR7 pro-drug with potential immunostimulating activity. Upon administration, ANA773 is metabolized into its active form, which binds to and activates TLR7, stimulating DCs and enhancing NK cell cytotoxicity. This activation results in the production of proinflammatory cytokines, including interferon alpha, and enhanced ADCC. TLR7 is a member of the TLR family, which plays a fundamental role in pathogen recognition and activation of innate immunity. Dosing is 400 to 800 mg PO QOD for 14 days of a 28-day cycle.
- AKT inhibitors:
  - Perifosine: A loading dose of 100 mg PO q6h is given on day 1 followed by daily dosing at 50, 100, or 150 mg for 20 days.
- PI3K Inhibitors:
  - Pilaralisib: Dose is 400 to 600 mg PO daily.
  - BKM120, BYL719, BEZ235, and XL147
- KRAS/MEK inhibitors:
  - Trametinib (Mekinist): This is used in KRAS mutated neuroendocrine cervical cancer. Dosing is 2 mg PO daily as monotherapy or in combination with dabrafenib (Taflinar) at 150 mg daily. It can also be used in BRAF^V600E/K-mutated melanoma or NSC lung or thyroid cancers.
  - Binimetinib (Mektovi): This can be used for LGSOCs. It is an MEK inhibitor dosed at 45 mg PO BID. It has been used in combination with encorafenib in BRAF^V600E or K-mutated melanomas.

- Folate receptor inhibitors
  - Farletuzumab: This is a mAb that binds to folate receptor alpha. The therapeutic index is present as folate receptor alpha is overexpressed in some tumor cells but absent in normal tissue. Dosing is 2.5 mg/kg IV weekly.
- Imatinib Mesylate (Gleevec): This inhibits the protein tyrosine kinase Bcr-Abl. Primary toxicities are nausea, vomiting, muscle cramps, skin rash, diarrhea, and heartburn, with a secondary toxicity of fluid retention. It is eliminated via the hepatobiliary system. Dosing is 400 mg/day PO for CML, and 600 mg/day for blast crisis CML or GIST.
- PARP inhibitors: These agents selectively bind to and inhibit PARP, inhibiting PARP-mediated repair of single- strand DNA breaks. PARP catalyzes posttranslational ADP-ribosylation of nuclear proteins and can be activated by single-stranded DNA breaks. PARP inhibition enhances the cytotoxicity of DNA-damaging agents and reverses tumor cell chemoresistance and radioresistance.
  - Olaparib: This is a small-molecule inhibitor of PARP1 and 2 with chemosensitizing, radiosensitizing, and antineoplastic activities. Dosing is 400 mg PO BID.
  - Veliparib: This is a PARP1 and 2 inhibitor with chemosensitizing and antitumor activities. Veliparib inhibits PARPs, thereby inhibiting DNA repair and potentiating the cytotoxicity of DNA-damaging agents. Dosing is 400 mg PO BID. It has the least PARP-trapping ability.
  - Rucaparib: This is a tricyclic indole PARP1 inhibitor with chemosensitizing, radiosensitizing, and antineoplastic activities. Rucaparib selectively binds to PARP1 and inhibits PARP1-mediated DNA repair. Dosing is 600 mg PO BID.
  - Niraparib: This is an inhibitor of PARP1 and 2, enhancing the accumulation of DNA strand breaks and promoting genomic instability and apoptosis. Dosing is 300 mg PO daily.
- CDK 4/6 inhibitors:
  - Palbociclib (Ibrance): This is an inhibitor of CDK 4/6 and works intranuclearly. Indication for treatment is for ER+/HER2- cancers. Dosing is 125 mg PO daily. It is usually given in combination with an aromatase inhibitor for a 28-day cycle for which palbociclib is taken for 21 days and the aromatase inhibitor (AI) for the full 28 days. Side effects are neutropenia and VTE.
- Epithelial cell adhesion molecules:
  - Catumaxomab (Removab): This is a rat–mouse hybrid mAb binding to antigens CD3 and EpCAM. It is used to treat malignant ascites and is administered IP. Dosing is 10, 20, 50, and 100 mcg given as a 6-hour IP infusion on days 0, 3, 7, and 10.

- Selective inhibitors of nuclear export compounds:
  - ○ Selinexor (Xpovio): binds to and inhibits the nuclear export protein XPO1. This leads to accumulation of tumor suppressor proteins in the nucleus, which is thought to reinitiate and amplify tumor suppressor function. This may then selectively induce apoptosis in cancer cells, while sparing normal cells. Dosing is 80 mg weekly PO.

Immunotherapies

Immunotherapy uses antibodies to block CTLA-4 and PD-1/PD-L1—they are checkpoint inhibitors. Normally, CTLA-4 is upregulated on the plasma membrane where it functions to downregulate T-cell function and induce T-cell arrest. Mice deficient in CTLA-4 die from fatal lymphoproliferation. PD-1 is a negative regulator of T-cell activity that limits T-cell activity when it interacts with PD-L1 and PD-L2. PD-1 inhibits effector T-cell activity within tissue and tumors. Antibodies that disrupt the PD-1 axis include those that target PD-1 and PD-L1.[8]

- **FANG vaccine:** This is a vaccine consisting of autologous tumor cells transfected with a plasmid expressing rhGM–CSF and bi-shRNA against furin, with potential immunostimulatory and antineoplastic activities. Upon intradermal vaccination GM–CSF protein recruits immune effectors to the site of injection and promotes antigen presentation. The furin bi-shRNAi blocks furin protein production. Decreased levels of furin lead to a reduction in the conversion of TGF beta into TGF beta1 and beta2 protein isoforms. In turn, as part of the negative feedback mechanism, reduced furin protein levels inhibit TGFbeta1 and TGFbeta2 gene expression, thereby further decreasing TGF levels. As TGFs are potent immunosuppressive cytokines, reducing their levels may activate the immune system locally and this can cause a cytotoxic T lymphocyte (CTL) response against the tumor cells.
- **Tremelimumab:** This is a human IgG2 (immunoglobulin G2) mAb directed against CTLA-4, with immune checkpoint inhibitory and antineoplastic activities. Tremelimumab binds to CTLA-4 on activated T-lymphocytes and blocks the binding of the antigen-presenting cell ligands B7-1 (CD80) and B7-2 (CD86) to CTLA-4, resulting in inhibition of CTLA-4-mediated downregulation of T-cell activation. This promotes the interaction of B7-1 and B7-2 with another T-cell surface receptor protein, CD28, and results in a B7-CD28-mediated T-cell activation that is unopposed by CTLA-4-mediated inhibition. This leads to a CTL-mediated immune response against cancer cells. CTLA-4, an inhibitory receptor and member of the immunoglobulin (Ig) superfamily, plays a key role in the downregulation of the immune system. Dosing is 15 mg/kg IV every 90 days.
- **Avelumab:** This is a human IgG1 mAb directed against PD-L1 protein, with immune checkpoint inhibitory and antineoplastic

activities. Upon administration, avelumab binds to PD-L1 and prevents the interaction of PD-L1 with its receptor PD-1. This inhibits the activation of PD-1 and its downstream signaling pathways. This may restore immune function through the activation of CTLs targeted to PD-L1-overexpressing tumor cells. In addition, avelumab induces an ADCC response against PD-L1-expressing tumor cells. PD-1, a cell surface receptor belonging to the Ig superfamily expressed on T cells, negatively regulates T-cell activation and effector function when activated by its ligand, and plays an important role in tumor evasion from host immunity. PD-L1, a transmembrane protein, is overexpressed in a variety of tumor cell types and is associated with poor prognosis. Dosing is 10 mg/kg IV every 2 to 3 weeks.

- **Pembrolizumab (Keytruda):** This is a humanized monoclonal IgG4 antibody directed against human cell surface receptor PD-1 with immune checkpoint inhibitory and antineoplastic activities. On administration, pembrolizumab binds to PD-1 and blocks the binding to and activation of PD-1 by its ligands, which results in the activation of T-cell-mediated immune responses against tumor cells. The ligands for PD-1 include PD-L1, overexpressed on certain cancer cells, and PD-L2, which is primarily expressed on APCs. Dosing is 2 mg/kg IV every 3 weeks, 200 mg every 3 weeks, or 400 mg every 6 weeks.

- **Nivolumab (Opdivo):** This is a fully humanized IgG4 mAb directed against the negative immunoregulatory PD-1 with immune checkpoint inhibitory and antineoplastic activities. Nivolumab binds to and blocks the activation of PD-1 by its ligands PD-L1 and PD-L2. This results in the activation of T cells and cell-mediated immune responses against tumor cells or pathogens. Nivolumab resulted in a 32% ORR in a phase III melanoma study compared to 11% for chemotherapy that included DTIC or carboplatin/paclitaxel. Dosing: Regimens may differ but is recommended at 3 mg/kg IV every 2 weeks.

- **Ipilimumab (Yervoy):** This is a CTLA-4 inhibitor. It is a recombinant human IgG1 mAb directed against the CTLA-4, with immune checkpoint inhibitory and antineoplastic activities. Ipilimumab binds to CTLA-4 expressed on T cells and inhibits the CTLA-4-mediated downregulation of T-cell activation. This leads to a CTL-mediated immune response against cancer cells. Ipilimumab was significant in melanoma patients for improving survival (2YOS; 18% vs. 5%). Dosing: Regimens may differ but a common therapy is 3 mg/kg IV every 3 weeks.[9]

- **Pidilizumab:** This is a humanized, IgG1 mAb directed against PD-1, with immune checkpoint inhibitory and antineoplastic activities. Pidilizumab binds to PD-1 and blocks the interaction between PD-1 and its ligands, PD-L1 and PD-L2. This prevents the activation of PD-1 and its downstream signaling pathways. This may restore immune function through the activation of NK cells and CTLs against tumor cells. Dosing varies but can be 1.5 mg/kg every 42 days.

- **Dostarlimab-gxly (Jemperli):** This is an anti PD-1 blocking mAb. Side effects are diarrhea, anemia, and constipation. Administration of doses one through four is 500 mg every 3 weeks. Subsequent dosing beginning 3 weeks after dose 4 (dose 5 onward): 1,000 mg every 6 weeks (2.2) IV over 30 minutes.

- **Balstilimab (AGEN2034):** This is a human IgG4 anti-PD-1 mAb that binds to PD-1, and functions as a PD-1 antagonist stimulating/activating T-cell receptor signaling and T-cell responsiveness to tumor-associated antigens. Dosing is 300 mg IV every 3 weeks (Figure 5.2).

- **Zalifrelimab (AGEN1884):** This is a CTLA-4-targeting human IgG1 mAb that antagonizes the inhibitory checkpoints of immune cell activation regulated by CTLA-4 signaling. Zalifrelimab has been shown to potentiate the activity of other immunomodulatory antibodies and to combine with PD-1 inhibition to elicit T cell-associated proliferative responses. Zalifrelimab has also shown activity and favorable tolerability as monotherapy to patients with PD-1-refractory solid tumors. It can be partnered with other immunotherapies as combination therapy. Dosing is 1 mg/kg once every 6 weeks as a single agent or in combination therapy.

- **Tisotumab vedotin:** This is an antibody-drug conjugate; it is a fully humanized mAb that binds to tissue factor, which is linked to a cytotoxic or antimitotic agent called MMAE. The complex is rapidly internalized and targets solid tumor cells and the complex is then sent to

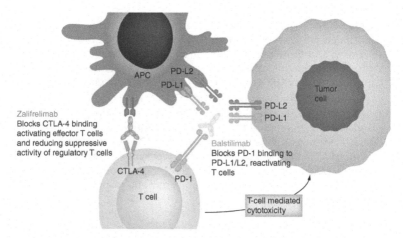

Figure 5.2 PD-1 and CTLA mechanisms.

Source: O'Malley DM, Randall LM, Jackson CG, et al. RaPiDS (GOG-3028): randomized Phase II study of balstilimab alone or in combination with zalifrelimab in cervical cancer. *Future Onc*. 2021;17(26). Available at https://www.futuremedicine.com/doi/10.2217/fon-2021-0529[10]

lysosomes for degradation. MMAE is subsequently released from the lysosome and further inhibits microtubule formation. Dosing is 2 mg/kg every 3 weeks via IV.

- **Cepilimab (Libtayo):** This is a mAb that targets checkpoint inhibitor PD-1 and blocks the interaction with PD-L1 and PD-L2 on T cells, inhibiting T-cell proliferation and cytokine production, thereby releasing the PD-1 pathway-mediated inhibition of the immune response and slowing tumor growth. Dosing is 350 mg IV every 3 weeks.
- **Anti-PD-L1:** Avelumab, atezolizumab, durvalumab
- **Anti-PD-1 inhibitors:** Nivolumab, pembrolizumab
- **Anti-CTLA4:** Ipilimumab

- **Adoptive Cell Therapy (ACT):** This involves infusion of autologous tumor-reactive T cells. This has been used in the treatment of some B-cell malignancies, cervical cancer, and metastatic melanoma. T-cell cultures generated from HPV-positive cancers and selected for HPV oncoprotein-reactive cultures were administered to patients. Treatment included lymphocyte-depleting conditioning chemotherapy regimen (cyclophosphamide 60 mg/kg IV daily for 2 days, fludarabine 25 mg/m^2 daily for 5 days), followed by HPV-TIL infusion IV as a single dose, and aldesleukin 720,000 IU/kg/dose IV boluses every 8 hours to a tolerance of a maximum of 15 doses. There was a 30% ORR. The magnitude of HPV reactivity the infusion produced, measured by interferon-gamma production, ELISPOT, or CD137 upregulation, was associated with clinical response.
- **Oregovamab:** This is a CA-125 specific murine mAb. Two mg are administered IV over 20 minutes at weeks 0, 4, 8, and then every 12 weeks until recurrence for up to 5 Y. A phase III trial failed to show prolongation of time to recurrence as maintenance mono-immunotherapy (10.3 months vs. 12.9 months for placebo with p = .29 log rank test).[11]
- **Abagovomab:** This is a murine mAb used as a surrogate antigen, and when administered, enables the immune system to identify and attack tumor cells displaying the CA-125 protein. It is administered as a 2-mg IV dose once every 2 weeks for 6 weeks, then once every 4 weeks for maintenance up to 21 months or until recurrence. A phase III study noted a measurable immune response but did not prolong RFS or OS.[12]

Treatment of Extravasation Injury
- **Cisplatin:** Thiosulfate should be injected into the skin site at 1/3 to 1/6 molar solution. For every 100 mg extravasated, 2 mL should be injected.

- **Doxorubicin:** Cold compresses should be applied immediately to the site for 60 minutes with consideration of an injection of 150 U hyaluronidase into the site. Cold topical DMSO can also be applied. This agent can cause extensive ulceration and treatment is debridement of the primary and recurrent ulcers.
- **Etoposide:** Consider an injection of 150 U of hyaluronidase into the site.
- **Mitomycin C:** Topical DMSO should be applied every 6 hours for 14 days.
- **Vinblastine:** Warm compresses should be applied immediately to the site for 60 minutes with consideration of an injection of 150 U of hyaluronidase into the site. Corticosteroids can also help if injected into the site.
- **Vincristine:** Warm compresses should be applied immediately to the site for 60 minutes with consideration of an injection of 150 U of hyaluronidase into the site.

Neutropenic Fever

Clinical judgment is recommended when determining which patients are candidates for outpatient management of neutropenic fever.[13] Using clinical criteria or a validated tool, such as the MASCC risk index, is helpful. Patients with febrile neutropenia should receive initial doses of empirical antibacterial therapy within 1 hour of triage and be monitored for ≥4 hours before discharge. An oral fluoroquinolone plus amoxicillin/clavulanate (or clindamycin, if penicillin allergic) is recommended as empiric outpatient therapy, unless fluoroquinolone prophylaxis was used before fever developed. Patients who do not defervesce after 2 to 3 days of an initial, empirical, broad-spectrum antibiotic regimen should be reevaluated and considered for inpatient treatment. Additional information is available at www.asco.org/supportive-care-guidelines and www.asco.org/guidelineswiki

Vaccinations in Cancer Patients

- Influenza inactivated virus: This is recommended annually for all patients older than 6 months except those receiving induction or consolidation chemotherapy for acute leukemia, those receiving anti-B-cell antibodies, administered 4 to 6 months after completion of chemotherapy.
- Pneumococcal conjugate 13 valent vaccine: This is recommended, starting 6 to 12 months after completion of therapy. Pneumococcal polysaccharide vaccine 23 should then be administered to adults and children more than 2 Y old and at least 8 weeks after the indicated dose(s) of pneumococcal conjugate 13 vaccine at minimum 12 months after completion of chemotherapy.

- Inactivated vaccines (DTaP [diphtheria, tetanus, and pertussis], Hib [Haemophilus influenzae type B], Hep A, and Hep B) may be given together at the same time but can be delayed in patients receiving more than 20 mg of prednisone daily.
- Zoster vaccine: This is recommended 24 months after completion of chemotherapy only if no ongoing immunosuppression and patient is seronegative for varicella (VSV).
- Vaccines administered during cancer chemotherapy should not be considered valid doses unless documentation of a protected antibody level.
- Live viral vaccines (MMR) should not be administered during chemotherapy. They can be administered starting 24 months after completion of chemotherapy and if the patient has no ongoing immunosuppression and is seronegative for MMR. Zoster and MMR can be given together.
- If patients are receiving anti-B-cell antibodies, vaccinations should be delayed at least 6 months (Table 5.1).

Table 5.1 Vaccine Recommendations During Chemotherapy

Inactivated Vaccine	Recommended Timing After Chemotherapy (Months)	Number of Doses
Influenza	4–6	1 annually
TDaP	6–12	3
Hep A	6–12	2
Hep B	6–12	2
Pneumococcal		
Conjugated 13-valent	6–12	3
Upon completion of Prevnar series, then pneumococcal polysaccharide vaccine 23	>12	1
Hib	6–12	3
Meningococcal conjugate	6–12	1
Live vaccines		
Zoster (VZV)	>24	1
MMR	>24	1–2

- COVID vaccinations:
  - These mRNA vaccinations and boosters have been deemed safe for use in cancer patients. Side effects include induration at injection site, myalgias, mild fever. Vaccination decreases serious disease status and hospitalization rates in cancer patients.

XRT

Radiation Types
There are different types of radiation currently used in medicine.

- X-rays are extranuclear radiation. They occur from the bombardment of an atom/target by another source—usually high-speed electrons.
- The alpha particle demonstrates cluster decay in which a parent atom ejects a defined daughter collection of nucleons. These have a typical kinetic energy of 5 MeV. Because of their relatively large mass, their +2 electric charge, and relatively low velocity, alpha particles are very likely to interact with other atoms and lose their energy. Their forward motion is effectively stopped within 5–11 cm of air or paper. This particle is the same as a helium-4 particle (two protons and two neutrons).
- Beta particles are high-energy, high-speed electrons emitted by certain types of radioactive nuclei. Beta particles are ionizing radiations. They are stopped by 1 cm of tissue. The production of beta particles is termed *beta decay*.
- Gamma particles are a form of ionizing radiation that originates from the decay of the nucleus of a radioactive isotope. Energies range from 10,000 (10^4) to 10,000,000 (10^7) electron volts.
- An isotope is one of two or more atoms having the same number of protons but a different number of neutrons. This makes the nucleus unstable. The atom then spontaneously decomposes/decays and excess energy is given off by emission of a nuclear electron or helium nucleus and radiation, to achieve a stable nuclear composition. Some of these isotopes include radium-226, cesium-137, iridium-192, cobalt-60, and gold-198.
- Electron energy comes from outside the nucleus. Electrons are used to treat tumors en face—close to the skin.

Definitions
- Roentgen is the amount of photon radiation that causes 0.001293 g of air to produce one electrostatic unit of positive or negative charge. It can also be defined as the amount of photon energy required to produce 1.61 × 1,012 ion pairs in 1 cm^3 of dry air at 0°C. It is a unit of exposure, not an amount of energy, that ionizing radiation imparts to matter.
- KERMA is the transfer of energy from photons to particles. Particles transfer this energy to tissue and this is defined as the *absorbed dose*.

- Rad: This is the amount of energy that radiation imparts to a given mass. A rad is a dose of 100 ergs (energy per gram) of given material. The SI unit for rad is the Gy, which is defined as a dose of one joule per kilogram. One joule equals 107 ergs, and one kilogram equals 1,000 grams, thus 1 Gy equals 100 rads.

- Relative biologic effectiveness (RBE) is the ratio of the dose required for a given radiation to produce the same biologic effect induced by 250 kV of x-rays.

- Isodose is a radiation dose of equal intensity to more than one body area usually visualized as a line on a graph showing body areas that receive equal doses of radiation.

- Skin-to-skin distance (SSD) is usually defined as 80 to 100 cm from the machine to the patient. Radiation is dosed at a fixed point from the patient and thus there needs to be standardization of distance for treatment.

- Isocenter is a fixed point on the patient around which treatment is rotated.

- Dmax is the point where the maximum amount of dose from one beam is deposited. The dose at Dmax is defined at 100%. The depths of Dmax for some common energies are 4 MV, 1.2 cm; 6 MV, 1.5 cm; 10 MV, 2.5 cm; and 18 MV, 3.2 cm.

- Percentage of depth dose is the change in dose with depth within the patient.

- Gross tumor volume (GTV): This refers to direct tumor volume by measurement. The GTV requires a high dose of radiation to treat the primary or bulky tumor. This dose is usually 80 to 90 Gy.

- Clinical target volume (CTV): This includes any region that has a high likelihood of harboring malignancy but appears clinically normal. The CTV requires a lower dose than GTV. This dose is usually around 45 to 54 Gy and is adequate to treat occult or microscopic disease.

- Planning target volume (PTV) is a margin added to account for organ motion and daily setup error.

Radiation Effects

There are two basic types of energy transfer that may occur when x-rays interact with matter:

- Ionization, in which the incoming radiation causes the removal of an electron from an atom or molecule, leaving the material with a net positive charge.

- Excitation, in which some of the x-ray's energy is transferred to the target material, leaving it in an excited (or more energetic) state.

There are three important processes that can occur when x-rays interact with matter. These processes are the photoelectric effect, the Compton effect, and pair production.

- The photoelectric effect produces energy in the eV to keV range. This type of radiation occurs when atoms absorb energy from light and emit electrons. This form of radiation is used for diagnostic x-rays and to simulate radiation treatment beams. Photoelectric absorption of x-rays occurs when the x-ray photon is absorbed, resulting in the ejection of electrons from the atom. This leaves the atom in an ionized state. The ionized atom then returns to the neutral state with the emission of an x-ray characteristic of the atom. Photoelectron absorption is the dominant process for x-ray absorption up to energies of about 500 keV.

- Pair production occurs when the x-ray photon energy is greater than 1.02 MeV. An electron and positron are created with the annihilation of the x-ray photon. Positrons are very short lived and disappear (positron annihilation) with the formation of two photons of 0.51 MeV energy. Pair production is of particular importance when high-energy photons pass through materials with high atomic numbers. This type of energy is not used clinically.

- The Compton effect occurs when an incident photon interacts with an outer electron. The energy that results is shared between the ejected electron and the scattered photon. Compton scattering is important for specimens with low atomic number. At energies of 100 keV to 10 MeV, the absorption of radiation is mainly due to the Compton effect. This type of energy is used for the radiation treatment of cancers. Photons are harvested from the decay of a source. First, the source has intrinsic decay. The electrons from this decay are used to bombard tungsten, causing the Compton effect. The resultant photon is the radiation we use in linear accelerator machines.

Energy Equivalences
- One Gy is equal to 1 J/kg of tissue.
- One Gy is equal to 100 cGy.
- One hundred rads are equal to 1 Gy.
- One rad is equal to 1 cGy.

Radiation Delivery
- External beam radiation is delivered using a linear accelerator machine. These machines deliver 4 to 24 MeV. Total radiation dose is administered via a daily divided dose called a *fraction*. Common daily doses/fractions are 1.8 to 2 Gy. A total dose of 90 Gy is needed to sterilize most tumors. Noncancerous tissues cannot tolerate this total dose from external beam radiation, so brachytherapy is needed to locally deliver radiation directly to the tumor.
  - Intensity modulated radiation therapy (IMRT) is a highly conformal dosing method that can minimize the dose to vital pelvic organs (bowel, bladder) while maximizing dose at risk of involved sites.

- ○ VMAT (volumetric) is similar to IMRT.
- ○ Boost: This refers to an extra dose to a defined area using IMRT, usually administered after the calculated primary dose.
- ○ Simultaneous integrated boost (SIB) is a tactic used to deliver higher doses to gross positive LN in a shorter time frame using IMRT, preserving normal tissues. A boost up to 2.2 Gy/fraction can occur.
- ○ Stereotactic body XRT can deliver focused high-dose EBXRT in one to five fractions to sites of metastatic disease. Re-irridation can use this technique.
- ○ Intra-operative (IOXRT): This technique uses a highly focused radiation beam to deliver a single high dose to a tumor bed or isolated unresectable disease during an open surgical procedure. The radiation uses electrons and brachytherapy.
- Brachytherapy is the local, and often internalized, delivery of radiation. For gynecologic cancers, radiation is often delivered using tandem and ovoids, vaginal cylinders, or interstitial needles. Brachytherapy is delivered at a low-dose or high-dose rate.
- ○ *LDR* is defined as 0.4 to 2 Gy/hr.
- ○ *HDR* is defined as a dose greater than 12 Gy/hr or greater than 20 to 250 cGy/min (12–15 Gy/hr). The dose conversion from LDR to HDR is 0.6.
- ○ HDR is more common now because of a number of patient-based reasons: Treatment time is shorter, treatment is delivered on an outpatient basis, there is no need for bed rest, there is better ability to retract the rectum for shorter periods of time, and therefore better patient acceptance and comfort. Clinically, there is better implant reproducibility and a greater degree of certainty that the sources will remain stable during treatment. The HDR applicators are less bulky, so patients with narrow vaginas do not necessarily have to be treated with interstitial implants. The smaller source size also allows for finer increments in source location and weighting and a better ability to shape the dose distribution.
- ○ Isotopes: Iridium-192 is the most commonly used isotope. The half-life of iridium is 74 days. Cesium-137 is no longer available, but its half-life is 30 Y. Cobalt-60 is also no longer used, but its half-life is 5.26 Y. Radium-226 has a half-life of 1,626 Y and has little use in modern radiation oncology.

Tumoricidal Basics

- Radiation dose is proportional to the time the patient is exposed to the dose. The dose is also proportional to the distance from the source (the inverse square law): $1/r^2$. Dosing used to be mg/hr based. It is now dosimetry based.
- In the log cell kill model, each dose—called a *fraction*—kills a fixed amount of cells. Radiation works by causing breaks in the DNA

backbone via one of two types of energy, a photon or a charged particle (an electron). This damage is either direct or indirect with ionization of the atoms that make up the DNA chain. Indirect ionization is the result of the ionization of water, forming free radicals, notably hydroxyl radicals, which then damage the DNA. Direct ionization is the result of electrons causing single-stranded DNA breaks. These single-stranded breaks need to be on opposing strands of DNA in close proximity to each other in order to create a DS break. Oxygen free radicals modify radiation damage making it irreparable. Oxygen is transported to tumors via the blood system, so adequate Hg levels are needed. Without oxygen, the cell survival curve shifts to the right.

- There are two cell survival/dose–response curves, the linear and the linear-quadratic. The linear "curve" is a straight line and this is represented by LDR. LDR is delivered over a protracted period of time and cell kill is by a single electron. The linear quadratic curve demonstrates cell kill caused by two breaks in the DNA from either the same electron or two different electrons. This cell survival curve is straight initially and then curves, representing HDR-type delivery.

- The linear quadratic equation is $-\ln S = \text{alpha}D + \text{beta}D2$. The alpha component is the nonpairable damage, whereas the beta component represents repairable damage. S is the surviving fraction of cells. The dose at which the cell kill is due to equal linear and quadratic components is called the *alpha beta ratio*.

- The BED is used as a guide to determine optimal dosing. The BED = $D[1 + d/(\text{alpha}/\text{beta})]$, where D is the total dose and d is the dose per fraction. Early side effects demonstrate an alpha/beta ratio of 10, whereas late side effects and tumor control assume an alpha/beta of 3.

- The cell can respond to radiation differently depending on its phase in the cell cycle. Late S phase is the most radioresistant phase and M phase is most radiosensitive. There are two possible outcomes after exposure to radiation: survival or death. If the cell survives there is cell-cycle arrest and DNA repair.

- There are three types of cell death. The first is apoptotic, which is ordered programmed cell death. A lot of tumors have mutations in apoptotic pathways and thus do not respond to apoptotic signals easily. The second type of cell death is mitotic. Mitotic death may take days. The third is senescence. Senescence occurs when cell proliferation is irreversibly arrested and death eventually ensues.

The Four Rs of Radiation

- Repair: Radiation in fractionated doses is not as lethal as if it were delivered in one high dose. Sublethal repair occurs when a certain percentage of cells are killed, and those that survive can repair their damage and continue to divide.

- Reassortment: Radiation kills cells best when they are in the late G2 and M phases, which are the most radiosensitive cycles. Other cycles are relatively radioresistant. After a dose of fractional radiation, the cells that were in the more radioresistant phases (and survived) reassort themselves into their next cell cycle. They then become more radiosensitive and when the next dose of radiation is delivered, they have a higher likelihood of death.

- Repopulation occurs when the surviving population of cells that are not lethally damaged divide and replace those that were killed.

- Reoxygenation occurs when the tumor generates new blood vessels to bring in a higher oxygen tension via Hg. Oxygen must be present during radiation to generate the free radical that yields DNA damage. Low oxygen tension makes cells more radioresistant.

Disease-Site Radiation Treatment

Cervical Cancer

Definitive radiation (nonsurgical primary treatment): All stages of cervical cancer can be treated with definitive XRT.

- Anatomical dosing is based on the paracervical triangle—the lateral vaginal fornices and the apex of the anteverted uterus. Dosing is directed at two common points. Point A is 2 cm superior and 2 cm lateral to the external cervical os. This correlates anatomically to where the ureter and the uterine artery cross. Point B is 2 cm superior and 5 cm lateral to the external cervical os. This point corresponds to the obturator LN basins. Point T is inside point A. It is 1 cm superior to the external cervical os and 1 cm lateral to the tandem; it receives a dose 2 to 3 x the dose to point A. Point P is located along the bony pelvic sidewall at its most lateral point and represents the minimal dose to the external iliac LNs. Point C is 1 cm lateral to point B and is approximate to the pelvic sidewall. Point H is an HDR point: It originates from a line that connects the mid-dwell position of the ovoids and intersects with the tandem. It then moves superiorly to the radius of the ovoids (to top of ovoids) + 2 cm, and then 2 cm perpendicularly. The vaginal surface is where the lateral radius of the ovoid and ring applicator falls. This receives a dose 1.4 to 2.0 x the point A dose.

- CT-based planning and conformal blocking is the current standard of care. Definitive dosing for cervical cancer prescribes a total dose to point A of 80 to 90 Gy with 60 Gy dosed to point B.
  - External beam radiation provides 45 to 50.4 Gy to point A via WP-XRT with a 15-Gy boost when appropriate.
  - Brachytherapy: The dose to point A is brought up from 50.4 Gy using external beam radiation to the total desired dose of 80 Gy in small- volume, and 85 to 90 Gy for large-volume tumors, Lower doses of 75-80 Gy can be considered for Stage 1A 1/2 tumors.

- If LDR is used, the brachytherapy dose is 50 to 60 cGy/hr with 40 Gy total given.
- If HDR is used, the dose is 30 Gy. The brachytherapy dose per HDR fraction to point A is 3 to 10.5 Gy. The total number of fractions is two to thirteen The number of fractions per week is one to three. The morbidity is lower for fractions less than 7 Gy. GOG protocols use 6 Gy × five fractions to point A. RTOG protocols allow more variation depending on the external beam radiation dose with brachytherapy fraction sizes of 5.3 to 7.4 Gy using four to seven fractions. Platinum-based chemotherapy should be used in the definitive management of cervical cancer.

  ○ Microscopic nodal disease demands an EBXRT dose of 45 to 50.4 Gy in 1.8 to 2 Gy daily fractions. 10- to 15-Gy boosts can be given to residual disease, bulky adenopathy, or the parametria.

  ○ Parametria: Doses needed to eradicate parametrial disease are recommended at 60 Gy.

  ○ Sequencing of brachytherapy with EBXRT is based on tumor size, patient anatomy, and practitioner discretion. For nonbulky disease, HDR is often integrated after 20 Gy of EBXRT around the second week of treatment. Alternatively, some deliver WP-XRT to 50.4 Gy followed by five HDR insertions.

- Brachytherapy most commonly uses the tandem and ovoid system. There are 48 dwell positions in the tandem. The radiation sources are usually spaced 2.5 to 5 mm apart. The dwell position is where the source is driven to stop. The longest tandem possible should be used. The tandem should be loaded so the sources reach the uterine fundus. This enables adequate distribution to the lower uterine segment, the paracervical tissues, and obturator LNs. The tandems have three curvatures (15°, 30°, and 45°); the greatest curvature is used in cavities measuring greater than 6 cm. A flange is added to the tandem after insertion into the uterine cavity and approximates the exocervix. The keel is then added and prevents rotation of the tandem after packing.

  ○ Vaginal ovoids come in four different sizes. The largest sized ovoid that the patient can tolerate is placed as far laterally and cephalad as possible. This gives the highest tumor dose possible. The mini-sized ovoid is 1.6 cm in diameter, the small is 2 cm in diameter, the medium is 2.5 cm in diameter, and the large is 3 cm in diameter. The mini does not have any shielding to protect the bladder. A wide separation of the ovoids is desired as this increases the dose to the pelvic sidewall. A 10-mg protruding source is recommended if the vaginal ovoids are separated by more than 5 cm. Optimal positioning is seen on the anterior–posterior (AP) view, with tandem midline and unrotated, the tandem is midway between the colpostats, the keel in close proximity to the gold seed marker fiducials placed in the cervical stroma, and the colpostats placed high in the vaginal fornices; on the lateral view, the tandem bisects the colpostat, there is sufficient anterior and posterior packing, and the tandem is equidistant from the sacral promontory and the pubis.

o The anterior bladder point is determined by placement of a Foley catheter with 7 mL of radiopaque material placed into the balloon. The balloon is then pulled down against the urethra, creating this point.

o The posterior rectal point is determined by packing the vagina with radiopaque packing and moving 5 mm posterior to that line.

o The vaginal surface dose should be kept below 140 Gy.

o Types of applicators:

  ▪ Fletcher-Suit and Henschke tandem and ovoids are commonly used. The Delclos applicator uses the mini ovoids. The Henschke applicator uses hemispherical ovoids, and the tandem and ovoids are fixed together. This creates an easier applicator for shallow vaginal fornices.

  ▪ The Fletcher-Suit and Delclos cylinders are used for narrow vaginas, when ovoids are contraindicated. They are also used to treat varying lengths of the vagina mandated by vaginal spread of disease. Cylinders vary in size from 2 to 4 cm in diameter.

  ▪ Ring applicators are an adaptation of the Stockholm technique. There are three sizes: The small is 36 mm, the medium is 40 mm, and the large is 44 mm diameter. It is important not to activate all positions in the ring, as this will increase the dosing to the bladder and rectum. Often, four dwell positions are activated on each side of the smallest ring, five dwell positions on each side of the medium ring, and six dwell positions on each side of the largest ring. Tandems are available in lengths of 2 to 8 cm and the tandem angles are available with 30°, 45°, 60°, and 90°.

  ▪ Interstitial applicators are used if there is a narrow or obliterated vagina, obliterated vaginal fornices, bulky or barrel-shaped cervical tumors, parametrial disease, vaginal disease, or if there is recurrent unresectable disease. This method of radiation delivery uses iridium-loaded stainless steel or plastic needles. There are a few different applicators. One is the MUPIT. Another is the Syed–Neblett template, which has three different templates consisting of 36, 44, or 53 needles. If LDR is used, the dosing is 60 to 80 cGy/hr with a total dose of 23 to 40 Gy over 2 to 4 days. If HDR is used, the dosing is 60% of the total LDR dose given in one to two fractions per day over 2 to 5 days. External beam radiation usually precedes implantation.

- In the postoperative posthysterectomy setting, patients can be broken into two risk categories: (a) those with intermediate-risk factors (LVSI, DOI, and tumor size), per GOG 92 and (b) those with high-risk factors (2+ positive LNs, lesion size >2 cm, margins ≤5 mm, positive margins, or parametrial involvement proven histologically) per GOG 109. WP EBXRT should be considered for those with intermediate-risk factors, and concurrent platinum-based chemotherapy in addition to WP EBXRT for those with high-risk factors. Some centers treat both groups with combination therapy. The adjuvant dose is 45 to 50.4 Gy EBXRT. The fields include the upper 3 cm of vaginal cuff, the parametria, and the internal and external iliac LN basins. If LN metastasis is documented, the upper border of the field should be increased to the next nodal basin or 7 cm higher than the involved LN and bulky LN should be boosted with an additional 10 to 15 Gy.

Uterine Cancer

- Brachytherapy for uterine cancer is commonly used in the adjuvant setting. Fletcher colpostats, or a variety of vaginal cylinders, are used. The upper one half to one third of the vagina is treated after a hysterectomy.

- When using Delclos or Burnett vaginal cylinders, treatment is to the upper 4 to 5 cm of the vagina. The dose distribution conforms to the shape of the cylinder. The dose is specified either at the mucosal surface or to 0.5 cm deep. Studies have shown that 95% of the vaginal lymphatics are located within 3 mm of the vaginal surface. The LDR dose is 80 to 100 cGy/hr to the surface and 50 to 70 cGy/hr if treated to 0.5 cm deep. Treatment to the vagina in the adjuvant setting is usually limited to a total HDR dose of 21 Gy in three doses of 7 Gy to the surface, or 5 Gy in six doses to 0.5 cm deep.

- Bulky stage II or IIIB uterine cancer should be preoperatively treated with XRT. Radiation is dosed at 85 to 90 Gy with 45 to 50.4 delivered by EBXRT and 21 to 30 Gy by brachytherapy.

- Medically inoperable uterine cancer is a rare occurrence. Radiation treatment is with the placement of double or triple intrauterine tandems, or Heyman–Simons capsules in combination with EBXRT. Total dosing follows that for the primary treatment of cervical cancer.

- Residual postoperative vaginal disease less than 0.5 cm may be treated with brachytherapy cylinders or ovoids to 45 or 50.4 Gy. If there is thicker residual vaginal disease, external beam or interstitial XRT is needed.

- Recurrent vaginal disease should be treated with EBXRT followed by brachytherapy. Doses over 80 Gy are usually needed. Recurrent pelvic disease can be treated with EBXRT.

- Indications for treatment in the adjuvant setting are based on stage and patient risk factors:

○ For HIR disease, patients are stratified by age and pathological risk factors to include G2/3, LVSI, or outer 1/2 to 1/3 myometrial involvement.

○ If there is cervical stromal involvement (stage II), a combination of EBXRT and brachytherapy is recommended.

○ For stage IIIA with adnexal metastasis, adjuvant EBXRT alone can give an 85% 5Y survival (YS). For stage IIIB parametrial or pelvic peritoneal disease, EBXRT with brachytherapy with/without chemotherapy can be considered. For stage IIIC, a combination of EBXRT and chemotherapy should be considered. Evidence supports the use of combined modality therapies as adjuvant therapies for patients with extrauterine disease.[14]

○ For early-stage patients with aggressive histology (serous, carcinosarcoma, or CC), XRT in combination with platinum-based chemotherapy has been used. For those with stage I disease, brachytherapy and consideration of chemotherapy are recommended. For those staged II or higher, EBXRT with chemotherapy is recommended.[15] Molecular subtyping is guiding some postoperative adjuvant therapy decisions as well.

Vulvar Cancer
- Indications for treatment are as follows:
  ○ FIGO stage IIIB and greater lesions: pelvic and groin LN basins
  ○ In the neoadjuvant setting in combination with platinum-based chemotherapy for select T2 and advanced T3/T4 lesions: If the patient has clinically negative or resectable groin LNs, pretreatment groin LN dissection can be considered. If all groin LNs are negative, patients can receive XRT to only the primary tumor otherwise primary tumor and groin LN basins are treated.
  ○ Adjuvant primary tumor-bed radiation can be considered if positive margin(s) are present after resection, and it is not feasible to resect further although this has not been shown to increase OS. Patients with close margins of 0.8 mm or less can also be counseled on adjuvant perineal radiation.
- Treatment: Radiation is prescribed to a total dose of 50.4 Gy in 1.8 Gy fractions 5 days/week in the adjuvant setting. Radiosensitizing platinum based chemotherapy is recommended. In select cases, doses can be boosted to 60 to 70 Gy. Brachytherapy can occasionally be prescribed as a boost. A 20-Gy boost to each groin can be delivered.
  ○ For unresectable T3/4 disease, 59.4 to 64.8 Gy in 33 to 36 fractions should be administered .
  ○ Patients should be simulated supine in the frog-leg position with a full bladder and with markers on the clitorus, anus, and urethra.
  ○ Inguinal femoral LN:
    ▪ Clinical/radiographic negative LN: 45–50Gy

- Positive but no extracapsular disease: 50–55Gy
- Positive with gross residual or unresectable disease: 60–70 Gy
  - Pelvic LN volumes should cover the external iliac/obturator, and internal iliac nodal regions with 7 mm of expansion.

Vaginal Cancer

- Treatment is indicated for all FIGO stages and definitively for stage II and higher. Treatment is usually a combination of EBXRT dosed at 45 to 50.4 Gy in 180-cGy fractions daily for 4 to 5 weeks, followed by brachytherapy or interstitial implants with an additional 21 to 30 Gy. Concurrent platinum-based chemotherapy should be considered. Coverage of groin and pelvic LN basins should be considered based on anatomic location of the primary tumor as well as imaging and pathologic (FNA) results.

Ovarian Cancer

- There are minimal uses for XRT for EOC. Isolated local recurrence or residual tumor after completion of chemotherapy are debatable indications.
- Historically, ovarian cancer was treated using the "moving strip" technique.
- For GCTs, radiation has a slightly higher indication. Dysgerminomas are highly radiosensitive and treatment can be considered for primary or recurrent disease.
- Sex cord stromal tumors can also benefit from XRT. This has been studied in recurrent granulosa cell tumors. There are data to support a 43% RR.[16]

Brain Metastasis

- Symptoms: Facial droop, CN II-X deficits, ataxia, arm drift, and expressive aphasia
- Evaluate and confirm with MRI, with and without contrast.
- Treatment: Decadron and WB-XRT for multiple metastases, Decadron and stereotactic radiation for solitary metastasis. Inpatient management is recommended for midline shift, herniation, or hemorrhage. Outpatient management is possible if the patient is compliant with support at home and has none of the preceding contraindications.
- Dosing:
  - WB-XRT: 30 Gy in 10 fractions is considered standard treatment per RTOG-6901 protocol in a palliative fashion.
  - Decadron: Mild symptoms: 4 to 8 mg/day. Moderate to severe symptoms from edema and intracranial pressure: 16 mg/day. Taper over a 2- to 7-week period based on symptom resolution. Side effects can include Cushing's syndrome, candidiasis,

psychiatric disorders, hyperglycemia, and peripheral edema. A common taper dose is 8 mg PO daily BID (based on severity) × 4 days, 4 mg PO BID for 4 days, then 2 mg/day until completion of radiation.

Design of External Beam Radiation Fields

- Four field box: The external beam fields are designed in a four-field box as AP/PA fields plus lateral fields. These are customarily outlined as 15 × 15 cm^2 for the AP/PA fields and 8- to 9-cm wide for the lateral fields. The intent of the four fields is to use narrow lateral beams to avoid some small bowel and a portion of the rectum posteriorly.

- CT or MRI based planning: CT- or MRI-based planning can accurately outline the radiation targets and simultaneously spare vital organs using mobile blocks called *collimators*. A collimator is a device that narrows a beam of particles and multiple collimators are used to vary the radiation fields. Radiation is dosed with a 0.7- to 1-cm expansion around the involved LN, bone, and muscle (CTV) except for the groin LN, where there should be a 2-cm margin. The PTV should have an additional 1-cm margin. In general, the principle of extending node treatment volume one nodal echelon proximal to the level of clinical involvement is a prudent guideline. IMRT is now being used in a significant number of centers to decrease side effects to vital structures. IMRT uses computer-controlled x-ray accelerators to distribute precise radiation doses to malignant tumors or specific areas within the tumor. The pattern of radiation delivery is determined using highly tailored computing applications.

Cervical Cancer
- Cervical cancer fields
  - CT-based planning is considered the standard of care using EBXRT. EBXRT volumes should cover gross disease, parametria, uterosacral ligaments, at least 3 cm of vaginal margin, presacral nodes, and other nodal basins involved or at risk. If negative LN are determined via surgical staging or imaging, the radiation volume should include all of the internal and external iliac, and the obturator LN basins. If bulky or residual tumor is present, or there were positive pelvic LN found at surgical staging, the radiation volume should cover the common iliacs as well, or the nodal basin above the highest involved LN. If common iliac or PA LN involvement is identified, extended-field pelvic and PA-XRT, up to the renal vessels (or even more cephalad), is advised.
  - **Conventional fields:** The superior border for nonbulky stage IB/IIA disease is S1/L5. For bulky or more advanced disease the border is L4/5. There are data to suggest that in 87% of patients the bifurcation of the common iliac vessels was above the L5 prominence.[17] Thus, it may be necessary to extend the upper field

border to L2/3. The inferior border is the mid or lower border of the obturator foramen or 3 to 4 cm below the most distal vaginal component of disease. It is important to cover the inguinal LN if the distal vagina is involved. The lateral borders are 2 to 2.5 cm lateral to the pelvic brim. The anterior border is the pubic symphysis. It may be necessary to extend this coverage to 2 cm anterior to the pubis in order to cover the external iliac arteries. The posterior border is conventionally set posterior to S2/S3. A study found that in stages IB and II, the most common inadequate margin was the posterior border at the S2/3 interface and there was no increase in rectal complications when the entire sacrum was included in the radiation field.[18] Some studies have shown that 79% of patients treated with conventional fields had inadequate coverage. CT-based planning was then able to cover 95% of patients appropriately.

- Midline blocks are used to increase the dose to the parametria or pelvic sidewalls while shielding the bladder, distal ureters, and rectosigmoid colon. Some customize the midline block at the 50% isodose line, which passes through point A. Some feather the block at specific isodose intervals. Most use rectangular blocks 4 to 5 cm in width, as this is the distance between the distal ureters. A margin of 0.5 cm lateral to the lateral ovoid surface is recommended in designing the width of the midline block.

- A parametrial boost of an additional 15 Gy is recommended if there is bulky parametrial disease or pelvic sidewall disease. This is done after completion of WP radiation.

- An LN boost is dosed at 15 Gy to enlarged or known positive LN. Data have shown that 16% of patients with biopsy-proven positive LN, treated with chemotherapy and radiation, have residual disease after 45 Gy even with a 15-Gy boost.[19]

- Extended-field radiation defines coverage of the PALN basins. The superior margin of this field is T12/L1 and the inferior margin is L4/5, laterally the spinous vertebral processes, and 2 cm anterior to the vertebrae.

○ IMRT: The TIME-C trial (RTOG-1203, NCT01672892) is comparing posthysterectomy patients receiving adjuvant XRT to evaluate GI toxicity in IMRT versus standard three-dimensional CT XRT.

Uterine Cancer
- Uterine cancer fields are as follows:
  ○ Conventional anatomic fields are superiorly the L4/5 interface, inferiorly the mid or lower obturator foramen, laterally 2 to 2.5 cm lateral to the pelvic brim, anteriorly the pubic symphysis, and posteriorly S2/3 of the sacrum. EBXRT covers the upper one half to two thirds of the vagina, the parametria, and the pelvic LNs.

Stage II cancers are recommended to have both external beam and brachytherapy.

- ○ CT-guided fields: This is the standard of care currently. XRT should target gross residual disease if present and cover the lower common iliac vessels, the internal and external iliac vessels, the parametia, the upper vagina/paravaginal tissue, the presacral LN (especially if stage II) with extended fields to cover the PALN basins if involved. The upper border of the extended PA fields should at least be to the level of the renal vessels.

- ○ Brachytherapy to the vaginal cuff alone can be given up to 50 Gy. If used in the adjuvant setting, HDR brachytherapy is usually dosed at 21 Gy, consisting of 7 Gy for three fractions to a vaginal depth of 0.5 cm or 6 Gy for five fractions—initiated as soon as the cuff is healed and no more than 12 weeks after surgery.

- External beam dosing: Adjuvant treatment of microscopic extrauterine disease should be 45 to 50.4 Gy with a 15-Gy boost to involved parametria or positive LN basins. Primary XRT for bulky stage II disease or definitive therapy in nonoperative candidates should total 75 to 80 Gy with combined EBXRT and brachytherapy.

- To decrease vital organ complications, the patient can be treated in the prone position with a full bladder or with use of a belly board.

Vulvar Cancer
- Vulvar cancer fields:
  - ○ Conventional fields: The superior field is no lower than the sacroiliac (SI) joints or higher than the L4/5 junction unless pelvic LN are involved; if so, the upper border should be raised to 5 cm above the most cephalad positive LN. The superior border should extend as a horizontal line at the level of the ASIS. The lateral border extends in a line connecting the femoral head and the ASIS with an additional 2-cm lateral margin. The medial border is 3 cm from the body's midline. The inferiolateral inguinal nodal border is parallel to the inguinal crease and inferior enough to encompass the inguinofemoral nodal bed to the intertrochanteric line of the femur, or 1.5 to 2 cm distal to the saphenofemoral junction. The inferior vulvar border should be inferiorly 2.5 cm below the ischial tuberosity or 2 cm below the most inferior portion of the primary vulvar tumor. A narrow posterior field is used with 15 to 18 MV and a wide anterior field is used with 6 MV and an additional 12 MV dose is prescribed to each groin. If the patient is thin and the depth of the inguinal vessels is less than 3 cm, an electron patch may be used. There is an 11% rate of femoral neck fracture or necrosis with these doses.

○ CT-based planning:
  ▪ Vulvar field: This is any gross vulvar disease plus any visible or palpable extension to the vagina. Bolus dosing should be used to adequately cover the superficial target volume.
  ▪ Groin field: This is, laterally, the inguinofemoral vessels to the sartorius and rectus femoris muscles medially, posteriorly to the vastus medialis muscle, and the pectineus muscle medially (or 3 cm medial to the vessels). The volume should be trimmed by 3 mm if there is no anterior skin involvement. The caudal extent is the top of the lesser trochanter of the femur and the anterior border is the sartorius muscle.
  ▪ The pelvic nodal: This includes the bilateral external iliac, obturator, and internal iliac nodal basins with 7 mm of symmetrical expansion, excluding bone and muscle. If pelvic nodes are involved, the upper border can be raised to 5 cm above the most cephalad positive node.
• Dosing: Doses are commonly 50.4 Gy in 1.8 Gy fractions daily. For unresectable disease, doses can be given to 59.4 to 64.8 Gy in 1.8 Gy fractions with a boost to 70 Gy if indicated.

Vaginal Cancer
The fields are similar to that of cervical cancer: These are, superiorly, the L5–S1 interface; inferiorly, to 2 cm below the lesion, and then 2 cm lateral to the pelvic brim. For lesions that include the lower one third of the vagina, the groins should be included. The lateral field margins should extend in a line connecting the femoral heads and the ASIS to include the inguinal nodes.

Ovarian Cancer
The fields are that of site-directed radiation or Whole abdomen radiation (WAR).

Whole Abdomen Radiation
WAR is not commonly given as adjuvant therapy. It can be given for salvage treatment. The total dose is 30 Gy in fraction sizes of 1.5 to 1.7 Gy/day. The field margins are 1 to 2 cm above the diaphragm superiorly (with heart shielding), 1 to 2 cm lateral to the peritoneal reflection, and inferiorly 2 cm below the inguinal ligament. Usually, WP-XRT follows with a dose of 45 to 50 Gy. The kidneys should be blocked at 15 Gy and the liver blocked at 25 Gy.

Radiation Effects
• The definition of an *early complication* is occurrence less than 3 months after completion of XRT. A *late complication* is defined as onset after 3 months. Late effects are usually due to capillary damage (endarteritis obliterans).

- **Skin toxicity** is usually delayed for 2 to 3 weeks. Most patients get moist desquamation about 2 weeks into treatment. There can also be erythema. Dry desquamation can occur after the fourth week. Toxicity is enhanced by actinomycin D and doxorubicin. Treatment is sitz baths, diarrhea control, calendula lotion, or Aquaphor cream, as well as sulfa-based barrier creams. The epidermis returns in 14 days. Late effects can be depigmentation and telangiectasias.

- **Vaginal toxicity** can be manifested with a yellow-white discharge due to mucositis. This can continue for 6 months. Treatment is with hydrogen peroxide douches, antibiotics, or hyperbaric therapy. Remember to rule out radiation necrosis and possible fistula—these complications may require a flap or even exenteration. The distal vagina is less tolerant, with a maximum dose of 80 to 90 Gy versus a maximum dose of 120 to 150 Gy for the proximal vagina. Narrowing and shortening of the vagina is a late effect and can occur in 80% of patients. Symptom is pain. Diagnosis is with examination. Treatment is with frequent intercourse, vaginal dilators, and estrogen cream. Neovaginal reconstruction is complicated with high rates of failure and potential fistula.

- **Urinary tract toxicity** can present with frequency, urgency, and dysuria from decreased bladder capacity. Pyridium may help.
  - Spasms can be relieved by smooth-muscle relaxants such as B&O suppositories or urospas. Always rule out infection. The UA can show radiation cystitis with WBC and RBC present, but without bacteria. Focal ulcerations, hyperemia, and edema occur at greater than 30 Gy. Above 60 Gy hematuria occurs due to telangiectasias.
  - Hemorrhagic cystitis occurs in 1% to 5%. Treatment is with continuous irrigation with normal saline, cautery ablation via cystoscopy, methylene blue instillation, formalin instillation, alum 2% instillation, hyperbaric oxygen, or Elmiron. Surgical diversion with a conduit is a last resort.
  - Ureteral stricture occurs at a rate of 2.5% at 20 Y. A unilateral stricture is more common. Symptoms include pain or an increasing BUN/creatinine level. Diagnosis is via laboratories, IVP, or CT imaging. Treatment is with stenting, dilation, or surgical resection and reanastomosis.

- **Fistula formation** can occur from the GI or urinary systems. Symptoms are spontaneous stool or urinary loss from an improper orifice. Diagnosis is with a full clinical examination, EUA with biopsies if necessary. A fistulogram, CT, MRI, or PET scan may be helpful.
  - Conservative management of bowel fistula is with NPO status, TPN, somatostatin 50 to 200 mcg SC TID, H2 blockers, Questran,

and tincture of opium BID (conservative management is rarely efficacious). Surgical intervention is with colostomy, repair, and excision of the fistulous tract.

○ Treatment of urinary fistula requires diagnosis of the location of the fistula, diversion with a Foley catheter or nephrostomy tube, and resection of the fistula and tract. A neobladder can be constructed as a last resort.

- **Bowel toxicity** is primarily diarrhea, which is due to shortened villi and loss of their absorptive function. The dose tolerance of the small bowel is 45 Gy, the large bowel is 70 to 75 Gy, and the anus is 60 to 65 Gy.

○ Acute radiation enteritis is demonstrated by watery diarrhea, which starts during the second or third week of treatment at about 20 Gy. There is increased flatulence and noisy bowel sounds. Treatment is with a low-residue diet, hydration, and antimotility agents. Somatostatin and bowel rest may be indicated. Chronic diarrhea is managed with dietary changes.

○ Small-bowel injury can occur as stricture or stenosis. It can present as a PSBO or a complete SBO. These occur in 5% of patients, with the terminal ileum and cecum being the most common site because they are anatomically fixed. Symptoms of a partial obstruction are delayed postprandial cramping, nausea, vomiting, and diarrhea. Diagnosis is with clinical examination or imaging with UGI and SBFT, or a CT scan. Treatment is with bowel resection and reanastomosis.

○ Malabsorption can occur from excess bile salts reaching the colon. These are cathartics, so treatment with cholestyramine may help.

○ Rectosigmoid toxicity can be symptomatic with a stricture causing a partial or complete LBO. Diverting colostomy may be a treatment of last resort.

○ Rectal toxicity can present with tenesmus, mucus production, pain, worsening of hemorrhoids, and proctitis. It occurs in 2% to 3% of patients. Treatment is with antispasmodics or steroid suppositories or enemas. Telangiectasia's can cause bleeding and ulceration. Treatment of these is with cortisone rectal suppositories, sulfasalazine enemas, mesalamine (Rowasa) suppositories BID for 6 weeks, and hyperbaric oxygen.

○ Gastric outlet obstruction can occur from progressive fibrosis and can even lead to perforation.

- **Ovarian failure** occurs between 2.5 and 6 Gy for the germ cell components, presenting as permanent sterility. The stromal support cells fail at 24 Gy. Attempts to prevent ovarian failure are occasionally successful. Options include midline oophoropexy (surgical placement behind the uterus), surgical transposition to the upper pelvis (with a 40%–71% rate of success), cortical stripping and cryopreservation, oocyte retrieval with cryopreservation, or in vitro fertilization and embryo cryopreservation.

- **Bone marrow toxicity** can present as follows:
  - ○ Pancytopenia. This occurs because 40% of the marrow is in the pelvis. Symptoms can include fatigue (anemia), increased susceptibility to infections (leukopenia), and bruising or bleeding (thrombocytopenia). Patients need weekly monitoring of the CBC.
  - ○ Insufficiency fractures can also occur. The tolerance for the femoral head is 45 Gy. Fractures most commonly occur in the sacrum, ileum, pubic bones, and acetabulum. Asymptomatic fractures occur at a rate of 34% to 39% and symptomatic fractures at a rate of 13%. Symptoms are the sudden onset of pain, which worsens with weight bearing. MRI is the best means for diagnosis. Treatment is surgical stabilization.
  - ○ The femoral neck can develop avascular necrosis. Treatment for this is hip replacement.
- **Liver toxicity** can present as follows:
  - ○ Veno-occlusive disease. This is due to platelet coagulation causing congestion and thrombocytopenia.
  - ○ Radiation hepatitis may occur and present with an elevated alkaline phosphatase 3 to 10 x normal. Small portions of the liver can receive up to 70 Gy. The whole liver should not receive more than 30 Gy.
- **Renal toxicity** usually manifests as a nephrotic syndrome. Toxicities present as HTN, leg edema, proteinuria, or a normocytic normochromic anemia. The kidney should not receive more than 18 to 20 Gy. To avoid toxicity, preferentially load 70/30 AP/PA and block the kidneys completely after 18 to 20 Gy.
- **Fetal toxicity:** In utero exposure of the fetus invariably occurs during the diagnosis and treatment of gynecologic malignancies in pregnancy. If treatment occurs at 1 to 2 weeks of pregnancy, the effect is all or nothing with spontaneous abortion, or continuation of pregnancy without effect. At 2 to 6 weeks, congenital anomalies and death can occur, with a 2-Gy dose yielding 70% mortality. At 6 to 16 weeks, growth retardation and intellectual disability occur with a risk of 40% per Gy. After 30 weeks, no gross malformations tend to occur. The risk of leukemia is increased if exposure is in the third trimester. The risk is about 6% per Gy. A dose less than 1 mGy is negligible. For the entire gestational period, there should be no more than 0.5 cGy exposure (Table 5.2).

Cervical Cancer and XRT Delivery Time

The prolongation of overall treatment time and timing of brachytherapy can impact the outcome of XRT. See Tables 5.3 and 5.4 for pelvic recurrence rate and survival by treatment time. Tables 5.3 and 5.4

Table 5.2 Radiation Tolerance of Organs

Organ	TD50 (Gy)
Bone marrow	5
Ovary	10
Kidney	25
Lung	30
Liver	50
Heart	60
Intestine	62
Spinal cord	60
Brain	65
Bladder	65

Table 5.3 Cervical Cancer Recurrence Rate Stratified by Radiation Treatment Duration

Stage	<7 weeks (%)	7–9 weeks (%)	>9 weeks (%)	p-Values
IB	7	22	6	$p < .01$
IIA	14	27	36	$p = .08$
IIB	20	28	34	$p = .09$
III	38	44	49	$p = .18$
III when point A dose >80 Gy	32	40	51	$p = .08$

Table 5.4 10Y Cause-Specific Survival by Treatment Time

Stage	<7 weeks (%)	7–9 weeks (%)	>9 weeks (%)	p-Value
IB	86	78	55	$p = .01$
IIA	73	41	48	$p = .01$
IIB	72	60	70	$p = .01$
III	42	42	39	$p = .43$
III (patient A dose >80 Gy)	46	44	37	$p = .016$

REFERENCES

1 Vay A, Kumar S, Seward S, et al. Therapy-related myeloid leukemia after treatment for epithelial ovarian carcinoma: an epidemiological analysis. *Gynecol Oncol.* 2011;123(3):456–460. doi: 10.1016/j.ygyno.2011.07.097

2 Hobohm U. Fever and cancer in perspective. *Cancer Immunol Immunother.* 2001;50(8):391–396. doi: 10.1007/s002620100216

3 Hurvitz SA, Park YH, Bardia A, et al. LBA14 neoadjuvant giredestrant (GDC-9545) + palbociclib (palbo) vs anastrozole (A) + palbo in post-menopausal women with oestrogen receptor-positive, HER2-negative, untreated early breast cancer (ER+/HER2– ebc): interim analysis of the randomised, open-label, phase ii coopera BC study. *Ann Oncol.* 2021;32:S1285–S1286. doi: 10.1016/j.annonc.2021.08.2086

4 Siena S, Sartore-Bianchi A, Di Nicolantonio F, et al. Biomarkers predicting clinical outcome of epidermal growth factor receptor-targeted therapy in metastatic colorectal cancer. *J Natl Cancer Inst.* 2009;101(19):1308–1324. doi: 10.1093/jnci/djp280

5 Monk BJ, Poveda A, Vergote I, et al. Anti-angiopoietin therapy with trebananib for recurrent ovarian cancer (TRINOVA-1): a randomised, multicentre, double-blind, placebo-controlled phase 3 trial. *Lancet Oncol.* 2014;15(8):S1470-2045(14)70244-X):799–808:. doi: 10.1016/S1470-2045(14)70244-X

6 Matei D, Sill MW, Lankes HA, et al. Activity of sorafenib in recurrent ovarian cancer and primary peritoneal carcinomatosis: a gynecologic oncology group trial. *J Clin Oncol.* 2011;29(1):69–75. doi: 10.1200/JCO.2009.26.7856

7 Coleman RL, Moon J, Sood AK, et al. Randomised phase II study of docetaxel plus vandetanib versus docetaxel followed by vandetanib in patients with persistent or recurrent epithelial ovarian, fallopian tube or primary peritoneal carcinoma: SWOG S0904. *Eur J Cancer.* 2014;50(9):S0959-8049(14)00248-2):1638–1648:. doi: 10.1016/j.ejca.2014.03.005

8 Stevanović S, Draper LM, Langhan MM, et al. Complete regression of metastatic cervical cancer after treatment with human papillomavirus-targeted tumor-infiltrating T cells. *J Clin Oncol.* 2015;33(14):1543–1550. doi: 10.1200/JCO.2014.58.9093

9 Postow MA, Callahan MK, Wolchok JD, et al. Immune checkpoint blockade in cancer therapy. *J Clin Oncol.* 2015;33(17):1974–1982. doi: 10.1200/JCO.2014.59.4358

10 O'Malley DM, Randall LM, Jackson CG, et al. RaPiDS (GOG-3028): randomized phase II study of balstilimab alone or in combination with zalifrelimab in cervical cancer. *Future Oncology.* 2021;17(26):3433–3443. doi: 10.2217/fon-2021-0529. https://www.futuremedicine.com/doi/10.2217/fon-2021-0529

11 Berek J, Taylor P, McGuire W, et al. Oregovomab maintenance monoimmunotherapy does not improve outcomes in advanced ovarian cancer. *J Clin Oncol.* 2009;27(3):418–425. doi: 10.1200/JCO.2008.17.8400

12 Sabbatini P, Harter P, Scambia G, et al. Abagovomab as maintenance therapy in patients with epithelial ovarian cancer: a phase iii trial of the AGO OVAR, COGI, GINECO, and geico--the MIMOSA study. *J Clin Oncol.* 2013;31(12):1554–1561. doi: 10.1200/JCO.2012.46.4057

13 Taplitz RA, Kennedy EB, Bow EJ, et al. Outpatient management of fever and neutropenia in adults treated for malignancy: American society of clinical oncology and infectious diseases society of America clinical practice guideline update. *J Clin Oncol.* 2018;36(14):1443–1453. doi: 10.1200/JCO.2017.77.6211

14 Klopp A, Smith BD, Alektiar K, et al. The role of postoperative radiation therapy for endometrial cancer: executive summary of an American society for radiation oncology evidence-based guideline. *Pract Radiat Oncol.* 2014;4(3):S1879-8500(14)00005-8):137–144:. doi: 10.1016/j.prro.2014.01.003

15 Kelly MG, O'malley DM, Hui P, et al. Improved survival in surgical stage I patients with Uterine Papillary Serous Carcinoma (UPSC) treated with adjuvant platinum-based chemotherapy. *Gynecol Oncol.* 2005;98(3):353–359. doi: 10.1016/j.ygyno.2005.06.012

16 Wolf JK, Mullen J, Eifel PJ, et al. Radiation treatment of advanced or recurrent granulosa cell tumor of the ovary. *Gynecol Oncol.* 1999;73(1):35–41. doi: 10.1006/gyno.1998.5287

17 Greer BE, Koh WJ, Figge DC, et al. Gynecologic radiotherapy fields defined by intraoperative measurements. *Gynecol Oncol.* 1990;38(3):421–424. doi: 10.1016/0090-8258(90)90084-x

18 Greer BE, Koh WJ, Stelzer KJ, et al. Expanded pelvic radiotherapy fields for treatment of local-regionally advanced carcinoma of the cervix: outcome and complications. *Am J Obstet Gynecol.* 1996;174(4):1141–1149. doi: 10.1016/s0002-9378(96)70656-7

19 Houvenaeghel G, Lelievre L, Rigouard A-L, et al. Residual pelvic lymph node involvement after concomitant chemoradiation for locally advanced cervical cancer. *Gynecol Oncol.* 2006;102(1):74–79. doi: 10.1016/j.ygyno.2005.11.037

6 Reproductive Function, Sexuality, and Pregnancy With Gynecologic Cancer

SEXUAL FUNCTION, FERTILITY, AND CANCER

Sexual Dysfunction

Sexual dysfunction is common in patients who are undergoing diagnosis of and treatment for gynecologic malignancies. This is due to pain, discomfort, bleeding, and/or psychological stress that may make intimacy difficult. Sexual disorders are typically not screened for effectively, thereby masking the problem. Even for patients in whom sexual dysfunction is identified, there is little support to manage the problem. Comprehensive screening questionnaires have been validated as effective screening tools for different sexual disorders.[1] Sexual disorders can be classified into four types: desire disorder, arousal disorder, orgasm disorder, and pain disorder.

- Pretreatment workup:
  - Evaluate patient for category of sexual disorder.
  - Discuss concerns related to specific cancer therapies, for example, surgical pain or altered anatomy, radiation-induced vaginal stenosis, menopausal symptoms related to surgery, radiation, or or chemotherapy.
  - Consider evaluation with the FSFI or the PROMIS Sexual Function Instrument.
  - Perform a physical exam: Note points of tenderness, vaginal atrophy, and anatomic changes associated with cancer surgeries or treatments. It is important to biopsy any suspicious lesions.
- Management: Guide treatment based on type of sexual disorder:
  - **Desire**
    - Chronic medical conditions, such as HTN, diabetes, anxiety, and depression can have a negative impact on desire and should be addressed.

- Surgical disfigurement may also be a factor in desire. For women with ostomies, the four-P's approach has been applied: prepare (adjust diet in preparation for intimacy to reduce GI problems), pouch (pouch covers are available in multiple different fabrics, including lace or silk), position (avoid positions that cause pressure on ostomy to prevent compression or spillage), and pleasure (communicate with the partner that the goal is pleasurable intimacy).[2]

- **Arousal and orgasm:** Treatment-induced menopause and altered gonadal function from XRT or chemotherapy are among factors that may contribute to a loss of arousal. In most hormonally sensitive cancers, systemic estrogen therapy has generally been contraindicated. However, for lower risk patients, topical estrogens have been found to be effective and relatively safe for the treatment of vaginal symptoms after menopause. Other nonhormonal therapies include vaginal moisturizers and lubricants. With regard to arousal, the prescription device Eros-CVD can be used to create gentle suction over the clitoris and has been proven beneficial in women with female arousal disorders, including those who have undergone treatment for cancer.

- **Pain:** Patients can experience pain during intercourse from vaginal foreshortening either due to surgery or XRT, or dryness from menopause or use of AIs. Patients may benefit from:

  - Along with the use of lubricants and possibly estrogen products, vaginal dilators can be used to lengthen and dilate the vagina.

  - One method to minimize dyspareunia may be positional changes.

  - Lidocaine 2% topical jelly applied to the vulva or vagina may reduce vulvodynia and dyspareunia.

  - Antidepressants and neuromodulators (gabapentin) can mitigate some pain symptoms, but caution should be used as they may also cause some arousal disorders.

  - Consider ospemifene for dyspareunia if the primary cancer was a nonhormone sensitive cancer.

- Encourage partner communication: Consider psychotherapy or sexual/couples counseling.

Pelvic Floor Dysfunction and Incontinence

In one review, the prevalence of any type of urinary incontinence (UI) in OC patients before treatment was about 50%, with 17% reporting vaginal bulging.[3] These approximated the rates for women without cancer. Posttreatment UI scores were not significantly different. Fecal incontinence was reported to affect 4% of patients preoperatively and 16% postoperatively. Fifty percent of women were sexually active after surgical treatment and reported high rates of dyspareunia (40%–80%) and vaginal dryness (60%–80%). Pelvic floor dysfunction (PFD) is common in women after OC management and rates are not different than the general population. There is a higher prevalence of UI and sexual dysfunction compared with bowel dysfunction.

- Brief sexual symptom checklist for women:
  - Are you satisfied with your sexual function?
  - How long have you been dissatisfied?
  - The problem(s) with your sexual function is:
    - Little or no interest in sex
    - Decreased genital sensation
    - Decreased vaginal lubrication
    - Difficulty obtaining orgasm
    - Pain during sex
    - Other
  - Which problem is the most bothersome?
  - Would you like to discuss it with your physician?

Ovarian Protection During Chemotherapy

Ovarian protection during chemotherapy has been investigated. Primary outcomes are resumption of menstruation and prevention of chemotherapy-induced ovarian failure, with pregnancy as a secondary outcome, if desired. Ovarian reserve is assessed by drawing FSH and AMH laboratories. Gonadal suppression with GnRH agonist treatment has not been shown to significantly protect ovarian function or affect resumption of menses after completion of chemotherapy; no protective effect was seen based on age, type of chemotherapy, type of malignancy, or GnRH analog type. There was no evidence that gonadal suppression protected any ovarian reserve parameters, including FSH, antral follicle count, or AMH levels.[4]

Fertility Preservation

- It is important to discuss the risk of infertility and fertility preservation options in patients anticipating cancer treatment as early as possible, before treatment starts. Document the discussion in the medical record (Table 6.1).
- At diagnosis, a baseline laboratory check for ovarian reserve should be assessed with FSH, LH, AMH, inhibin B levels, and US assessment of antral follicle counts.
- Refer those patients who express an interest, or are ambivalent about fertility preservation, to reproductive specialists.
  - Present both embryo and oocyte cryopreservation.
  - Discuss ovarian transposition if WP-XRT.

Table 6.1 Chemotherapeutic Drugs and Risk of Infertility

Definite	Chlorambucil
	Cyclophosphamide
	L-Phenylalanine mustard
	Nitrogen mustard
	Busulfan
	Procarbazine
Probable	Doxorubicin
	Vinblastine
	Cytosine arabinoside
	Cisplatin
	Nitrosoureas
	Amsacrine
	Etoposide
Unlikely	MTX
	Fluorouracil
	Mercaptopurine
	Vincristine
Unknown	Bleomycin

- Surgical manipulation/transposition of the ovaries should be performed close to the initiation of XRT due to potential remigration of the ovaries to the pelvis.
- Inform patients there are insufficient data on GnRH analogs as a fertility preservation method.
- Inform patients of conservative surgical options:
  - Radical trachelectomy is used for cervical cancer patients with 1A2 to 1B1 tumors less than 2 cm in diameter, negative frozen section ECC, non–high-risk histology, and variably with invasion less than 1 cm. The ConCerv trial showed a 3.5% recurrence rate and a 5% rate of positive LN in women with 2009 stage 1A2-1B1 who underwent conization or simple hysterectomy with sentinel or complete LND. Data on more conservative simple trachelectomy with P/PA-LND is pending (SHAPE trial).
  - Ovarian cystectomy can be considered for early ovarian cancers/LMP tumors—albeit with a higher risk of recurrence.
  - Completion hysterectomy BSO can also be considered after completion of childbearing for early-staged ovarian cancers, medically treated stage I uterine cancers, and stage 1A1 cervical cancers treated with conization.

- For children: Use established methods of fertility preservation (oocyte cryopreservation) for postpubertal minor children, with patient assent, if appropriate, and parent or guardian consent.

- Ovarian tissue cryopreservation and transplantation: Harvesting of oocytes can be rapidly stimulated and is cycle-day independent now. Ovarian stimulation protocols using aromatase inhibitors may reduce the concern for stimulation of ER-positive cancers (gynecologic and breast).

- Pregenetic screening: If a patient is known positive for a pathogenic then embryo screening can be recommended.

- In patients of reproductive age with intact reproductive organs, birth control should be administered due to the high risk of teratogenicity from cytotoxic chemotherapeutics as well as biologics.[5]

- Cervical cancer exclusive of neuroendocrine and adenoma malignum:
  - Stage IA1:
    - LVSI absent: CKC (preferably) or LEEP with 3-mm negative margins is adequate therapy. If margins on the CKC are positive, repeat CKC should be performed. Consideration of simple trachelectomy if fertility is desired is another option. Recurrence rates are less than 0.5% and 5YS is comparable to hysterectomy rates at 99%.
    - LVSI present: Cone biopsy with negative 3-mm margins with a P-LND and consideration of PA-LND can be performed. SLND is also a possibility. A radical trachelectomy with P-LND can also be considered. Recurrence rates can increase to 9% if LVSI is present.
  - Stage IA2:
    - Radical trachelectomy and P-LND with/without PA-LND
    - Consideration of CKC/LEEP with negative 3 mm margins; if positive margins: repeat CKC or simple trachelectomy with P-LND with/without PA-LND or
  - Stage IB1: A radical trachelectomy with P-LND with/without PA-LND can be considered. The standard maximum tumor size is <2 cm. This should not be offered to those with high-risk pathology. Some studies have shown outcomes in patients with larger tumor sizes, but the risk of needing adjuvant therapies was 64% and subsequent infertility follows.
    - For stage 1A2–IB2, a 94% 5Y DFS and 97% OS was seen in CKC with laparoscopic PLND approaches. Better pregnancy outcomes were reported by Cao et al with a vaginal approach at 39.5 versus 9.8%, but the recurrence rate was higher in the vaginal approach group. For tumor sizes >2cm, NACT, followed

by radical abdominal trachelectomy, has been proposed but with a much higher rate of recurrence: ducumented at 17%.

- For those in need of pelvic radiation: ovarian transposition, uterus-sparing XRT, and at times, uterine transposition remote from the radiation field has been performed. A laparoscopic approach noted an 88.6% success rate for ovarian transposition and preservation of ovarian function.

- Uterine cancer Stage 1
  - Consideration of hysteroscopic resection (minimal outcome data available) of the tumor has been proposed. Patients with G 1 disease without LVSI and MRI imaging demonstrating no MI are candidates. This should be followed by PO or IUD progestin hormonal therapy.

  - Hormonal therapy alone or in combination with hysteroscopic resection: PO high-dose progestins (megestrol acetate 320 mg/day or MPA 600 mg divided doses daily) or a high-dose IUD for 3 to 6 months have been used (or combination PO Megace at 160 mg QD and high dose IUDO). Repeat endometrial sampling should occur at 3 to 6 months. If regression is demonstrated, the patient can attempt conception. If persistence or progression is demonstrated at 6-12 months, a hysterectomy with staging as appropriate should be recommended.

  - Ovarian preservation with egg retrieval and in vitro fertilizaton followed by embryo transfer to a gestational carrier can be offered to those wanting biological children. Ovarian preservation alone for prevention of early-onset menopause is also documented. Some literature now documents the safety of ovarian preservation at the time of staging a hysterectomy. Counseling is recommended if ovarian preservation is considered. Early age of onset of uterine cancer can signal a genetic syndrome (HNPCC, which has a 10% chance of ovarian cancer) and other studies have documented a 25% rate of adnexal pathology in younger patients. Without a BSO, comprehensive surgical staging is not complete and there is always the risk of undiagnosed adnexal pathology. Consider salpingectomy if ovarian preservation is performed. CV risk factors can be modifiable, whereas cancer cannot. Consider hyperstimulation and egg retrieval with cryopreservation and a gestational surrogate if fertility is desired.
    - Uterine transplantation can be discussed although this has mainly been offered to patients with congenital reproductive tract anomalies and is still "investigational," having been performed at one or two selected academic centers via study protocols.

- Ovarian cancer: Consider hyperstimulation and egg retrieval with cryopreservation of the unaffected ovary.

- ○ Early-stage (IA–IB disease) invasive epithelial, borderline, germ cell, sex cord, or stromal tumors:
    - Consider ovarian cystectomy or USO with staging to include LND, staging biopsies, omental biopsy.
    - For LMP tumors with both ovaries involved yet complete resection is deemed obtainable, an ovarian cystectomy can be considered. LMPs that were early stage had a fatal recurrence rate of 0.5% and a spontaneous pregnancy rate of 54%. In advanced stage LMPs, the spontaneous pregnancy rate was 34% with a fatal recurrence rate of 2%.
    - For invasive EOC stage IA–IB, USO with comprehensive staging, including LND, has been shown to be safe. But for G 3 and stages IC: long-term outcomes and safety are not apparent.[6]
    - If the patient was initially unstaged:
        - □ Low-risk GCT: Observe and treat upon identification of recurrence.
        - □ For epithelial, high-risk germ cell, sex cord, or stromal tumors: Consider staging surgery followed by recommended adjuvant therapies.
  - ○ Advanced stage: Perform surgical debulking in additon to recommended adjuvant therapies.
- Controlled ovarian hyperstimulation for egg retrieval prior to chemo/radiotoxic treatment or surgical removal has evolved to include a random start (rather than traditional follicular-phase start). Letrozole use with embryo freezing in endometrial and breast cancer patients avoids the estrogenic drive for ovarian stimulation, which may adversely affect oncologic outcomes in estrogen-sensitive tumors. Ovarian tissue cryopreservation with autotransplantation can also be considered if there is no time for controlled ovarian hyperstimulation.

XRT and Fertility
- The ovaries are the most radiosensitive organs, with only 5 to 15 Gy of XRT causing sterility.
- Age does play a role in the risk of infertility with XRT. The older a woman is when receiving XRT to the ovaries, the higher her risk of ovarian failure.
- Operative procedures performed to protect the ovaries from XRT include midline oophoropexy (moving the ovaries behind the uterus) or transposition above the pelvic brim.
- Other efforts used to protect the ovaries from XRT damage are pelvic shielding/uterus sparing XRT.

- Cortical stripping with cryopreservation, oocyte retrieval with cryo-preservation, in vitro fertilization with embryo cryopreservation, or oophorectomy with cryopreservation and subsequent reimplanta-tion of ovarian tissue are all additional strategies used for fertility preservation.

Notable Studies
EIN and Endometrioid Cancer: In this study, 4,007 women aged ≤45 Y diagnosed with endometrial cancer or EIN were reviewed between 2000-2014. Pregnancy events were identified.[7] Of patients, 76.9% (*n* = 3,189) received standard surgical management with hysterec-tomy. Of 818 patients initially treated with progestins, 397 (48.5%) subsequently underwent hysterectomy, and 421 (51.5%) did not. Patients who received progestin therapy were younger than those who had hysterectomy (median age, 36 vs. 41 Y; p <.001). Those who were diagnosed with EIN had an association of a greater likelihood to receive progestin therapy (*p* <.0001). For the 421 patients who received progestin therapy alone, 92 patients (21.8%; 92/421) had 131 pregnancies of which 49 resulted in live births (live birth rate, 11.6%). For the 397 patients treated with progestin therapy followed by hysterectomy, 25 patients (6.3%; 25/397) had 34 pregnancies with 13 live births before hysterectomy. The median age of patients who experienced a live birth following diagnosis during the study period was 36 Y. Among patients who experienced any pregnancy event, 54% of patients used some form of fertility treatment. Median time from diagnosis to live birth was 756 days. Those who were treated with progestins were more likely to experience a live birth if they employed assisted fertility services (OR, 5.9; 95% CI: 3.4–10.1; p <.0001).

- Molecular subtype influences response to fertility sparing treat-ment in uterine cancer.[8] Fifty-seven EMB specimens obtained before hormone therapy were evaluated, and patients were classi-fied according to the PRoMisE molecular subtypes (MSI [microsat-ellite instability], POLE [polymerase ε], NSM/WT-p53, and abnormal p53). The primary endpoint was the RR after hormone therapy. The CRR was 75.4% after hormone therapy overall. Patients with MSI had a significantly lower CRR or PRR than wtp53 (44.4% [95% CI: 4.0–85.0] vs. 82.2% [95% CI: 71.0–94.0]; p = .018) and 6-month CRR (11.1% [95% CI: 0.2–37.0] vs, 53.3% [95% CI: 38.0–68.0]; *p* =.010). For patients who are MSI, four underwent immediate hysterec-tomy because of treatment failure and three received an upstaged diagnosis after hysterectomy. Thus, the PRoMisE molecular classi-fication has prognostic significance in the fertility-sparing manage-ment of endometrial cancer.

CANCER IN PREGNANCY

- Cancer occurs in one woman per every 1,000 live births, with approximately 4,000 cases of concurrent pregnancy and maternal malignancy each year. The most common cancer in pregnancy is breast cancer. The most common cancer of the female reproductive system in pregnancy is cervical cancer.
- If cancer is diagnosed prior to 22 to 24 weeks' gestation, the patient can decide to terminate the pregnancy (legalities dependent on state laws).
- If a malignancy is diagnosed after fetal viability, treatment can be delayed until the late second trimester, third trimester, or after delivery, depending on the specific clinical situation.

XRT in Pregnancy

- XRT has different effects on a fetus depending on the stage of fetal development at the time of radiation exposure.
- At preimplantation, the effects are "all or nothing," meaning that XRT will either kill the embryo or not affect it at all, although there are recent reports of increased rates of fetal malformations with XRT prior to implantation.
- Organogenesis occurs 8 weeks after fertilization. The main fetal effect of XRT during organogenesis is IUGR, but a wide array of congenital structural deformities can occur. With doses of greater than 1 Gy, morphologic anomalies and intellectual delay may develop.
- The main effect of XRT in the fetal stage is resultant cognitive impairment. The CNS is the most sensitive until about 25 weeks. IUGR can also occur with doses greater than 0.5 Gy.
- The recommended maximum dose of XRT during pregnancy is 0.5 Gy (Table 6.2). The threshold for fetal damage is 100mGy.
- There are three principal sources of XRT exposure to the fetus during maternal XRT: photon leakage through the treatment head of the machine, scatter XRT emanating from the imaging equipment, and internal scatter within the mother from the treatment beams. Fetal XRT exposure can be reduced by external shielding, but internal scatter cannot be modified.
  - Imaging modalities:
    - X-rays with abdominal shielding are allowed yielding minimal radiation exposure to the fetus of <0.1mGy.
    - CT is not recommended but can be performed when necessary with IV iodinated contrast.
    - MRI without contrast is determined to be safe in pregnancy and the benefit is enhanced visualization of deep soft tissue structures without ionizing radiation. MRI using gadolinium is

Table 6.2 Fetal Radiation Dose per Radiologic Exam Type

Type of Examination	Fetal Dose Range in cGy
CXR	0.00006
KUB	0.15–0.26
Lumbar spine	0.65
Pelvis	0.2–0.35
Hip	0.13–0.2
IVP	0.47–0.82
Upper GI series	0.17–0.48
Barium enema	0.18–1.14
Mammography	0.00001
CT head	0.007
CT upper abdomen	0.04
CT pelvis	2.5
99-Tc bone scan	0.15
KUB	00000

not recommended due to risk of stillbirth or fetal death as well as rheumatologic and skin problems.

- PET scans can be used with proper hydration and bladder catheter placement to reduce fetal exposure.
- Whole-body diffusion-weighted MRI could replace PET with equal efficacy for nodal and distant metastasis detection, and lower rates of AEs to the fetus.
- SLN mapping using 99-T is contraindicated for cervical cancer, but not for vulvar cancer. ICG SLN mapping data is insufficient to report recommendations or risk at this time.
- Therapeutic radiation treatment: Any use will deliver a significant dose to the fetus and any therapeutic dose will cause fetal death.

Chemotherapy in Pregnancy

- The background rate of fetal anomalies for all pregnancies is 2% to 3%. The risk of anomalies with chemotherapy in the first trimester is 6% using single-agent drug regimens and 17% with combination therapies. If folate antagonists are excluded, the risk is reduced to 6%.

- Chemotherapeutic agents commonly used during pregnancy are vinca alkaloids, doxorubicin, and cisplatin. Alkylators, such as cisplatin and doxorubicin, can carry a 14% risk of fetal anomalies in the first trimester and 4% in the second trimester. Vinca alkaloids are particularly useful during the first trimester and do not cross the placenta. Doxorubicin can be used in the first trimester of pregnancy. The MDR1 P-glycoprotein is found in higher amounts of the endometrium and placenta. MDR1 may provide protection for the fetus. Cisplatin can cause a 50% risk of IUGR, bilateral neonatal hearing loss, or leukopenia. Antimetabolites can cause cranial nasal dystocia, auditory malformations, micrognathia, and limb deformities.
- Chemotherapy: should preferably be delayed until after 14 weeks' GA when platinum (carboplatin preferentially due to fetal ototoxicity with cisplatin), taxanes, etoposide, bleomycin and anthracyclines can be used. Bevacizumab should be avoided as should other targeted therapies.
  - Dosing should be based on actual weight—dosing regimens are the same as nonpregnant protocols.
    - Chemotherapy should be discontinued at >35–36 weeks' GA to allow for a 3-week period for cytopenias to resolve before delivery. Due to maternal myelosuppression and nadirs of blood components, there are increased risks of infection, and decreased wound healing for procedures such as episiotomy and cesarean section.

Surgical Management in Pregnancy
- Locoregional anesthesia is preferred.
- Timing of surgery is preferred in the (early) second trimester.
- The left lateral tilt is advised when positioning for surgery.
- Minimally invasive approaches have been shown to have fewer fetal AEs, shorter operative times, shorter LOS, and fewer preterm contractions.
  - MIS can cause more hypercapnia, uterine perforation, reduced uterine blood flow due to the use of CO_2 and insufflation pressures. Recommendations are to keep surgical length less than 120 minutes and keep insufflation pressures between 10 to 13 mmHg.
- Fetal cardiotocography/monitoring is not feasible during pelvic surgery.
- Care should be taken with perioperative medicines that cross the placental-blood barrier.
- There are increased risks for maternal aspiration from relaxed esophageal tone in pregnancy due to progesterone, and rapid sequence intubation is recommended.

Cervical Cancer in Pregnancy

- Cervical cancer occurs in approximately 1.4 to 4.6 cases per 100,000 pregnancies.[9]

- Pregnant patients are 3.1 times more likely to be diagnosed with stage I disease versus nonpregnant patients. There is no difference in survival in pregnant versus nonpregnant patients. Treatment of preinvasive lesions can be delayed until after delivery as the progression of dysplasia to a higher grade postpartum is 7%.

- Cervical cancer in pregnancy has not shown to have adverse maternal/fetal oncologic outcomes.

- Cervical cancer in pregnancy is diagnosed via cervical biopsy of gross lesions or colposcopic-directed biopsy of lesions at risk of invasion. ECC is contraindicated during pregnancy.

- Conization is indicated if there is persistent severe cervical dysplasia suggestive of an invasive lesion, minimal stromal invasive disease found on cervical biopsy, or if invasive disease cannot be ruled out by colposcopy and biopsy alone.

- In the first trimester, 24% of patients undergoing cervical conization experienced fetal loss,[10] with a 10% loss in the second trimester.[11] In the third trimester, conization was complicated by high blood loss but no loss of pregnancy. Another report[12] detailed a 9% risk of hemorrhage and a 4% risk of delayed bleeding. There may be an increased rate of preterm deliveries.

- CKC is possibly better than LEEP in pregnancy because it is easier to control the size of the specimen with a CKC. Furthermore, a loop is difficult to pass through the more edematous cervix, which occurs with pregnancy. A coin-shaped biopsy is preferred in pregnant patients rather than a cone-shaped biopsy.

- Timing of the conization should be between 14 and 20 weeks' gestation. Placement of a McDonald cerclage at the time of a cervical excision procedure can be considered. Cervical length should be assessed at intervals after conization and before 24 weeks—if limited residual cervical length (<2.5 cm), a cerclage chould be considered.

Management of Cervical Cancer in Pregnancy

- Desirous of pregnancy preservation:
  - Stage IA1 with no LVSI: A conization can fully treat the cancer.
  - Stage 1A1 with LVSI—Stage IB1:
    - < 22 weeks' IUP: A staging LND should be performed initially and can be performed up to 22 weeks' IUP.
    - > 22 weeks: If GA is more than 22 weeks, treatment delay until the postpartum period can occur, or consideration of NACT can be implemented. NACT can continue until 35 weeks' IUP.

- Stage IB2
  - If <22 weeks' IUP there are 2 options:
    - Pelvic LND f/b chemotherapy or surveillance until postpartum treatment initiation, or
    - NACT with surgical staging after tumor response; if pelvic LN are positive, pregnancy termination is recommended. If patients refuse, NACT should proceed.
  - If > 22 weeks' IUP, NACT only can be implemented.
  - Stage IB3 and higher: NACT should be implemented if pregnancy preservation is desired.
- If pregnancy is not desired/is to be terminated:
  - Stages IA2–IB2:
    - First to early-second trimester: A radical hysterectomy with fetus in situ
    - Late second trimester: A radical hysterectomy after hysterotomy and removal of fetus.
    - Chemoradiation can always be administered instead of surgical management.
  - Stage IB3 and higher:
    - First trimester: Chemoradiation should be initiated with fetus in situ.
    - Second trimester: Chemoradiation should begin after hysterotomy and fetal removal.
- Progression of cancer during pregnancy is rare. Treatment delay can be considered for early-stage cancers diagnosed after 20 weeks. Longer delays that allow a pregnancy, 20 weeks to proceed to term are controversial.
- Spontaneous abortion occurs at doses of 40 Gy. 27% of patients do not pass the conceptus spontaneously and require evacuation. In patients with advanced-stage cancers, near term, a short delay is permissible, followed by radiotherapy within 2 to 3 weeks of delivery.
- The mode of delivery of pregnant patients with cervical cancer is controversial.
  - Vaginal delivery may be possible with small-volume tumors or in patients previously treated by conization.
  - Cesarean delivery can decrease the risk of hemorrhage and obstructed labor, especially in cases in which there is a large friable tumor. If a cesarean section is performed, a classical cesarean hysterotomy should be made. This can be followed by radical hysterectomy and/or ovarian transposition. A cesarean that is planned and timed is better than an unplanned delivery because of the possibility of hemorrhage and need for emergent hysterectomy, likely eliminating the opportunity for staging.

- Vaginal metastasis or recurrence has been reported. There have been 10 cases of episiotomy-site recurrence in women who have had vaginal deliveries. Fourteen percent of patients who had a cesarean section had local metastasis following delivery compared to 59% of patients who delivered vaginally. Some studies showed decreased survival with vaginal delivery (75% vs. 55% for cesarean delivery).[13]

Ovarian Neoplasms in Pregnancy

- Ovarian neoplasms are detected at 0.2 to 3.8 cases/100,000pregnancies.[14] Most ovarian masses found in pregnancy are simple ovarian cysts, with approximately 70% resolving by the second trimester. Surgical evaluation is indicated in the second trimester if the mass persists and is greater than 6 to 8 cm, rapidly increasing in size, or complex. Torsion can occur in 5% to 15% of pregnant patients and often occurs during the time when the uterus is rapidly growing (the first 16 weeks of pregnancy) or during postpartum uterine involution. Seventeen percent of these masses can cause obstruction of labor, necessitating cesarean delivery. Surgical treatment, if indicated, is usually unilateral cystectomy. If malignant, a USO with staging procedure and cytoreduction is indicated.
- Malignancy is found in 2% to 6% of adnexal masses. Most ovarian cancers in pregnancy are found at stage I, likely due to incidental early detection during fetal US.
- A tumor marker that remains unchanged during pregnancy is LDH. CA-125 has limited usefulness in pregnancy because it is nonspecific and levels can fluctuate throughout pregnancy.
- GCTs are the most common ovarian neoplasms found during pregnancy and mature teratomas are the most common histologic type.
  - Dysgerminoma is the most common malignant GCT and comprises about 30% of all ovarian malignancies found during pregnancy. They are bilateral in 10% to 15% of cases. Because these neoplasms can rapidly increase in size, they can cause pain, incarcerate in the pouch of Douglas, and torse.
  - In a study of pregnant patients with dysgerminoma, obstructed labor occurred in 33% of patients and fetal death occurred in 24%.[15]
  - Treatment of dysgerminomas is primarily surgical. At minimum, a USO is performed along with ipsilateral pelvic and PA-LND, and staging biopsies.
  - In patients with advanced dysgerminoma, adjuvant chemotherapy is indicated.
  - The rate of recurrence is approximately 10% for disease confined to one ovary.

- Immature teratomas (IT)s and endodermal sinus tumors are other GCTs that can occur in pregnancy. Treatment is primarily surgical and fertility preserving surgery is usually feasible.
- All patients with nondysgerminoma tumors except for stage IA G 1 IT should receive adjuvant chemotherapy. Regimens include bleomycin, etoposide, cisplatin and vinblastine.
- Sex cord stromal tumors, such as granulosa cell tumors and Sertoli–Leydig tumors, are uncommon during pregnancy, but when they do occur, they are associated with rupture, hemoperitoneum, and labor dystocia. Treatment is surgical, with staging and fertility preserving surgery.
- EOCs diagnosed during pregnancy have the same prognosis as in nonpregnant patients. Surgical staging should be performed. The administration of chemotherapy during the second and third trimesters is feasible if indicated for advanced disease.
- Surgical evaluation up to GA of 22 weeks' IUP can be performed to include omentectomy, appendectomy, and peritoneal biopsy as well as LND in addition to USO. If comprehensive staging is limited due to uterine size/access to the pelvis, postpartum restaging should occur. If the GA is > 22 weeks' IUP, treatment postponement to the postpartum period can be considered. If advanced-stage cancer is identified via biopsy, consideration of pregnancy termination in the first trimester can occur. If termination is declined, platinum-based chemotherapy should proceed and cytoreductive surgery should occur early in the postpartum period when R0 disease status can be obtained.
- Ovarian tumors of LMP are usually found as stage I and clinical outcomes are favorable. If found unexpectedly, staging can occur after delivery.

Other Gynecologic Cancers in Pregnancy
- Other gynecologic malignancies are quite rare during pregnancy:
- Vaginal cancer:
  ○ Symptoms/signs include a vaginal mass and abnormal vaginal discharge or bleeding.
  ○ Treatment is with chemoradiation.

- Vulvar cancer:
  ○ May present with symptoms of vulvar irritation and pruritus, or with a visible mass.
  ○ Radical vulvectomy with uni or bilateral LND can be performed and 99-T can be used at the lowest dose available with the surgical procedure occurring < 2 hours after injection. Removal of the involved LN also removes the 99-T. SPECT-CT should not be performed and indigo carmine should not be used due to

anaphylaxis. Patients diagnosed in the third trimester can delay treatment until postpartum. If SLN is/are positive, then full LND should be performed and termination of pregnancy or early delivery should be advised followed by EBXRT. If preoperative inguinal FNA shows LN + at the time of diagnosis, EBXRT in a timely fashion should occur and termination of pregnancy in the first or second trimester is recommended.

  ○ Cesarean section is recommended in the third trimester to prevent wound complications unless a well-healed small wound was present and there is no potential for dystocia from introital scarring.

- Endometrial cancer associated with pregnancy is usually diagnosed postpartum. The prognosis is usually favorable as most tumors are focal and well differentiated.

Obstetric Care

- This should be coordinated with maternal–fetal medicine specialists.
- A definitive estimated gestational age should be performed via US as early as possible.
- A comprehensive fetal anatomy scan should be performed at 18 to 20 weeks' IUP.
- Standard maternal–fetal vitamins and supplements should be taken.
- Standard genetic screening should occur at benchmarked times.
- Surgery during pregnancy: Fetal monitoring before and after surgery should occur. If uterine manipulation is undertaken, tocolytic use can be considered.
- Interval growth scans for assessment for IUGR and morphologic anomalies in patients receiving chemotherapy are indicated every 4 weeks. Antenatal monitoring via Doppler US followed by non stress tests when viability is reached, is indicated.
- Evaluation of fetal anemia via peak systolic velocity of middle cerebral artery blood flow is useful, especially when using platinum agents.
- Delivery is indicated after 37 weeks and fetal lung maturity (FLM) can be assessed if early. If preterm delivery is inevitable, steroids should be administered.

Delivery Management

- Mode of delivery for those with cervical cancers is usually via cesarean given the risk of tumor laceration and hemorrhage, tumor dystocia, or episiotomy-site implantation of tumor cells ,which yields fatal results. Avoidance of a low transverse site incision for cervical cancer patients is necessary to avoid transposition of cancer cells to the abdominal wound and hemorrhage from the neovascularization of the tumor. Cesarean radical hysterectomy can be performed as well after delivery of the baby, general anesthesia is used for the hysterectomy portion. LND or SLND can be done at the same time. Cesarean section is also recommended for vulvar cancer patients. Those patients with completely excised cervical or ovarian cancers can attempt vaginal delivery if no oncologic contraindications are present at the time of delivery.

- Prophylaxis for VTE is recommended with heparin or derivatives.
- Initiation or continuation of chemotherapy/radiation can be started immediately after vaginal delivery and 1 week after cesarean section.
- The placenta should be sent to pathology for evaluation of metastasis and neonatal evaluation should be comprehensive.
- Breastfeeding is contraindicated for women who are on active chemotherapy regimens to avoid medication transmission to the baby through breast milk. Breastfeeding is also contraindicated for those on targeted therapies. Time from last administration to initiation of breastfeeding should be 3 weeks or more.
- Birth control should be offered/advised and hormonal contraceptive options reviewed in concordance with the tumor receptor status.
- Management of patients with radical trachelectomy[16]
  - Periconceptional counseling: Discussion should be held regarding a high risk of infertility as well as a high risk of both early-pregnancy loss and PTD.
  - A cerclage should have been placed at the time of the trachelectomy. The presence of a Saling procedure should be evaluated.
  - Cervical cytology: Should be checked before, early in, and after pregnancy to detect cancer recurrence.
  - Screening and treatment for infection: Bacterial vaginosis should be evaluated at least monthly. It is recommended that women avoid vaginal sexual intercourse between 14 and 34+ weeks' of gestation.
  - First-trimester pregnancy loss: Expectant management without D&C is indicated for early miscarriage.
  - Second trimester loss: Women should undergo cesarean section to avoid laceration of the residual cervix and/or removing the cerclage.
  - Frequency of prenatal visits:
    - Monthly until 20 weeks
    - After 20 weeks: Every 2 weeks
      - Residual cervical length should be measured using TVUS at each visit after 18 weeks. A short cervical length (<13 mm) measured at 21 to 23 weeks' of gestation predicts PTD before 34 weeks.
    - After 28 weeks: Weekly

- ○ Prophylaxis:
  - Bed rest is not routinely advised. If abnormal vaginal bleeding and short cervical length occur, admission with tocolytic administration for antenatal steroids and magnesium neuroprotection is standard of care.
  - Antibiotics are not routinely recommended.
  - Use of fetal fibronectin to predict PTD or PPROM is unclear.
  - Efficacy of vaginal progesterone use to prevent PTD is unclear.
- ○ Delivery:
  - Timing:
    - □ Delivery at 37 weeks is recommended or 3 weeks after last chemotherapy.
    - □ If there are higher risk factors, such as PTL and bleeding, timing after 34 weeks is acceptable. Fetal lung maturity determination after corticosteroid administration is recommended if GA is <37 weeks.
  - Method:
    - □ Cesarean section (CS):
      - A transverse incision in the lower uterus is recommended except for cervical cancer patients.
      - A classical CS or high-transverse CS can be considered. but is associated with higher blood loss and sequalae in future pregnancies.
- ○ Postpartum: Retained products of conception, endometritis, and lochimetria are all concerns due to the narrowed cervical canal. The cerclage should be left intact at the time of the CS.

REFERENCES

1. Quirk F, Haughie S, Symonds T. The use of the sexual function questionnaire as a screening tool for women with sexual dysfunction. *J Sex Med.* 2005;2(4):469–477. doi: 10.1111/j.1743-6109.2005.00076.x
2. Perez K, Gadgil M, Dizon DS. Sexual ramifications of medical illness. *Clin Obstet Gynecol.* 2009;52(4):691–701. doi: 10.1097/GRF.0b013e3181bf4b4c
3. Pizzoferrato A-C, Klein M, Fauvet R, et al. Pelvic floor disorders and sexuality in women with ovarian cancer: a systematic review. *Gynecol Oncol.* 2021;161(1):S0090-8258(21)00086-X):264–274:. doi: 10.1016/j.ygyno.2021.01.026
4. Elgindy E, Sibai H, Abdelghani A, et al. Protecting ovaries during chemotherapy through gonad suppression: a systematic review and meta-analysis. *Obstet Gynecol.* 2015;126(1):187–195. doi: 10.1097/AOG.0000000000000905
5. Loren AW, Mangu PB, Beck LN, et al. Fertility preservation for patients with cancer: American society of clinical oncology clinical practice guideline update. *J Clin Oncol.* 2013;31(19):2500–2510. doi: 10.1200/JCO.2013.49.2678
6. Taylan E, Oktay K. Fertility preservation in gynecologic cancers. *Gynecol Oncol.* 2019;155(3):S0090-8258(19)31532-X):522–529:. doi: 10.1016/j.ygyno.2019.09.012

7. Harrison RF, He W, Fu S, et al. National patterns of care and fertility outcomes for reproductive-aged women with endometrial cancer or atypical hyperplasia. *Am J Obstet Gynecol.* 2019;221(5):S0002-9378(19)30687-8):474:. doi: 10.1016/j.ajog.2019.05.029

8. Chung YS, Woo HY, Lee J-Y, et al. Mismatch repair status influences response to fertility-sparing treatment of endometrial cancer. *Am J Obstet Gynecol.* 2021;224(4):S0002-9378(20)31175-3):370:. doi: 10.1016/j.ajog.2020.10.003

9. Amant F, Berveiller P, Boere IA, et al. Gynecologic cancers in pregnancy: guidelines based on a third international consensus meeting. Ann Oncol. 2019;30(10):1601–1612. doi:10.1093/annonc/mdz228

10. Averette HE, Nasser N, Yankow SL, et al. Cervical conization in pregnancy. Analysis of 180 operations. *Am J Obstet Gynecol.* 1970;106(4):543–549. doi: 10.1016/0002-9378(70)90039-6

11. Hannigan EV. Cervical cancer in pregnancy. *Clin Obstet Gynecol.* 1990;33(4):837–845. doi: 10.1097/00003081-199012000-00019

12. Robinson WR, Webb S, Tirpack J, et al. Management of cervical intraepithelial neoplasia during pregnancy with LOOP excision. *Gynecol Oncol.* 1997;64(1):153–155. doi: 10.1006/gyno.1996.4546

13. Jones WB, Shingleton HM, Russell A, et al. Cervical carcinoma and pregnancy. A national patterns of care study of the american college of surgeons. *Cancer.* 1996;77(8):1479–1488. doi: 10.1002/(SICI)1097-0142(19960415)77:8<1479::AID-CNCR9>3.0.CO;2-7

14. Amant F, Berveiller P, Boere IA, et al. Gynecologic cancers in pregnancy: guidelines based on a third international consensus meeting. *Ann Oncol.* 2019;30(10):S0923-7534(19)60973-7):1601–1612:. doi: 10.1093/annonc/mdz228

15. Karlen JR, Akbari A, Cook WA. Dysgerminoma associated with pregnancy. *Obstet Gynecol.* 1979;53(3):330–335.

16. Kasuga Y, Ikenoue S, & Tanaka M, Ochiai D. Management of pregnancy after radical trachelectomy. *Gynecologic Oncology.* 2021;162. 10.1016/j.ygyno.2021.04.023.

7 Survivorship Care for Gynecologic Malignancies

SURVEILLANCE RECOMMENDATIONS

Surveillance Guidelines

- At completion of primary surgery/adjuvant therapy or initial definitive treatment, patients should be counseled regarding the purpose of follow-up.
- History and physical examination should include a vaginal speculum examination, bimanual exam, and rectal examination. There is no evidence for the regular use of most imaging or laboratories; these should only be obtained guided by patient symptoms or physical exam findings. Pap smears of the vaginal cuff are not recommended in patients with a history of endometrial cancer. It is not recommended to perform colposcopy for Pap tests that are LSIL or less in women with a history of cervical cancer.[1]
- Screening for significant anxiety and depression symptoms should be included and psychosocial support should be offered at each visit.
- Referral for palliative care for women with advanced or relapsed gynecologic cancer is important for QOL. Avoidance of unnecessary treatments at the end of life reduces patient and family discomfort.
- In addition to cancer-specific follow-up, all women should have a PCP who provides them with routine healthcare assessments to include HTN, breast cancer screening, and bone density assessment. On discharge from oncologic care, women and their PCPs should receive specific information on which symptoms to be aware of and to seek additional assessment for.

Uterine Cancer

- Low Risk disease (include: stage I, grades 1 to 2): Surveillance should include a history, physical exam, and pelvic exam with visual inspection of the vaginal cuff. The time interval is every 6 months for 1 to 2 Y, then annually. Pap smears are not recommended.

- High-risk disease surveillance includes those with stage I, G 3 disease, stage II and higher—all grades. Surveillance should include a history, physical exam, and pelvic exam with visual inspection of the vaginal cuff. Time interval is every 3 months for 2 Y, every 6 months up to Y 5, then annually. Pap smears are not recommended.

Ovarian and Tubal Cancer

- Surveillance should include a history, physical exam, and pelvic exam with visual inspection of the vaginal cuff. The time interval is every 3 months for 2 Y, every 6 months up to Y 5, then annually.
- Genetic testing should be performed on all HGSTOC patients for *BRCA1/2* and other identified associated genes.
- Women with GCTs should have laboratory testing to include the tumor marker that was elevated at the time of presentation.
- Cost of surveillance in ovarian cancer: An additional $26 million will be needed to identify the 5% of women with recurrence seen only on CT. Of patients, 95% had either elevated CA-125 or office visit findings at the time of recurrence. The surveillance cost for the U.S. ovarian cancer population for 2 Y after diagnosis and surgery is $32.5 billion using NCCN guidelines and $58 billion if one CT scan is obtained.[2]
- **Rustin guidelines**: The EORTC 55955 reported that there was no evidence of a survival benefit with early treatment of relapse on the basis of an elevated CA-125 concentration alone, and therefore the value of routine measurement of CA-125 in the survival care of patients with ovarian cancer who attain a CR after first-line treatment. Thus, relevant therapy, not timing, is vital.[3]

Cervical Cancer, Vulvar, and Vaginal Cancer

- Surveillance should include a history, physical exam, and pelvic exam with visual inspection of the vaginal cuff. The time interval is every 3 months for 2 Y, every 6 months up to Y 5, then annually.
- Vaginal screening with cytology alone should be done no more than annually ASCUS and LSIL should not usually be further assessed with colposcopy.
- Well-woman care should include smoking cessation.

Melanoma Patients

Melanoma patients: The previous recommendations do not apply and follow-up should be guided by the current literature associated with cytotoxic, biologic, and immunotherapies[4,5] (Tables 7.1–7.4).

Table 7.1 Endometrial Cancer Surveillance Recommendations

Variable		Months			Y		
		0–12	12–24	24–36	3–5	>5	
Review of symptoms and physical examination	Low risk (stage IA G 1 or 2)	Every 6 months	Yearly	Yearly	Yearly	Yearly	
	Intermediate risk (stage IB–II)	Every 3 months	Every 6 months	Every 6 months	Every 6 months	Yearly	
	High risk (stage III/IV, serous or CC)	Every 3 months	Every 3 months	Every 6 months	Every 6 months	Yearly	
Pap test/ cytologic evidence		Not indicated	Not indicated	Not indicated	Not indicated	Not indicated	
CA-125		Insufficient data to support routine use	Insufficient data to support routine use	Insufficient data to support routine use	Insufficient data to support routine use	Insufficient data to support routine use	
Radiographic imaging (CXR, PET/CT, MRI)		Insufficient data to support routine use	Insufficient data to support routine use	Insufficient data to support routine use	Insufficient data to support routine use	Insufficient data to support routine use	
Recurrence suspected		CT and/or PET scan; CA-125	CT and/or PET scan; CA-125	CT and/or PET scan; CA-125	CT and/or PET scan; CA-125	CT and/or PET scan; CA-125	

Table 7.2 EOC Surveillance Recommendations

| Variable | Months | | | | Y | |
	0–12	12–24	24–36	3–5	>5
Review of symptoms and physical examination	Every 3 months	Every 3 months	Every 4–6 months	Every 6 months	Yearly
Pap test/cytologic evidence	Not indicated	Not indicated	Not indicated	Not indicated	Not indicated
CA-125	Optional	Optional	Optional	Optional	Optional
Radiographic imaging (CXR, PET/CT, MRI)	Insufficient data to support routine use	Insufficient data to support routine use	Insufficient data to support routine use	Insufficient data to support routine use	Insufficient data to support routine use
Recurrence suspected	CT and/or PET scan; CA-125	CT and/or PET scan; CA-125	CT and/or PET scan; CA-125	CT and/or PET scan; CA-125	CT and/or PET scan;CA-125

Table 7.3 Nonepithelial Ovarian Cancer (Germ Cell and Sex-Cord Stromal Tumors) Surveillance Recommendations

Variable		Months			Y		
		0–12	12–24	24–36	3–5	>5	
Review of symptoms and physical examination	GCTs	Every 2–4 months	Every 2–4 months	Yearly	Yearly	Yearly	
	Sex-cord stromal tumors	Every 2–4 months	Every 2–4 months	Every 6 months	Every 6 months	Every 6 months	
Serum tumor markers	GCTs	Every 2–4 months	Every 2–4 months	Not indicated	Not indicated	Not indicated	
	Sex-cord stromal tumors	Every 2–4 months	Every 2–4 months	Every 6 months	Every 6 months	Every 6 months	
Radiographic imaging (CXR, CT, MRI)	GCTs	Not indicated unless tumor marker normal at initial presentation	Not indicated unless tumor marker normal at initial presentation	Not indicated	Not indicated	Not indicated	
	Sex-cord stromal tumors	Insufficient data to support routine use	Insufficient data to support routine use	Insufficient data to support routine use	Insufficient data to support routine use	Insufficient data to support routine use	
Recurrence suspected		CT scan, tumor markers	CT scan, tumor markers	CT scan, tumor markers	CT scan, tumor markers	CT scan, tumor markers	

Table 7.4 Cervical, Vulvar, and Vaginal Cancer Surveillance Recommendations

Variable	Months				Y	
	0–12	12–24	24–36	3–5	>5
Review of symptoms and physical examination	Every 6 months	Every 6 months	Yearly	Yearly	Yearly
	Low risk (early stage, treated with surgery alone, no adjuvant therapy)				
High risk (advanced stage, treated with primary chemotherapy/XRT or surgery plus adjuvant therapy)	Every 3 months	Every 3 months	Every 6 months	Every 6 months	Yearly
Pap test/cytologic evidence	Yearly	Yearly	Yearly	Yearly	Yearly
Recurrence suspected	CT and/or PET scan	CT and/or PET scan	CT and/or PET scan	CT and/or PET scan	CT and/or PET scan

Survivorship Guidelines

A patient is considered a cancer survivor from the time of diagnosis, through the rest of her life.

- Care of the survivor should include the following: Prevention and surveillance of new and recurrent cancers, and assessment of late psychosocial and physical effects. Intervention for consequences of cancer and treatment include late effects of treatment, medical comorbidities, psychologic distress, and financial and social concerns. Coordination of care between PCPs and specialists is necessary to ensure that all of the survivor's health needs are met.
    - An annual periodic assessment is recommended to determine any needs and necessary interventions. This assessment is to include current disease status, performance status, medication review, medical comorbidity management, and potential reversible causes for any symptoms due to prior treatment.
    - Symptom review should include assessment of the following:
        - Cardiac toxicity: Assess for SOB, chest pain, paroxysmal nocturnal dyspnea, especially if there is a history of anthracycline or Trastuzumab administration.
        - Anxiety and depression: Is patient bothered more than half the day with little interest or pleasure in doing things, does she have days feeling down, depressed, or hopeless, or not being able to control or stop worrying?
        - Cognitive function: Is there difficulty multitasking or paying attention, difficulty remembering things, or is the thought process slower?
        - Fatigue: Is there persistent fatigue despite a good night's sleep and does the fatigue interfere with usual activities?
        - Pain: Is there any pain score that should be documented?
        - Sexual function: Are there any concerns regarding sexual function or activity in the patient or with the partner, and are these concerns causing distress personally or within the relationship?
        - Sleep: Are there problems falling asleep or staying asleep? Is there excessive sleepiness? Is snoring a problem? Does the partner notice sleep apnea?
        - Healthy lifestyle: Is regular physical activity worked into each day? Is a healthful diet eaten each day?
        - Vaccination: Seasonal flu vaccine and other indicated vaccinations are recommended.
- Secondary malignancies may occur in survivors due to genetic predisposition, environmental exposures, prior oncologic therapy (XRT, alkaloid cytotoxic therapy). Screening for secondary malignancies should be shared between the PCP and the oncology providers.

- Specific toxicities:
  - Cardiac:
    - Causes: Often due to anthracycline, can be induced by receptor-targeted therapies (trastuzumab), chest irradiation (left-sided breast or mantle XRT), and can take up to 10 Y to become evident
    - There are four stages:
      - Stage A:
        - Cardiac risk factors are present but no structural heart disease. Risk factors are HTN, dyslipidemia, family history of cardiomyopathy, age greater than 65, smoking, obesity, alcoholism, comorbid cardiac diseases (atrial fibrillation, CAD, baseline structural heart disease, and personal history of rheumatic fever), and diabetes.
        - Pretreatment workup: Thorough clinical screening for heart failure should occur within 1 Y of completion of anthracycline therapy. An echocardiogram should be obtained.
        - Treatment: Primary prevention with early detection is suggested. Diet, exercise, BP control, cholesterol-lowering medications, and consideration of cardiac remodeling/cardioprotective agents need to be considered.
      - Stage B:
        - Structural heart disease is present but there are no signs or symptoms of heart failure: Patients may have LVH, LV diastolic dysfunction, asymptomatic valvular disease, or a previous MI.
        - Pretreatment workup: Follow suggestions as in stage A with referral to cardiologist for further diagnosis and management.
      - Stage C:
        - Signs and symptoms of heart failure are present with underlying structural heart disease.
        - Management: Refer to cardiologist for further diagnosis and management.
      - Stage D:
        - Signs and symptoms: Advanced structural heart disease with significant symptoms of heart failure are present at rest despite maximal medical therapy and interventions.
        - Management: Refer to cardiologist for further diagnosis and management.

○ Pain:

- Pretreatment workup: Quantify, qualify, and determine the etiology and pathophysiology of the pain. It is important to discuss with the patient goals for comfort and function, and determine whether it is a specific cancer pain syndrome.

- Pain types: Determine the type of pain: neuropathic from neuromas or nerve transection; postsurgical pain from amputation, neck dissection, mastectomy, and thoracotomy; musculoskeletal pain: myalgias, arthralgias, bone pain, and myofascial pain ; GI discomfort: SBO, PSBO, chronic diarrhea, or constipation; pelvic pain or urinary pain from surgery, XRT, hydronephrosis, or infection.

- Management is with physical therapy, pelvic floor exercise, dorsal column stimulation for chronic cystitis or pelvic pain. Neuromodulating SSRIs/SNRIs, or gabapentin can be used in addition to biofeedback. Massage therapy may be an additional resource. Additional means of pain modification can be use of NSAIDs, narcotics, bowel regimen, a low roughage/low residue diet, and hydration. Surgical options, when appropriate, are to bypass, stent, or divert bowel obstructions.

- It is important to ensure there is no recurrent tumor with imaging and biopsy.

- The best means to reduce the risk of chronic pain due to treatment is optimal control of acute pain. This is achieved through use of a distress screening tool prior to office visits, assessment and triage, and working with OB/GYN and family medicine to deliver the highest level of care.

- SNPs in apolipoprotein 3r and catechol-O-methyltransferase genes are the most common changes associated with cognitive dysfunction.[6]

○ Lymphedema: The etiology is usually from LND but may be from XRT, scarring, or tumor obstruction. Referral to a lymphedema specialist is indicated with assistance from compression garments, progressive resistance training, physical therapy with range- of-motion exercises, and manual lymphatic drainage.

- Anxiety and depression:

○ Mood Disorders

- General anxiety disorder or adjustment disorder with anxious mood:

    □ Symptoms are excessive anxiety that is difficult to control that involves sleep disturbances, restlessness, muscle tension, irritability, difficulty concentrating, and easy fatigue.

    □ Management: Refer for counseling for consideration of medical management.

- Panic disorder: Acute onset of at least four of the following:

- □ Palpations, sweating, chills or hot flashes, trembling or shaking, sensation of SOB, chest pain or discomfort, nausea, dizziness, out-of- body experience/being detached from self, fear of dying, fear of losing control, and paraesthesias
- □ Management: Refer for counseling and consideration of medical management.
- PTSD:
  - □ Inclusion criteria: Patient experiences recurrent intrusive memory of the trauma or recurrent dreams of the event, avoidance of stimuli associated with the trauma, numbing of general responsiveness, inability to recall traumatic events, feeling of detachment from body, restricted range of emotion, sense of foreshortened future. Increased arousal can manifest as hypervigilance, exaggerated startle, irritability, difficulty concentrating, and sleep disturbance.
  - □ Management: Refer for counseling and consideration of medical management.
- Obsessive-compulsive disorder:
  - □ Inclusion criteria: Patient experiences recurrent persistent thoughts, impulses, or images that cause marked distress that the person attempts to suppress with some thought or action. This often manifests as repetitive behaviors or mental acts that a person is compelled to perform in response to the obsession, to reduce stress or prevent some unrealistic dreaded event.
  - □ Management: Refer for counseling and consideration of medical management.
- Major depressive disorder:
  - □ Inclusion criteria: Patient experiences depressed mood or a loss of interest or pleasure in daily activities for more than 2 weeks and this mood represents a change from the person's baseline. There is impaired function in social, occupational, and educational activities. Five of nine of the following specific symptoms must be present nearly every day: depressed mood or irritability present most of the day, nearly every day, as indicated by either subjective report (e.g., feels sad or empty) or observation made by others (e.g., appears tearful); decreased interest or pleasure in most activities most of each day; significant weight change (5%) or change in appetite; change in sleep with either insomnia or hypersomnia; change in activity with either psychomotor agitation or retardation; fatigue or loss of energy; feelings of worthlessness or excessive or inappropriate guilt; concentration is diminished or more

indecisiveness is present; there is suicidal ideation (SI) either with SI thoughts or a suicide plan.

◻ Management: Refer for counseling and consideration of medical management versus admission if SI is present.

○ Nutrition and weight management: Weight gain after cancer diagnosis and treatment is common. Strategies to prevent weight gain should be discussed. Weight gain can exacerbate risk or functional decline, comorbidity, and possible cancer recurrence or death, and reduce QOL. Nutritious weight gain for underweight patients should be encouraged. Weight maintenance for normal-weight patients should also be encouraged.

▪ Principles of weight loss: Limit foods that are high in calories and low in nutrients; substitute high-calorie foods with energy-dense foods such as vegetables, fruits, soups, whole grains; use portion control, smaller plates, and one-serving limits; and routinely evaluate food labels. There is no evidence to support the use of weight-loss supplements in cancer survivors.

▪ Principles of weight gain: Evaluate appetite changes and eating patterns.

○ If appetite stimulants are indicated:

▪ Megace 40 mg daily: Take care due to possible increased risk of VTE.

▪ Mirtazapine 15 mg daily (Remeron): This is also an antidepressant.

○ Assess cancer treatment effects (surgery, XRT): GI dysmotility, swallowing and dysphagia, oropharyngeal anatomic changes, and bowel dysfunction can all contribute to lower PO intake or GI absorption.

○ For ovarian cancer and WP-XRT survivors: Low-fiber nonbulky-vegetable diets (minimizing lettuce and cruciferous vegetables) can be encouraged. Be mindful of GI tract reconstruction/anastomoses.

○ Comorbidities that may limit exercise or modify metabolism are CV disease, arthritis, DM, renal disease, liver disease, mood disorders, thyroid disease, GI disease, medication use, and dental health.

Hormone Replacement

RRBSO is recommended for *BRCA1/2* mutation carriers to prevent ovarian cancer. In a prospective cohort study of 872 *BRCA1* mutation carriers from 1995 to 2017 who had a mean follow-up of 7.6 Y, carriers of *BRCA1* mutation with no personal medical history of cancer who underwent bilateral oophorectomy were followed for incident breast cancer. The mean (*SD*) age of women was 43.4 (8.5) Y. In this study, 92 (10.6%) incident breast cancers were diagnosed. HRT use after oophorectomy was not associated with an increased risk of breast cancer, (HR, 0.97; 95% CI: 0.62–1.52; p =.89) when examining forever use versus no use of HRT. When evaluating the effects of estrogen versus combination HRT, a difference was found. At 10-Y follow-up, the cumulative incidence of breast cancer for those who used estrogen alone was 12% versus 22% for those who used combination estrogen plus progesterone (AD, 10%; LR *p* = .04).[7]

REFERENCES

1. Salani R, Backes FJ, Fung MFK, et al. Posttreatment surveillance and diagnosis of recurrence in women with gynecologic malignancies: Society of Gynecologic Oncologists recommendations. *Am J Obstet Gynecol.* 2011;204(6):466–478. doi: 10.1016/j.ajog.2011.03.008

2. Armstrong A, Otvos B, Singh S, et al. Evaluation of the cost of CA-125 measurement, physical exam, and imaging in the diagnosis of recurrent ovarian cancer. *Gynecol Oncol.* 2013;131(3):S0090-8258(13)01191-8):503–507:. doi: 10.1016/j.ygyno.2013.09.017

3. Rustin GJS, van der Burg MEL, Griffin CL, et al. Early versus delayed treatment of relapsed ovarian cancer (MRC OV05/EORTC 55955): a randomised trial. *Lancet.* 2010;376(9747):1155–1163. doi: 10.1016/S0140-6736(10)61268-8

4. Elit L, Reade CJ. Recommendations for follow-up care for gynecologic cancer survivors. *Obstet Gynecol.* 2015;126(6):1207–1214. doi: 10.1097/AOG.0000000000001129

5. Rimel BJ, Burke WM, Higgins RV, et al. Improving quality and decreasing cost in gynecologic oncology care. Society of Gynecologic Oncology recommendations for clinical practice. *Gynecol Oncol.* 2015;137(2):S0090-8258(15)00666-6):280–284:. doi: 10.1016/j.ygyno.2015.02.021

6. Shapiro CL. Cancer survivorship. *N Engl J Med.* 2018;379(25):2438–2450. doi: 10.1056/NEJMra1712502

7. Kotsopoulos J, Gronwald J, Karlan BY, et al. Hormone replacement therapy after oophorectomy and breast cancer risk among BRCA1 mutation carriers. *JAMA Oncol.* 2018;4(8):1059–1065. doi: 10.1001/jamaoncol.2018.0211

8 Palliative Care

PALLIATIVE CARE PATHWAYS

Palliative Care

Palliative care is an area of healthcare that specifically focuses on relieving and preventing the suffering of patients from diagnosis onward. It facilitates effective communication between the patient and practitioner, and it supports the goals of cure, life prolongation, QOL, or acceptance of death. These efforts are not initially end-of-life care but can facilitate discussion. It is also helpful in determining code status and signing of POLST form. Discussion can provide effective management of expectations, treatment-associated toxicities, financial toxicities, and channels for supportive care within the medical field and/or community.

- The ultimate goal is to provide the best possible QOL for people facing the pain, symptoms, and stress of serious illness. It is appropriate throughout all stages of an illness. It can be provided along with treatments that are meant to cure.

- Palliative therapies not only improve a patient's QOL, but also have been shown to extend life. In a study of patients with metastatic non–small- cell lung cancer, patients were randomized to receive either early palliative care integrated with standard oncologic care or standard oncologic care alone. Despite the fact that fewer patients in the early palliative care group than in the standard care group received aggressive end-of-life care (33% vs. 54%, $p = .05$), median survival was longer among patients receiving early palliative care (11.6 vs. 8.9 months, $p = .02$).[1]

- Palliative surgical or medical intervention can relieve symptoms and lead to less pain for the patient. In these instances, correction of the terminal disease is not anticipated or achieved. Approximately 10% of procedures are performed for palliative intent, not cure.

- Financial toxicity: A study showed a significant cost savings to patients and the system with early enrollment and usage of hospice care, without any decrease in QOL.

Hospice

Hospice care is palliative care that typically occurs when a patient is considered to be terminal, or within 6 months of death.

End-of-Life Discussion

It can be quite difficult discussing the implications of a life-threatening illness with a patient and family. There are a few things to keep in mind when discussing terminal disease and end-of-life care:

- Hope is important, but is not a plan.
- Emotions run high. Negative emotions, such as fear, anxiety, frustration, and depression, are common and are manifested in a variety of ways by patients and their caregivers.
- Respect is important. Healthcare providers should listen to and honor the perspectives and choices of patients and their families.

Multidisciplinary Approach

A multidisciplinary approach is important.

- Effective palliative care involves a team approach. This involves the patient and her physician and may also include palliative care physicians; specialists; general practitioners; nurses; nursing assistants or home health aides; social workers; chaplains; and physical, occupational, and speech therapists.

Communication

Communication is the most important factor in terminal care.

- Timing of discussion: Soon after the diagnosis of advanced or recurrent cancer, options for palliative care should be discussed.
- Ensure that legal documents are drawn up: These include a living will, power of attorney, and advance directive/POLST.
- Specific issues to address with the patient: Discuss the need for ventilatory support, TPN, the need for emergent surgery, interventional procedures for relief of acute symptoms, invasive procedure endpoints and indications, DNR consent, timing for discontinuation of supportive measures, location for death (hospital vs. home).
- Ask–Tell–Ask Method
  - Ask the patient or family what their awareness and knowledge of the disease and disease status is. Tell the patient/family what the current clinical situation and prognosis is. Ask for feedback so you can assess their understanding and interpretation.[2]

Delivering Bad News

Spikes Method
This approach uses a six-step protocol.

- Step 1: Set up the interview: Arrange for privacy, involve significant others and family, sit down, connect with the patient and family, minimize interruptions (phone/pager on vibrate).
- Step 2: Assess the patient's perception: What is your understanding of your situation?
- Step 3: Obtain the patient's invitation: How would you like me to give you information about your test results?
- Step 4: Knowledge and information given to the patient: Provide a warning: "I'm afraid I have bad news." Ensure the appropriate level of comprehension and vocabulary of the patient. Avoid excessive bluntness. Give the information in small bites and assess the patient's understanding at each step.
- Step 5: Address the patient's emotions with empathetic response: Observe and identify the patient's emotion; let the patient know you have identified the emotion.
- Step 6: Strategy and summary: Establish a plan to address the patient's goals of care and QOL as well as fears. Frankly discuss expectations and goals for both patient and loved ones.

Management of Specific Symptoms

- Dyspnea: Causes and treatment options
    - Pneumonia: antibiotics and pulmonary hygiene
    - Lymphangitic tumor: diuretics, glucocorticoids
    - Pneumonitis, XRT or chemotherapy induced: glucocorticoids
    - PE: anticoagulation, IVC filter
    - Pleural effusion: Indwelling catheter, thoracentesis, VATS, pleurodesis (bleomycin, talc, tetracycline)
    - Airway obstruction by tumor or adenopathy: XRT, glucocorticoids, stent
    - Bronchoconstriction: COPD/asthma: bronchodilators, glucocorticoids
    - Retained or excess secretions: anticholinergic drugs
    - Massive ascites causing SOB: paracentesis with or without indwelling catheter
    - Anxiety manifested as hyperventilation: anxiolytics, behavioral therapy
    - Additional measures: facial cooling with fan, chest physical therapy
    - Consider supplemental oxygen, but this does not always correlate with symptomatic resolution.
    - Systemic opioids
- Anorexia: Reversible causes: constipation, pain, medications, hypercalcemia, mucositis, and bowel obstruction; treatments: gastrokinetic agents such as metoclopramide, low-dose corticosteroids,

progestone agents (Megace), antidepressants (Remeron), cannabinoids such as dronabinol, palliative surgery with bowel diversion

- Nausea: 60% of patients have nausea and vomiting, usually resulting from various receptors triggered in the GI tract. It is important to rule out cerebral metastasis. Other causes are uremia, electrolyte imbalances, and hypercalcemia. Treatment: Use antiemetics at optimal dosing and route of administration, use scheduled around-the-clock dosing, and add second agent when monotherapy fails rather then switch agents.
  - Dopamine antagonist: Consider chlorpromazine 6.25 mg PO/IM/IV every 8 hours, prochlorperazine PO/PR/IM/IV 10 to 50 mg every 4 to 8 hours, metoclopramide 5 to 20 mg PO/IV every 2 to 8 hours, haloperidol 0.5 to 1 mg q8ho PO/IV.
  - Anticholinergic: Clopalamine transdermal 1.5 mg q3d; hydroxyzine 6.25 to 25 mg qHS
  - H1 antihistamine: Diphenhydramine PO/IV/IM 12.5 to 50 mg q6h; promethazine PO/IM 12.5 to 25 mg q8h
  - 5HT3 antagonist: Ondansetron PO/IV/SL 4 to 20 mg every 4 to 8 hours; dolasetron 100 mg PO q24h; granisetron 2 mg PO q24h; palonosetron 0.01 mg/kg IV q24h, transdermal 3.1 mg q24h, IV 0.25 mg q24h
  - Steroids: Dexamethasone PO/IV 4 to 24 mg daily
  - Cannabinoids: Dronabinol 7.5 to 15 mg PO every 3 to 4 hours
  - Benzodiazepines: Lorazepam IV/PO 0.5 to 2 mg q4-h
- Malignant ascites: Treatment: Paracentesis, indwelling (pleurX) drains. Diuretics may relieve ascites associated with portal HTN from hepatic metastasis. VEGF targeting agents can reduce ascites as well.
- Malignant bowel obstruction:
  - Types: Mechanical: from tumor obstruction; compressive: from external ascites compression; functional: from carcinomatosis coating the surface of the bowel obstructing peristalsis
  - Treatment:
    - Conservative management involves use of a NGT, IVF, bowel rest, NPO status, pain and nausea control. Steroids may reduce bowel edema (decadron 4 mg q6 hours), and octreotide may reduce secretions.
    - Surgical: Surgery to release bowel adhesions or monofocal tumor; resection with reanastomosis, bypass or diversion and ostomy, bowel stent, G/J-tube, or hospice. The addition of TPN is expensive and can add an average of 4 to 6 weeks of life.
- Constipation: This can be disease related, or a side effect of antiemetics or opioids. Treatment: Use stool softeners, osmotic agents,

stimulants, lubricants, and enemas. Bulking agents are not as helpful.

- Terminal hemorrhage: This is defined as rapid blood loss that is internal or external with volume depletion. It occurs in 3% to 14% of patients.
  - It can be classified by cause:
    - Anatomic from tumor invasion or erosion into blood vessels or organs
    - Generalized due to coagulopathy or thrombocytopenia
    - Mixed
  - Common sites are GI, GU, and respiratory.
  - Treatment: Volume resuscitation, correction of the underlying coagulopathy, consider IR embolization of proximal vessel(s). Specific site indications:
    - Vaginal bleeding: Attempt to control with vaginal packing with or without Monsels solution, XRT, IR arterial embolization, endoscopic cautery, surgical ligation of large vessels, excision of bleeding tissue.
    - Hemorrhagic cystitis: Can be treated with CBI, cystoscopic coagulation, instillation of 1% alum, methylene blue, or formalin instillation, which is 80% effective but should be used as a last resort.
    - Palliative measures: Apply pressure, use dark towels and suction, consider sedatives. Midazolam is rapid acting and is given IV or SC 2.5 to 5 mg every 10 to 15 minutes.
- Bone metastasis: Treat with NSAIDs; directed XRT; absorptive XRT with strontium; bisphosphonates; or Denosumab, which is a human mAb that binds to and neutralizes the receptor activity of NKB ligand, protecting bone from demineralization. If pathologic fracture is identified, bone-stabilizing surgery may be indicated.
- Hypercalcemia: Diagnosis is a serum calcium level above 10.2 adjusted for albumin. Treatment is IVF, bisphosphonates, calcitonin 2 to 8 IU/kg SC or IM q12h; consider administration of furosemide.
- Brain metastasis: Headache is present in 40% to 50% of patients. Seizures occur in 10% to 20%. Nausea, vomiting, visual changes, and gait disturbance (cerebellar) are other symptoms. First-line therapy is steroids, 4 to 8 mg/day of dexamethasone, followed by XRT 48 hours after onset of steroids. For patients with one to three lesions and good control of systemic disease, targeted XRT or stereotactic radiosurgery can be considered. If stable systemic disease with good treatment options, consultation with neurosurgery for possible resection can also be considered. For patients with one to three lesions and poor control of systemic disease, WB-XRT is

recommended. If four or more lesions are present or there is unresectable disease, WB-XRT is also recommended. WB-XRT is delivered in 10 fractions of 3 Gy for a total of 30 Gy, or 15 fractions of 2.5 Gy to a maximum of 37.5 Gy.

- Delirium: Common causes are medications, infection, electrolyte abnormalities, hypoxia, uremia, liver failure, urinary retention, and uremia.
  - Subtypes
    - Hypoactive subtype: May exhiibit as lethargy, sedation, psychomotor retardation, hypoxia, metabolic disturbances, hepatic encephalopathy.
    - Hyperactive subtype: Symptoms are agitation, restlessness, hyperactivity, hallucinations, delusions. These symptoms should be correlated with alcohol or drug withdrawal, or potential adverse effects of medication.
    - Mixed subtype
  - Treatment
    - Nonpharmacologic treatment involves orientating the patient to what is familiar and to family presence, not using restraints, and ensuring use of eye glasses and hearing aids.
    - Medications include haloperidol, chlorpromazine. Olanzapine and risperidone are alternatives to haloperidol. If irreversible hyperactive delirium, lorazepam 1 mg every 3 minutes as needed.
- Fatigue occurs in 60% to 90% of patients, especially those undergoing chemotherapy. Commonly associated symptoms are pain, depression, and insomnia. Most pharmacologic agents have not been found to be statistically beneficial, including antidepressants, coQ10, L-carnitine, or CNS stimulating agents. Yoga has been the only identified exercise regimen to show improvements in fatigue.
- Insomnia occurs in 30% to 50% of patients. Treatment can be pharmacologic as well as behavioral:
  - Pharmacologic
    - Consider benzodiazepines (lorazepam, temazepam) and nonbenzodiazepine hypnotics (zolpidem, zaleplon, eszopiclone). These can be associated with lower QOL indices and increased severity of symptoms. Therefore, they should be used in combination with nonpharmacologic measures and for the shortest time possible.
    - Consider hormonal and herbal products, including melatonin and ramelteon.
    - Antidepressants, including trazodone, mirtazapine, and paroxetine, have been tried. There was no improvement in insomnia but some improvement was shown in depression scores.

- ○ Cognitive behavioral therapy, including stimulus control, sleep restriction, relaxation training, sleep hygiene education, and cognitive therapy, can be recommended as first-line therapy. In a randomized trial, yoga demonstrated improvements in sleep quality.
- Chemotherapy-induced neuropathy: Different prescription and OTC medications to treat neuropathy have been tried, all without much success, to include ALA, neurontin, and carnitine.
- Agonal breathing and sounds: Can be treated with glycopyrolate 0.1 to 0.2 mg IV or SC q4h, atropine 0.4 mg SC every 15 minutes, or scopolamine 1.5-mg patch.
- Pain: Assess and manage per the WHO pain ladder. Additional potential interventions are use of anticonvulsants, antidepressants, muscle relaxants, and corticosteroids.
  - ○ Acute pain syndromes are partially reversible: Chemotherapy can induce some of these symptoms as can recent surgery or XRT.
    - Oxaloplatin
      - □ Symptoms: Cold-induced paresthesias and muscle cramping
      - □ Prevention: IV calcium and magnesium supplementation; GSH may also be beneficial.
    - Paclitaxel
      - □ Symptoms: diffuse aching in joints within 3 days of administration that resolves at 7 days.
      - □ Prevention: Consider ALA and ALC.
        - ALA dosing: 600 mg IV once weekly for 3 to 5 weeks, then 1,800 mg PO daily
        - ALC dosing: 1 gm PO TID for 8 weeks
    - Treatment for these and other acute pain syndromes: Pregabalin titrated to target dose of 150 mg PO TID, venlafaxine 50 mg 1 hour before oxaliplatin infusion and venlafaxine ER 37.5 mg PO BID days 2 to 11, duloxetine titrated to target dose of 60 mg PO daily for 12 weeks, acupuncture.
  - ○ Chronic pain: 33% of patients have chronic pain after curative-intent treatment.
    - Arthralgias are common in women taking aromatase inhibitors.
    - Surgical pain occurs as phantom pain, neuroma or scar pain, nerve injury pain, or postreconstruction pain.
    - XRT pain includes plexopathies, peripheral nerve entrapment, myelopathy, pelvic pain, osteoradionecrosis, myofascial fibrosis, restricted range of motion, dermatitis, enteritis,

cystitis, proctitis, pelvic fractures, secondary malignancies, and fistula.

- Treatment: antidepressants to include tricyclic antidepressants (TCA), SSRIs, and serotonin-norepinephrine reuptake inhibitors (SNRIs); pregabalin and gabapentin; topical lidocaine; NSAIDS; opioids; interventional nerve blocks, intrathecal therapy, joint injection, implantable devices, and vertebroplasty exercise and physical therapy/occupational therapy should be incorporated into treatment. Psychological interventions and massage can be included.[3]

Active Dying (Transitioning)

Patients will have increased somnolence, increased oral secretions from the inability to swallow, a decreased appetite, potential delusions and/or hallucinations, body temperature fluctuation, decreased urinary output, apnea, agonal breathing, and skin mottling.[4]

Ethical Issues

When the wishes of a patient contradict the physician's management desires and compromise cannot be attained, transfer of care to another physician may be appropriate.

The involvement of a hospital ethical committee may be appropriate at times.

Ethical Guidelines
- Nonmaleficence
- Beneficence
- Autonomy
- Justice

Medical futility: After having an open discussion with the patient about the terminal disease and realistic expectations, the physician needs to determine when it is advisable to move from an aggressive therapeutic approach to supportive care. The pathway for withdrawal of care, once a decision has been made, is as follows:

- Obtain informed consent.
- Plan for the procedure and potential side effects.
- Address the patient's distress.
- Move the patient to an appropriate setting.
- Use adequate sedation.
- Document the procedure.
- Review the outcomes.

Notable Studies

Patients were retrospectively assessed between 2005 to 2012 who had received grater than 12 months of continuous Medicare coverage before death due to ovarian cancer: The study demographics were 1,788 (77%) White, 359 (15%) Hispanic, 158 (7%) Black, and 26 (1%) other. Of these patients, 1,756 (75%) enrolled in hospice prior to death but only 1,580 (68%) died in hospice; 176 (10%) of 1,756 patients unenrolled and died without hospice; 346 (20%) unenrolled from hospice multiple times. The median amount paid by Medicare during the last 6 months of life was $38,530 for those in hospice compared to $49,942 if never enrolled in hospice (p <.0001) and was higher for Black and Hispanic patients compared to White patients. Thirty percent of hospice unenrolled patients and 40% of multiply enrolled hospice patients received at least one life-extending or invasive care procedure following unenrollment from hospice.[5]

REFERENCES

1. Temel JS, Greer JA, Muzikansky A, et al. Early palliative care for patients with metastatic non-small-cell lung cancer. *N Engl J Med.* 2010;363(8):733–742. doi: 10.1056/NEJMoa1000678

2. Paek B. I see you, I hear you-only then, I speak. *Obstet Gynecol.* 2021;137(5):892–893. doi: 10.1097/AOG.0000000000004346

3. Pachman DR, Barton DL, Swetz KM, et al. Troublesome symptoms in cancer survivors: fatigue, insomnia, neuropathy, and pain. *J Clin Oncol.* 2012;30(30):3687–3696. doi: 10.1200/JCO.2012.41.7238

4. Landrum LM, Blank S, Chen L, et al. Comprehensive care in gynecologic oncology: the importance of palliative care. *Gynecol Oncol.* 2015;137(2):S0090-8258(15)00674-5):193–202:. doi: 10.1016/j.ygyno.2015.02.026

5. Taylor JS, Zhang N, Rajan SS, et al. How we use hospice: hospice enrollment patterns and costs in elderly ovarian cancer patients. *Gynecol Oncol.* 2019;152(3):S0090-8258(18)31356-8):452–458:. doi: 10.1016/j.ygyno.2018.10.041

9 Statistics and Reference Material

STATISTICS

Definitions

- General definitions
  - Variable: Anything that is manipulated in an experiment
  - Independent variable: Something that is varied by and under the control of the experimenter.
  - Dependent variable: This is a variable that responds to manipulation.
  - Nominal variable: This is a variable in a named category, for example, sex, diagnosis.
  - Ordinal variable: This refers to a set of ordered categories, for example, stages of cancer are ordered, but the significance between each step is not known.
  - Interval variable: This is a measurement variable that is used to define values measured along a scale, with each point placed at an equal distance from one another. For example: temperature, age.
  - Ratio is the comparison of two quantities of the same units that indicates how much of one quantity is present in the other quantity.
  - Parametric: Refers to data that follow a normal distribution.
  - Nonparametric: Refers to data that do not follow a normal distribution (nominal and ordinal).
  - Incidence: This is the current number of new events/population at risk determined during same time interval.
  - Prevalence: Refers to the total number of events/population at risk. Prevalence should be more than the incidence.
- Measures of central tendency
  - Mode: This is the value most often reported.

- ○ Median: This represents the value with half the responses below and half above (nonparametric).
- ○ Mean: This is the average of all values.
- Measures of dispersion
  - ○ Standard deviation (*SD*) of the mean is the square root of the variance. The smaller the *SD*, the less each score varies from the mean: 1 *SD* = 68%, 2 *SD* = 95.5%, 5 *SD* = 99%.
  - ○ Variance is the average of the squared differences from the mean (value of point − mean)^2/total number of data points.
  - ○ Range is the difference between the highest value and the lowest value.
  - ○ Percentile is where the result lands out of 100.

Methods Used to Analyze Data

There are two methods used to analyze data. Descriptive statistics communicate results, but do not generalize beyond the sample. Inferential statistics communicate the likelihood of these differences occurring by a chance combination of unforeseen variables.

- Null hypothesis: By statistical convention, it is assumed that the speculated hypothesis is always wrong and that the observed phenomena simply occur by chance. It is this hypothesis that is to be either nullified or not nullified by the test. When the null hypothesis is nullified, it is possible to conclude that data support the alternative hypothesis.
- Significance level: The extent to which the test in question shows that the "**speculated hypothesis**" has or has not been nullified is called its *significance level*; the higher the significance level, the less likely it is that the phenomena in question could have been produced by chance alone.
- Statistics for inference (hypothesis) testing:
  - ○ Confidence intervals (CIs) are used to indicate the reliability of an estimate. The CI is calculated by 1-alpha.
  - ○ Standard error (*SE*) is used to help determine whether the result is true or occurs more by chance. SE = SD/square root of sample size. The SE can either be systemic, where the wrong measure is taken each time, or random, where the answer is different each time the experiment is run.
  - ○ Margin of error refers to the amount the results are expected to change from one experiment to another.
  - ○ CLT states that if the sample size is sufficiently large (*n* >10), the mean will normally distribute regardless of the original distribution. This theory allows the parametric assessment of nonparametric data.

○ z-test compares the sample mean with the known population mean.

- Sensitivity: Sensitivity relates to the test's ability to identify positive results. The sensitivity of a test indicates the proportion of people who have the disease who test positive for it. For example, a sensitivity of 100% means that the test recognizes all actual positives—that is, all sick people are recognized as being ill. Thus, in contrast to a high-specificity test, a negative result in a high-sensitivity test is used to rule out the disease.

  This can be written as follows:

  Sensitivity = Number of true positives/number of true positives + number of false negatives or

  True positives/all positive with disease

  If a test has high sensitivity, then a negative result would suggest the absence of disease.

- Specificity: Specificity relates to the ability of the test to identify negative results. The *specificity* of a test is defined as the proportion of patients who do not have the disease who will test negative for it. This can also be written as follows:

  Specificity = Number of true negatives/number of true negatives + number of false positives or

  True negatives/all negative with disease

  The specificity states the ability of a test to determine whether the patient who tests negative does not have the disease.

- PPV: This test reflects the probability that the person with the positive test has the underlying condition being tested for.

- NPV: This test reflects the proportion of subjects with a negative test result who are correctly diagnosed. A high NPV means that when the test yields a negative result, it is most likely correct in its assessment (Table 9.1).

Table 9.1 Sensitivity, Specificity, PPV, and NPV

	Disease positive	Disease negative
Positive test	A	B
Negative test	C	D
Sensitivity—True positives/all with disease		A/(A + C)
Specificity—True negatives/all without disease		D/(B + D)
PPV		A/(A + B)
NPV		D/(C + D)

Table 9.2 Relationship Between Truth/Falseness of the Null
Hypothesis and Test Outcomes

	Null Hypothesis (*H0*) Is True	Null Hypothesis (*H0*) Is False
Reject null hypothesis	Type I error FP	Correct outcome TP
Fail to reject null hypothesis	Correct outcome TN	Type II error FN

- Type I error: This occurs when one rejects the null hypothesis (*H0*) when it is true. A type I error may be compared to a false positive. The rate of the type I error is called the size of the test and denoted by the Greek letter α (alpha). It usually equals the significance level of a test. In the case of a simple null hypothesis, α is the probability of a type I error. If the null hypothesis is composite, α is the maximum of the possible probabilities of a type I error. The rate of a type I error is related to the CI ($1 - \alpha = $ CI).

- Type II error: This occurs when one fails to reject a false null hypothesis. A type II error may be compared to a false negative. The rate of the type II error is denoted by the Greek letter β (beta) and is related to the power of a test ($1 - \beta = $ power). See Table 9.2.

  FP rate (α) = Type I error = 1 – Specificity = FP/(FP + TN)

  FN rate (β) = Type II error = 1 – Sensitivity = FN/(TP + FN)

  Power = Refers to the chance of detecting a difference that is really there = $1 - \beta$.

  CI = Refers to the chance that a true value lies within the specified interval (1–alpha).

  Confidence level = Refers to the chance that, with repeated sampling, the range of values contains the actual parameter.

  Likelihood ratio positive = Sensitivity/(1 – specificity)

  Likelihood ratio negative = (1 – sensitivity)/specificity

- Alpha is the cutoff for the p value.

- p-value: Refers to a measure of the strength of the evidence against the null hypothesis.

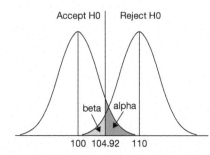

- One- and two-tailed tests: If the distribution from which the samples are derived is considered to be normal, Gaussian, or bell shaped, then the test is referred to as a one- or two-tailed *t*-test.
    - A one-tailed test evaluates samples that fall within the curve and are excluded if they fall into one of the tails of the curve. For an *SD* of 95%, the full 5% falls into the single tail of the curve.
    - A two-tailed test evaluates samples that fall within the curve and are only excluded if they fall into either one of the tails of the curve. For an *SD* of 95%, 2.5% falls into each tail. It is recommended that most statistical analysis should be two tailed.
    - A test is called *two tailed* if the null hypothesis is rejected for values of the test statistic that fall into either tail of its sampling distribution, and it is called *one sided* if the null hypothesis is rejected only for values of the test statistic falling into one specified tail of its sampling distribution.
    - If the test is performed using the actual population mean and variance, rather than an estimate from a sample, it would be called a one- or two-tailed *z*-test.
- *Power* is affected by the significance criterion, the magnitude of effect, and the sample size. The beta level is usually set at 0.2. Thus, the power by convention is usually 0.8. There are two ways to perform a power analysis: a priori and posthoc. A priori (before) is the means to estimate for a sufficient sample size. Posthoc (after) analysis is usually not recommended.
    - To decrease the amount of type I error, the alpha level can be reduced (e.g., from 0.05 to 0.01).
    - To decrease the amount of type II error, the sample size can be increased, the effect size can be changed, or the significance criterion can be changed.
- Attributable risk: This refers to the risk of disease or death in a population exposed to some factor of interest minus the risk of those not exposed.

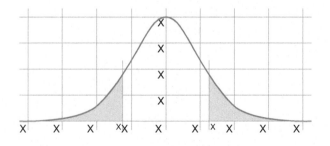

Receiver Operating Characteristic

The receiver operating characteristic (ROC) is the graphical plot of the sensitivity (on the y-axis), or the true positive rate, versus 1 – specificity (on the x-axis), or the false positive, for a binary classifier system as its discrimination threshold is varied. The ROC can also be represented equivalently by plotting the fraction of true positives out of all positives (TPR = true positive rate) versus the fraction of false positives out of the negatives (FPR = false positive rate). It reflects the accuracy of the test. The area under the ROC curve is closely related to the Mann–Whitney U test, which tests whether the positives are ranked higher than the negatives. For an optimal test, all data points should fall into the upper left quadrant.

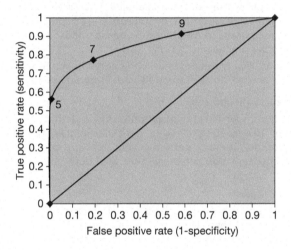

Endpoints of a Study

Endpoints of a study are important for evaluation of PFS, OS, and clinical response. It is necessary to choose good primary endpoints to reflect the effectiveness of the experimental therapy. Surrogate endpoints are often chosen instead because of proposed study length, study cost, and known etiologic associations with the primary endpoint.

Phases of Trials

The following are the four phases of trials:

- A phase I trial is a dose-limiting trial. Doses of drugs are tested until a maximum tolerated dose is determined. When 50% to 75% of patients have an adverse event (DLT), the dose one level less than the DLT dose is chosen as the MTD. The MTD is chosen as the dose to proceed with to the next phase of the trial.
- A phase II trial assesses the activity and toxicities of the drug chosen at the MTD in relation to the disease of interest.

- A phase III trial assesses efficacy. There are two types of phase III trials: the noninferiority trial and the equivalency trial.
  - The noninferiority trial evaluates two drugs to ensure their outcomes are similar (e.g., cisplatin vs. carboplatin with paclitaxel in ovarian cancer).
  - The equivalency trial evaluates an augmentation in care (adding platinum to XRT for cervical cancer vs. XRT alone).
  - The randomized controlled trial is the most expensive type of study. It takes a large amount of time to complete, needs a large number of subjects (150 in each arm to reduce the type II error), is prospective, provides the best level of evidence, and is the only type of trial to prove causality. Two factors can be chosen for study design: either hypothesis based (efficacy/noninferiority/equal) or outcome-of-interest based (efficacy or application in everyday practice).
- A phase IV trial is the postmarketing surveillance trial that ensures the drug is working appropriately with stated benefits.

Randomization Techniques
There are a number of randomization techniques that can be applied: simple/coin toss, sequential digits, permuted blocks, stratified blocks, dynamic randomization, systemic nth; cluster, census, matching, restriction, quota, volunteer, cross-over, split body, and factorial.

Eligibility Criteria
Eligibility criteria are the criteria used to determine which patients to enroll in a study. These criteria serve four functions: scientific benefit, safety, logistic considerations, and regulatory considerations.

Bias and Confounding
To avoid bias or confounding, patients and/or investigators can be blinded, masked, adjusted for specific factors, randomized, the sample size can be increased, a placebo can be used, and factors can be restricted or matched.

Trial Safety, Review, and Ethics
- The DSMB is responsible for quality control, administrative capacities, and endpoint monitoring. The knowledge of any benefit or harm tends to accumulate over time and the DSMB monitors the safety and efficacy of the trial impartially. It can also perform an interim analysis for safety and outcomes.
- An IRB was mandated in 1974 to be established locally for all government-funded research.
- Human subject rights have been established in two main doctrines. The Belmont Report (1979) outlines respect for persons, justice,

and beneficence. The Nuremberg Code (1949) outlines human subject rights to include that participation in the study be voluntary, the study be worthwhile, the study be unavailable by other means, the current state of knowledge is obtained from animals and cannot be obtained further from animal studies, there will be avoidance of unnecessary suffering, no deaths are to be expected, the risk is consistent with study benefits, appropriate precautions are taken for the study, the study is planned and reported by qualified persons, consent is ongoing, assessment of risks and benefits are ongoing, and the study is to be terminated if the risk of injury is imminent.

Types of Trials

Trials can be broken up into the following types:

- Prospective and retrospective types. The prospective trials include randomized controlled trials and cohort trials. The retrospective trials include the case control and cross sectional trials.
- Another way to look at trials is randomized trials versus observational trials. The observational trials are the cohort trials, the case control trials, the ecologic trials, case series, and the case report.
- Umbrella trials: Umbrella studies are designed to test the impact of different drugs on different mutations in a single cancer type. The trial design can help to facilitate patient screening and accrual, and is quite suitable for trials examining low-prevalence diseases. The primary features of umbrella trials are as follows:
  - The inclusion of multiple treatments and multiple biomarkers within the same protocol
  - A design that allows for randomized comparisons
  - A design that can have flexible biomarker cohorts and can add/drop biomarker subgroups
- Basket trials: Basket studies are designed to test the effect of a single drug on a single mutation in a variety of cancer types. They provide a unique way of merging the traditional clinical trial design with rapidly evolving genomic data that facilitate the molecular classification of tumors. Basket trials can also screen multiple drugs across many cancer types. A basket design provides evidence for pairing a drug with a validated biomarker in a specific tumor.

Trial Evaluation

- Validity is described in two fashions. External validity means the study results apply to the entire population. Internal validity means the study results apply specifically to those individuals studied.
- Symmetry means that all things between groups are similar.
- Confounding is the distortion of the effect of one risk factor by the presence of another.

- Bias is any process or effect that produces results that differ systematically from the truth.
  - Nondifferential bias means that the biases are the same in all study groups.
  - Differential bias means that the biases are different between groups.
  - There are a number of types of bias. Confounding bias is the systematic error in which there is failure to account for the effect of one variable on others. Ecological bias is the systematic error in which the group average is applied to individuals. Measurement bias occurs when the measurement methods consistently differ between groups. Screening biasoccurs when the disease is picked up earlier in the latent period by screening, but this screening does not affect the course of the disease. Reader bias is error of interpretation by reader inference. Sampling bias occurs when study design or execution produces errors in sampling. Zero time bias occurs when unintended differences exist from the beginning of the study, at enrollment.

Survival Analysis

Survival analysis: There are two main types of survival analysis.

- The time series analysis is the parametric analysis.
- The Kaplan–Meier analysis is nonparametric and allows right censoring. Kaplan–Meier analysis is used because all patients cannot start the study at the same time, there is withdrawal or loss to follow-up, patients die, and the study must end.
- The log-rank test compares the survival curves of two or more groups. It is a nonparametric test.
- The Cox regression proportional hazards test allows analysis of several risk factors affecting survival. It is a nonparametric test as well.
- The Wilcoxon rank sum test can be used when no censoring occurs.

Causality

Causality: There are a number of criteria used to judge causality. There must be validity to the study, strength in the study, plausibility (there is current biological support), consistency (the study can be replicated), a temporal relationship, a dose response, and alternative explanations have been ruled out.

WHO Screening Guidelines

WHO screening guidelines are in place to provide support for optimization of screening tests. These include: the disease history is understood, the disease is an important health problem, there is a latent stage to the disease, there is a test for the disease and it is sensitive, there is treatment for the condition, facilities are available for diagnosis and treatment, the cost to diagnosis is low and acceptable to the patient, there is an agreed policy on who to treat, and the screening is a continuous process.

Parametric Versus Nonparametric Testing

- Parametric testing means that there was random sampling, there is a normal distribution, the two populations are independent, there are quantitative variables (interval or ratio), and the variances of the normal distributions are equal. Parametric tests include the z-test (which tests the means of the populations), the one-sided t-test, the t-test, the paired t-test, and the unpaired t-est. Also included are the analysis of variance (ANOVA; which measures differences between two or more groups), the analysis of covariance (ANCOVA; which measures the difference between two or more groups and combines regression), the FANCOVA (which is the factorial ANOVA and allows comparison between two or more groups with each variable having at least two levels).

- Nonparametric tests are qualitative and measure associations. These tests include the binomial test, the sign test, the Wilcoxon test, the Mann–Whitney U test, the Fishers test, the chi-square test, the Kruskal–Wallis test, and the Friedman test.

To Quantify Associations

To quantify associations, three types of tests are commonly used. The Pearson's test is for parametric data. The Spearman's rank correlation is for nonparametric data. Kendall's correlation is often used to document concordance.

Means of Magnitude

Means of magnitude tests refers to three ratios.

- The OR is used in case control and logistic regression. It can be calculated as ad/bc. It indicates the risk of an event happening. It can be reversed and 1/OR indicates the event-free survival.

- The RR is used in cohort and randomized controlled trials. It can be calculated as exposed/unexposed, or a/a + b/c/c + d. The RR is cumulative over the entire study period, or the patients' or samples' life span.

- The HR is the ratio of hazards and equals the probability of an event in the treatment group divided by the probability of event in the control group over a unit of time.

Univariate Versus Multivariate Testing

- The univariate test evaluates data on a single variable. It facilitates more advanced analysis and is the first step in looking at data analysis.

- The multivariate test looks at more than one variable at a time. This test can reduce a large number of variables to a smaller number of factors for data modeling. It can select a subset of variables based on which original variables have the highest correlation with the principle of interest. It validates a scale by demonstrating that items load on the same factor.

Table 9.3 compares parametric tests to nonparametric tests for specific indications.

Surrogate Endpoints

Surrogate endpoints in tubo-ovarian cancer are now accepted outcomes. OS as a mandated primary endpoint has many problems, including size, length, expense, and clinical relevance. OS remains the most objective clinical trial endpoint, but as survival increases and new cytotoxic, targeted, and immunologic therapies are emerging, OS may become less clinically relevant. A composite endpoint is integration of multiple endpoints into a single metric (OS, RR, toxicity, etc.). For trial endpoints, ineffective therapy is an RR less than 10%. Effective therapy has an RR of 25%. Safety/toxicity, duration of response, number of CR, should also be evaluated.[1]

ICER

The ICER is a statistic used in cost-effectiveness analysis to summarize the cost-effectiveness of a healthcare intervention. It is defined by the difference in cost between two possible interventions, divided by the difference in their effect. It represents the average incremental cost associated with one additional unit of the measure of effect. The ICER can be estimated as: $ICER = (C_1 - C_0)/(E_1 - E_0)$ where C_1 and E_1 are the cost and effect in the intervention group and where C_0 and E_0 are the cost and effect in the control group. Costs are usually described in monetary units, whereas effects can be measured in terms of health status or another outcome of interest. A common application of the ICER is in cost–utility analysis, in which case the ICER is synonymous with the cost per QALY gained.

REFERENCE MATERIAL

Surveillance Visit Checklist: Checklist for Surveillance of Gynecologic Malignancies

Patient name _____

Visit date _____

Disease site and stage _____

Date of diagnosis/surgery _____

Date treatment completed _____

Table 9.3 Parametric Versus Nonparametric Tests

Goal	Measurement (from Gaussian Population)	Rank, Score, or Measurement (from Non-Gaussian Population)	Binomial (Two Possible Outcomes)	Survival Time
Describe one group	Mean, SD	Median, interquartile range	Proportion	Kaplan–Meier survival curve
Compare one group to a hypothetical value	One sample t-test	Wilcoxon test	Chi-square or binomial test	
Compare two unpaired groups	Unpaired t-test	Mann–Whitney U test	Fisher's test (chi-square for large samples)	Log-rank test or Mantel–Haenszel
Compare two paired groups	Paired t-test	Wilcoxon test	McNemar's test	Conditional proportional hazards regression
Compare three or more unmatched groups	One-way ANOVA	Kruskal–Wallis test	Chi-square test	Cox proportional hazard regression
Compare three or more matched groups	Repeated-measures ANOVA	Friedman test	Cochrane Q	Conditional proportional hazards regression

(continued)

Table 9.3 Parametric Versus Nonparametric Tests *(continued)*

Goal	Measurement (from Gaussian Population)	Rank, Score, or Measurement (from Non-Gaussian Population)	Binomial (Two Possible Outcomes)	Survival Time
Quantify association between two variables	Pearson correlation	Spearman correlation	Contingency coefficients	
Predict value from another measured variable	Simple linear regression or nonlinear regression	Nonparametric regression	Simple logistic regression	Cox proportional hazard regression
Predict value from several measured or binomial variables	Multiple linear regression or multiple nonlinear regression		Multiple logistic regression	Cox proportional hazard regression

Source: From GraphPad Software, Inc. All rights reserved. Copyright 2017, used with permission.

- Symptoms review and treatment side effects
- Pain (abdominal or pelvic, hip or back)
- Abdominal bloating
- Vaginal bleeding (also rectum, bladder)
- Weight loss
- Nausea and/or vomiting
- Cough or shortness of breath
- Lethargy/fatigue
- Swelling of abdomen or leg(s)
- Sexual dysfunction
- Neuropathy
- Fatigue

Physical examination

- General physical examination
- Lymph node assessment (axillary, supraclavicular, and inguinal)
- Pelvic examination (vulvar, vaginal speculum, bimanual, and rectovaginal exam)

    Tumor markers _____

Disease Status
- No evidence of disease
- Suspect recurrence
- Radiographic imaging _____
- Biopsy _____
- Refer to gynecologic oncologist _____

Routine health maintenance
Breast cancer screening:

- Yearly clinical breast examination _____
- Mammogram _____
- Every 1 to 2Y starting with ages 40 to 49Y, then yearly
- Colon cancer screening
- Colonoscopy or flexible sigmoidoscopy _____
- Every 5 to 10Y beginning at the age of 45Y

Genetic Screening
- Not indicated
- Recommended/completed _____

Menopausal Assessment
- Osteoporosis prevention

- ○ Calcium (1,200–1,500 mg) and vitamin D (800 IU)
- ○ Bone mineral density testing: begin at the age of 65 Y or sooner if on glucocorticoid therapy (WHO criteria can be used for reference)
- Smoking cessation
- Weight maintenance (exercise, diet)

Gynecologic Oncology Referral Parameters

Endometrial Cancer

- Biopsy-confirmed endometrial cancer of any grade

Pelvic Mass
- Presence of, or concern for, advanced disease
  - ○ Omental caking—Imaging-guided biopsy can be helpful.
  - ○ Pleural effusion—Cytology from thoracentesis can be helpful.
  - ○ Ascites—Cytology from paracentesis can be helpful.
  - ○ Elevated tumor marker(s): ACOG recommends referral for a pre-menopausal CA-125 greater than 200 and postmenopausal CA-125 greater than 35.
- A clinically suspicious pelvic mass:
  - ○ Simple and larger than 8 to 10 cm
  - ○ Larger than 4 cm and:
    - Fixed
    - Nodular
    - Bilateral
    - Excrescences
    - Solid components
- Premenarchal girls with a pelvic mass
- Postmenopausal women with a suspicious mass or elevated tumor markers as above. ACOG recommends referral for a CA-125 above 35.
- Perimenopausal women with a persistent suspicious ovarian mass, particularly when associated with an elevated CA-125
- Young patients who have a pelvic mass and elevated tumor markers (CA-125, AFP, hCG, LDH)
- A suspicious pelvic mass found in a woman with a significant family or personal history of ovarian, breast, or other cancers (one or more first-degree relatives)

Cervical Cancer
- Biopsy-confirmed (conization or directed) invasive carcinoma

- Women with suspicious cervical lesions should be biopsied before referral.

Vaginal Cancer
- Biopsy-confirmed invasive vaginal cancer
- Women with suspicious vaginal lesions should be biopsied before referral; suspicious lesions include:
  - Nonhealing ulcers
  - Bartholin's gland: Persistent cysts in women over 40
  - Exophytic lesions

Vulvar Cancer
- Biopsy-confirmed invasive vulvar cancer
- Women with suspicious vulvar lesions should be biopsied before referral. These suspicious lesions include:
  - Nonhealing ulcers
  - Areas of chronic pain or pruritus
  - Areas of pigment change
  - Grossly enlarged lesion
- Depending on practitioner's comfort level:
  - Women with multifocal, complex, and/or recurrent VIN 3
  - Women with Paget's disease of the vulva

Gestational Trophoblastic Disease
- Referral should occur after evacuation of the molar pregnancy if there is evidence of persistent trophoblastic disease/GTD:
  - GTD (low or high risk)
  - Choriocarcinoma
  - Placental site trophoblastic tumor
  - Epithelioid trophoblastic tumor

If there is evidence of metastatic disease at initial diagnosis, referral should occur immediately.

Performance Status Scales
Gynecologic Oncology Group /Eastern Cooperative Oncology Group[1]
0: Asymptomatic (fully active, able to carry on all pre-disease activities without restriction)
1: Symptomatic but completely ambulatory (restricted in physically strenuous activity but ambulatory and able to carry out light or sedentary work)
2: Symptomatic, less than 50% in bed during the day (ambulatory, capable of all self-care, unable to carry out any work activities; up and about more than 50% of waking hours)

3: Symptomatic, greater than 50% in bed, but not bedbound (capable of limited self-care, confined to bed or chair 50% or more of waking hours)
4: Bedbound (completely disabled; cannot perform any self-care; totally confined to bed or chair)
5: Dead

Karnofsky Performance Status Scale Rating Criteria (%)
100: Normal; no complaints; no evidence of disease
90: Able to carry on normal activity; minor signs or symptoms of disease.
80: Normal activity with effort; some signs or symptoms of disease
70: Cares for self; unable to carry on normal activity or do active work.
60: Requires occasional assistance, but is able to care for most personal needs.
50: Requires considerable assistance and frequent medical care. Unable to care for self; requires equivalent of institutional or hospital care; disease may be progressing rapidly.
40: Disabled; requires special care and assistance.
30: Severely disabled; hospital admission is indicated although death is not imminent.
20: Very sick; hospital admission is necessary; active supportive treatment is necessary.
10: Moribund; fatal processes are progressing rapidly.
0: Dead

Adverse Event Grading

- CTCAE (ctep.cancer.gov/reporting/ctc.html)

Response Evaluation Criteria in Solid Tumors
Tumor response is measured via RECIST guidelines version 1.1, 2009.[3] These are the WHO criteria for measuring tumor response.

Definition of Disease
- Measurable disease: This refers to the presence of at least one measurable lesion. If the measurable disease is restricted to a solitary lesion, its neoplastic nature should be confirmed by cytology/histology.
- Measurable lesions: These are lesions that can be accurately measured in at least one dimension with LD ≥20 mm using conventional techniques or ≥10 mm by spiral CT scan.
- Nonmeasurable lesions: These are all other lesions, including small lesions (LD <20 mm with conventional techniques or <10 mm with spiral CT scan), that is, bone lesions, leptomeningeal disease, ascites, pleural/pericardial effusion, inflammatory breast disease,

lymphangitis cutis/pulmonis, cystic lesions, and also abdominal masses that are not confirmed and followed by imaging techniques.

- All measurements should be taken and recorded in metric notation, using a ruler or calipers. All baseline evaluations should be performed as closely as possible to the beginning of treatment and never more than 4 weeks before the beginning of treatment.

- The same method of assessment and the same technique should be used to characterize each identified and reported lesion at baseline and during follow-up.

- Clinical lesions are considered measurable only when they are superficial (e.g., skin nodules and palpable lymph nodes). For the case of skin lesions, documentation by color photography, including a ruler to estimate the size of the lesion, is recommended.

Method of Measurement

- CT and MRI are currently the best available and reproducible methods to measure selected target lesions. Conventional CT and MRI should be performed with cuts of 10 mm or less in slice thickness. Spiral CT should be performed using a 5-mm contiguous reconstruction algorithm.

- Lesions on CXR are acceptable as measurable lesions when they are clearly defined and surrounded by aerated lung. However, CT is preferable.

- When the primary endpoint of the study is objective response evaluation, US should not be used to measure tumor lesions.

- The utilization of endoscopy and laparoscopy for objective tumor evaluation is not widely accepted.

- Tumor markers alone cannot be used to assess response. If markers are initially above the upper normal limit, they must normalize for a patient to be considered in complete clinical response when all lesions have disappeared.

Baseline Documentation of "Target" and "Nontarget" Lesions

- All measurable lesions up to a maximum of two lesions per organ and five lesions in total, representative of all involved organs, should be identified as target lesions and recorded and measured at baseline.

- Target lesions should be selected on the basis of their size (lesions with the LD) and their suitability for accurate repeated measurements (either by imaging techniques or clinically).

- A sum of the LD for all target lesions will be calculated and reported as the baseline sum LD. The baseline sum LD will be used as the reference by which to characterize the objective tumor response.

- All other lesions (or sites of disease) should be identified as nontarget lesions and should also be recorded at baseline. Measurements of these lesions are not required, but the presence or absence of each should be noted throughout follow-up.

Response Criteria
- Target lesions
  - CR = disappearance of all target lesions.
  - PR = 30% decrease in the sum of the LD of target lesions, taking as reference the baseline sum LD.
  - PD = 20% increase in the sum of the LD of target lesions, taking as reference the smallest sum LD recorded since the treatment started or the appearance of one or more new lesions.
  - SD = small changes that do not meet the preceding criteria.
- Nontarget lesions
  - CR = disappearance of all nontarget lesions and normalization of tumor marker level.
  - SD = persistence of one or more nontarget lesion(s) or/and maintenance of tumor marker level above the normal limits.
  - PD = appearance of one or more new lesions and/or unequivocal progression of existing nontarget lesions.
  - SD = small changes that do not meet these criteria.

Best Overall Response
- Evaluation of "best overall response": The best overall response is the best response recorded from the start of the treatment until PD/recurrence (taking as reference for PD the smallest measurements recorded since the treatment started).
  - Patients with a global deterioration of health status requiring discontinuation of treatment without objective evidence of disease progression at that time should be classified as having "symptomatic deterioration." Documentation of objective progression after discontinuation of treatment should occur.
  - When it is difficult to distinguish between residual disease and normal tissue and evaluation of CR depends on this determination, it is recommended that the residual lesion be fine-needle aspirated/biopsied to confirm status.

Confirmation of Response
- To achieve PR or CR status, changes in tumor measurements must be confirmed by repeat assessments that should be performed at least 4 weeks after the criteria for response are first met.
- The goal of confirmation of objective response is to avoid overstating the observed response rate.
- For SD, follow-up measurements must have met SD criteria at least once after study entry with a minimal interval, usually not less than 6 to 8 weeks.

Duration of Overall Response
The duration of overall response is measured from the time criteria are met for CR or PR (whichever status is recorded first) until the first date that PD is objectively documented, taking as reference for PD the smallest measurements recorded since the treatment started.

Duration of Stable Disease
- SD is measured from the start of the treatment until the criteria for disease progression are met, taking as reference the smallest measurements recorded since the treatment started.
- The clinical relevance of the duration of SD varies for different tumor types and grades. Therefore, it is highly recommended that the protocol specify the minimal time interval required between two measurements for determination of SD. This time interval should take into account the expected clinical benefit that such a status may bring to the population under study.

Immune Response RECIST Criteria
- Measurement of immune-related response criteria (irRC) tumor burden: Tumor burden is measured by combining "index" lesions with new lesions. With irRC, new lesions represent a change in overall tumor burden. The irRC retained the bidirectional measurement of lesions that had originally been set for the WHO/RECIST 1.1 Criteria.
- Assessment of immune-related response. In the irRC, an immune-related complete response (irCR) is the disappearance of all lesions, measured or unmeasured, and the appearance of no new lesions; an immune-related partial response (irPR) is a 50% drop in tumor burden from baseline; and immune-related progressive disease (irPD) is a 25% increase in tumor burden from the lowest level recorded. All else is considered immune-related stable disease (irSD).[4]

Common Chemotherapy Protocols and Dosing
For common protocols and dosing, see Table 9.4.

Useful Formulas

- The Cockcroft–Gault equation provides an estimate of creatinine clearance (CrCl) based on age, weight, sex, and serum creatinine without the need for a 24-hour urine collection.

$$\text{CrCl} = \frac{[(140 - Age) \times Weight(kg)] \times 0.85}{[0.72 \times SerumCr(mg/dL)]}$$

- The Calvert formula calculates the carboplatin dosing using the GFR from the Crockcroft–Gault equation: Dose (mg) = target AUC × (GFR + 25). The AUC is usually set from 5 to 7 for untreated patients and 4 to 6 for previously treated patients.

- The Jelliffe formula is good for adult patients with normal muscle mass who are not on hemodialysis. This calculation is not applicable to patients less than 18 Y old, with serum creatinine less than 0.6 mg/dL, weight less than 35 or more than 120 kg, unstable creatinine, muscle mass less than 70% or more than 130% of normal.

$$CrCl \text{ (female)} = 0.9 \{[98 - 0.8 \times (A-20)]/SCr \text{ (mg/dL)}\}$$

where A = age in Y; CrCl = creatinine clearance in mL/min/1.73 m^2. The patient's BSA must be determined. The CrCl value obtained by the equation must be multiplied by (BSA/1.73) to obtain the patient's CrCl in absolute terms (i.e., mL/min). Weight is in kilograms and height is in centimeters.

- For BSA, the most widely used formula is the Du Bois formula:

$$BSA \text{ (m}^2\text{)} = 0.007184 \times W^{0.425} \text{ kg} \times H^{0.725} \text{ cm}$$

A commonly used and simple calculation is the Mosteller formula:

$$BSA = \text{Square root of } (W \times H/3,600) = 0.016667 \times W0.5 \times H0.5$$

- The fractional excretion of sodium can help determine prerenal, intrinsic, or postrenal disease:

$$FENa = (UNa \times SCr)/(SNa \times UCr) \times 100$$

A value below 1% indicates prerenal disease.

A value above 2% or 3% indicates acute tubular necrosis or other kidney damage.

- Serum osmolality = $2[Na] + [K] + BUN/2.8 + Glu/18$

Normal is 280 to 295 mOsm/kg.

- Fe deficit = $1,000 + (15-Hgb) \times (kg \text{ weight})$

Normal is 2 g.

- A-a Gradient = $PAO_2 - PaO_2$. The $PAO_2 = (FiO_2 \times (760 - 47)) - (PaCO_2/0.8)$

Normal is 5 to 10 mmHg; or less than current age in Y/4 + 4.

- Corrected serum Na: measured sodium + 0.016 × (serum glucose in mg/dL − 100)

Table 9.4 Common Chemotherapy Protocols

IV paclitaxel/carboplatin	Paclitaxel 175 mg/m^2 IV, Day 1
Cycle length 21 d	Carboplatin AUC 5–6 IV, day 1
	or
	Paclitaxel 80 mg/m^2, days 1, 8, and 15
	Carboplatin AUC 5–6 IV, day 1
	or
	Paclitaxel 80 mg/m^2 IV, days 1, 8, and 15
	Carboplatin target (AUC of 2) IV, days 1, 8, and 15
IV paclitaxel, IP cisplatin, paclitaxel	IV paclitaxel (135 mg/m^2 over 24 hr) on day 1
Cycle length 21 d	IP cisplatin (100 mg/m^2 in a liter of normal saline) on day 2
	IP paclitaxel (60 mg/m^2) on day 8
	Alternative outpatient schedule:
	IV paclitaxel (175 mg/m^2 over 3 hr) on day 1 followed by IP cisplatin (100 mg/m^2 in a liter of normal saline) on day 1
	IP paclitaxel (60 mg/m^2) on day 8
	Dose reduction of IP cisplatin can be to 75 mg/m^2
Carboplatin desensitization	Carboplatin target (AUC of ____/dose) (= _____ mg) to be infused as four separate infusions (dilutions):
	Dose 1—1:1,000 dilution IVPB over 60 min
	Dose 2—1:100 dilution IVPB over 60 min
	Dose 3—1:10 dilution IVPB over 60 min
	Dose 4—remaining carboplatin IV over 60 min
Carboplatin, liposomal doxorubicin	Doxorubicin, liposomal 30 mg/ m^2 IV
Cycle length 28 d	Carboplatin AUC of 5 IV
Carboplatin, docetaxel	Docetaxel 100 mg/m^2 IV, day 1

(continued)

Table 9.4 Common Chemotherapy Protocols *(continued)*

Cycle length 21 d	Carboplatin AUC 5–6 IV, day 1
Carboplatin, gemcitabine	Carboplatin AUC 5 IV, day 1
Cycle length 21 d	Gemcitabine 1,000 mg/m² IV, days 1, 8
Doxorubicin, liposomal	Doxorubicin, liposomal 40 mg/m² IV
Cycle length: 28 d	
Cisplatin with XRT	Cisplatin 40 mg/m² IV (maximum of 70 mg/dose)
Cycle length 7 d	
Cisplatin, paclitaxel, bevacizumab	Cisplatin 50 mg/m² IV
Cycle length 21 d	Paclitaxel 175 mg/m² IV
	Bevacizumab 15 mg/Kg IV
Cisplatin, topotecan	Topotecan 0.75 mg/m² IV; give on days 1, 2, and 3 of each cycle
Cycle length 21 d	Cisplatin 50 mg/m² IV; give on day 1 of each cycle
Topotecan	Topotecan 1.25–1.5 mg/m³ IV over 30 min on days 1–5 of each cycle
	Cycle length 21 d
	or
	Topotecan 4 mg/m² IV, days 1, 8, 15
	(cycle length 28 d)
Gemcitabine	Gemcitabine 1,000 mg/m² IV, days 1, 8
Cycle length 21 d	
Olaparib	400 mg PO BID continuously may be used as monotherapy for advanced ovarian cancer with deleterious or suspected deleterious germline *BRCA* mutations in patients who have been treated with three or more prior lines of chemotherapy
Methotrexate	Methotrexate 0.4 mg/kg/d IV or IM, days 1–5
Cycle length 14 d	or

(continued)

Table 9.4 Common Chemotherapy Protocols *(continued)*

	Methotrexate 1 mg/kg IM, days 1, 3, 5, and 7 plus folinic acid 15 mg PO 30 hr after each MTX dose on days 2, 4, 6, and 8
Actinomycin D	Actinomycin D 12 mcg/kg IV, days 1–5
Cycle length 14 d	or
	Actinomycin D 1.25 mg/m^2 IV
EMACO	Etoposide 100 mg/m^2 IV over days 1 and 2 of each cycle
Cycle length 14 d	Methotrexate 100 mg/m^2 IV push, day 1 of each cycle
	Methotrexate 200 mg/m^2 IV by continuous infusion over 12 hr; give immediately after methotrexate injection on day 1 of cycle
	Leucovorin 5 mg tabs—three tablets PO every 12 hr for 2 days, starting 24 hr after beginning of methotrexate days 1 and 2
	Actinomycin D 0.5 mg IV push, days 1 and 2 of each cycle
	Day 8
	Vincristine 1 mg/m^2 (maximum of 2 mg/dose) IV, day 8 of each cycle
	Cyclophosphamide 600 mg/m^2 IV, day 8 of each cycle
BEP	Bleomycin: 15–20 units/m^2 IV (maximum 30 units), days 1, 8, 15
Bleomycin, Etoposide, Cisplatin	Etoposide: 100 mg/m^2 IV, days 1–5
Cycle length: 21 d	Cisplatin: 20 mg/m^2 IV, days 1–5
VPB	Vinblastine: 0.15 mg/kg on days 1 and 2 Bleomycin: 15 units/m^2/wk starting day 2, Cisplatin 100mg/m2 on day 1 for 4–5 cycles
Vinblastine, Cisplatin, Bleomycin,	

(continued)

Table 9.4 Common Chemotherapy Protocols *(continued)*

Cycle length 21 d	
VAC	Vincristine: 1–1.5 mg/m² on day 1, actinomycin D: 0.5 mg/d × 5 days, cyclophosphamide: 150 mg/m²/d
Vincristine, actinomycin, cyclophosphamide	
Cycle length 28 d	
POMB-ACE	POMB
Cisplatin, vincristine, methotrexate, bleomycin	Day 1: vincristine 1 mg/m² IV, methotrexate 300 mg/m² 12-hr infusion
Atinomycin, cyclophosphamide, etoposide	Day 2: bleomycin 15 mg IV 24-hr infusion, folinic acid rescue to start 24 hr after methotrexate 15 mg every 12 hr for 4 doses
	Day 3: bleomycin 15 mg IV 24-hr infusion
	Day 4: cisplatin 120 mg/m² IV 12-hr infusion with IVF and 3 g magnesium
	ACE
	Days 1–5: etoposide 100 mg/m²/d
	Day 3–5: actinomycin D 0.5 mg IV
	Day 5: cyclophosphamide 500 mg/m² IV
OMB	Day 1: vincristine 1 mg/m² IV, methotrexate 300 mg/m² IV 12-hr infusion
Vincristine, methotrexate, bleomycin	Day 2: bleomycin 12 mg IV 24-hr infusion, folinic acid rescue to start 24 hr after start of methotrexate 15 mg every 12 hr IV for four doses
Initiate with two courses of POMB followed by ACE. POMB alternates with ACE until biochemical remission, then alternate ACE with OMB. Interval between courses 9 and 11 days.	Day 3: bleomycin 15 mg IV 24-hr infusion

REFERENCES

1. Herzog TJ, Alvarez RD, Secord A, et al. SGO guidance document for clinical trial designs in ovarian cancer: a changing paradigm. *Gynecol Oncol.* 2014;135(1):3–7. doi: 10.1016/j.ygyno.2014.08.004

2. Oken MM, Creech RH, Tormey DC, et al. Toxicity and response criteria of the Eastern Cooperative Oncology Group. *Am J Clin Oncol.* 1982;5(6):649–655.

3. Eisenhauer EA, Therasse P, Bogaerts J, et al. New response evaluation criteria in solid tumours: revised RECIST guideline (version 1.1). *Eur J Cancer.* 2009;45(2):228–247. doi: 10.1016/j.ejca.2008.10.026

4. Wolchok JD, Hoos A, O'Day S, et al. Guidelines for the evaluation of immune therapy activity in solid tumors: immune-related response criteria. *Clin Cancer Res.* 2009;15(23):7412–7420. doi: 10.1158/1078-0432.CCR-09-1624

Abbreviations

5-FU	5-fluorouracil
5YS	5-year survival
A/C	assist-control
AABB	American Association of Blood Banks
ABC	ATP binding cassette
ABG	arterial blood gas
ACE	angiotensin-converting enzyme
ACOG	American Congress of Obstetricians and Gynecologists
ACP	American College of Physicians
ACS	acute coronary syndrome
ACT	adoptive T-cell therapy
Act-D	dactinomycin
ACTION	Adjuvant Chemotherapy in Ovarian Neoplasms
AD	absolute difference
ADCC	antibody-dependent cellular cytotoxicity
ADH	antidiuretic hormone
ADLs	activities of daily living
AEs	adverse events
AFFIRM	Atrial Fibrillation Follow-up Investigation of Rhythm Management
AFP	alpha fetoprotein
AGC	atypical glandular cells
AGO	arbeitsgemeinschaft gynaekologische onkologie
AGUS	abnormal glandular cells of unknown significance
AHM	anti-Müllerian hormone
AIS	adenocarcinoma in situ
AJCC	American Joint Committee on Cancer
ALA	alpha-lipoic acid
ALC	acetyl-l-carnitine
ALI	acute lung injury
ALK	anaplastic lymphoma kinase
ALTS	ASCUS/LSIL Triage Study
AML	acute myeloid leukemia
ANC	absolute neutrophil count
ANCOVA	analysis of covariance
ANOVA	analysis of variance

AP/PA	anterior–posterior/posterior–anterior
APD	abdominal peritoneal disease
aPTT	activated partial thromboplastin time
ARB	angiotensin receptor blockers
ARDS	acute respiratory distress syndrome
ASA	acetylsalicylic acid
ASA score	American Society of Anesthesiologists Score
ASC	atypical squamous cells
ASC-H	atypical squamous cells, cannot exclude high grade
ASC-US	atypical squamous cells of undetermined significance
ASCCP	American Society of Coloscopy and Cervical Pathology
ASD	atrial septal defect
ASIS	anterior superior iliac spine
AST	aspartate transaminase
ATCH	adrenocorticotropic hormone
ATHENA	Addressing the Need for Advanced HPV Diagnostics
ATP	adenosine triphosphate
AUB	atypical uterine bleeding
AUC	area under the curve
AURELIA	Avastin Use in Platinum-Resistant Epithelial Ovarian Cancer
AV	atrioventricular block
BED	biologically equivalent dose
BEE	basal energy expenditure
BEP	bleomycin, etoposide, cisplatin
BER	base-excision repair
BID	twice a day
BiPAP	bilevel positive airway pressure
bi-shRNAi	bifunctional short hairpin RNAi
BMI	body mass index
BMP	basic metabolic panel
BNP	brain natriuretic peptide
BOOST	bevacizumab ovarian optimal standard treatment
BOT	borderline ovarian tumors
BP	blood pressure
BRRS	Bannayan-Riley-Ruvaicaba syndrome
BSA	body surface area
BSE	bovine spongiform encephalopathy
BSO	bilateral salpingo-oophorectomy
BUN	blood urea nitrogen
CA-125	cancer antigen-125
CABG	coronary artery bypass graft
CAH	complex atypical hyperplasia
CAP	cisplatin, doxorubicin, cyclophosphamide
CBC	complete blood count
CBI	continuous bladder irrigation

CCC	clear cell carcinoma
CCR	complete clinical response
CCRT	continuous renal replacement therapies
CCU	critical care unit
CD	cisplatin, doxorubicin
CDC	Centers for Disease Control and Prevention
CDP	cisplatin, doxorubicin, paclitaxel
CEA	carcinoembryonic antigen
CER-T	chimeric endocrine receptor T-cell
cfDNA	cell-free DNA
CHAMOCA	cyclophosphamide, hydroxyurea, actinomycin D, methotrexate, vincristine, leucovorin, doxorubicin
CHF	congestive heart failure
CHIP	clonal hematopoiesis of indeterminate potential
CI	confidence interval
CIN	cervical intraepithelial neoplasia
CIR	cumulative incidence rate
CIS	carcinoma in situ
CIWA	Clinical Institute Withdrawal Assessment
CKC	cold knife cone
CKMB	creatine kinase-MB
CM	complete mole
CML	chronic myeloid leukemia
CMP	comprehensive metabolic panel
CMV	continuous mandatory ventilation
CN	cranial nerve
CNS	central nervous system
CO	cardiac output
COPD	chronic obstructive pulmonary disease
CPAP	continuous positive airway pressure
CPH-I	Copenhagen Index
CPK	creatine phosphokinase
CPR	complete pathological response
CR	complete response
CRC	colorectal cancer
CrCl	creatinine clearance
CRRT	continuous renal replacement therapy
CS/PHTS	Cowden Syndrome/PTEN Harmatoma Syndrome
CSS	cancer-specific survival
CT	computed tomography
CTC	common toxicity criteria
CTCAE	Common Terminology Criteria for Adverse Events
CTLA-4	cytotoxic T-lymphocyte-associated antigen 4
CTV	clinical target volume
CUSA	Cavitron ultrasonic surgical aspiration
CV	cardiovascular
cva	costovertral angle

CVA	cerebrovascular accident
CVP	central venous pressure
CXR	chest x-ray
DC	dendritic cells
D&C	dilation and curettage
DBP	diastolic blood pressure
dDAVP	desmopressin
DES	diethylstilbestrol
DESKTOP	Descriptive Evaluation of Preoperative Selection KriTeria for OPerability
DFI	disease-free interval
DFS	disease-free survival
DHEA	dehydroepiandrosterone
DHEAS	dehydroepiandrosterone sulfate
DHFR	dihydrofolate reductase
DIC	disseminated intravascular coagulation
DKA	diabetic ketoacidosis
DLCO	carbon monoxide diffusion capacity test
DLL4	delta-like ligand-4
DLT	dose-limiting toxicity
DM	diabetes mellitus
DMSO	dimethyl sulfoxide
DNR	do not resuscitate
DOAC	direct oral anticoagulants
DOI	depth of invasion
DOR	duration of response
DP	disease progression
DS	double-stranded
DSMB	Data Safety Monitoring Board
DSS	disease-specific survival
DTIC	dacarbazine
DVIN	differentiated-type VIN
DVT	deep vein thrombosis
EBL	estimated blood loss
EBXRT	external beam radiation therapy
ECC	endocervical curettage
ECOG	European Cooperative Oncology Group
EDM	exonuclease domain mutations
EF	ejection fraction
EFS	event-free survival
EGD	esophagogastroduodenoscopy
EGFR	epidermal growth factor receptor
EIA	enzyme immunoassay
EIN	endometrial intraepithelial neoplasia
EKG	electrocardiogram
ELISA	enzyme-linked immunosorbent assay
ELISPOT	enzyme-linked immunospot assay

EMA-CO	etoposide, methotrexate, actinomycin D–cyclophosphamide, and vincristine
EMACO	etoposide, methotrexate, actinomycin D, cyclophosphamide, and vincristine
EMA-EP	etoposide, methotrexate, actinomycin D–etoposide, cisplatin
EMB	endometrial biopsy
EMS	endometrial stripe
EOC	epithelial ovarian cancer
EORTC	European Organisation for Research and Treatment of Cancer
EP	etoposide, cisplatin
ER	estrogen receptor
ERAS	enhanced recovery after surgery
ERT	estrogen replacement therapy
ESRD	end-stage renal disease
ESS	endometrial stromal sarcomas
ETT	epithelioid trophoblastic tumor
EUA	examination under anesthesia
FAK	focal adhesion kinase
FANCOVA	factorial analysis of variance
FAP	Familial adenomatous polyposis
FDA	Food and Drug Administration
FDG	fludeoxyglucose
FEV	forced expiratory volume
FFP	fresh frozen plasma
FGFR	fibroblast growth factor receptor
FLT-3	fms-like tyrosine kinase 3
FIGO	International Federation of Gynecology and Obstetrics
FISH	fluorescence in situ hybridization
FN	false negative
FNA	fine-needle aspiration
FP	false positive
FRC	functional residual capacity
FRHM	familial recurrent hydatidiform mole
FSFI	Female Sexual Function Instrument
FSH	follicle-stimulating hormone
FUDR	floxuridine
G	grade
GC	gemcitabine-cisplatin
GCIG	Gynecologic Cancer Inter Group
GCSF	granulocyte colony stimulating factor
GCTs	germ cell tumors
GFR	glomerular filtration rate
GI	gastrointestinal
GIS	gastrointestinal anastomosis
GIST	gastrointestinal stromal tumor

GMC	gracilis myocutaneous flap
GMCSF	granulocyte-macrophage colony-stimulating factor
GnRH	gonadotropin-releasing hormone
GOG	Gynecologic Oncology Group
GSH	glutathione
GST	glutathione S-transferase
GTD	gestational trophoblastic disease
GTN	gestational trophoblastic neoplasia
G-tube	gastrostomy tube
GTV	gross tumor volume
GU	genitourinary
Gy	gray
HE4	human epididymis protein 4
H&E	hematoxylin and eosin stain
HAART	highly active antiretroviral therapy
HBOC	hereditary breast and ovarian cancer
hCG	human chorionic gonadotropin
Hct	hematocrit
HDR	high-dose rate
HER2	human epidermal growth factor receptor 2.
HERS	HIV Epidemiology Research Study
HFU	hospital-based follow-up
Hg	hemoglobin
HGFR	hepatocyte growth factor receptor
HGSC	high-grade serous carcinoma
HGSTOC	high-grade serous tubo-ovarian cancer
HIPEC	hyperthermic intraperitoneal chemotherapy
HIR	high intermediate risk
HLA	human leukocyte antigen
HNPCC	hereditary nonpolyposis colon cancer
HPF	high-power field
HPL	human placental lactogen
HPV	human papillomavirus
HR	hazard ratio
HRd	homologous recombination deficient
HRp	homologous recombination proficient
HRT	hormone replacement therapy
HSIL	high-grade squamous intraepithelial lesion
HSV	herpes simplex virus
HTN	hypertension
HTR	hemolytic transfusion reaction
HUS	hemolytic uremic syndrome
IBD	inflammatory bowel disease
ICC	invasive cervical cancer
ICE	ifosfamide, cisplatin, etoposide
ICER	incremental cost-effectiveness ratio
ICG	indocyanine green

ICON	International Collaborative Ovarian Neoplasm
IDS	interval debulking surgery
IHC	immunohistochemistry
IHD	ischemic heart disease
IM	intramuscular
IMA	inferior mesenteric artery
IMV	intermittent mandatory ventilation
IMRT	intensity-modulated radiation therapy
IMXRT	intensity-modulated radiation therapy
INH	isoniazid
INR	international normalized ratio
IOXRT	intraoperative radiation therapy
IP	intraperitoneal
IQR	interquartile range
IRB	institutional review board
IRR	incidence rate ratio
irCR	immune-related complete response
irPD	immune-related progressive disease
irPR	immune-related partial response
irRC	immune-related response criteria
irSD	immune-related stable disease
ISSVD	International Society for the Study of Vulvar Diseases
IT	immature teratoma
ITCs	isolated tumor cells
ITT	intention-to-treat
IUGR	intrauterine growth restriction
IUD	intrauterine device
IUP	intrauterine pregnancy
IV	intravenous
IVC	inferior vena cava
IVF	intravenous fluid
IVP	intravenous pyelography
JGOG	Japanese Gynecologic Oncology Group
JP	Jackson-Pratt
JVD	jugular venous distension
JVP	jugular venous pressure
KERMA	kinetic energy related to mass
KUB	kidneys, ureters, bladder
LACC	Laparoscopic Approach to Cervical Cancer
LAST	lower anogenital squamous terminology
LBO	large-bowel obstruction
LD	longest diameter
LDH	lactate dehydrogenase
LDR	low-dose rate
LEEP	loop electrosurgical excision procedure
LEER	laterally extended endopelvic resection
LFS	Li-Fraumeni syndrome

LFT	liver function test
LGSC	low grade serous carcinoma
LGSOC	low-grade serous ovarian cancer
LH	luteininzing hormone
LIWS	low intermittent wall suction
LLO	*listeriolysin O*
LMP	low-malignant potential
LMS	leiomyosarcoma
LMW	low molecular weight
LMWH	low-molecular weight heparin
LN	lymph node
LND	lymph node dissection
LOH	loss of heterozygosity
LOS	length of stay
LP	likely pathologic
LPF	low-power field
LR	lactated Ringer's
LS	Lynch Syndrome
LSIL	low-grade squamous intraepithelial lesion
LV	left ventricular
LVAD	left ventricular assist device
LVEF	left ventricular ejection fraction
LVI	lymphovascular invasion
LVSI	lymphovascular space invasion
mAb	monoclonal antibody
MAC	methotrexate, actinomycin D, cyclophosphamide
MASCC	Multinational Association for Supportive Care in Cancer
MAP	mean arterial pressure
MAPK	mitogen-activated protein kinase
MBP	mechanical bowel preparation
MCT	mature cystic teratoma
MD	minimal disease
MDR	multidrug resistance
MDS	myelodysplastic syndromes
METS	metabolic equivalents
MI	myometrial invasion
MIS	minimally invasive surgery
MMAE	monomethyl auristatin E
MMMTs	mixed Müllerian mesodermal tumors
MMR	measles, mumps, rubella
MMRd	mismatch repair deficient
MMRp	mismatch repair proficient
MODS	multiple organ dysfunction syndrome
MPA	medroxyprogesterone acetate
MRI	magnetic resonance imaging
MS	multiple sclerosis

MSI	microsatellite instability
MTD	maximum tolerated dose
MTHFR	methylenetetrahydrofolate reductase
MTIC	monomethyl triazeno imidazole carboxamide
mTOR	mammalian target of rapamycin
MTP	massive transfusion protocol
MTX	methotrexate
MUDPILES	methanol, uremia (chronic renal failure), diabetic ketoacidosis, propylene glycol, (infection, iron, iso-niazid, inborn errors in metabolism), lactic acidosis, ethylene glycol, salicylates
MUGA	multigated acquisition
MUPIT	Martinez universal perineal interstitial template
MVP	mitral valve prolapse
NACT	neoadjuvant chemotherapy
NASBA	nucleic acid sequence–based amplification
NCCN	National Comprehensive Cancer Network
NCDB	National Cancer Data Base
NCI	National Cancer Institute
NCIC	National Cancer Institute of Canada
NE	not-estimable
NFT	no further treatment
NGT	nasogastric tube
NICD	Notch intracellular domain
NIF	negative inspiratory force
NK	natural killer
NKB	neurokinin B
NMBA	neuromuscular blocking agent
NNRTI	non-nucleoside reverse transcriptase inhibitor
NOS	not otherwise specified
NOVEL	New Ovarian Elaborate
NPBC	non-platinum based chemotherapy
NPO	nothing by mouth
NPV	negative predictive value
NRTI	nucleotide reverse transcriptase inhibitor
NS	not statistically significant
NSAID	nonsteroidal anti-inflammatory drug
NSC	non–small-cell
NSE	neuron-specific enolase
NTG	nitroglycerin
NTRK	neurotrophic tyrosine receptor kinase
O/E	observed-to-expected ratio
OC	ovarian cancer
OCP	oral contraceptive pills
OCSI	ovarian cancer symptom index
OR	odds ratio
ORR	overall response rate

OS	overall survival
OTC	over-the-counter
OTT	optimal treatment time
PA	para-aortic
PA-XRT	para-aortic radiation therapy
PAC	premature atrial contraction
PALN	para-aortic lymph node
PALND	para-aortic lymph node dissection
PAOP	pulmonary artery occlusion pressure
PAP	Papanicolaou
PAP diastolic	diastolic pulmonary arterial pressure
PAP mean	mean pulmonary arterial pressure
PAP systolic	systolic pulmonary arterial pressure
PARP	poly (ADP-ribose) polymerase
PARP-i	poly (ADP-ribose) polymerase inhibitors
PAS+	periodic-acid-Schiff positive
PAWP	pulmonary artery wedge pressure
PC	peritoneal cytology
PCA	patient-controlled analgesia
PCC	prothrombin complex concentrate
PCN	percutaneous nephrostomy
PCP	*pneumocystis pneumonia*
PCR	polymerase chain reaction
PCWP	pulmonary capillary wedge pressure
PD	progressive disease
PD-1	programmed cell death protein 1
PDA	patent ductus arteriosus
PDGFR	platelet-derived growth factor receptor
PDS	primary debulking surgery
PE	pulmonary embolus
PEEP	positive end-expiratory pressure
PEF	peak expiratory flow
PEG	polyethylene glycol
PET	positron emission tomography
PFI	progression-free interval
PFS	progression-free survival
PFT	pulmonary function test
PFTC	primary fallopian tube cancer
PHTS	PTEN hamartoma tumor syndrome
PI	predictive index
PI3K	phosphoinositide-3 kinase
PICC	peripheral inserted central catheter
PLCO	prostate, lung, colon, and ovarian cancer
PI-R	platinum-resistant
PJ	Peutz–Jeghers syndrome
PLAP	placental alkaline phosphatase

PLD	pegylated liposomal doxorubicin
PLND	pelvic lymph node dissection
PLUMSEEDS	paraldehyde, lactate, uremia, methanol, salicylates, ethylene glycol, ethanol, diabetic ketoacidosis, starvation
PMPB	postmenopausal bleeding
PO	orally/per os
POD	postoperative day
POISE	Perioperative Ischemic Evaluation Study
POLST	physician orders for life sustaining treatment
POLE	polymerase epsilon
POMB-ACE	cisplatin, vincristine, methotrexate, bleomycin, actinomycin D, cyclophosphamide, etoposide
PPE	palmar plantar erythema
P PA-LND	pelvic and para-aortic lymphadenectomy
PPV	positive predictive value
PR	partial response
PRBC	packed red blood cells
PRoMisE	Proactive Molecular Risk Classifier for Endometrial Cancer
PS	pressure supported
PSBO	partial small-bowel obstruction
PSTT	placental site trophoblastic tumor
PT	prothrombin time
PTCA	percutaneous transluminal coronary angioplasty
PTD	preterm delivery
PTSD	posttraumatic stress disorder
PTT	partial thromboplastin time
PTU	propylthiouracil
PTV	planning target volume
PVB	cisplatin, vinblastine, bleomycin
PVC	premature ventricular contractions
PVD	peripheral vascular disease
PVI-FU	prolonged venous infusion of 5-FU
PVR	post void residual
QALY	quality-adjusted life year
QID	four times a day
QOL	quality of life
RA	room air
Rad	radiation absorbed dose(s)
RAM	rectus abdominis myocutaneous flap
RBBB	right bundle branch block
RBC	red blood cells
RBE	relative biologic effectiveness
RECIST	response evaluation criteria in solid tumors
RFLP	restriction fragment length polymorphism
RFS	recurrence-free survival

rhGM-CSF	recombinant human granulocyte macrophage-colony stimulating factor
RM	restricted means
RMI	risk of malignancy index
RMST	restricted mean survival time
ROCA	risk of ovarian cancer algorithm
ROMA	risk of ovarian malignancy algorithm
ROS1	c-ros oncogene 1
RR	response rate
RRBSO	risk-reducing bilateral salpingo-oophorectomy
RRSO	risk-reducing salpingo-oophorectomy
RTK	receptor tyrosine kinase
RTOG	Radiation Therapy Oncology Group
SBE	subacute bacterial endocarditis
SBFT	small-bowel follow through
SBO	small-bowel obstruction
SBP	systolic blood pressure
SC	subcutaneous
SCC	squamous cell carcinoma
SCD	sequential compression device
SCIA	superficial circumflex iliac artery
SCTAT	sex cord tumor with annular tubules
SD	standard deviation
SE	standard error
SEE-FIM	Sectioning and Extensively Examining the FIMbriated End
SEER	Surveillance Epidemiology and End Results
SEPA	superficial external pudendal artery
SEPAL	Survival Effect of Para-Aortic Lymphaenectomy
SG	specific gravity
SGO	Society of Gynecologic Oncology
SI	sacroiliac
SIADH	syndrome of inappropriate antidiuretic hormone secretion
SIL	squamous intraepithelial lesion
SIMV	synchronized intermittent mandatory ventilation
SIRS	systemic inflammatory response syndrome
SIS	saline infusion sonography
SCJ	squamocolumnar junction
SL	sublingual
SLL	second-look laparotomy
SLN	sentinel lymph node
SLND	sentinel lymph node dissection
SMA	superior mesenteric artery
SO	sarcomatous overgrowth
SOB	shortness of breath

SOCQER	Surgery in Ovarian Cancer Quality of life Evaluation Research study
SOFA	sequential organ failure assessment
SPECT	single-photon emission CT
SPECT/CT	single-photon emission computed tomography with CT
SRA	serotonin release assay
SSD	source to skin distance
SSI	surgical site infection
STDs	sexually transmitted diseases
STEMI	ST elevation myocardial infarction
STIC	serous tubal intraepithelial carcinoma
STS	soft tissue sarcoma
STSG	split thickness skin grafts
STUMP	smooth muscle tumor of uncertain malignant potential
SVR	systemic vascular resistance
SVT	superficial vein thrombosis
TA	thoracoabdominal
TACO	transfusion-associated circulatory overload
TAH	total abdominal hysterectomy
TAP	paclitaxel, doxorubicin, cisplatin
TB	tuberculosis
TBW	total body water
TC	paclitaxel and carboplatin
TCA	tricyclic antidepressant
TCG	paclitaxel, carboplatin, and gemcitabine
TE	thromboembolism
TG	triglycerides
TGF	transforming growth factors
TH-BSO	total hysterectomy bilateral salpingo-oophorectomy
TIA	transient ischemic attacks
TID	three times a day
TIL	tumor-infiltrating lymphocyte
TKI	tyrosine kinase inhibitor
TLR5	toll-like receptor 5
TLR7	toll-like receptor 7
TN	true negative
TNM	tumor, node, metastasis
TOC	tubo-ovarian cancer
TolR	Tol-receptor death ligand
TP	true positive
TPN	total parenteral nutrition
TRALI	transfusion-related acute lung injury
TSH	thyroid-stimulating hormone
TRUST	Trial of Radical Upfront Surgical Therapy
TTP	time to progression

TTF-1	thyroid transcription factor-1
TVUS	transvaginal ultrasound
UA	urinalysis
UAD	upper abdominal disease
UFH	unfractionated heparin
UGI	upper gastrointestinal
UI	urinary incontinence
UKCTOCS	U.K. Collaborative Trial of Ovarian Cancer Screening
UNC	ureteroneocystostomy
US	ultrasound
USS	ultrasound screening
USO	unilateral salpingo-oophorectomy
UTI	urinary tract infection
UTROSCT	uterine tumor resembling ovarian sex-cord tumor
UU	ureteroureterostomy
UUS	undifferentiated uterine sarcoma
V/Q	ventilation/perfusion
VAC	vincristine, doxorubicin, cyclophosphamide
VAIN	vaginal intraepithelial neoplasia
VAP	ventilator acquired pneumonia
VATS	video-assisted thoracic surgery
VCB/CT	vaginal cuff brachytherapy followed by paclitaxel/ carboplatin chemotherapy
VE-cadherin	vascular cadherin–endothelial cadherin
VEGF	vascular endothelial growth factors
VEGFR	vascular endothelial growth factor receptor
VIA	visual inspection with acetic acid
VIN	vulvar intraepithelial neoplasia
VIP	etoposide, ifosfamide, cisplatin
VMAT	volumetric modulated arc therapy
VPB	vinblastine, cisplatin, bleomycin
VSD	ventricular septal defect
VTE	venous thromboembolism
VUS	variants of uncertain significance
WAR	whole abdominal radiotherapy
WB-XRT	whole brain radiation therapy
WBC	white blood cell
WHO	World Health Organization
WIHS	Women's Interagency HIV Study
WP	whole pelvic
WP-XRT	whole pelvic radiation therapy
WT	wild type
XRT	radiation therapy
Y	year
YS	year survival

Index